Routledge Revivals

Science and Football

I0891097

First published in 1988, this book contains edited and revised papers presented at the first World Congress of Science and Football.

Held under the auspices of the International Council of Sport, Science, and Physical Education, the Congress was a unique gathering of international scientists researching into football and practitioners professionally involved in the many football codes. American football, soccer, rugby league, rugby union, Australian rules, Gaelic football and national variations of these games are all covered in depth, in both amateur and professional systems.

Nutrition, biomechanics, equipment, physiology, sociology, psychology, coaching, management, training, tactics, strategy are among the main subject areas the contributors cover. With over 22 countries represented and with players, managers and coaches involved as well as academics the book represents a truly international, comprehensive and practical picture of contemporary football.

Science and Football

Proceedings of the first World Congress of
Science and Football
Liverpool, 13-17th April 1987

Edited by
T. Reilly,
A. Lees,
K. Davids
and
W. J. Murphy

Routledge
Taylor & Francis Group

First published in 1988
by E. & F. N. Spon Ltd

This edition first published in 2011 by Routledge
2 Park Square, Milton Park, Abingdon, Oxon, OX14 4RN

Simultaneously published in the USA and Canada
by Routledge
711 Third Avenue, New York, NY 10017

Routledge is an imprint of the Taylor & Francis Group, an informa business

Publisher's Note
The publisher has gone to great lengths to ensure the quality of this reprint but points out that some imperfections in the original copies may be apparent.

Disclaimer
The publisher has made every effort to trace copyright holders and welcomes correspondence from those they have been unable to contact.

A Library of Congress record exists under LC control number: 97664065

ISBN 13: 978-0-415-50911-4 (hbk)

Science and Football

EDITED BY
T. Reilly
A. Lees
K. Davids
and
W. J. Murphy

PROCEEDINGS OF THE
FIRST WORLD CONGRESS OF
SCIENCE AND FOOTBALL
LIVERPOOL 13-17TH APRIL 1987

LONDON NEW YORK
E. & F. N. SPON

First World Congress of Science and Football
Liverpool, 13–17 April 1987

Organized from Liverpool Polytechnic
and held at the Albert Dock, Liverpool

Organizing Committee

A. Carroll
P. Chambers
K. Davids
W. J. Murphy
R. Jones
D. Shaw
P. Sutcliffe
D. Wright

Congress Organizers

T. Reilly and A. Lees
Department of Sport and Recreation Studies
Liverpool Polytechnic
Byrom Street
Liverpool L3 3AF

Promotions and Administration
Ms Helen Latham

First published in 1988 by E. & F. N. Spon Ltd
11 New Fetter Lane, London EC4P 4EE

Published in the USA by E. & F. N. Spon
29 West 35th Street, New York NY 10001

Printed in Great Britain by St. Edmundsbury Press
Bury St. Edmunds, Suffolk

ISBN 0 419 14360 2

British Library Cataloguing in Publication Data

World congress of science and football
(1st : 1987 : Liverpool, England)
Science and football
1. Football. Physiological aspects
I. Title II. Reilly, Thomas
612'.044
ISBN 0-419-14360-2

Contents

Preface

It was our privilege to organize the First World Congress of Science and Football held at the Albert Dock, Liverpool, in April 1987. The broad aim of the Congress was to bring together those scientists whose research work is directly related to football and practitioners of football interested in obtaining current information about its scientific aspects. The Congress attempted to bridge a gap between research and practice so that scientific knowledge about football could be communicated and later applied.

The theme of football was broadly interpreted to embrace all codes, amateur and professional, including soccer, rugby union, rugby league, American football, Australian Rules and Gaelic football. The intention was to provide a forum where the common threads, in research and practice, among these games could be debated. Existence of common factors between games has been demonstrated in recent years, for example, when Australian Rules and Gaelic footballers have competed in 'compromise rules football' and when rugby union and rugby league, soccer and American football officials have shared their stadia.

The idea of organizing the First World Congress of Science and Football was first mooted by Professor Jan Clarys, Secretary General of the World Commission on Sports Biomechanics. His proposal to base the Congress at Liverpool was enthusiastically adopted by the authorities of Liverpool Polytechnic who provided substantial back-up and support for its organization. From the outset the encouragement from the offices of the International Council of Sport Science and Physical Education, who provided patronage and set the Congress within its calendar of events, was invaluable. Within the UK the Congress was supported by the British Association of Sports Sciences.

The city of Liverpool was an appropriate choice of venue for an inaugural conference with the stated aims. It is regarded as one of the world's capital cities of soccer with Everton and Liverpool football clubs being located in the heart of the city: both clubs offered substantial support to the Congress.

Besides, the North West of England is the major area of popularity for rugby league whilst rugby union too has a strong foothold in the region. Liverpool is conveniently near to Eire to provide a fair representation of Gaelic football: the homes of American football and Australian Rules football were more remote, but both codes were well represented. The footballing bodies who supported the Congress in principle at the outset – the Football League, EUFA, English Rugby Football Union, Rugby League Association, Gaelic Athletic Association and Western Australian Rules Association – provided the necessary moral support for the Congress to realize its aims.

The formal oral lectures at the Congress were complemented by interactive sessions – posters, seminars, workshops and demonstrations. The workshop and seminar sessions addressed practical issues and provided an opportunity for delegates to discuss problems in a relatively informal manner with a panel of experts. It is our regret that the information from these sessions could not be collated into a volume such as this, nevertheless we wish to acknowledge the enormous contributions that were made in these sessions to the success of the Congress. Separate topics and contributors were:– Nutrition (Don MacLaren, Ira Jacobs and Bjorn Ekblom), mental preparation (John Syer), surfaces (J. Roberts, B. Hall and B. Williams), football in the community (Joe Patton, Eric Dunning and Alan Sefton), refereeing (Toshio Asami, Geraint Davies and Ron Campbell), management (David Oxley, David Weldrick, Malcolm Cook and Egil Olsen) and match analysis (Mike Hughes). Inspector Keith Wilkinson conducted a valuable workshop on 'football crowd control' and Brian Macasskey (Chicago Bears) addressed the topic 'Coaching and training in American Football'. There was also a workshop on 'preventive football medicine' (Jan Ekstrand and Dennis Wright) to complete a one-day 'football medicine' strand of the Congress. The fundamentals of Australian Rules, Gaelic football and American football were explained by Brian Douge, David Weldrick and Brian Macasskey respectively, in seminar sessions on the opening afternoon so that delegates unfamiliar with these games could acquire a basic understanding of them.

A more concrete demonstration of the football codes was provided at the exhibition games held during the Congress. One afternoon was set aside so that skills and training practices of the various codes were employed. Liverpool FC hosted the demonstrations of soccer and Gaelic football at its renowned Anfield ground. A typical soccer training session was conducted by the professional staff at Liverpool FC. This was followed by a highly entertaining exhibition of Gaelic football skills, orchestrated by Frank Fahey from Hollymount, and a 9-a-side match between the visiting Hollymount (Co. Mayo) team who had travelled from Eire and the local Gaelic football team, John Mitchells (Liverpool). The rugby demonstrations took place at Waterloo Rugby Union Football Club. The Rugby Union session conducted by David Shaw introduced novel modifications to the game, such as mini-rugby and 'new-image' rugby. In conjunction with this was the demonstration of Rugby League, supervised by Phil Larder, using the current national league championship winners, Wigan RFLC. For many of the delegates who hailed from 45 different countries, these insights into football practice were important.

For promotion and administration of the Congress we are indebted to Helen Latham: without her unstinting devotion to duty the Congress would not have approached the heights it attained. In the months before and during the Congress participants recognized that Helen formed the hub of the organizational machinery and appreciated the calm competence with which their requests were met. Behind the scenes the work of Celia Latham, Elsie Lucas and Leanne Carney was important. The Secretariat was supported during the Congress by the students of Sports Science, Languages, Outdoor and Physical Education, all from Liverpool Polytechnic. We are deeply indebted to our colleagues within the Department of Sport and Recreation Studies at the Polytechnic who boosted our morale on the odd occasion it began to wane.

From the opening addresses at the Albert Dock by Mr John Smith CBE (Chairman, The Sports Council), Mr Philip Carter, CBE (President, Football League), Dr Ken Ridings (Rectorate, Liverpool Polytechnic) and Professor Walter Dufour (representing the World Commission on Sports Biomechanics and ICSSPE) – to the Congress banquet at Goodison Park, home of Everton FC, it was rewarding to see the dreams of the organizing committee being realized. The closing addresses by Dr F. H. Sanderson (Head of Department of Sport and Recreation Studies of Liverpool Polytechnic) and Professor J. M. Greep (University of Maastricht, Netherlands) looked forward to the Second World Congress to be held at Maastricht in 1991. This will ensure that the achievement at Liverpool, the first occasion in which representatives of all the football codes convened in a meeting of minds, will be continued and extended in the future.

Thomas Reilly and Adrian Lees
Congress Organizers

Introduction

There is a wealth of evidence to show that football in one form or another was played in various cultures many centuries ago. There seems to be an atavistic urge in the apparently trivial pursuit of kicking a football around a field. The emergence of organized football can be traced to the latter half of the nineteenth century. Since then the various football codes have become highly professional in their outlook and in their promotions.

From the early years of this century there has been a rich legacy of descriptive literature about football, its joys and raptures, its despairs and disappointments. Later, more incisive analysis of the games has produced a heritage of tactical insights from which training and coaching theories have evolved. In contemporary football much effort is spent in forecasting match outcomes, promoting football teams and the games' image, analysing trends in match play and conducting post-mortems after unexpected defeats. In the world of football fanatics all contributors to the discussion are self-acknowledged experts and agreement in debates is rare.

The worlds of football and of science seem at face value to be poles apart: the former revolves around intuition and emotion, the latter is concerned with facts and verifiable observations. Nevertheless there is increasing awareness among football practitioners that information from scientific endeavours can contribute both to the understanding and solution of problems that confront them. This kind of knowledge can be helpful to the football manager, coach, trainer, medical staff, player and/or match official. This volume contains papers presented at the First World Congress on Science and Football at Liverpool, April 13th–17th, 1987. The Congress itself contained 10 keynote address, 9 workshop sessions, 9 seminars, 9 posters and 113 formal communications. Manuscripts of the presentations were subjected to 'peer review' and where necessary revised and edited. For a variety of reasons it was not possible to publish all of the papers: hopefully those that are published here provide a reasonable flavour of the Congress programme and exemplify the many ways in which 'science' and 'football' may be linked. We regret that we could not include material submitted after our deadlines, as we had to provide a camera ready copy to the publishers in a reasonable time after the Congress.

The contents are organized into sections or parts, the main division being on a disciplinary basis. This includes not only the scientific disciplines but also medical and management/coaching aspects. Where it was thought appropriate, papers were grouped according to topics which on occasions transcended disciplinary boundaries.

The editors are indebted to those contributors who responded promptly to our queries and quibbles, and at short notice checked the word-processed typescript. We thank also those individuals who willingly acted as referees but who must remain anonymous.

We are grateful also for the encouragement and support of editorial and production staff at the publisher's office. The camera ready copy was prepared at Liverpool Polytechnic to ensure uniformity of typeface among the contributions. That the volume reached completion at all was due to the competence and patience of Margaret, Mary, May, Sue and Val in the Typing Pool who had to endure our endless insistence on instant attention while the book was in preparation.

T. Reilly
A. Lees
K. Davids
W. J. Murphy

Part I

Common threads: opening keynote address

FOOTBALL: THE COMMON THREADS BETWEEN THE GAMES

Brian Douge
West Australian Football League Inc., Subiaco Oval, Subiaco, W.A.,
P.O. Box 275, West Australia 6008, Australia.

Introduction

American Football, Australian Rules football, Gaelic football, Rugby League, Rugby Union and soccer are sports which have tremendous spectator appeal. Each of these football codes attracts 60 000 - 120 000 spectators to its major championship matches. The fans are attracted to football for a variety of reasons ranging from traditional rivalry between teams to an appreciation of skills.

American Football, Rugby League and Rugby Union are codes which have a similar appearance. Players in these codes adopt 'front-line' positions prior to the commencement of each play, use throwing and running as the primary methods for transporting the ball, only kick the ball on a few specific occasions, employ body tackling as a major skill and are involved in stop and start passages of play which last between 5-90s. Soccer, Australian Rules and Gaelic football while being very different from the above mentioned three codes, have similar characteristics. Players in these codes adopt positions which are dispersed over the playing surface, use kicking as the primary method for transporting the ball, tend to pass the ball rather than run with it, use limited body tackling and are involved in relatively continuous play.

A computerised literature search highlighted an extreme variation in the number of investigations in each football sport. For example in the area of injury, there were 5400 studies conducted in American Football and only one study in Gaelic football. The apparent neglect of Gaelic football in this paper is not necessarily due to a lack of commitment to this particular code. It is rather due to the non-appearance of relevant material in the international sports medicine literature.

All codes are sensitive to the need to reduce the number of playing hours lost through injury. At all levels, the loss of a key player through injury results in a reduction in the competitiveness of a team (Ekstrand et al., 1983) and a high injury rate deters prospective participants.

Unfortunately because of the nature of football there is a relatively high risk of injury compared to other sports. Of 1652 sports injuries reported in three casualty departments in Brisbane, Australia in 1980, 35 sports were represented. Altogether 63% of cases occurred in either Australian Rules, Rugby League, Rugby Union or soccer: the figures could be due to the popularity of football as a sporting activity. Sixty percent of these injuries occurred during competition and 11% during training (Smithers and Myers 1985). Of 4673 sports injuries at Ulleval Hospital in Oslo (Norway) 35% were caused by football (Maehlum and Daljord, 1984).

The risk of injury is at one end of the spectrum of deterrents and attractions for football participants. At the other end of the spectrum are the highly attractive external and internal elements of football which encourage participants to ignore the injury risk.

This paper attends to those common elements of the football codes which have:-

(i) captured the interest and attention of players and spectators, and
(ii) prompted scientific investigation.

Common attractive components of football codes

Passing

Visual examination reveals that despite the varying methods used to project the ball, there are several similarities in the passing strategies adopted by each football code. Some of the common strategies include:-

(i) short quick passing to create an opening in defence:
(ii) long direct and indirect passing to develop space and provide an opportunity to increase the forward momentum of the team;
(iii) placing the ball to the receiver's advantage, thus limiting any possibility of interception by a defender;
(iv) supportive running to provide the ball carrier with planned or reactionary passing options;
(v) the prevalence of automated responses which are interwoven with necessarily creative and impulsive passes;
(vi) passing the ball with the intent of developing optimal ball and team momentum;
(vii) the adoption of situationally specific passing strategies.

Evasion

Evasion is evident in most team sports. However, the need to optimise evasion skills is accentuated in football codes, particularly in American Football, Australian Rules, Rugby League and Rugby Union.

In each of these codes, the distance a player may run with the ball is not restricted. One of the most exciting sights at any football match is a solo run with the ball, knowing that the ball carrier is the only player who can be tackled.Some of the common evasion strategies include:-

(i) false body movement (e.g. eyes and hip) to deceive the opponent into thinking that the ball carrier is committed to a path other than the intended path;
(ii) use of acceleration and speed;
(iii) selective use of peripheral vision;
(iv) effective use of sidestepping, swerving and turning skills:
(v) automated evasive responses to tackler strategies;

(vi) support for the evading ball carrier is provided by team-mates who either block the path of opponents or provide passing options. The availability of passing options enables the ball carrier to use a fake pass as part of the evasion strategy.

Catching

Catching the ball is a dominant skill in American Football, Australian Rules, Rugby League, Rugby Union, and Gaelic football. In soccer catching is restricted to the goalkeeper and therefore is not a dominant skill; nevertheless, it is extremely important.

Some of the common catching strategies include:-

(i) in American Football, Rugby League, Rugby Union and soccer - protecting the ball by clutching it to the body as soon as possible. In Australian Rules and Gaelic football the ball is most often held in the hands after a catch to permit quick disposal;

(ii) catching the ball in outstretched hands when being closely checked by an opponent;

(iii) moving to meet the ball at the catcher's optimal height and speed;

(iv) catching the ball in two hands rather than one;

(v) developing quick reflexive catching skills to cope with unpredictable ball movement;

(vi) selectively attending to the ball visually despite the possible risk of injury due to the aggressive posture of another catcher or a tackler.

Contact

Contact is permitted in American Football, Australian Rules, Rugby League and Rugby Union, however in soccer and Gaelic football intentional contact is prohibited. In all codes, the evaluation of the degree of contact in relation to the contact rules is typically dependent upon the interpretation of the umpire or referee.

Some of the common contact strategies include:-

(i) moving into situations of possible collision with maximum momentum;

(ii) mauling an opponent when tackling;

(iii) performing the tackling skill in such a way that the risk of head and neck injury is minimal;

(iv) deliberately using contact which is outside the rules of the game;

(v) accepting the prevalence of unintentional contact and the possible resulting injury;

(vi) using contact as a means of controlled and uncontrolled aggression.

Kicking

Kicking is the unifying factor between all of the codes. While kicking is common to the codes, all codes have produced methods of kicking unique to their game. In all codes a moving or stationary ball may be kicked off the ground, kickers may be in a situation where being tackled while kicking is either permitted or prohibited, and points are scored by kicking the ball between and/or under goal posts.

Some of the common kicking strategies include:-

- (i) punt kicking to gain maximum distance and positional advantage. It is typically used to convert a highly defensive situation into a possible offence;
- (ii) adopting an angular approach when having a free kick for goal or for maximum distance;
- (iii) using various minor adjustments to foot contact to produce a range of effective kicks for specific situations;
- (iv) guiding the ball onto the foot with the hand.

Unpredictability

The relatively large number of players in each of the football games, combined with the high injury risk, enhances the possibility for every team to 'have their day' and win. Some of the common components of the codes which produce unpredictability include:-

- (i) misdirected passing which often results from pressure by an opponent;
- (ii) the shape of the ball in Australian Rules, American Football, Rugby League and Rugby Union;
- (iii) varying playing surfaces;
- (iv) encouragement of players to be creative and develop initiative;
- (v) a large playing area permitting the development of optional plays;
- (vi) varying permutations and combinations of team line ups and strategies.

Common Areas of Scientific Investigation

The following tables (Tables 1-8) identify some of the common research areas between the codes. Unfortunately, due to time constraints, the vast array of investigations from which facts can be gleaned, and the limited access to some codes (Gaelic football, Rugby League and American Football), the Tables are representative rather than exhaustive.

On most occasions, the data relate to professional teams and depict the findings of a series of studies in each area. The rugby data are typically from Rugby Union. Most of the American Football data come from investigations conducted between 1975-1980, while data for the other codes eminate mostly from research conducted in the 1980's.

Some of the common areas of investigation include body composition, physiology of performance, time and motion, yearly programmes, injuries, modifications, kicking, spectator and/or player violence. There are other common areas of investigation. In psychology, for example, other than the reports that different personalities tend to play in different positions in teams, no information was found to suggest that common threads exist between the codes.

Body Composition and Physiology of Performance

Players in Australian Rules and American Football can be up to 193cm tall, while some soccer players are only 167cm tall. Overall American Football (190.2cm) has the tallest players, Australian Rules (183cm) and Rugby (183cm) players have the same height and soccer (176cm) has the shortest players on average. American Football (197kg) has the heaviest players and soccer (76kg) the lightest. Despite Australian Rules (93kg) having heavier individuals than Rugby (88kg), the average weight of Rugby players (84kg) is heavier than that of Australian Rules players (80kg).

Table 1. Height, weight and $\dot{V}O_2max$ of football players

	Height (cm)	Weight (kg)	$\dot{V}O_2max$ (ml kg^{-1} min^{-1})	Source
Soccer	167-186* $\bar{x}$ 176	74-86* $\bar{x}$ 76	59-63	Ekblom, 1986 Raven et al., 1976 Rhodes et al., 1986
Rugby	176-187 $\bar{x}$ 183	81-88 $\bar{x}$ 84	54-60*	Maud, 1983 Burke et al., 1983 Bell, 1980
American Football	182-193 $\bar{x}$ 190.2	85-117* $\bar{x}$ 107	45-53*	Wilmore et al.,1976 Adams et al., 1982 Burke et al., 1983
Australian Rules Football	176-193* $\bar{x}$ 183	79-93* $\bar{x}$ 80	64	Dawson, 1985 Ackland et al.,1984

*Extreme range caused by the varying demands of specific player positions in the game.

Australian Rules (64 ml kg^{-1} min^{-1}) and soccer players (59-63 ml kg^{-1} min^{-1}) have the highest $\dot{V}O_2max$, indicating a requirement for continuous effort of a reasonable intensity. American Football (45-53 ml kg^{-1} min^{-1}) has the lowest $\dot{V}O_2max$ which is only minimally above the average population.

Table 2. Age, lean body weight and body fat of football players

	Age (years)-	L.B.W. (kg)	%Fat	Somatotype	Source
Soccer	25.6	67-75 x 68	8-13 x 9.5		Withers, 1982 Raven et al.,1976 Raven et al.,1976 Rhodes et al.,1986 Maud and Shultz 1984
Rugby	28.1	71-77 x 76	9-13 x 12	Endo- Mesomorph	Maud and Shultz 1984 Williams et al. Bell, 1980
American Football	24.6	77-96 x 91	9-18 x 16	Endo- Mesomorph	Wilmore et al.,1976 Burke et al., 1983 Bloomfield, 1979
Australian Football	24.3	x 79	8-14 x 10	Mesomorph	Dawson, 1985 Douge, 1978

The average ages for the elite in soccer (25.6), American Football (24.6), and Australian Rules (24.3) are very similar. In Rugby the players seem to be older, mean age being 28.1 years.

Despite Rugby players (84 kg) being heavier than Australian Rules players (80 kg, see Table 1) the lean body weight (LBW) of Australian Rules players (79 kg) is heavier than Rugby players (76 kg). Australian Rules, American Football and Rugby players are all essentially mesomorphs with American Football and Rugby players having a significant endomorphic component. It would be logical also to predict mesomorphy as the dominant characteristic body type of soccer players.

Unfortunately the extreme variance in percent body fat values resulting from the use of various non-compatible techniques and formulae detracts from the validity of comparisons between the codes. The percent body fat values in Table 2 are those obtained either from the use of the Durnin and Womersley (1974) procedure or from averaging a variety of scores reported in a particular code.

Soccer (9.5%) and Australian Rules (10%) players have similar percent body fat content. While individual players in American Football and Rugby (9%) are relatively lean, overall the Rugby players (12%) and American Football (16%) are fatter than players in the other codes.

Table 3. Flexibility, 40 yard sprint, vertical jump and bench press of footballers. (Mean values are given with range in parentheses)

	Flex-ibility (cm)	40 yard Sprint	Vertical Jump (cm)	Bench Press (kg)	Source
Soccer	41	5.0	56 (53-59)	73	Reilly, 1979 Raven et al., 1975 Rhodes et al., 1986 Ekblom, 1986
Rugby	44		54 (51-57)	86	Maud, 1983 Maud and Shultz, 1984
American Football	46 (41-49)	4.75		138	Wilmore et al.,1976 Crews and Meadows, 1978
Australian Rules	42	5.05	57 (52-62)	82	Dawson, 1985 Parkin, 1982 Douge, 1978

Traditionally power athletes have been more flexible than aerobic athletes. One could suggest that power athletes have more rigorous flexibility routines because of the demands of their sport.

This notion is supported by the data in Table 3 where the least flexible sports, soccer (41 cm) and Australian Rules (42 cm), have the slowest 40 yard sprint times, 5.0 s and 5.05 s respectively, and the most flexible sport, American Football (46 cm), has the fastest 40 yard sprint time, 4.75 s.

In Australian Rules and soccer, players are required to jump explosively to either catch or head the ball. It is not surprising therefore to find that soccer (56 cm) and Australian Rules players (57 cm) have the highest vertical jumps amongst the various football codes.

The significant variance in the players' upper body strength reflects the relative demands of each code and the difference in the size of players between the codes. The American Football players (138 kg) are much stronger than those in the other codes. Rugby (86 kg) and Australian Rules (82 kg) are very similar. Understandably because soccer is primarily a non-tackle (upper body tackling) game, the upper body strength of the players (73 kg) is relatively low.

Table 4. Mean and maximum heart rate (HR) and $\mathring{V}E$ of footballers in match-play. (Ranges are given in parentheses)

	Mean HR (beats min^{-1})	Max. HR (beats min^{-1})	$\dot{V}$ (ℓ min^{-1})	Source
Soccer	157	188	167 (154-181)	Reilly, 1986 Ekblom, 1986 Raven et al.,1975 Rhodes, 1986
Rugby	161	184	175	Maud, 1983 Morton, 1978
American Football		182	155 (143-174)	Wilmore, 1976
Australian Rules				Hahn et al.,1979

The mean game heart rates (HR) during match-play in soccer (157 beats min^{-1}), Rugby (161 beats min^{-1}) and Australian Rules (161 beats min^{-1}) are almost identical. Maximum HR values mirror the relative aerobic contributions of each code. Soccer (188 beats min^{-1}) and Australian Rugby (186 beats min^{-1}) are the highest HR values, while the more anaerobic game of American Football (182 beats min^{-1}) has the lowest maximum HR during competition.

Knowing that the average age of the rugby players is four years older than the other codes, it could be assumed that the 184 beats min^{-1} for Rugby is a similar percentage of maximum HR to the other codes. Also the low aerobic component in American Football could explain the low $\dot{V}E$ (155 l min^{-1}) despite the greater size of the players.

Soccer (167 l min^{-1}) and Rugby (175 l min^{-1}) have high ventilation values, thus reflecting the relatively aerobic demands of the games. The higher $\dot{V}E$ for Rugby could be explained by the greater size of the players (see Table 1).

The following areas of physiological investigation are identified as currently prominent in one or more of the football codes:-

(i) Blood analysis - lactate, glycogen, protein, haemoglobin (Hb), haematocrit, glucose, triglyceride, cholesterol, serum ferritin;

(ii) Muscle fibre configuration;

(iii) Anaerobic power and capacity;

(iv) Aerobic energy yield during play - % $\dot{V}O_2$ max.

(v) Energy expenditure for each physical involvement, e.g. exertional costs of changes in directional modes of running (Reilly and Bowen, 1984) and dribbling (Reilly and Ball, 1984).

(vi) Heat dissipation, fluid replacement and weight loss;

(vii) Muscle torque - muscle balance, rehabilitation using isokinetic equipment;

(viii) Phosphate recovery evaluation and training.

According to the parameters in Table 5, the movement of players in Australian Rules and soccer is almost identical. Of the 11195 m covered by soccer players, 26.3% involves walking, 44.6% jogging and 18.9% striding-sprinting. Australian Rules players cover 10633 m comprising 27% walking, 58% jogging and 20% striding-sprinting.

Rugby players (5800 m) cover far less distance with a much larger portion sprinting (34%) and walking (37%). The amount of time players have the ball as a percent of the total game time in Rugby, soccer and Australian Rules is 1.3%, 1.9% and 1.7% respectively. It should be remembered that there is a pronounced division of labour in Rugby and so some players will walk much more than sprint.

Table 5. Time and motion study of footballers

	Soccer		Rugby		Australian Rules Football	
Distance covered in Game (m)	11 195 (Withers 1982)		5800 (Morton 1978)		10 633 (Hahn et al.,1979)	
Mode of travel % of total distance						
Walking	26.3		37.0		27.0	
Jogging	44.6		28.0		58.0	
Stride-Sprint	18.9		34.0		20.0	
% Distance/Time covered in Sprint mode	5%	6.0m	56%	10 s*	30%	5 m
	50%	18.0m	85%	15 s*	57%	10 m
	80%	32.0m	5%	30 s*	78%	20 m
	90%	44.0m			89%	30 m
	95%	55.0m			95%	40 m

* Rugby sprinting was measured as an amount of time in the sprint mode.

In soccer and Australian Rules, nearly all (95%) of the sprinting is over distances of less than 60 m. The majority of sprints are less than 20 m, 78% in Australian Rules and over 50% in soccer. In Rugby, the majority of sprints last considerably longer than in soccer or Australian Rules. Assuming that a 10 s sprint is equivalent to approximately 60-70 m, then in Rugby only 56% of the sprints are less than 60-70 m.

The energy expenditures for Rugby and Australian Rules have been determined from an assessment of training and game heart rates and types of training activity. The training patterns in these games exhibit a typical weekly rhythm (Fig. 1).

The weekly cycles of energy expenditure for Rugby, Soccer and Australian Rules are very similar. Rugby and Australian Rules are identical and soccer tends to be less demanding on Sunday and more demanding on Wednesday. This reflects the build-up tapering and recovery days framed around week-end (Saturdays) competition.

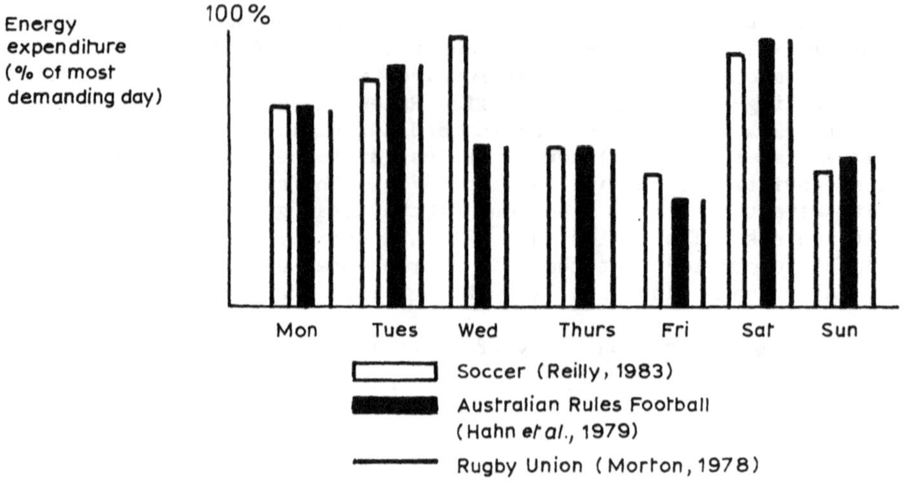

Figure 1. Typical weekly rhythm in expenditure of energy among the various football codes

Yearly Programme

The components of the yearly programme for each code are basically the same. Identified in Table 6 are the specific activities which make up the yearly programme of all football codes. The emphasis placed on specific activities varies markedly between the codes.

Table 6. Components of the yearly programme for players of Australian Rules, Soccer, American Football and Rugby

1. Running - continuous, fartlek, long-slow interval - short-fast interval, specific speed and agility;
2. Resistance work - strength endurance, strength, power, specific power;
3. Body circuits and flexibility routines;
4. Individual skills;
5. Game and team skills, offence and defence;
6. Patterns of play drills;
7. Minor games.

Kicking

Biomechanical analysis has necessarily resulted in a common set of performance criteria for the basic kicks in each code. There are times in each code when a relatively immobile ball is kicked.

Common technical suggestions arising from research in soccer (Block, 1982) and soccer, Australian Rules and Rugby (Bloomfield et al., 1979; Elliott et al., 1980) are:-

(i) 45° approach with slight forward lean;
(ii) leg adduction of kicking leg on second last step to cater for trunk rotation;
(iii) explosive final step;
(iv) externally rotate non-kicking hip;
(v) support foot 15-20cm to the side of the ball, transverse arch crosses imaginary ball bisection;
(vi) internally rotate kicking leg during kick: trunk rotation begins simultaneously with right (kicking leg) hip extension and right knee flexion;
(vii) left knee eccentric contraction to absorb body weight;
(viii) right knee leads foot to ball;
(ix) as right knee passes over the ball, it is forcefully extended and foot plantar-flexed; left arm adducts across chest to prevent excessive left shoulder rotation and keep shoulders parallel to goal line;
(x) deceleration by eccentric knee flexion, external rotation, extention and abduction at hip joint.

Marking and catching

The following brief summary of an investigation by Walsh (1980) reveals an area of research requiring attention in each code although it does not identify a common research thread in football. More importantly perhaps, it reveals an approach to catching which should be emphasised in each code.

The advantages of side-on approach vs front approach to catching a football are:-

(i) it is easier to assess vertical flight characteristics;
(ii) it is easier to assess ball velocity;
(iii) greater accuracy in predicting the flight of the ball over last 6-7m due to maximal disparity of two retinal images;
(iv) late entry into opponent's visual field;
(v) increased capacity for hip rotation to contribute to height of jump.

Spectator and Player Violence in Football

All football codes comment on the prevalence of violence on and off the playing field. The following quotations represent attempts to explain the characteristics of football which promote violence.

'Extreme reactions are more likely when the spectator is a strong supporter and more predisposed to biased perception; the spectator is a member of a group which endorses aggressive behaviour; the spectator is part of a large, noisy, chanting, densely-packed standing crowd; the spectator observes rough contact, aggressive, combative sports, or the spectator's team suffers an unexpected defeat' (Glencross, 1978).

A second view was presented by Silva (1983):-

'...the more 'physical' the participation, the longer one had been involved in sport, or the higher the competitive level of participation, the more legitimate rule violating behaviour was perceived... ...in order to enhance continuation in organised sport, male athletes (especially in contact and collision sports) must learn and follow expectancies for normative rule violating behaviour'

According to McIntosh (1979);-

'70% of professional players and 54% of amateur players believe players in position to score should be brought down unmercifully. Also condoned are toughness, deception, dishonesty and anger'.

The roots of violence among players and spectators may be more complex then apparent in these explanations. The phenomenon of soccer hooliganism is considered in detail elsewhere in this volume by Dunning and co-workers.

Injuries

Head and neck injuries are common to all codes. American Football and Rugby (26%) have reported similar percentages of head and neck injuries as have soccer (12%) and Australian Rules (13%).

Table 7. Football, head and neck injuries

	%	Comments
Soccer	12	From 1964-1980 (Biener, 1982)
	5.2	Youth soccer (Schmidt-Olson et al., 1985)
Rugby	22	Period of 20 years (O'Connell, 1954)
	26	From 1980-1983, Youth (Sparks, 1981)
	18.9	Adult-student Rugby (Reilly and Hardiker, 1981)
Australian	10.2	One season (Wiklund et al., 1985)
Football	13.0	One season (Jeffries and Dawson, 1979)
American	29.0	8 years of College football (Albright et al., 1985) 40000 players treated for head and neck injuries in school football in 1976 (Underwood, 1978).

The types of head and neck injuries that are common to each code are soft tissue damage, concussion, fractured teeth, fractured nose, fractured maxilla, fractured mandible and fractured vertebra. When fatalities in American Football were examined there were on average 19 deaths per 100 000 participants every year from 1960-1978 (Mueller and Blyth, 1979).

It should be noted that mouthguards are encouraged in all codes (Upson, 1982). Additionally American Football team owners made helmet blocking or 'ramming' illegal in 1979 (Cushing, 1979).

Table 8 reveals the most common injury sites in each code. In soccer (53%), Rugby (38%) and Australian Rules (62%) most injuries occur to the lower limb. It should be noted that knee braces are mandatory for 25 year olds in the U.S.F.L.

Injuries to the knee pervade each code, Rugby (15%), soccer (25%), American Football (24%) and Australian Rules (10%). Ankle injuries are dominant in soccer (23%), Rugby (16%) and Australian Rules (18%).

All codes report that minimal injury occurs prior to puberty and that veterans suffer the least injury among professional players. The most susceptible age group to injury in all codes is the 15-24 year olds (La Cava, 1964; Mueller and Blyth, 1979: Jeffries and Dawson, 1979).

The most common types of injury are contusions: soccer (30%), Rugby (33%), Australian Rules (35%). The next most common injury is sprains, accounting for 41% of injuries in soccer and 27% in Australian Rules.

The most common cause of injury is the tackle: soccer (47%), Rugby (53%), Australian Rules (22%). In Rugby and Australian Rules, contact contributes to 75% and 71% of injury respectively.

A possible source of injury in football is the surface on which the game is played. Stevenson and Anderson (1981) investigated 32 teams playing on artificial turf and 32 teams on natural turf playing touch football. Twice as many injuries were recorded in the artificial turf teams compared to the natural turf teams. On the basis of this study it seems that grass is preferable to synthetic surfaces on safety criteria.

Injury reduction in football

Authorities in American Football, Australian Rules, soccer and Rugby all advocate early mobilisation, isokinetic testing and isokinetic exercise for the rehabilitation and reduction of hamstring and ligament tears (Heiser et al., 1984 and Sandor et al., 1986). To enhance safety in children's football, certain modifications of the adult form of the game may be made. To produce an attractive, safe and enjoyable sporting environment for children to learn the skills of football, the codes have independently identified common strategies. There is agreement on the need to maximise activity and safety, eliminate game complications and reduce stoppages and contact.

Methods include:- reducing the size of field, having less players per team, varying the ball size, shape and texture, shortening the game time, and rotating the players through different positions.

These suggestions have arisen from research work in Rugby by Docherty and Morton, (1980); in soccer by McIntosh, (1979); in Australian Rules by Gibson, (1977); and in American Football and soccer by Rokosz, (1981).

Overview

There are several common threads between the games. This review highlights those common threads which are specific to football. In particular, threads which have captured the interest and attention of players and spectators and have prompted scientific investigation

Table 8. Injury site in football
Percentage of injuries occurring at the site on the body which is most prone to injury and common to each code of football

	Ankle	Knee	Lower limb	Thigh	Comment	Source
Soccer	20–23%	14–25%	53%	Not significant	10 year olds – 1.88% 19 year olds – 8.74%	McCarroll et al., 1984 Biener, 1982 Schmidt-Olsen et al.,1985 Ekstrand et al.,1983
Rugby	6–16%	12–15%	32–38%	Not significant	14 year olds-less injury 12 year olds-minimal injury	Sparks, 1981 Sparks, 1981 Reilly, 1981 Sidney, 1983
American Football	Not significant	24%	Not significant	Not significant	12 year olds and veterans have less injury	Ryan et al., 1986 Mueller and Blyth, 1979 Underwood, 1978
Australian Rules Football	12–18%	10%	62%	21–23%	Novices are twice as vulnerable to injuries as veterans	Aaron, 1985 Jeffries and Dawson, 1979

N.B. Detroit Lions (American Football) had 21 knee operations in one season.

Table 9. Major cause and type of injury in football

	Contusion	Sprain	Tackle	Contact	Source
Soccer	10–30%	27–41%	47%	Not significant	La Cava, 1964 McCarroll et al., 1984 Schmidt-Olsen, 1985 Ekstrand et al., 1983
Rugby	14–33%	Not significant	46–53%	75%	Sparks, 1981 Sidney, 1983
Australian Rules Football	35%	27%	22%	71%	Aaron, 1985 Jeffries and Dawson, 1979
American Football – In one year injured:		1 000 000 in 20 000 high schools 70 000 in 900 colleges 100% of NFL players			Underwood, 1978 Heisen et al., 1984

have been described.

The interrelationship of many components of each code necessarily encourages the transfer of expertise and knowledge from one football code to the other. There are already examples of the cross fertilisation of ideas in the areas of kicking technique, tackling, protective equipment, rehabilitation, strategy and others. Football coaches, umpires, players, trainers, administrators and researchers should enthusiastically pursue knowledge from all football codes.

References

Aaron, W. and Whitford K. (1985) A survey of injuries in Australian Rules Football in one season. Shenton Park Sports Clinic: Unpublicised Report.

Ackland, T., Dawson, B. and Roberts, C. (1984) Pre-season fitness profile of Australian football players and umpires. Sports Coach, 8, 43-48.

Adams, J., Mottola, M., Bagnall, K.M. and McFadden, K.O. (1982) Total body fat content in a group of professional football players. Sports Sci., 7, 36-40.

Albright, J.P., McAuley, E., Martin, R., Gowley, E.T. and Foster, D.T. (1985) Head and neck injuries in college football: an eight year analysis. J.Sports Med., 13, 147-152.

Bell, W. (1980) Body composition and maximal aerobic power of rugby union forwards. J. Sports Med. Phys. Fit., 20, 447-451.

Biener, K. (1982) Sportunfeele bei Einzelsportorten (Sport accidents in different forms of sport). Sozialund Praeventimedizin, 27, 16-18.

Block, P. (1982) Video analysis may reduce soccer injuries. (Incorrect kicking techniques). Physician and Sportsmed., 10, 29-32.

Bloomfield, J. (1979) Modifying human physical capacities and/or technique to suit performance. Sports Coach, 3, No. 2.

Bloomfield, J., Elliott, B.C. and Davies, C.M. (1979) Development of the soccer kick, a cinematographical analysis. J. Human Mov't. Stud., 5, 152-159.

Burke, L.M., Read, R.S.D. and Gollan, R.A. (1983) Australian rules football: an anthropometric study of participants. Unpublished report.

Crews, T.R. and Meadows, W.J. (1978) Analysis of reaction time, speed and body composition of college football players. J. Sports Med. Phys. Fit., 18, 169-174.

Cushing, D. (1979) N.F.L. expands roughness rules. Physician Sportsmed., 7, 17-18.

Dawson, B. (1985) Physical and physiological characteristics of eight league footballers. Sports Coach, 9, 33-36.

Docherty, D. and Morton, A.R. (1980) Mini-Rugby - a modified game for skill and action. Sports Coach, 4, 8-12.

Douge, B.M. (1978) Testing in Australian rules football. Sports Coach, 6, No. 1.

Durnin, J.V.G.A. and Womersley, J. (1974) Body fat assessed from total body density and its estimation from skinfold thickness: measurements in 481 men one woman aged 16 to 72 years. Brit. J. Nutr., 32, 77-97.

Ekblom, B. (1986) Applied physiology of soccer. Sports Med., 3, 50-60.
Ekstrand, J., Gillquist, J., Moller, M., Oberg, B. and Liljedahl, S. (1983) Incidence of soccer injuries and their relation to training and team success. Amer. J. Sports Med., 11, 63-67.
Elliott, B.C., Bloomfeld, J. and Davies, C.M. (1980) Development of the punt kick: a cinematographical analysis. J. Human Mov't. Stud., 6, 142-150.
Gibson, B. (1977) Participation in junior Australian Rules football. Sports Coach, 15-25.
Glencross, D. (1978) Spectators and sport. Sports Coach, 2, No. 2.
Hahn, A., Taylor, N., Hunt, B., Woodhouse, T. and Schultz, G. (1979) Physiological relationships between training activities and match play in Australian Football rovers. Sports Coach, 3, No. 3.
Heisen, T.M., Weber, J., Sullivan, G., Clare, P. and Jacobs, R.R. (1984) Prophylaxis and management of hamstring muscle injuries in intercollegiate football players. Amer. J. Sports Med., 12, 368-370.
Jeffries, A.O. and Dawson, G.M. (1979) A study of injuries to League footballers in Australian Rules football. Unpublished report, University of Western Australian.
La Cava, G. (1964) The prevention of accidents caused by sport. Paper presented at the International Congress of Sport Sciences, Tokyo.
Maehlum, S. and Daljord, O.A. (1984) Acute sports injuries in Oslo: a one year study. Brit. J. Sports Med., 18, 181-185.
McCarroll, J.R., Meaney, C. and Sieber, J.M. (1984) Profile of youth soccer injuries. Physician Sportsmed., 12, No. 2.
McIntosh, P. (1979) Fair play: The player's view, in P. McIntosh (Ed.), Fair play, London: Heinemann. 1979.
Maud, P.J. (1983) Physiological and anthropometric parameters that describe a rugby union team. Brit. J. Sports Med., 17, 16-23.
Maud, P.J. and Shultz, B.B. (1984) The U.S. national rugby team: a physiological and anthropometric assessment. Phys. Sportsmed., 12, 86-99.
Milburn, L.J. and Kerlan, R.(1976) Football pros' strengths - and c.v. weakness - charted. Physician Sportsmed., 4, 45-54.
Morton, A.R. (1978) Applying physiological principles to rugby training. Sports Coach, 2, 4-9.
Mueller, F.O. and Blyth, C.S. (1979) Catastrophic head and neck injuries. Physician Sportsmed., 7, 71-74.
O'Connell, T.C.J.(1954) Rugby football injuries and their prevention: a review of 600 cases. J. Irish Med. Ass., 34-20.
Parkin, D. (1982) Fitness appraisal in Australian Football. Sports Coach, 6, 40-44.
Raven, P.B., Gettman, L.R., Pollock, M.L. and Cooper, K.H. (1976) A Physiological evaluation of professional soccer players. Brit. J. Sports Med., 10, 209-216.
Reilly, T. (1981) Sports Fitness and Sports Injuries. London: Faber and Faber.
Reilly, T. (1983) Observations on fitness and training for soccer. Soc. Nat. Inst. Sport J., 6, 3-11.

Reilly, T. (1986) Fundamental studies in soccer. In: Beitzage zun Sportspielforshaung. Sportwissenschaft und Sportpracis. (edited by R. Andresen) pp. 114-120. Hamburg: Verlag Ingrid Czwalina.
Reilly, T. and Ball, D. (1984). The net physiological cost of dribbling a soccer ball. Res. Quart. Exerc. Sport, 55, 267-271.
Reilly, T. and Bowen, T. (1984). Exertional costs of changes in directional modes of running. Percept. Motor Skills, 58, 149-150.
Reilly, T. and Hardiker, R. (1981) Somatotype and injuries in adult student rugby football. J. Sports Med. Phys. Fit., 21, 186-191.
Rhodes, E.C., Potts, J.E.,. Mosher, R.E., McKenzie, D.C. and Franks, I.M. (1986) Physiological profiles of the Canadian olympic soccer team. Can. J. Appl. Sports Sci., 11, 31-36.
Rokosz, F.M. (1981) Modification of team sports rules. Paper presented at the Annual Convention of the American Alliance for Health, Physical Education, Recreation and Dance, (Boston, M.A.).
Ryan, A.J., Grant, T.T., Rosenfled, R.T., Rovewze, G.D. and Schottenfeld, M. (1986) Knee braces to prevent injuries in football. Physician Sportsmed., 14, 108-112, 115-118.
Sandor, S.M., Hart, J.A.L. and Oakes, B.W. (1986) Case study rehabilitation of a surgically repaired medical collateral knee ligament using a limited motion cast and isokinetic exercise. J. Orthop. Sports Phys. Therapy, 7, 154-158.
Schmidt-Olsen, S., Bünemann, L.K.H., Lade, V. and Brassoe, J.O.K. (1985) Soccer injuries of youth. Brit. J. Sports Med., 19, 161-164.
Sidney, (1983) Schoolboy rugby union injuries. A Survey Conducted by the Australian School's Rugby Union A.S.R.U. Report.
Silva, J.M. (1983) The perceived legitimacy of rule violating behaviour in sport. J. Sports Psychol., 5, 438-448.
Smithers, M. and Mayers, P.T. (1985) Injuries in sport. A prospective casualty study. Med. J. Austr., 142, 457-461.
Sparks, J.P. (1981) Half a million hours of rugby football. Brit. J. Sports Med., 15, 30-32.
Stevenson, M.J. and Anderson, B.D. (1981) Effects of playing surfaces on injuries in college intramural touch football. J. Nat. Intramural Recr. Sports Ass., 5, 59-64.
Underwood, J. (1978) An unfolding tragedy. Sports Illustrated, 49, 69-82.
Upson, N. (1982) Dental injuries and the attitudes of rugby players to mouthguards. Brit. J. Sports Med., 16, 241-244.
Walsh, W.D. (1980) Marking skill in Australian football front - on versus side-on approach to the ball. Sports Coach, 4, 37-40.
Wiklund, M., Wan, A. and Whitford, K. (1985) A survey of injuries in Australian rules football in one season. Unpublished report.
Williams, C., Reid, E.M. and Coutts, R. (1973) Observations on the aerobic power of University Rugby players and professional soccer players. Brit. J. Sports Med., 7, 390-39.
Wilmore, J.H., Parr, R.B., Haskell, W.H., Costill, D.L., Milbun, W. and Kerlan, R.K. (1976) Football pro's strength and weakness charted. Physician Sportsmed., 4, 45-54.
Withers, R.T. (1982) Fitness for Soccer. In: Soccer Fundamentals. N.S.W.: A.H. and A.W. Reed Pty Ltd.

Part II

Nutrition

NUTRITION FOR THE ELITE FOOTBALLER

Ira Jacobs
Defence and Civil Institute of Environmental Medicine, 1133 Sheppard Avenue West, Downsview, Ontario, Canada, M3M 3B9.

Introduction

No single topic addressed by the various papers in the proceedings of this conference will guarantee success for the footballer or for any other competitive athlete or coach. The purpose of this paper is to present the football practitioner with the results of nutrition studies which, if properly applied, should enhance the potential for players to perform at their physical optimum. The majority of the discussion will centre around the consumption of carbohydrate since it is the only macronutrient the availability of which has been shown to be associated with enhanced or impaired exercise performance.

Fuel Availability and Exercise

Newsholme and Leech (1983) have calculated the duration of time during which an average sized man (65 kg body weight, 12% body fat) could either run at a marathon pace (84 kJ min^{-1}) or walk (6.4 km h^{-1}, 21.7 kJ min^{-1}) using only one of the body's available fuel stores (Table 1). In contrast with such theoretical calculations, the transduction of the chemical energy in these fuel supplies into mechanical work by muscle tissue depends on simultaneous contributions by all of the fuel reserves. The energy demands of sedentary activities are covered approximately equally by the catabolism of fat and carbohydrate; the contribution of carbohydrates increases as the intensity of exercise increases until almost the entire energy demand of maximal intensity exercise of a 30-60 s duration is met by carbohydrate metabolism. Although protein metabolism probably contributes significantly more to energy metabolism than previously believed (Lemon et al., 1984) Table 1 demonstrates that it is unlikely that the body's stores of protein and/or fat would be depleted to the extent that the capacity to transduce energy to the working muscles would be impaired. Thus, the only fuel store which appears to be relatively scarce is the store of carbohydrate, stored as glycogen in the liver and skeletal musculature. The following sections will describe how glycogen availability relates to the capacity to perform exercise of various intensities and what happens to muscle glycogen levels during actual soccer matches.

Table 1. Fuel reserves in average man

Fuel store	Reserve g	Reserve kJ	Fuel sufficient for Walking days	Fuel sufficient for Running min
Adipose tissue	9000	337000	10.8	4018
Liver glycogen	90	1500	0.05	18
Muscle glycogen	350	6000	0.20	71
Circulating glucose	20	320	0.01	4
Body protein	8800	150000	4.8	1800

Modified from Newsholme and Leech (1983).

Muscle Glycogen and Physical Performance

The introduction of the percutaneous needle biopsy technique (Bergström, 1962) to study muscle metabolism during exercise not only confirmed classical earlier experiments (Christensen and Hansen, 1939) demonstrating that endurance exercise performance is enhanced after a carbohydrate-rich diet, but also documented a direct association between such performance and the amount of glycogen stored in the exercising muscles before beginning exercise (Ahlborg et al., 1967; Bergström et al., 1967; Hermansen et al., 1967). These studies also demonstrated that muscle glycogen stores could be severely reduced by either hard exercise or by several days of a carbohydrate-poor diet, and that a carbohydrate-rich diet would cause increased intramuscular glycogen stores and improve endurance exercise performance in a controlled laboratory setting. Karlsson and Saltin (1971) were the first to apply these findings in a field setting when they demonstrated that each of 10 runners completed a 30 km cross-country run in less time after a carbohydrate-rich diet than after their normal diet. All of these findings provided the basis for the carbohydrate-loading diet that is today practised by many endurance runners, such as marathoners, during the week before competition. The reader is referred to Åstrand (1967) and Sherman et al. (1981) for in-depth discussion of such dietary procedures.

Although the studies referred to above relate primarily to high intensity endurance exercise lasting longer than 45-60 min, many competitive sporting activities demand maximal intensity exercise for a duration ranging from only a few seconds to a few minutes. Many team sports in particular require that the athlete perform both endurance and sprint exercise at various times during a game. The rate of glycogen utilization increases exponentially with increases in exercise intensity (Saltin and Karlsson, 1971) so the question arises as to the effects on maximal intensity, short term exercise performance when muscle glycogen levels are very depleted. Recent studies suggest that strength and muscular endurance are impaired after hard exercise which induces glycogen depletion (Jacobs et al., 1981; Maughan and Poole, 1981; Heigenhauser et al., 1983; Young and Davies, 1984; Greenhaff et al., 1987), but it is difficult in these studies to separate out the effects of glycogen depletion from the effects of the hard exercise used to induce the glycogen depletion. More recent studies have clarified this picture somewhat and it seems that dynamic and static muscular strength are impaired even two to three days after hard exercise, even if glycogen levels are restored to near normal levels (Young and Davies, 1984; Sherman et al., 1984; Jacobs, 1987). There is evidence to suggest, however, that this impairment is more marked when muscle glycogen levels are low (Young and Davies, 1984; Jacobs, 1987).

Besides the decreased strength and/or muscular endurance, there is also a biochemical indicator of whether or not the rate of energy transferred from glycogen breakdown to enable the muscles to perform work is impaired when glycogen levels are low. During maximal intensity exercise of a short duration the end-product of glycogen breakdown is high levels of lactic acid. Although lactic acid, or lactate as it exists in muscle tissue or blood, has negative connotations associated with muscular fatigue, the ability to perform high intensity, short term exercise is dependent on the muscle's ability to derive energy from this particular metabolic pathway. In a series of studies where exercise and dietary manipulations induced glycogen depletion and associated impairments of strength (Jacobs, 1981a), muscle lactate levels after maximal intensity exercise lasting about 1 min were also significantly lower when compared to a control trial (Jacobs, 1981b). These studies and others (Karlsson, 1971; Klausen and Sjogaard, 1980) suggest that if glycogen concentrations are lower than about 50% of normal resting levels significant impairments occur in the musculature's ability to transduce energy from the breakdown of glycogen to lactate.

In summary of this section, evidence has been presented that intramuscular glycogen availability is crucial for optimal performance of not only endurance exercise, but also short term, sprint type exercise.

Glycogen and Football

The relatively high intensity at which competitive soccer is played (Reilly and Thomas, 1976) is, per se, evidence of the fact that muscle glycogen fuels a large proportion of the energy demands. Further indirect evidence is found in the high blood lactate concentrations measured during competitive matches (Ekblom, 1986). Ekblom (1986) also showed that lactate levels were higher in players playing in more elite divisions, suggesting that the intensity of play, and thus the importance of glycogen is higher in these divisions than in more recreational divisions.

Table 2 lists the results of studies in which direct measurements of changes in muscle glycogen during a soccer match have been reported. This table confirms that glycogen is indeed depleted quite markedly after competitive soccer, but also that the muscle glycogen levels 24 h after a match may not be fully restored. This latter finding can be partially explained on the basis of a lack of awareness of the importance of sufficient nutritional carbohydrate consumption, because an analysis of the dietary records of world class soccer players showed that only 47% (596 g) of the total calories consumed were carbohydrates (Jacobs et al., 1982). This is significantly less than the 55-60% of total calories, or over 650 g of carbohydrate, that would be advised for elite athletes of this body size.

Table 2. Thigh muscle glycogen relative to pre-game values

Reference	When	Glycogen concentration (%pre-game value)
Karlsson, 1969 cited in Ekblom, 1986	post-game	30%
Saltin, 1973	post-game	10%
Jacobs et al.,1982 Jacobs et al.,1982 (pre-game value estimated)	post-game 24 h post-game	43% 63%
Leatt and Jacobs, 1986 Leatt and Jacobs,this volume	post-game 19 h post-game	52%

From Table 2 and the data of Ahlborg et al. (1967) and Bergström et al. (1967), it is possible to estimate the impairment in endurance exercise performance associated with the glycogen values observed in soccer players at the end of a match. The extent of the expected impairment at the end of a match could range from below 40% to 70% of what endurance performance is normally. The day after a competitive match, the glycogen values reported in Table 2 suggest that endurance exercise performance would still not be restored to its normal level.

Do these expected performance impairments actually occur in a game situation? Saltin (1973) described a study in which one team of players performed hard exercise to induce glycogen depletion the day prior to a match. Film analyses revealed that the players who were glycogen depleted when they began the game covered significantly less ground during the match than the control team. Additionally, the control team sprinted at maximal speed during 20-25% of the playing time in contrast to the glycogen depleted team which sprinted less than 5% of the playing time.

In summary, the physical demands of football are such that glycogenolysis is the major metabolic pathway by which energy is transferred to the exercising muscles. Glycogen in the leg musculature is significantly depleted by competitive matches and restoration of glycogen stores to optimal pre-game values may not occur because of the frequency of games and/or training, or a lack of awareness of the importance of carbohydrates for the restoration of muscle glycogen stores.

Nutritional Strategies

The potential consequences for athletes of not consuming sufficient carbohydrates is exemplified in a study in which the subjects exercised for two hours on three consecutive days (Costill et al., 1971). When carbohydrates comprised 70% of their caloric intake the subjects were able to restore their leg muscle glycogen stores during the 24h between exercise bouts. On another occasion when carbohydrates made up only 40% of the consumed calories the subjects were not able to restore their glycogen stores and the result was that they commenced each day of exercise with progressively lower glycogen stores. By the last day, the pre-exercise glycogen levels were extremely depleted and the expected performance impairments would be very marked if the subjects had been asked to exercise maximally. This study by Costill et al. (1971) is important because the exercise schedule is not all that different from that of football players who may train two or three times in addition to one or two competitive matches a week during their peak season.

The relatively extreme carbohydrate loading technique practiced by endurance cyclists and runners is not feasible for football players who would have to go through drastic exercise and dietary manipulations once or twice weekly during their competitive season, in contrast to the runner or cyclist who competes on a relatively less frequent basis. The replenishment of glycogen stores should not, however, be a difficult problem because the rate of restoration is a direct function of the quantity of carbohydrates consumed. A daily intake of at least 600 g of carbohydrates, comprising about 65-70% of total energy consumption, should ensure adequate daily restoration of glycogen stores during peak season (Costill et al., 1981). Compare this suggestion with the 47% carbohydrate intake reported for one elite European soccer team (Jacobs et al., 1982) and the requirement for nutritional counselling becomes obvious.

In terms of the rate of replenishment of muscle glycogen stores, the consumption of either simple sugars or more complex starches results in similar values over a 24 h period (Costill et al., 1981). In other words, it does not really matter from this perspective if the carbohydrates are consumed as sugar in tea or in the form of pasta or cereals; there may be other nutritional benefits associated with the consumption of starches,but with regard to glycogen restoration rate either simple or complex sugars are equally effective.

The timing of carbohydrate ingestion on the day of a game can be crucial. On the day of a competition it is recommended that the last full meal be consumed three to four hours before the game and that it be a light meal consisting primarily of carbohydrates. Since carbohydrates are more easily digested than fats or proteins, they would leave less residue in the stomach by game time. If carbohydrates are consumed between 30-60 min before exercise there is a danger that the exercise will result in high levels of insulin being secreted or will enhance the effect of this hormone (Costill et al., 1977; Foster et al., 1979; Hargreaves et al., 1984). The end effect could be that more sugar is taken up from the blood and more glycogen is utilized during exercise than is normally the case; both of these actions may impair rather than optimize the conditions for the body to perform exercise (Costill et al., 1977; Foster et al., 1979). This matter is still not clear, however, because of recent findings which demonstrated no greater glycogen utilization nor any performance impairment when a solid carbohydrate candy bar was eaten 30 min before exercise (Devlin et al., 1986). In contrast to the above, liquid or solid carbohydrate consumed just prior to or during exercise may enhance subsequent performance (Coyle et al., 1983; Neufer et al., 1987).

Fluid Balance

Soccer players may lose between one to five percent of their body weight by sweating during a match (Mustafa and Mahmoud, 1979; Kirkendall, 1985; Ekblom, 1986). The decrease in plasma volume that occurs with such sweat loss is associated with significant endurance performance impairments (Saltin, 1964), although the effects on explosive power and muscular endurance are minimal (Jacobs, 1980).

Unfortunately, the human thirst mechanism is not an adequate indicator of a physiological state of dehydration. In order to delay the onset of such dehydration players should be encouraged to drink during breaks in a match and to drink more than thirst dictates after a match to ensure adequate rehydration. Studies of the rate at which various types of fluids are emptied from the stomach have indicated that cooler solutions empty more rapidly than do warmer solutions and that more concentrated solutions empty more slowly than less concentrated solutions (Costill and Saltin, 1974; Foster et al., 1980; Seiple et al., 1983).

This latter finding is relevant considering the results of studies referred to above which showed that the ingestion of liquid carbohydrate within 15 min before or during exercise may prolong the time to exhaustion during endurance exercise, perhaps by using circulating glucose as an energy subtrate and delaying or retarding the rate of muscle glycogen utilization (Coyle et al., 1983; Neufer et al., 1987). Leatt and Jacobs (1986) recently reported that muscle glycogen depletion was less in players who drank 500 ml of a 7% glucose polymer solution 15 min before a match and again at half time, than in players who only drank water. In light of the earlier discussion of the relationship between glycogen synthesis and the quantity of consumed carbohydrates, it might be tempting to suggest drinking a concentrated glucose solution before exercise. As mentioned above, however, a strong concentration would result in a reduced rate of delivery of the glucose to the blood stream in comparison with a less concentrated drink. A 10-15% sugar concentration is a suggested guideline to ensure that sufficient amounts of glucose reach the blood stream quickly enough to be of potential benefit in situations where muscle glycogen levels are likely to be extremely depleted. Drinking copious amounts of such a solution after a match or training session will serve dual purposes of more rapidly restoring both fluid balance and glycogen stores (for review, see Lamb and Brodowicz, 1986).

Micronutrients

The need for supplementary electrolytes such as sodium, potassium or magnesium, added to fluids ingested during or after matches is debatable. The quantity of electrolytes lost in sweat during a high intensity exercise (Costill, 1978; Saltin, 1978) is easily regained by consuming a couple of well balanced meals. Even the growing belief that a dietary iron deficiency per se impairs performance has been recently shown to be unfounded (Celsing et al., 1986). Vitamin deficiencies, however, can present real performance and health hazards if the athlete is not made aware of the importance of a balanced diet (van der Beek, 1985). It was recently demonstrated that even a period as short as three weeks of eating a diet consisting of normally consumed foodstuffs can result in performance impairments associated with reduced tissue vitamin concentrations (van der Beek et al., 1987).

Conclusion

Competitive football demands exercise at a relatively high intensity for a prolonged duration as well as maximal intensity, sprint-like exercise performed intermittently throughout a match. The rate at which the energy required to meet these demands must be supplied, dictates that the musculature is highly dependent on its stores of glycogen. Exhaustion of these stores impairs the athlete's ability to perform up to his/her potential. This paper has attempted to enhance awareness of the quantity of carbohydrates one must consume to ensure that sufficient muscle glycogen stores will be available at the beginning of a match so that skill and physical fitness, not fuel availability, will decide the winner.

References

Ahlborg, B., Bergström, J., Brohult, J., Ekelund, L.-G., Hultman, E. and Maschio, G. (1967) Human muscle glycogen content and capacity for prolonged exercise after different diets. Forsvarsmedicin, 3, 85-100.

Åstrand, P.-O. (1967) Diet and athletic performance. Fed. Proc., 26, 1772-1777.

Bergström, J. (1962) Muscle electrolytes in man. Scand. J. Clin. Lab. Invest., Suppl. 68.

Bergström, J., Hermansen, L., Hultman, E. and Saltin, B. (1967) Diet, muscle glycogen and physical performance. Acta Physiol. Scand., 71, 140-150.

Celsing, F., Blomstrand, E., Werner, B., Pihlstedt, P. and Ekblom, B. (1986) Effects of iron deficiency on endurance and muscle enzyme activity in man. Med. Sci. Sports Exerc., 18, 156-61.

Christensen, E.H. and Hansen, O. (1939) Arbeitsfahigkeit und Ernahrung. Scand. Arch. Physiol., 81, 160-171.

Costill, D.L. (1978) Muscle water and electrolytes during acute and repeated bouts of dehydration. In: Nutrition, Physical Fitness and Health (edited by J. Parizkova and V.A. Rogozkin), pp.98-116. Baltimore: University Park Press.

Costill, D.L., Bowers, R., Granam, G. and Sparks, K. (1971) Muscle glycogen utilization during prolonged exercise on successive days. J. Appl. Physiol., 31, 834-838.
Costill, D.L., Coyle, E., Dalsky, G., Evans, W., Fink, W. and Hoopes, D. (1977) Effects of elevated plasma FFA and insulin on muscle glycogen usage during exercise. J. Appl. Physiol., 43, 695-99.
Costill, D.L. and Saltin, B., (1974) Factors limiting gastric emptying during rest and exercise. J. Appl. Physiol. 37, 679-83.
Costill, D.L., Sherman, W.M., Fink, W.J., Maresh, C., Witten, M. and Miller, J.M. (1981) The role of dietary carbohydrates in muscle glycogen resynthesis after strenuous running. Amer. J. Clin. Nutr., 34, 1831-1836.
Coyle, E.F., Hagberg, J.M., Hurley, B.F., Martin, W.H., Ehsani, A.A. and Holloszy, J.O. (1983) Carbohydrate feeding during prolonged strenuous exercise can delay fatigue. J. Appl. Physiol., 55, 230-35.
Devlin, J.T., Calles-Escandon, J. and Horton, E.S. (1986) Effects of pre-exercise snack feeding on endurance cycle exercise. J. Appl. Physiol., 60, 980-985.
Ekblom, B. (1986) Applied physiology of soccer. Sports Med., 3, 50-60.
Foster, C., Costill, D.L. and Fink, W.J. (1979) Effects of pre-exercise feedings on endurance. Med. Sci. Sports Exerc., 11, 1-5.
Foster, C., Costill, D.L. and Fink, W.J. (1980) Gastric emptying characteristics of glucose and glucose polymer solutions. Res. Quart. Exerc. and Sport, 51, 299-305.
Greenhauf, P.L., Gleeson, M. and Maughan, R.J. (1987) The effects of dietary manipulation on blood acid-base status and the performance of high intensity exercise. Eur. J. Appl. Physiol., 56, 331-37.
Hargreaves, M., Costill, D.L., Coggan, A. and Nishibata, I. (1984) Effect of carbohydrate feeding on muscle glycogen utilization and exercise performance. Med. Sci. Sports Exerc., 16, 219-22.
Heigenhauser, G.J.F., Sutton, J.R. and Jones, N.L. (1983) Effect of glycogen depletion on the ventilatory response to exercise. J. Appl. Physiol., 54, 470-74.
Hermansen, L., Hultman, E. and Saltin, B. (1967) Muscle glycogen during prolonged severe exercise. Acta Physiol. Scand., 71, 129-139.
Jacobs, I. (1980) The effects of thermal dehydration on performance of the Wingate Anaerobic Test. Int. J. Sports Med., 1, 21-24.
Jacobs, I. (1981a) Lactate, muscle glycogen and exercise performance in man. Acta Physiol. Scand., Suppl. 495.
Jacobs, I. (1981b) Lactate concentrations after short, maximal exercise at various glycogen levels. Acta Physiol. Scand., 111, 465-469.
Jacobs, I. (1987) Influence of carbohydrate stores on maximal human power output. In: Exercise - Benefits, Limits and Adaptations (edited by D. Macleod, R.J. Maughan, M. Nimmo, T. Reilly and C. Williams), pp. 104-115. London: E and F.N. Spon Ltd,
Jacobs, I., Kaiser, P. and Tesch, P. (1981) Muscle strength and fatigue after selective glycogen depletion in human skeletal muscle fibers. Eur. J. Appl. Physiol., 46, 47-53.
Jacobs, I., Westlin, N., Karlsson, J., Rasmusson, M. and Houghton, B.

(1982) Muscle glycogen and diet in elite soccer players. Eur. J. Appl. Physiol., 48, 297-302.
Karlsson, J. (1971) Lactate in working muscle after prolonged exercise. Acta Physiol. Scand., 82, 123-30.
Karlsson, J. and Saltin, B. (1971) Diet, muscle glycogen and endurance performance. J. Appl. Physiol., 31, 203-206.
Kirkendall, D.T. (1985) The applied sports science of soccer. Physician Sportsmed., 13, 53-9.
Klausen, K. and Sjøgaard, G. (1980) Glycogen stores and lactate accumulation in skeletal muscle of man during intense bicycle exercise. Scand. J. Sports Sci., 2, 7-12.
Lamb, D.R. and Brodowicz, G.R. (1986) Optimal use of fluids of varying formulations to minimize exercise-induced disturbances in homeostasis. Sports Med., 3, 247-74.
Leatt, P.B. and Jacobs, I. (1986) Effects of glucose polymer ingestion on muscle glycogen utilization during a soccer match. Med. Sci. Sports Exerc. 18 (Suppl.), 56.
Lemon, P., Yarsheski, K.E. and Dolny, D.G. (1984) The importance of protein for athletes. Sports Med., 1, 474-484.
Maughan, R.J. and Poole, D.C. (1981) The effects of a glycogen-loading regimen on the capacity to perform anaerobic exercise. Eur. J. Appl. Physiol., 46, 211-219.
Mustafa, K.Y. and Mahmoud, N.E.A. (1979) Evaporate water loss in African soccer players. J. Sports Med. Phys. Fit., 19, 181-3.
Neufer, P.D., Costill, D.L., Flynn, M.G., Kirwan, J.P., Mitchell, J.B. and Houmard, J. (1987) Improvements in exercise performance: effects of carbohydrate feedings and diet. J. Appl. Physiol., 62, 983-988.
Newsholme, E.A. and Leech, A.R. (1983) Biochemistry for the Medical Sciences. New York: John Wiley and Sons.
Reilly, T. and Thomas, V. (1976) A motion analysis of work-rate in different positional roles in professional football match-play. J. Human Mov't. Stud., 2, 87-97.
Saltin, B. (1964) Aerobic and anaerobic work capacity after dehydration. J. Appl. Physiol., 19, 1114-1118.
Saltin, B. (1973) Metabolic fundamentals in exercise. Med. Sci. Sports, 5, 137-46.
Saltin, B. (1978) Fluid, electrolyte and energy losses and their replenishment in prolonged exercise. In Nutrition, Physical Fitness and Health (edited by J. Parizkova and V. Rogozkin), pp. 76-97. Baltimore: University Park Press.
Saltin, B. and Karlsson, J. (1971) Muscle glycogen utilization during work of different intensities. In: Muscle Metabolism During Exercise (edited by B. Pernow and B. Saltin), pp.289-99. New York: Plenum Press.
Seiple, R.S., Vivian, V.M., Fox, E.L. and Bartels, R.L. (1983) Gastric-emptying characteristics of two glucose polymer-electrolyte solutions. Med. Sci. Sports and Exerc., 15, 366-69.
Sherman, W.M., Armstrong, L.E., Murray, T.M., Hagerman, F.C., Costill, D.L., Staron, R.C. and Ivy, J.L. (1984) Effect of a 42.2 km footrace and subsequent rest or exercise on muscular strength and work capacity. J. Appl. Physiol., 57, 1668-73.
Sherman, W.M., Costill, D.L., Fink, W.J. and Miller, J.M. (1981)

Effect of exercise-diet manipulation on muscle glycogen and its subsequent utilization during performance. Int. J. Sports Med., 2, 114-118.
van der Beek, E.J. (1985) Vitamins and endurance training: food for running or faddish claims? Sports Med., 2, 175-197.
van der Beek, E.J., van Dokkum, W., Schrijver, J., Wedel, M. and Gaillard, A.W.K. (1987) Impact of restricted vitamin intake on functional performance in man. Submitted for publication.
Young, K. and Davies, C.T.M. (1984) Effect of diet on human muscle weakness following prolonged exercise. Eur. J. Appl. Physiol., 53, 81-85.

EFFECT OF GLUCOSE POLYMER SUPPLEMENTATION ON PERFORMANCE OF SOCCER PLAYERS

Donald T. Kirkendall, Carl Foster, Joseph A. Dean, John Grogan and Nancy N. Thompson
Cleveland Clinic Foundation, Cleveland, Ohio and Mount Sinai Medical Center, Milwaukee, Wi., U.S.A.

Introduction

Studies of the effects of nutrition on athletic performance have been directed mainly towards endurance sports. It has been shown that exercise can be maintained for longer when preceded by a high carbohydrate diet (Christensen and Hansen, 1939), and that muscle glycogen depletion is a common antecedent of fatigue during prolonged exercise. Enhancement of pre-exercise muscle glycogen improves both endurance (Bergstrom et al., 1967) and anaerobic (Maughan and Poole, 1981) performance. A recent approach to enhancing carbohydrate intake has been the use of glucose polymers which have favourable gastric emptying characteristics (Foster et al., 1980; Seiple et al., 1984), improve endurance performance (Coyle et al., 1983) and may (Leatt and Jacobs, 1986) or may not (Coyle et al., 1986) slow the rate of muscle glycogen depletion.

An extension of these studies would be to explore dietary effects on performance in team sports. Certainly, team sports involve a far larger number of athletes than do endurance sports. In the literature, only one reference to the use of a 'glucose syrup' in a team sport - soccer (Muckle, 1973) - was found. The literature indicates that soccer is a glycogen-depleting activity (Agnevik, 1970; Saltin, 1973) that requires a change of speed or direction every 5-6 s (Reilly and Thomas, 1976). Sprints average about 15 m approximately every 90 s (Reilly and Thomas, 1976), while players run at a 'cruise' or sprint once every 30 s (Reilly and Thomas, 1976). In addition, the training and ad libitum dietary habits of soccer players hinder full repletion of muscle glycogen (Jacobs et al., 1982). Lastly, work rate, particularly during the latter stages of the game, is affected by pre-game muscle glycogen levels (Saltin, 1973).

Our intent was to determine whether use of a glucose polymer would affect work rate during soccer matches. The study was done under field conditions designed to simulate actual scheduling dilemmas. The question was whether an acute use of a carbohydrate supplement might affect the course of a single outdoor match (Study I) or of an indoor tournament (Study II).

Methods

Two separate settings were investigated. One studied outdoor play (Study I) with a relatively acute design to determine whether performance during the course of a single regulation game could be affected. The other (Study II) evaluated indoor play to determine whether recovery between games could be enhanced.

Study I (outdoor play)
The subjects (n = 10) were from a regionally ranked collegiate men's outdoor team. On average they were 20.8 (± 1.7) years of age, 173.9 (± 4.6) cm tall and 74.0 (± 5.8) kg in weight. Two unrestricted games were played (Tuesday and Thursday) on a full field (110 m x 70 m), with 9 men (including the goalkeeper) a-side and the teams being of equal strength. The diet preceding each game and between the two games was ad libitum. Light training occurred on the day preceding and the day between the test days.

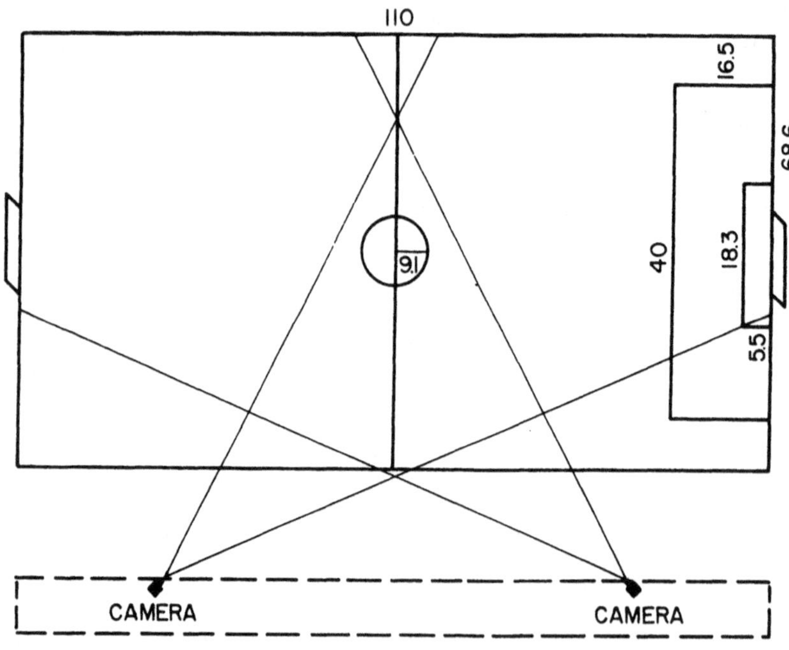

Figure 1. Two fixed-position camera alignment for taping outdoor soccer

The game was taped using two fixed position cameras (Figure 1). Distances and intensities were estimated according to the method of Reilly and Thomas (1976). Intensities were described as walking, jogging, cruising ('running with manifest purpose and effort'), and sprinting. One recorder reduced the data. Three 5 min segments were taped each half. The data were then extrapolated to a 90 min game.

No correction was made for the untaped portions of the field.

Players were randomly (and in double blind fashion) divided into a placebo (aspartame sweetened 'Kool-Aid') and experimental ('Exceed High Carbohydrate Source', Ross Laboratories, Columbus, OH) group. The conditions were reversed for the second game. A quantity of 400 ml of either solution was consumed both immediately before the game and during the interval. Approximately 125 g of carbohydrate was consumed in the experimental condition.

Study II (indoor play)

The subjects were selected from a local club level amateur soccer team. On average they were 33.6 (± 3.4) years of age, 177.7 (± 3.2) cm in height and 77.2 (± 11.5) kg in weight. The day prior to each trial was taken as a rest day with no exercise. Two full indoor games (each game = 2 x 24 min) were played. The games were separated by one hour and were played on a standard pitch size (70 x 39 m). One week later the two-game 'tournament' was repeated with reversed dietary conditions. The teams were 5 men each (no goalkeeper and only 2 substitutes). No shots from outside the penalty area (7.5 x 9 m) were allowed. This permitted reasonable play patterns without the necessity of using a goalkeeper.

The first game for each day served as the control game. During the one hour pause, each player consumed the placebo or experimental drink (400 ml, 23% CHO) as in Study I.

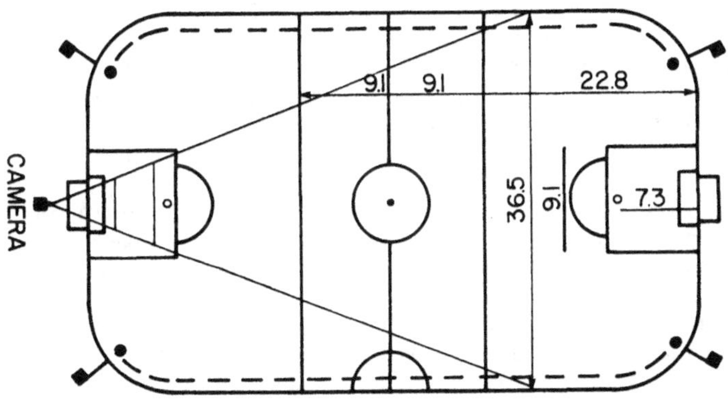

Figure 2. One fixed-position camera alignment for taping indoor soccer

The games were taped by a single fixed position camera which pictured 58% of the field (Figure 2). Data for the entire duration of each game were reduced as in Study I and extrapolated to estimate full field distances. Reliability of the method was in excess of 0.90 (Figure 3). The unit of analysis was a ratio of the total distance covered in the experimental versus the control by each half (Study I) or game (Study II). The positional movement intensities (walking, jogging) were summed as were strategic movement intensities (cruising, sprinting).

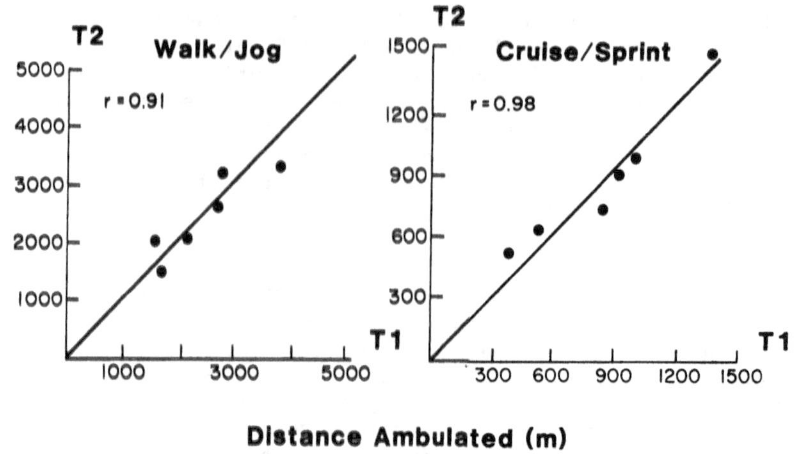

Figure 3. Reliability of the data reduction method

Three-day diet recalls were collected and analyzed by a commercial nutritional data base (Anjon Nutrition Systems, South Bend, IN). Values were compared using paired t-tests. Differences were considered significant at a P value less than or equal to 0.05.

Results

The distance ratios are presented in Figures 4 (Study I) and 5 (Study II). In Study I, the differences between distance ratios for 1st and 2nd half were not significant for the positional intensities (walk+jog). The distance ratio for the strategic intensities (cruise + sprint) and total distance was significantly greater for the 2nd half of the 'supplement' trial compared to the placebo trial ($P < 0.05$).

In Study II (Figure 5), there were no significant differences between dietary conditions for positional movements or total distance. However, during the "supplement" game, movement at strategic intensities was significantly increased ($P < 0.05$).

Dietary recalls (Study II) showed that the caloric intake (Study II) averaged 2316 kcal (9695 kJ) per day. This comprised 262 g carbohydrate per day which was 44% of the total dietary intake.

Discussion

The total distance (7200-7300 m) covered in the outdoor games was a little less than that previously reported (Reilly and Thomas, 1976). The small difference was probably due to the inability to tape the full field due to camera location. Corrected for the percentage of the playing surface filmed (82.7%), the total estimated distance (8706-8827 m) compares well with other reports (Reilly and Thomas, 1976). The mean distance of 2656 m per game during Study II is the only value available on this style of indoor soccer. Because

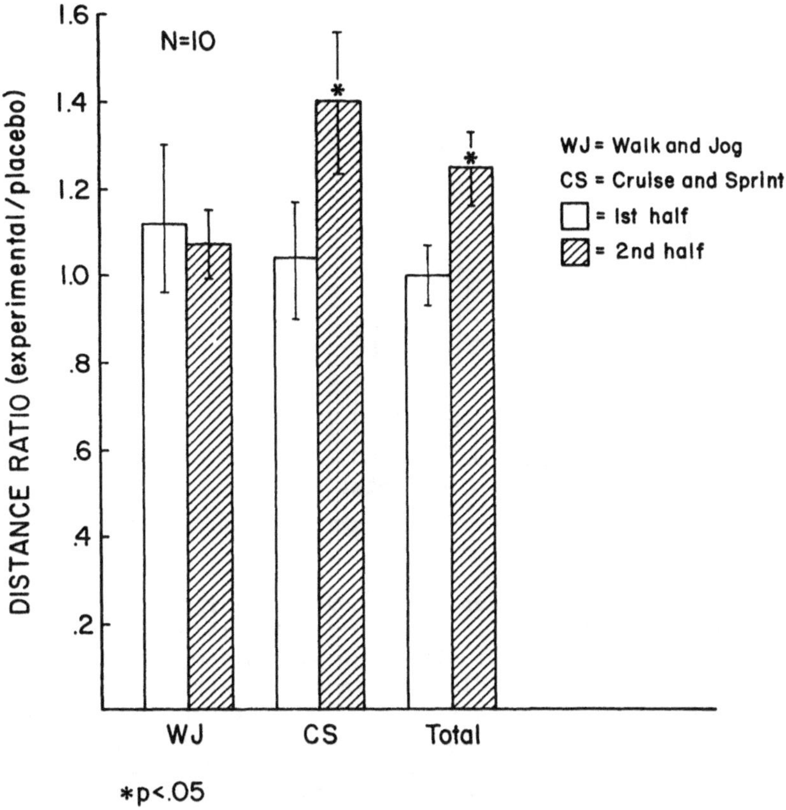

Figure 4. Distance ratio (Study I) by half and intensity (Mean ± SE)

of modifications in rules, these indoor games appeared as a small field outdoor game. This represents a different pattern of play to that played professionally in the U.S. (MISL) which makes extensive use of 'dasher boards' and frequent substitution. Thus, it is possible that the distances observed in Study II vary from the American professional game.

The distance ratios from the indoor games (Study II - Figure 5) showed that there was minimal difference in the total distance covered between conditions. However, the outdoor game (Study I) showed nearly a 25% greater total distance ratio during the second half (Figure 4, $P < 0.05$). There were no significant differences in either Study I or II in the distance ratios for the positional (walk+jog) intensities (Figures 4 and 5). The major difference was the significantly greater distance ratio at strategic intensities for the 2nd half (Study I) or the 2nd game (Study II). The distance ratio was over 40% higher for the 'supplement' game.

There are at least three reasons for the enhanced performance observed following the dietary interventions employed in this

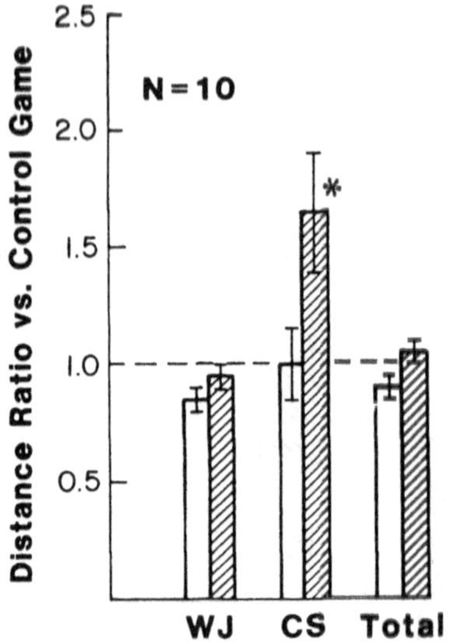

Figure 5. Distance ratio (Study II) by game and intensity (Mean ± SE)

study. First, low values for muscle glycogen will limit aerobic performance (Sherman and Costill, 1984). Saltin (1973) has demonstrated that soccer players with high pre-game muscle glycogen concentration covered 13% more distance than counterparts with low pre-game values. This pattern was particularly evident during the second half of play. Players with high pre-game muscle glycogen covered 27% of the total game at a walk and 24% at maximal speed. The low glycogen group covered 50% of the distance at a walk and only 15% at maximal speed.

Second, diet and activity on the days preceding the game will affect pre-game glycogen levels. Costill et al. (1971) showed that a mixed diet will not replenish muscle glycogen overnight following heavier than usual exertion. Jacobs et al. (1982) observed a low total caloric intake with less than 50% of energy from carbohydrate in soccer players following a game. Consequently, muscle glycogen was still low (at 73 mM kg^{-1}) 48 hours later, when another game might normally be scheduled. This may be why the subjects of both Saltin (1973) and Agnevik (1970) demonstrated pre-game glycogen levels that were about 25% below what might be considered normal (Åstrand and Rodahl, 1977). The subjects of Jacobs et al. (1982) were 41% below that expected for sedentary individuals (125 mM kg^{-1}). The dietary habits of our subjects indicated a similar dietary pattern.

Third, use of glucose polymers to enhance carbohydrate intake has been associated with improved endurance performance (Coyle et al., 1983, 1986; Hargreaves et al., 1984). The mechanism by which pre-exercise carbohydrate ingestion improves work output has not been clarified. Hargreaves et al. (1984) suggested that the elevated circulating blood glucose effectively delayed the depletion of glycogen during cycle ergometry. Leatt and Jacobs (1986), in a field trial of polymer use in soccer, have shown greater glycogen depletion in the control versus the polymer condition. Conversely, Coyle et al. (1986) have demonstrated that glycogen depletion is not delayed during exhaustive cycling accompanied by the CHO supplementation. Rather, the increased exercise duration was supported by circulating glucose.

Exhaustion from endurance performance at 70-80% of $\dot{V}O_2$ max has been shown to be related to glycogen levels below 25 mM kg^{-1} (Sherman and Costill, 1984). Saltin's (1973) pre-game high and low glycogen groups showed 32 and 6 mM kg^{-1} respectively at intermission. So, under ordinary circumstances, the second half of most soccer games is likely to be played under glycogen depleted circumstances. Accordingly, it is hardly surprising that distances run during the second half of soccer games are usually less than during the first half (Reilly and Thomas, 1976). This may be why the first half of the game (Study I) or game pair (Study II) was unaffected by carbohydrate ingestion. If we can assume that the players in this study had muscle glycogen levels consistent with subjects in other studies, then 1st half (or 1st game) work should not have been affected because muscle glycogen levels were not low. However, the 2nd half (or 2nd game) work would be expected to be influenced by exogenous carbohydrate supplementation.

The question may arise as to possible glycogen replenishment in the one hour interval in Study II. Some glycogen repletion has been shown to occur in the early recovery period (Costill et al., 1981; Hermansen and Vaage, 1977). Ivy (1986) has shown that if carbohydrate was ingested immediately after exercise, there was significantly greater muscle glycogen resynthesis than if carbohydrate was ingested 2 hours post-exercise.

These results suggest that the improvement in work performance in soccer observed in this study may be attributable to two mechanisms. In the outdoor trial, the supplement may have elevated blood glucose to spare glycogen, as suggested by Leatt and Jacobs (1986) or offer an alternative fuel source once glycogen has been depleted (Coyle et al., 1986). In the indoor trial, the one hour break between games may have allowed for some glycogen replenishment. The data of Ivy et al. (1983) lend support to this suggestion.

The results of this investigation support the concept that acute dietary inverventions with a glucose polymer previously shown to be effective in enhancing endurance performance (Coyle et al., 1983, 1986; Hargreaves et al., 1984), may be useful during team sports such as soccer. This result was not only observable under the two common strategic variations used in this investigation, but is also consistent with responses predictable from known principles of glycogen metabolism.

Acknowledgements

This study was supported by a grant from Ross Laboratories, Columbus, Ohio. The authors wish to acknowledge the helpful comments of Keith Wheeler, Ph.D.

References

Agnevik, G., Fotboll. (1970) Iddrottsfysiologi Rapport, Nr 7, Stockholm: Trygg-Hansa.

Åstrand, P.O. and Rodahl, K. (1977) Textbook of Work Physiology. New York: McGraw-Hill.

Bergstrom, J., Hermansen, L., Hultman, E. and Saltin, B. (1967) Diet, muscle, glycogen and physical performance. Acta. Physiol. Scand., 71, 190-150.

Christensen, E.H. and Hansen, O. (1939) Respirotorischer Quotient and 02 Aufnahme. Scand. Arch. Physiol., 81: 180-189.

Costill, D.L., Bowers, P., Branam, G. and Sparks, K. (1971) Muscle glycogen utilization during prolonged exercise on successive days. J. Appl. Physiol., 31, 824-838.

Costill, D.L., Sherman, W.M., Fink, W.J., Maresh, C., Witten, M. and Miller, J.M. (1981) Role of dietary carbohydrates in muscle glycogen resynthesis after strenuous running. Amer. J. Clin. Nutr., 34, 1831-1836.

Coyle, E.F., Coggan, A.R., Klemment, M.K. and Ivy, J.L. (1986) Muscle glycogen utilisation during prolonged strenuous exercise when fed carbohydrate. J. Appl. Physiol., 61, 165-172.

Coyle, E.F., Hagberg, J.M., Hurley, B.F., Martin, W.H., Ehsani, A.A. and Holloszy, J.O. (1983) Carbohydrate feeding during prolonged strenuous exercise can delay fatigue. J. Appl. Physiol. Respirat. Environ. Exerc. Physiol., 55, 230-235.

Foster, C., Costill, D.L. and Fink, W.J. (1980) Gastric emptying characteristics of glucose and glucose polymer solutions. Res. Quart. Exerc. Sport, 51, 299-305.

Hargreaves, M., Costill, D.L., Coggan, A., Fink, W.J. and Nishibata, I. (1984) Effect of carbohydrate feedings on muscle glycogen utilisation and exercise performance. Med. Sci. Sports Exerc., 16, 219-222.

Hermansen, L. and Vaage, O. (1977) Lactate disappearance and glycogen synthesis in human muscle after maximal exercise. Am. J. Physiol., 233, E422-E429.

Ivy, J.L. (1986) Muscle glycogen repletion following exercise. Paper presented at American College of Sports Medicine Annual Meeting, Indianapolis, In.

Ivy, J.L., Miller, W., Dover, V., Goodyear, L.G., Sherman, W.M., Farrell, S. and Williams, H. (1983) Endurance improved by ingestion of glucose polymer supplement. Med. Sci. Sport. Exerc., 15, 466-471.

Jacobs, I., Wrestlin, N., Karlsson, J., Rasmusson, M. and Houghton, B. (1982) Muscle glycogen and diet in elite soccer players. Europ. J. Appl. Physiol., 48, 297-302.

Leatt, P.B. and Jacobs, I. (1986) Effects of glucose polymer ingestion on muscle glycogen utilisation during a soccer match. Med. Sci. Sports Exerc., 18 (2-suppl), 86.

Maughan, R.J. and Poole, D.C. (1981) Effects of a glycogen loading regimen on the capacity to perform anaerobic exercise. Eur. J. Appl. Physiol., 46, 211-219.

Muckle, D. (1973) Glucose syrup ingestion and team performance in soccer. Brit. J. Sports Med., 7, 340-343.

Reilly, T. and Thomas, V. (1976) A motion analysis of work-rate in different positional roles in professional football match-play. J. Human Mov't. Stud., 2, 87-89.

Saltin, B. (1973) Metabolic fundamentals in exercise. Med. Sci. Sports, 5, 137-146.

Seiple, R.S., Vivian, V.M., Fox, E.L. and Bartels, R.L. (1984) Gastric emptying characteristics of two glucose polymer electrolyte solutions. Med. Sci. Sports Exerc., 15, 366-369.

Sherman, W.M. and Costill, D.L. (1984) The marathon: dietary manipulation to optimize performance. Amer. J. Sports Med., 12, 44-51.

EFFECT OF A LIQUID GLUCOSE SUPPLEMENT ON MUSCLE GLYCOGEN RESYNTHESIS AFTER A SOCCER MATCH

Peter B. Leatt and Ira Jacobs
University of Toronto, and the Defence and Civil Institute of Environmental Medicine, Toronto, Canada.

Introduction

It is now well established that an adequate supply of muscle glycogen is required to maintain high intensity exercise performance. At exercise intensities ranging from 70 - 80% of maximal aerobic power ($\dot{V}O_2$max), exhaustion of the exercising muscles will occur after approximately 90 min when the muscles' glycogen stores are almost totally depleted (Bergstrom et al., 1967). Published data reveal that the physiological demands of soccer approximate similar exercise intensities. Radiotelemetry has shown that during a soccer match a player's average heart rate is high and may frequently approach maximum (for review see Ekblom, 1986). The mean distance a player covers during a match is reported to range from 8.7-11.5 km (Ekblom, 1986). It is important to note that a total of almost 1 km may be covered in short intermittent sprints (Reilly and Thomas, 1976), because the rate of muscle glycogen utilization is known to increase greatly as the level of exercise intensity rises (Saltin and Karlsson, 1971).

In team sports such as soccer, players are required to train and compete at regular intervals. Clearly it is important for a professional soccer player to have large glycogen stores in order to maintain optimum physical performance. However, it has been shown that the resynthesis of muscle glycogen in professional soccer players following competitive match-play can be extremely slow, requiring more than a 48 h recovery period (Jacobs et al., 1982). The cause of this very slow resynthesis was not apparent.

An adequate intake of dietary carbohydrate is necessary to permit glycogen resynthesis following exercise. This has been demonstrated by Hermansen et al. (1967), who showed that if glycogen- depleted subjects consumed a diet very low in carbohydrate for a few days, they were unable to resynthesize significant amounts of muscle glycogen. The present study employed a glucose polymer supplement to raise the carbohydrate intake of some of the subjects. It was hypothesized that the subjects who consumed the glucose solution would, by virtue of their higher carbohydrate intake, have a greater muscle glycogen resynthesis than a control group who ingested a placebo.

Methods

Subjects were recruited from the Canadian National Youth Soccer Team. Ten subjects, with a mean age of 19.1 years, volunteered to participate in the study after giving written informed consent. The subjects were divided into two equal groups, balanced for playing position. This was done because the physical demands of soccer may vary according to the positional role (Reilly and Thomas, 1976).

All subjects took part in an 11-a-side soccer match played between members of the Canadian National Youth team and the full National team. Immediately following the game a muscle biopsy was obtained from each volunteer. The subjects in the experimental group (n=5) were each given five bottles, each containing 500 ml of a tasteless 7% glucose polymer solution (Polycose$^{(R)}$, Ross Laboratories) flavoured with a non-caloric artificial sweetener. The subjects in the control group (n=5) also received five bottles containing water flavoured with the same sweetener.

After the muscle biopsy each subject consumed one drink and was instructed to take the remaining four away and to drink them in addition to his normal dietary intake before returning the next day for the second biopsy. Dietary intake of macronutrients was recorded by each subject during the recovery period using two-dimensional visual food portion charts (Posner et al., 1981). The subjects were individually instructed about the use of these charts in recording their dietary intake. Approximately 19 h later the subjects returned for the second biopsy. Dietary record sheets were checked and each subject was individually interviewed to ensure that all nutritional intake had been recorded. One subject from the control group was unable to return for the second biopsy and his results have been excluded from all calculations. Glycogen was assayed on freeze-dried muscle tissue samples and is expressed as glucose units measured after hydrolysis in hydrochloric acid (Karlsson, 1971).

Results

Following the 19 h recovery period muscle glycogen concentration had risen by only 50 and 18 mmol kg^{-1} dry weight in the experimental and control groups, respectively (Table 1). There were no significant differences in muscle glycogen concentration between the two groups either after the soccer match or 19h later. The change in muscle glycogen was also not significantly different between the two groups and the amount of glycogen synthesized was very small.

Table 1. Muscle glycogen concentrations (m mol kg^{-1}) in the vastus lateralis muscle of soccer players immediately after and 19 hours after a game

Group		Post Game	19h Recovery	Increase
Experimental (n=5)	Mean	253	303	50
	SD	65	28	
Control (n=4)	Mean	287	306	19
	SD	30	29	

Further analysis of the data revealed that there was a highly significant negative correlation between the post-game glycogen level and the change in muscle glycogen during the recovery period ($r=-0.88$, $P<0.001$), i.e. those players with the lowest muscle glycogen at the end of the match experienced the greatest glycogen resynthesis. This relationship was not statistically correlated with the dietary carbohydrate intake during this period.

Dietary analysis revealed that the consumption of carbohydrate during the recovery period, including the drinks, was 536 g in the experimental group and 397 g in the controls. However, there were no significant differences between the two groups for the total carbohydrate, fat, or protein consumption (Table 2).

Table 2. Analysis of dietary intake during the 19 h recovery period

Group		Fat		Protein		Carbohydrate		Energy
		(g)	(%)	(g)	(%)	(g)	(%)	(kJ)
Experimental	Mean	97	26	95	11	536	65	14499
	SD	45	7	40	3	209	9	5513
Control	Mean	156	39	103	13	397	48	15151
	SD	97	8	30	3	131	6	7248

Discussion

The justification for supplementing the diet with a glucose solution is that the rate of glycogen synthesis can be drastically reduced by a diet deficient in carbohydrate (Bergstrom et al., 1967). The intention in this study was to raise the total carbohydrate consumption of the experimental group by such a degree that the supply of substrate would not be a limiting factor for glycogenesis. Although there was no significant difference between the two groups in the total carbohydrate consumption, the results clearly show that the subjects' diets contained sufficient carbohydrate to enable a far greater glycogen resynthesis than was observed.

Many studies have demonstrated a rapid muscle glycogen resynthesis following exercise. For example, glycogen supercompensation has been demonstrated within 24 h in subjects consuming 500 g (Bergstrom et al., 1967) or 575 g of carbohydrates (Gollnick et al., 1972). However, the time required for complete resynthesis may vary from 12 h (Maehlum, 1978) to 46 h (Piehl et al., 1974). More importantly, we observed no clear relationship between carbohydrate intake and muscle glycogen resynthesis. It would seem therefore that there are factors other than the carbohydrate intake that affect the rate of glycogen resynthesis.

Saltin (1973) investigated the effect of low muscle glycogen on the work rate of soccer players. It was clear from this study that players who began the soccer match with low glycogen levels covered a smaller total distance and sprinted far less than players who began with a normal glycogen level. Furthermore, laboratory studies have shown that low glycogen will not only restrict physical endurance (Bergstrom et al., 1967), but will also reduce the ability to perform high intensity exercise (Jacobs, 1981).

Following the soccer match in the present study, the subjects had not reduced their muscle glycogen to levels as low as those commonly reported following exhaustive exercise in laboratories. However, this is not unexpected since players in a team sport such as soccer are self-paced and may therefore reduce their work output when tired. In contrast, a subject exercising on a laboratory ergometer would be encouraged to continue until physically exhausted. The post-match glycogen values in the present study were similar to figures reported by Jacobs et al. (1982) following a professional soccer match.

The relatively high muscle glycogen levels following the soccer match may have been at least partly responsible for the subsequent slow resynthesis. There is a well documented relationship between muscle glycogen synthesis and the absolute muscle glycogen concentration. Exercise induced glycogen depletion stimulates the enzyme glycogen synthase (Bergstrom et al., 1972; Maehlum et al., 1977), thus increasing the rate of glycogen formation. Associated with this reduction in muscle glycogen is an increase in the rate of glucose transport into the muscle cell (Richter et al., 1982; Fell et al., 1982). The increased action of insulin appears to be dependant on the intensity and duration of the prior exercise bout. If the exercise does not reduce the glycogen content sufficiently, then the insulin sensitivity is not affected (Maehlum and Pruett, 1973). These findings may well explain in part the strong correlation between the post-game muscle glycogen level and the amount of subsequent glycogen synthesis which was observed in this and another study with soccer players (Jacobs et al., 1982). This further supports the role of muscle glycogen concentration per se in the control of glycogen resynthesis.

Despite these points a significant resynthesis of glycogen would still be expected, given a rest period of approximately 19 h and a quite large carbohydrate intake. To the authors' knowledge none of the subjects took part in any exercise during the recovery period. However, Bonen et al. (1985) have shown that even light work requiring only 20% $\dot{V}O_2$max can cause further glycogenolysis during the post-exercise recovery period.

In conclusion, a glucose polymer supplement did not increase the rate of muscle glycogen resynthesis following soccer match-play. Furthermore, the rate of resynthesis was extremely slow. This could not be explained by a lack of carbohydrate in the diet. It would seem therefore that some other unknown factor(s) restricted the rate of restoration of the glycogen stores.

Acknowledgment

The authors acknowledge the enthusiasm and willingness to participate in this study by the coaches and players of the Canadian National teams. This work was supported by a grant from Sport Canada.

References

Bergstrom, J., Hermansen, L., Hultman, E. and Saltin, B. (1967) Diet, muscle glycogen and physical performance. Acta Physiol. Scand., 71, 140-150.

Bergstrom, J., Hultman, E., and Roch-Norlund, A.E. (1972) Muscle synthetase in normal subjects. Scand. J. Clin. Lab. Invest. 29, 231-236.

Bonen, A., Ness, G.W., Belcastro, A.N. and Lee, K. (1985) Mild exercise impedes glycogen repletion in muscle. J. Appl. Physiol: Respir. Envir. Exerc. Physiol., 58, 1622-1629.

Ekblom, B. (1986) Applied physiology of soccer. Sports Med., 3, 50-60.

Fell, R.D., Terblanche, S.E., Ivy, J.L., Young, J.C. and Holloszy, J.O. (1982) Effect of glycogen content on glucose uptake following exercise. J. Appl. Physiol: Respir. Envir.and Exerc. Physiol., 52, 434-437.

Gollnick, P.D., Piehl, K., Saubert IV, C.W., Armstrong, R.B. and Saltin, B. (1972) Diet, exercise, and glycogen changes in human muscle fibres. J. Appl. Physiol., 33, 421-425.

Hermansen, L., Hultman, E. and Saltin, B. (1967) Muscle glycogen during prolonged severe exercise. Acta Physiol. Scand., 11, 129-139.

Jacobs, I. (1981) Lactate, muscle glycogen and exercise performance in man. Acta Physiol. Scand. Supplementum, 495.

Jacobs, I., Westlin, N., Karlsson, J. and Rasmusson, M. (1982) Muscle glycogen and elite soccer players. Eur. J. Appl. Physiol. Occup. Physiol., 48, 297-302.

Karlsson, J. (1971) Lactate and phosphagen concentrations in working muscle of man. Acta Physiol. Scand., Supplementum, 358.

Maehlum, S. (1978) Muscle glycogen synthesis after a glucose infusion during post-exercise recovery in diabetic and non diabetic subjects. Scand. J. Clin. Lab. Invest., 38, 349-354.

Maehlum, S. and Pruett, E.D.R. (1973) Muscular exercise and metabolism in male juvenile diabetics II. glucose tolerance after exercise. Scandinavian J. Clin. Lab. Invest., 32, 149-153.

Maehlum, S., Hostmark, A. and Hermansen, L. (1977) Synthesis of muscle glycogen during recovery after prolonged severe exercise in diabetics and non-diabetic subjects. Scand. J. Clin. Lab. Invest., 37, 309-316.

Piehl, K. (1974) Time course for refilling of glycogen stores in human muscle fibres following exercise-induced glycogen depletion. Acta Physiol. Scand., 90, 297-302.

Posner, B.M. and Morgan, J.L. (1981) Dietary Instruction Manual, The Use of the 2D Food Portion Visual. Newton: Nutrition Consulting Enterprises.

Reilly, T. and Thomas, V. (1976) A motion analysis of work-rate in different positional roles in professional football match-play. J. Human Mov't. Stud., 2, 87-97.

Richter, E.A., Garetto, M., Goodman, N. and Ruderman, N. (1982) Muscle glucose metabolism following exercise in the rat: increased sensitivity to insulin. J. Clin. Invest., 69, 785-793.

Saltin, B. and Karlsson, J. (1971) Muscle glycogen utilization during work of different intensities. In Muscle Metabolism During Exercise (edited by B. Pernow and B. Saltin), pp.289-299. New York: Plenum Press.

Saltin, B. (1973) Metabolic fundamentals in exercise. Med. Sci. Sports, 5, 137-146.

Part III

Physiology of match-play

THE PHYSIOLOGICAL LOAD IMPOSED ON SOCCER PLAYERS DURING REAL MATCH-PLAY

D. Van Gool, D. Van Gerven and J. Boutmans
Instituut voor Lichamelijke Opleiding, Tervuursevest 101, 3030 Leuven (Heverlee), Belgium.

Introduction

To get a correct impression of the physiological load imposed on soccer players during competitive soccer, the observations have to be made during real match-play. According to Reilly and Thomas (1976) the total distance covered gives a general idea of the physiological load associated with soccer match-play. Published results vary from 3360 m (Winterbottom, 1954), over 4834 m (Knowles and Brooke, 1974), over 8680 m (Reilly and Thomas, 1976), 9790 m (Winkler 1983), 10112 m (Whitehead, 1975), 10332 m (Van Meerbeek et al., 1983), 10631 m (Van Cauter and Vrijens, 1984), 11527 (Withers et al., 1982) to 13260 m (Ohashi, 1979). More information is available when the intensity of the movement activities is taken into account. Until now the division of the total distance into discrete movement activities is mostly based on subjective feelings of the observer (Van Cauter and Vrijens, 1984).

More specific physiological parameters can be considered. Oxygen uptake can be measured when expired air is sampled in Douglas bags or in other respiratory devices (Seliger et al., 1970). Based on the linear relationship between oxygen uptake and heart rate during a standardised exercise test in the sub-maximum area (Berggren and Christensen, 1950; Åstrand, 1952; Monod, 1967), heart rate may be used for estimating oxygen uptake. Heart rate may also be used on its own as an indicant of the total stress (Maxfield, 1971). The concentration of lactate in blood samples taken after each half must be considered carefully as an index of the contribution of the anaerobic lactic energy deliverance systems during match-play (Agnevik, 1970; Cochrane and Pyke, 1976; Hollman et al., 1981; Dressel et al., 1984). In most of the studies cited only one parameter was observed at a time, observations being made on different players in different games or on only one player during a single game.

The aim of this study was to determine the physiological load imposed on 7 soccer players under real match-play conditions by employing a number of parameters. These included movement behaviour, heart rate and estimated oxygen uptake.

Methods

Subjects

All measurements were made during a friendly game between the soccer teams of the K.U. Leuven and Birmingham University (score 7-0). The observed players (aged 19 - 23 years) were members of the Belgian University team and they played in a team configuration known as '4-4-2'.

Measuring distance covered

A complete soccer game was filmed using a 16 mm camera with a film-speed of five images per second. The camera was placed on top of a 57 m high building located near the field. This enabled recording of the total field in each image and so all outfield players could be observed during the same game.

The film was projected on an 'x-y' coordinated system and analysed using the Mutoh Drafting and Digitizing Machine CX 3000. This unit was connected with a computer system and the measured coordinates were stored on a floppy disk. The Mutoh system measured with an accuracy of 0.1 mm.

The system measured the coordinates in 'film display units' (mm) and those coordinates had to be transformed to 'real field units' (m) using translation and rotation factors. This transformation procedure was described in detail by Vanhille (1983).

Each second, all the players were positioned and the distance between two successive points was calculated using the formula:-

$$D = \sqrt{(x_1 - x_2)^2 + (y_1 - y_2)^2}$$

D = the distance between two points

$x_1 y_1$ = the coordinates of point 1

$x_2 y_2$ = the coordinates of point 2

The speed of movement was also calculated using the method of Usui and Amidror (1983). The first derivative of the running distance was calculated and expressed in m s^{-1}.

Movement categories were formed based on the results of a pilot study where the subjective feelings were coupled with objective measurements based on movement speed. During a pilot study 24 footballers were asked to traverse a distance of 30 m in different ways during which the exact running time was recorded. Thus, the speed of movement could be calculated. Movements were divided according to intensity into walking, jogging, cruising and sprinting. Other movements, such as running and walking backwards and sideways or dribbling, were not considered as separate categories because they could not be observed on the film display. To draw a clear distinction between the categories an arbitrary scaling was set up, taking the experimental results into account. Table 1 shows the definitive movement categories with the corresponding speeds.

Table 1. Minimum and maximum speed for each movement category

STANDING STILL	0	1.3					$m\ s^{-1}$
WALKING		1.3	2.04				$m\ s^{-1}$
JOGGING			2.04	4.89			$m\ s^{-1}$
CRUISING				4.89	6.93		$m\ s^{-1}$
SPRINTING					6.93	8.15	$m\ s^{-1}$
	0	16	25	60	85	100%	

It may be surprising that there is also a category 'standing still'. This is due to the fact that the minimum speed in the category 'walking' was 1.31 $m\ s^{-1}$. Each movement with a speed less than 1.31 $m\ s^{-1}$ was deemed to belong to the category 'standing still'.

The discrete movement activities 'standing still plus walking' were considered as low intensity activities, 'jogging' as medium intensity activity and 'cruising plus sprinting' as high intensity activities.

Recording heart rate

Heart rate was recorded on 7 players using a radio telemetric system (Siemens Telecust 36E2). The methodology for intermittent recording of heart rate has been described by Van Gool et al. (1983).

Estimating oxygen uptake

All subjects performed a maximal stress test on a treadmill until exhaustion. The modified Taylor protocol (constant speed of 11.2 km h^{-1}, inclination increased by 2.5% every 3 min) was employed. Individual linear regression equations relating heart rate and $\dot{V}O_2$ were calculated. Oxygen uptake could be estimated from the heart rate measurements during the game using these formulae.

Results

The results for each of the players are shown for first and second halves in Tables 2 and 3 respectively. The mean total distance covered was 10225 (± SD = 580)m, for the 7 players. Of the total distance covered 42.9% was at a low intensity, 42.6% at medium intensity and 7.5% at high intensity. During the first half the players covered 444 m more than in the second half. Mean heart rate during the first half was 169 beats min^{-1}; for the second half the mean value was 165 beats min^{-1}. This corresponds respectively to 86.7% and 84.4% of the maximal heart rate. During the match the players were working at about 75% of their maximal aerobic

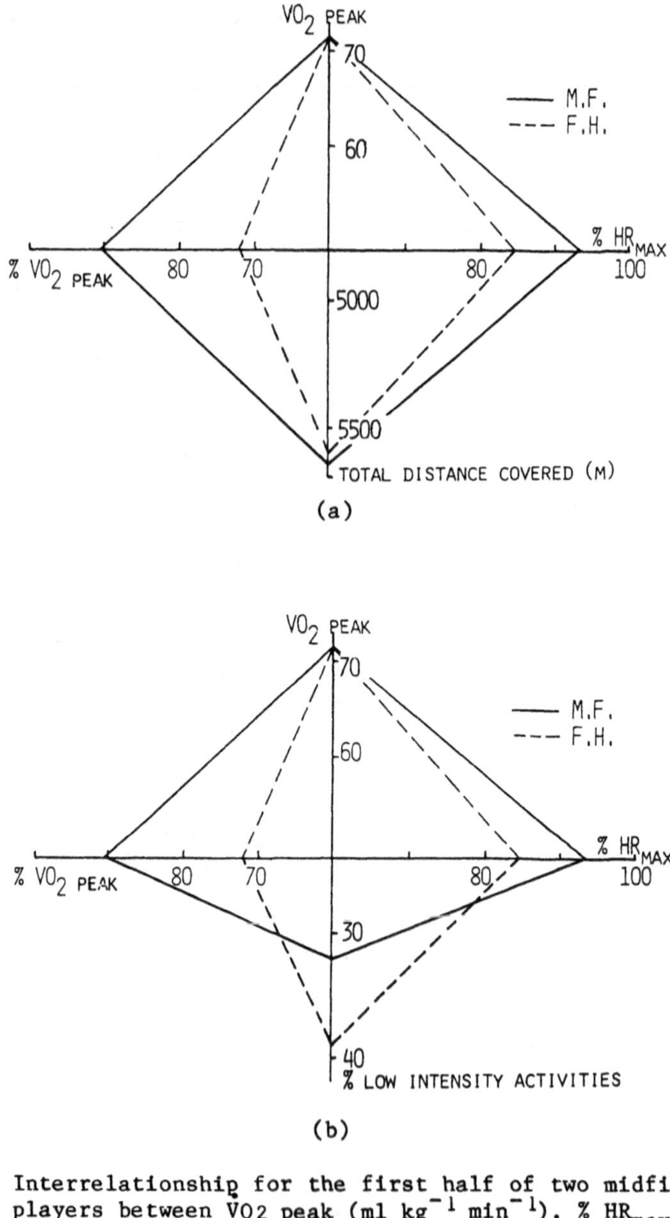

Figure 1. Interrelationship for the first half of two midfield players between $\dot{V}O2$ peak (ml kg^{-1} min^{-1}), % HR_{max}, % $\dot{V}O2$ peak and (a) total distance covered, (b) % of total distance covered by low intensity activities

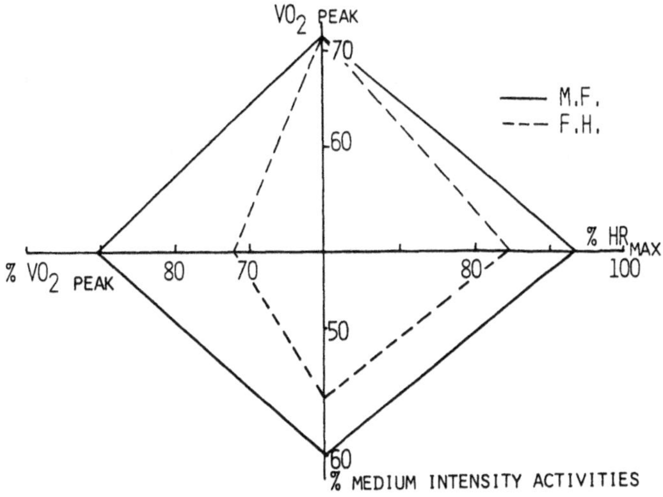

(c)

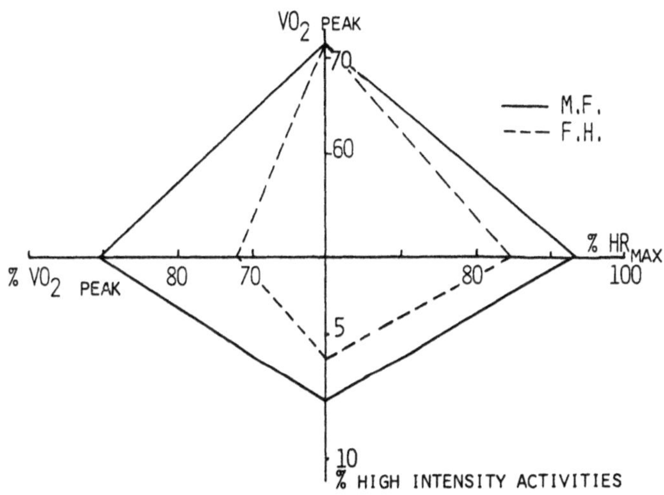

(d)

Figure 1. Interrelationship for the first half of two midfield players between $\dot{V}O_2$ peak (ml kg^{-1} min^{-1}), % HR_{max}, % $\dot{V}O_2$ peak and (c) % $\dot{V}O_2$ total distance covered by medium intensity activities (top), (d) % $\dot{V}O_2$ total distance covered by high intensity activities (bottom)

Table 2. Mean values for oxygen uptake, heart rate, and distance covered for each player during the first half. Peak $\dot{V}O_2$ values are also included

		J.W. (d)	M.M. (d)	M.F. (m)	D.G. (m)	F.H. (m)	B.L. (a)	E.L. (a)	$\bar{X}$	SD
Laboratory										
peak $\dot{V}O_2$ (ml kg^{-1} min^{-1})		58.0	68.0	71.0	67.0	71.0	66.5	63.5	66.4	4.5
Field										
HR (beats min^{-1})		170	170	182	160	163	170	166	169	7.1
% HR_{max}		86.8	87.9	93.6	84.5	84.5	85.7	83.9	86.7	
$\dot{V}O_2$ (ml kg^{-1} min^{-1})		46.6	54.9	63.7	50.2	50.9	48.9	47.7	51.8	5.9
% $\dot{V}O_2$ peak		80.3	80.7	89.7	74.9	71.7	73.5	75.1	78.0	
Distance Covered										
Total	m	5376	5283	5659	5262	5596	4906	5259	5355	249
Low intensity	m	2190	2307	1811	2207	2175	2494	2189	2196	204
	%	41	44	32	42	39	51	42	41	
Medium intensity	m	2763	2623	3414	2641	3096	1807	2779	2732	496
	%	51	50	60	50	55	37	53	51	
High intensity	m	423	353	434	414	325	605	291	407	103
	%	8	6	8	8	6	12	5	8	

(d) = defender, (m) = midfield player, (a) = attacker

Table 3. Mean values for oxygen uptake, heart rate, and distance covered for each player during the second half

		J.W. (d)	M.M. (d)	M.F. (m)	D.G. (m)	F.H. (m)	B.L. (a)	E.L. (a)	$\bar{X}$	SD
Field										
HR (beats min^{-1})		162	158	181	155	167	167	167	165	8.4
% HR_{max}		82.1	81.9	93.3	82.2	86.3	84.1	84.2	84.9	
$\dot{V}O_2$ (ml kg^{-1} min^{-1})		42.9	46.8	63.4	47.4	53.1	47.0	48.0	49.8	6.4
% $\dot{V}O_2$ peak		74.0	68.8	89.3	70.7	74.8	70.7	75.6	74.8	
Distance Covered										
Total	m	4346	4799	5242	4970	5400	4487	4988	4890	380
Low intensity	m	2229	2171	2028	2013	2313	2279	2280	2187	123
	%	51	45	39	40	43	51	46	45	
Medium intensity	m	1889	2442	2688	2624	2649	1659	2420	2339	404
	%	44	51	51	53	49	37	48	48	
High intensity	m	228	186	526	333	438	549	288	364	143
	%	5	4	10	7	8	12	6	7	

(d) = defender, (m) = midfield player, (a) = attacker

capacity. Consequently playing soccer was deemed to be highly demanding in terms of distance run, heart rate and oxygen uptake.

The relations between peak oxygen uptake (ml kg^{-1} min^{-1}), distance covered, heart rate and estimated oxygen uptake (expressed as % of the maximum values) were examined. Table 2 and Table 3 show the values and Figure 1 illustrates the relations. The first half results of two midfield players (M.F. and F.H.) are illustrated and these will be discussed in detail.

First of all, the values of the physiological parameters are compared with the results of the total distance covered (Fig. 1a). As both players had the same peak oxygen uptake (71 ml kg^{-1} min^{-1}) and covered about the same distance (5600 m) there is a clear difference in the extent that the players were taxing their maximal aerobic capacity.

Player M.F. was found to be working at 93% of his maximal heart rate and at 90% of his $\dot{V}O_2$ peak. The corresponding values for the other player (F.H.) were 84.5% and 71.7% respectively. So the total distance covered in the first half gives no indication of the extent to which the players were using their maximal aerobic capacity. This statement may be explained when the distance covered in each of the discrete movement activities (expressed as a percent of the total distance covered) is taken into account (Fig. 1b,1c,1d). It is noted that the results of this comparison have to be seen in the light of the relation between the physiological parameters and the total distance covered. Figure 1b shows that player F.H. covered 39% of the total distance in low intensity activities, while player M.F. covered only 32% of the total distance at the low intensity.

If the values of the physiological parameters for both players are plotted against the medium and high intensity activities (expressed as a percent of the total distance covered) (Figure 1c,1d), player M.F. scores the higher in comparison with player F.H.

These results explain why this player (M.F.) had to load his maximal aerobic capacity to a greater degree than player F.H. Player M.F. could be described as the 'toiler' of the team. Player F.H., who had the same value for $\dot{V}O_2$ peak, and who covered as much distance as the other player, seemed to cover this distance more by low and medium intensity activities. He was not required to tax his maximum aerobic power to such an extent as player M.F. This player can be described as a midfield player who is almost continually in motion but who allows his team-mates to do the intensive work.

Conclusions

The physiological load imposed on soccer players when playing a real match, seems to be high. The study of the relations between the parameters showed that the total distance covered does not reflect the extent that players were using their maximal aerobic capacity. Nevertheless, the total distance in combination with the running distances in each of the discrete movement categories (expressed as a percent of the total distance covered) can help to explain the extent that each player taxes his maximal aerobic power when playing a game. The relation varied between the individual players and so no general outline was found. The physiological measurements suggest that the mean training intensity should be high (approximately 75% of $\dot{V}O_2max$) to prepare the players for real match-play conditions.

References

Agnevik, G. (1970) Fotboll, Idrottsfysiology (Rapport 7). Stockholm: Trygg-Hansa.

Åstrand, P.O. (1952) Experimental studies of physical working capacity in relation to sex and age. Kopenhagen: Munksgaard, pp 171.

Berggren, G. and Christensen, E.H. (1950) Heart rate and body temperature as indices of metabolic rate during work. Arbeitsphysiol., 14, 255-260.

Cochrane, C. and Pyke, F. (1976) Physiological assessment of the Australian soccer squad. Aust. J. Health, Phys. Ed. and Recr., 73, 21-25.

Dressel, A., Hach, F. and Weicker, H. (1984) Trainingspraktische Konsequenzen aufgrund einer metabolische Beurteilung bei Fussballspielern. Leistungssport, 14, 27-32.

Hollmann, W., Liesen, H., Mader, A., Heck, H., Rost, R., Dufaux, B., Schürch, P., Lagerström, D. and Föhrenbach, R. (1981) Zur Höchst- und Dauerleistungsfähigkeit der deutschen Fussball-Spitzenspieler. Deutsche Zeitschrift für Sportmedizin, 32, 113-120.

Knowles, J.E. and Brooke, J.D. (1974) A movement analysis of player behaviour in soccer match performance. Paper presented at the 8th Conference, British Society of Sports Psychology (Salford).

Maxfield, M.E. (1971) The indirect measurements of energy expenditure in industrial situations. Amer. J. Clin. Nutr., 24, 1126-1138.

Monod, H. (1967) La validité des mesures de fréquence cardiaque en ergonomie. Ergonomics, 10, 485-537.

Ohashi, J. (1979) Een poging tot de analyse van de bewegingen van voetballers tijdens een wedstrijd. Proceedings Nikon University, Tokyo: Nikon University, 33-38 (vertaling uit Japans).

Reilly, T. and Thomas, V. (1976) A motion analysis of work-rate in different positional roles in professional football match-play. J. Human Mov't. Stud., 2, 87-97.

Seliger, V., Navara, M. and Pachlopnikova, V. (1970) Der energetische Metabolismus im Verlauf des Fussballspiels. Sportarzt und Sportmedizin, 21, 114-118.

Usui, S. and Amidror, I. (1983) Digital differentiation filter for biological signal processing; In: Biomechanics VIII-B (International Series on Biomechanics 4b; International Congress of Biomechanics 8, Nagoya, 1982 (edited by H. Matsui and K. Kobayashi), pp 1207-1214. Champaign, Illinois: Human Kinetics.

Van Cauter, C. and Vrijens, J. (1984) Onderzoek naar de fysieke belasting van voetballers tijdens een competitiewedstrijd. Tijdschrift voor Lichamelijke Opvoeding, 91, 2-7.

Van Gool, D., Van Gerven, D. and Boutmans, J. (1983) Heart rate during a soccer game: a new methodology. J. Sports Sci., 1, 154.

Vanhille, L. (1983) Analyse van spelstructuren. (Leuven: K.U. Leuven; Doctoraatsproefschrift Lichamelijke Opleiding).

Van Meerbeek, R., Van Gool, D. and Janssens, P. (1983) De afstand afgelegd tijdens een voetbalwedstrijd. Hermes (Leuven), 16, 15-24.

Whitehead, N. (1975) Conditioning for Sports. East Ardsley, Wakefield: EP Publishing.

Winkler, W. (1983) Spielerbeobachtung bei Fussballspielen im Zusammenhang mit Spielerpositionen, Spielsystem und Laufbelastung. Leistungsfussball, 21, 63-68.

Winterbottom, W. (1954) Voetballen. Antwerpen: De Vlijt, pp271.

Withers, R.T., Maricic, Z., Wasilewski, S. and Kelly, L. (1982) Match analysis of Australian professional soccer players. J. Human Mov't. Stud., 8, 159-176.

SPORTSMEDICAL MEASUREMENTS OF PERFORMANCE IN SOCCER

G. Gerisch, E. Rutemöller and K. Weber
Deutsche Sporthochschule Köln, Institut für Sportspiele, Carl-Diem-Weg 2, D-5000 Köln 41, West Germany.

Introduction

Soccer is a branch of sport with a profile of complex requirements. Because of the variety of factors affecting motor and mental abilities, as well as the effects of the opposing and supporting players on behaviour during play, it is difficult to recognize and rank the impact of single, interfering components within the whole. Such judgement, however, is of major practical interest, because by these means many important disclosures for the planning and practice of training can be made, and at the same time a reliable basis is provided for a valid performance diagnosis and prognosis (Fig. 1).

The multiple demands in a soccer game cannot be adequately simulated in the laboratory. The conduct of field studies for clarifying the structure of play and determining the demands of games faces many methodological, instrumental and organisational problems. An elegant diagnosis of isolated or complex components of performance in games requires a clear description of the desired form of demand; such a diagnosis requires a test mode with a high fidelity to the particular sport.

The planning, realization and evaluation of training processes cannot be made without the most exact determination of the loading intensity in practice and competition. Here the relation between anaerobic-alactacid and aerobic energy metabolism is of central concern in the development and optimization of physical performances. For this reason the focus of the present work is on the determination of lactate levels in the blood, and other indices of aerobic and anaerobic endurance.

Field studies and tests in conjunction with the determination of lactate levels in sports serve two main purposes:-

(i) objective statements can be made regarding the current individual competition and about the appropriate loading in training;

(ii) the observations are sport-specific and the demand on aerobic capacity can be estimated independent of motivation.

Next to the high sensitivity of the blood lactate levels towards various forms of energy supply to the working muscle, the determination of the lactate level has further advantages. These are the convenience for frequent repeatability and problem-free blood

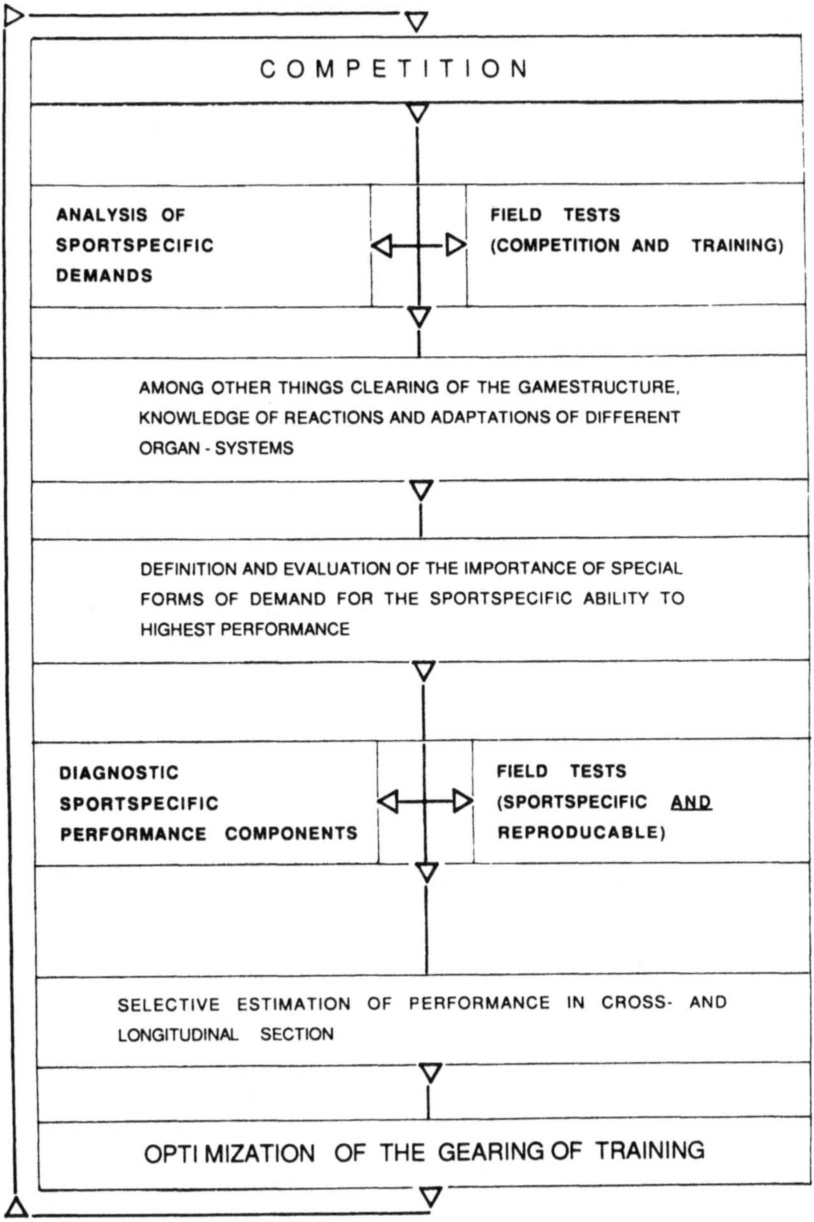

Figure 1. Field studies and tests within the aegis of sport-specific training and competition

sampling, especially as only a 20 µl sample is required. The information on the blood lactate concentration has its limits, however. It needs to be critically appraised, especially when the physical demands are complex, as for instance in the game of soccer. The simultaneous determination of other parameters from the intermediate metabolism, such as glucose, glycerin, carbamide (urea), alanine and the catecholamines, adrenaline and noradrenaline, may be helpful.

The observation and recording of the sport specific structural requirements (i.e. distance covered and velocity of motion, detailed lists of actions with and without the ball, effective time of play) are necessary to match the physiological data with the match-play requirements. This enables conclusions relevant to the practice of sport games to be derived from the synopsis of the test results.

Methods

The following performance diagnosing measures were employed in both field and laboratory conditions:-

(i) determination of blood lactate levels (n = 37) and length and speed of distances covered in 4 championships matches of the top amateur league (Oberliga Nordrhein, n = 24);

(ii) determination of blood lactate concentrations of two teams in two experimental matches (n = 22) - man-to-man covering, and secondly zone coverage;

(iii) determination of the aerobic capacity in the subjects of both field studies as a supporting measure to guarantee a well-founded interpretation of the data collected in competition.

Results

The average blood lactate levels of single soccer teams (excluding the goalkeeper) varied between 4-6 mM (Table 1) in championship games. The standard deviations indicate regular occurrences of peak lactate of about 7-8 mM. This is within the acidosis zone, which does not only cause subjective feelings of 'leaden legs', but according to Liesen (1983) leads to a deficit in technical, tactical functions even in top level soccer and hockey. These limitations to technique after high metabolic demands have been confirmed experimentally in tennis players and handball players.

From a purely metabolic viewpoint it is understandable if the team coach substitutes early on those players, who had extremely high, or low lactate values and at the same time were either incapable of fulfilling the more complex coordination tasks, or those who because of their poor running performance (with or without the ball) did not prove supportive to the team. The substituted players are indicated in Table 2. Therefore the question arises whether fine controls of lactate levels during training and competition could convey useful information to the players as well as the coaches, so that the players are able to employ their performance potential more economically over the whole playing-time. This information might additionally support the timing of the substitution of players. From

Table 1. Median (± SD) values of 4 soccer matches at the highest level of play in amateurs (without the goalkeeper)

Top amateur League (amateurs)			Lactate mM 1st half	Lactate mM 2nd half
1.12.84	WSV - Xanten	n = 10	5.15 ± 2.55	4.36 ± 2.47
15.12.84	FC K(A) - WSV	n = 10	5.65 ± 1.30	6.05 ± 2.96
	FC K(A) - WSV	n = 9	4.27 ± 2.24	4.57 ± 2.46
11.5.85	WSV - FC K(A)	n = 10	7.22 ± 2.69	4.63 ± 1.57
	WSV - FC K(A)	n = 10	5.52 ± 2.02	3.84 ± 1.07
19.5.85	WSV - SW Essen	n = 10	3.79 ± 1.26	4.61 ± 2.74
1984/85	4 games	n = 59	5.58 ± 2.01	4.68 ± 2.16

Table 2. Blood lactate levels ($\bar{x}$ ± SD) of all field players at the end of each half-time within the championship match of the top amateur league

1. FC Köln (A) 15.12.84			
Players	Lactate mM 1st half	Lactate mM 2nd half	
2	6.35	6.15	
3	6.80	12.40	out 69'
4	5.55	2.20	out 79'
5	6.30	5.75	
6	5.55	6.85	
7	5.30	2.75	
8	2.20	7.65	
9	5.85	6.10	
10	6.25	4.45	
11	6.40	3.90	
12	-	7.55	in 69'
14	-	6.95	in 79'
$\bar{x}$	5.65	6.06	
SD	1.30	2.69	

a systematic observation of players it becomes clear how playing position, tactical purpose, the total distance covered and the distribution of effort influence the quality and quantity of typical actions in soccer. It becomes clear also how they influence the maximum speed and length of distances run. We found considerable differences in the length of distance run and the intensity levels designated 2 (2-5 m s^{-1}) and 3 (5 m s^{-1}). The distance determination of an amateur league team made up of midfield players ($n = 14$) and offensive players ($n = 5$) amounted to an average of barely under 10 000 m ($\bar{x} \pm SD = 9050 \pm 969$) for three championship matches. Within the total distances midfield and offensive players averaged about 1500 m at a tempo classed as level 3.

The findings for distance covered and lactate levels (Table 3) make plain how important and necessary it is to have a differentiated training programme within a team in order to build up strong points and eliminate weak points. Little attention is in fact given to this in day-to-day practice.

Table 3. Blood lactate rates of various players with different tactical assignments

Top amateur league (amateurs)		Playing position	Lactate mM		
			1st half	2nd half	E 3'*
15.12.84 1.FC K	4	'man-to-man defence'	5.55	2.20	1.80
2:3 (1.0) WSV	8	'water-carrier'	9.90	9.70	8.40
11.5.85 WSV	3	Libero	7.10	6.45	4.90
3:1 (1.0) 1.FCK	5		2.10	2.10	1.90

*3 min after the end of play

As determined in a standardized laboratory treadmill test (Fig. 2), an elevated 'anaerobic-aerobic' threshold enables teams with superior general endurance to reach higher speeds and therefore put the pressure on opponents during competition. Conversely, weaker endurance players must shorten their running distances and reduce the intensity in order to prevent a collapse in performance. This applies above all to the tactical assignment in 'man-to-man-coverage'. It is therefore not surprising to find drastic differences in lactate level when two teams with different endurance capacities compete in 'man-to-man' contest (Fig. 3). The blood lactate levels of the same players were far more compatible when players were assigned to 'zone-coverage' (Fig. 4). At the same time we found a reduction of average blood lactate levels. In comparing zone coverage, other experts also found a smaller difference in performance between the two teams (Hollman et al., 1981); this proves so even in games with closer final scores. The inferior team, which was mainly made up of experienced former national league players, could at most compensate for its deficits in areas such as endurance by more economical runs and a 'clever' style of play.

Implications for Training

It is possible to derive fundamental ideas on endurance and speed training from the empirical findings relating to blood lactate levels during training and competition and our analysis of distance covered. The following goals should be aimed for:-

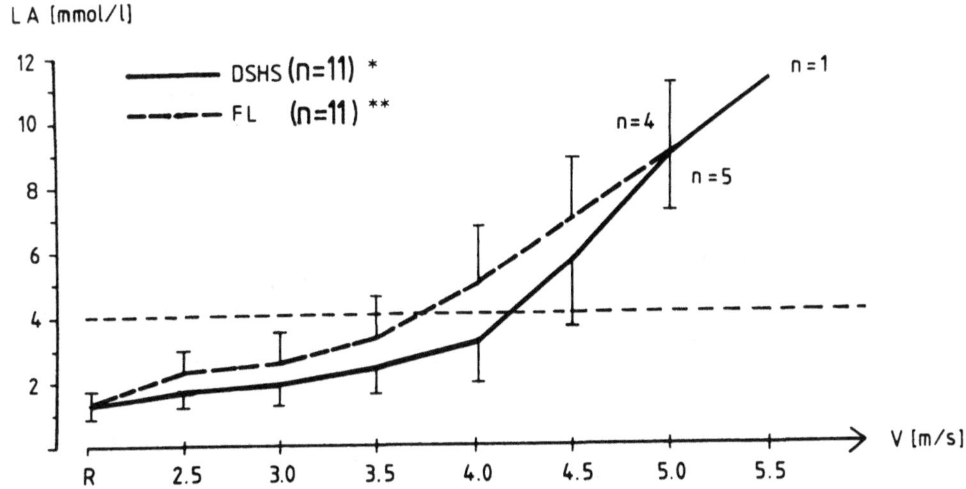

Figure 2. Comparative description of the blood lactate levels of two different teams during a steady rise in loading on the treadmill

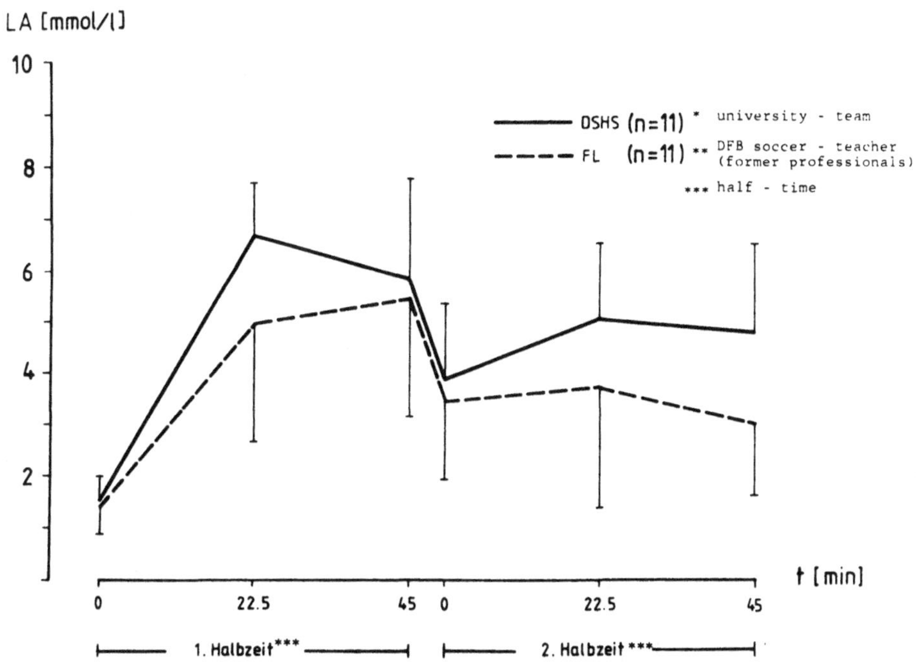

Figure 3. Blood lactate levels of two soccer teams (without goal-keepers) during the given tactical assignment – 'man-coverage'

(i) Raising the general aerobic endurance
This includes development of high fatigue-resistance in maximal speeds during the entire game; ability to recover quickly during play following several highly intense sprints, or following counter-attacks over extended distances; quick and thorough recovery during competition (including half-time intermission), after individual competitions and after intense training.

(ii) Increase of the anaerobic alactacid capacity
This necessitates an improvement in speed of irregular sprints and in shots: this applies foremost to sprint or double sprints over 5-30 m distances (possibly culminating with a shot or goal or precise pass)

(iii) Raising of the aerobic endurance efficiency on the one hand and increase of dynamic (explosive) power on the other with the exclusion of negative reciprocal effects.

(iv) Optimal transfer of the training goals to the specific demands of soccer competition (with or without the ball).

A high quality base of endurance is fundamental for a successful development of the training goals listed. It is the basis for other major forms of motor demand (i.e. strength, speed) and at the same time is an indispensable requirement for extensive training. A

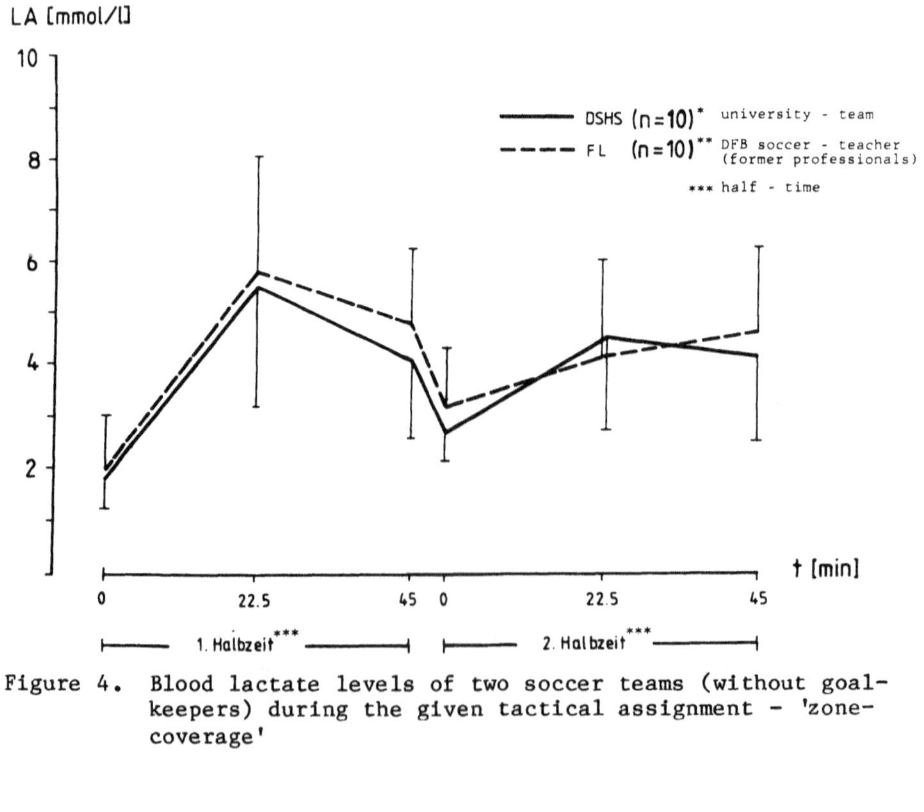

Figure 4. Blood lactate levels of two soccer teams (without goal-keepers) during the given tactical assignment - 'zone-coverage'

systematically developed endurance training programme for soccer players therefore begins with basic endurance training, which then in a second phase (in an uninterrupted flow) is taken over by a soccer specific competitive endurance training.

In closing we summarize those implications which are not in unison with the present regular training practice in professional soccer. Firstly the extent and intensity of training needs to take account of individual and team-tactical aspects. Secondly, soccer players need a systematic endurance training programme for the improvement of their basic endurance capacity and for the optimization of their recovery. Thirdly, typical speed-endurance training with high superacidosis - for example, through 'tempo' sprints or intensive interval training - should be reduced to a sport-specific speed training within primarily the anaerobic range on the one hand, and an endurance training primarily within the aerobic range on the other.

Of course, during the realization of these demands, it is extremely important not to neglect or negatively influence other important training objectives from technical or tactical areas. The daily extent of training should also not be greatly increased. Free capacity, however, exists for the new winter-break - introduced by the DFB for the German national league (Bundesliga) - and for the transition period after the championship round. These periods of time especially should be put to use, instead of remaining as a passive regeneration period as is usual in soccer.

References

Hollmann, W., Liesen, H., Mader, A., Heck, H., Rost, R., Dufaux, B., Schürch, J., Lagerström, D. and Föhrenbach, R. (1981) Zur Höchst- und Dauerleistungsfähigkeit der deutschen Fussball-Spitzenspieler. Dtsch. Ztschr. Sportmed., 32, 113-120.

Liesen, H. (1983) Schnelligkeitsausdauer im Fussball aus sportmedizinischer Sicht. Fussballtraining, 1, 27-31.

WORK INTENSITY DURING SOCCER TRAINING AND MATCH-PLAY

Hans Christian Rohde and Torben Espersen
Institute of Physical Education, Odense University, DK-5230 Odense, M., Denmark.

Introduction

To a certain extent technical and tactical aspects of soccer must be trained during physical conditions similar to those found during matches, if the training aim is to be effective. The purpose of this paper is to compare the physical work load of soccer training to that encountered during real 1st Division matches. This comparison is based on heart rate (HR) and lactate measurements obtained during soccer training and soccer games. The present results are part of a large project, which also involved tests on maximal oxygen uptake and interval running tests in the laboratory.

Methods

Subjects

Six players from a Danish first division team were chosen for the investigation. They were all informed about the testing procedure and gave a verbal agreement to participate. The players' position on the team were:- forward (n=1), midfield (n=3) and defence (n=2). The mean (±SD) age and body weight were 26±4 years and 73.0±5.2kg, respectively.

Procedures

The physiological parameters measured were heart rate (HR) and lactate concentration in aterialized blood. The HR was measured continuously (5 s samples) with the Sports Tester PE 3000 (Polar Electro, Finland). The equipment consisted of an electrode belt with a transmitter, which records the ECG and sends electro-magnetic signals to a receiving watch, incorporating a microcomputer, which stores the HR values as well as the time.

The belt was strapped around the chest approximately at the height of the lower third of the sternum. The watch was placed in a small pocket in the waistband. The electrode belt weighed 46 g (1.64 oz.), the transmitter 40 g (1.43 oz), the receiver (microcomputer) 48 g (1.71 oz).

Blood samples for measuring the concentration of lactate were taken between 1 and 1.5 min after the activity stopped and before any warm-down period. The samples were taken from a fingertip. The blood was collected in a glass containing heparin crystals. A 100 µl sample of blood was used, mixed with 500 µl of perchloric acid. The samples were kept chilled to 0°C and later centrifuged in the laboratory. Here the blood serum was frozen. The lactate concentration was later analyzed according to a photoenzymatic method (Boehringer).

The measurements were performed during training and during 1st division competitive matches. One week of training consisted of 6 x 1.5 hours from Monday to Thursday. Training on the day the measurements were made was meant to be the most intense for the week, according to the coach.

Every training session consisted of a 20 min warm-up and usually 3 practice games, each lasting about 20 min. The HR measurements were obtained in 30 practice games. Total number of measurements, n = 104 in 10 training sessions. Lactate samples were obtained in 15 practice games.

The HR measurements in the competitive matches were obtained for one half at a time for each player; during the 4 competitive matches, a number of subjects were measured, giving a total of 18 measurements (Table 2) (total n = 18 4 matches). The lactate samples were obtained before the match, during the half time and after the match from the players who had their heart rates measured.

Data processing

The data stored in the watch were transferred via an interface to a computer. Curves were then printed with HR as a function of the time. These curves were analysed at two levels:- (i) HR max (HR max - 15 beats min^{-1}), (ii) (HR max - 15 beats min^{-1})- (HR max - 50 beats min^{-1}). These two levels were separately decided in accordance with the subjects' results measured earlier during discontinuous running tests on a treadmill. These tests, were performed 5 times during the experimental period (13.2.86 - 21.6.86). They were used to measure the recovery time from running. The speed corresponded to HRmax - 15 beats min^{-1} (2 min workperiods: 8 times) and the duration of the recovery was measured as the time for HR to drop 50 beats min from the maximal value.

Maximal heart rate (HRmax) was ascertained during a direct measurement of $\dot{V}O_2$ max while running on a treadmill. Expired air was collected in Douglas bags and dried samples were analyzed on a Beckmann LB2-CO2 analyser and a Servomex 02 analyser. The volume of expired air was measured in a spirometer. These tests were taken five times during the experimental period. The HR recordings between HR max and HR max - 15 beats min^{-1} (High intensity) as well as between HR max - 15 beats min^{-1} and HR max - 50 beats min^{-1} (Medium intensity) were examined for their durations and for the average HR. The analyses were made either from actual HR transcriptions or from HR-curves measured by planeometry.

An average (±SD) of all players in each practice game was found as well as a total average (±SD) of all practise games. An average for every competitive match as well as an overall average (±SD) of all matches was calculated.

The total averages of training and competition were compared and the percentage difference was tested for statistical significance

(Student's t-test). The lactate values were treated in a similar manner for both practice games and competitive matches. The HR as a percent of the maximal value was found according to the formula:- (mean HR-resting HR x 100)/(HR max - resting HR). The resting heart rates were estimated to be 60 beats min for all players.

Results

The player's training intensity in the medium zone was 74% of HR max for 68% of the training time. In comparison the competitive match-play intensity was 77% for 66% of the match time. Only for 4% of the training time were the HR values in the high interval range. The mean training intensity was then 91% of HR max. During the competitive matches these values were 26% for duration and 91% for exercise intensity in the high intensity zone. Results for training and match-play are given in Table 1 and Table 2 respectively.

The measurements of blood lactate concentration showed average values during training at 3.3 mM and 1.8 mM after training (Table 3). The total average for training was 2.7 mM ($\pm$ SD = 1.6; n = 28). For the competitive matches the average after the first half was 5.1 mM and after the match 3.9 mM (Table 4). The total average for the matches was 4.4 mM ($\pm$SD = 1.9; n = 22).

Discussion

It is common to use heart rate as a measure of the physical work-load 'in the field.' Technically this is not complicated and it causes hardly any inconvenience to the subject. In sports with close contact (e.g. soccer) it is important that the equipment is small and light and without danger to the subject. The present equipment fulfils these requirements.

Generally a linear relationship exists between HR, work-rate and oxygen uptake, but at near maximal work-loads the linearity between HR and $\dot{V}O_2$ is not always seen (Astrand and Rodahl, 1977: p.189 and p.455). In this case we assume a linearity between HR and work-rate so that HR reflects the actual work-load. However, HR can be influenced by stress, which the competition may induce. One may, therefore, expect that part of the HR response during a competition can be caused by emotional stress. To what extent the high physical work loads will neutralize the effects of stress is not known, but it seems likely that it occurs to some extent (Astrand and Rodahl, 1977: p.460).

The major component of the physical load in soccer is running. One may ignore the phases of ball-touching, because they comprise only a very small part of the whole match.

It is difficult to set a limiting standard for the physical condition a soccer player must have. The physical, psychological, tactical and technical skills are all interrelated in a complex pattern (Von Hollmann et al., 1978). Whether or not technical and tactical skills will be optimized in a training situation cannot be determined directly as the question is concerned with subjective capacities. The physical work load of training, however, is

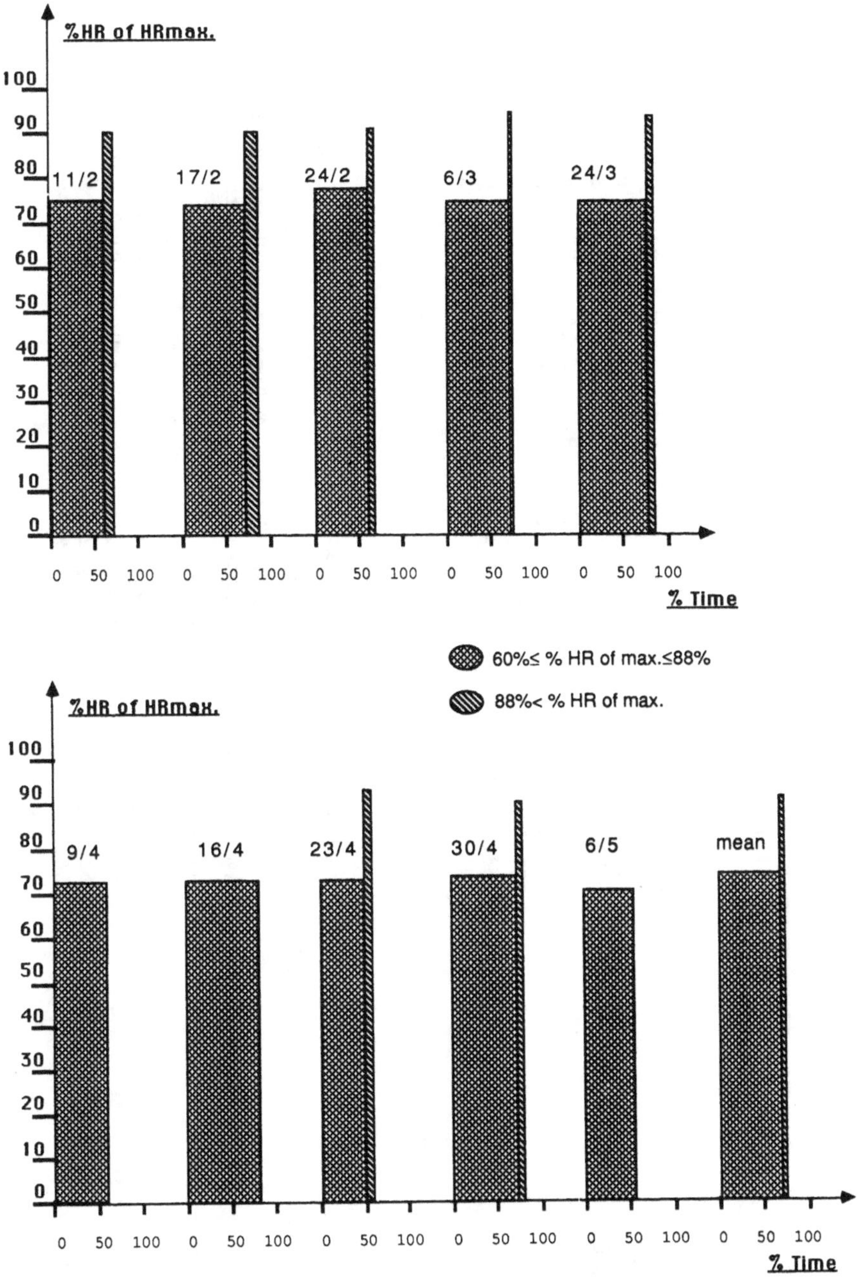

Figure 1. Heart rate (% HRmax) as a function of the time (% of training session time) in which the players have been in the medium and high intervals during training

Table 1. Heart rate measurement as % of HR max for the ten training sessions (mean ± SD)

Date	Subjects	Measurements	% Time (medium int)	Heart Rate beats min^{-1}	% Time (high int)	Heart Rate beats min^{-1}
11.2.86	5	15	67.5 ± 18.8	75.0 ± 5.7	11.1 ± 12.9	90.2 ± 1.2
17.2.86	2	6	74.2 ± 17.6	73.3 ± 4.0	15.3 ± 17.9	90.4 ± 1.8
24.2.86	4	8	63.4 ± 17.5	77.4 ± 3.4	5.3 ± 7.4	90.8 ± 0.4
6.3.86	5	13	74.9 ± 26.3	74.9 ± 4.9	0.4 ± 0.9	94.7 ± 5.4
24.3.86	3	12	83.0 ± 12.8	74.6 ± 3.7	0.7 ± 2.4	93.3 ± 0
9.4.86	4	11	60.0 ± 16.3	72.4 ± 3.8	•	•
16.4.86	5	12	80.5 ± 18.3	73.2 ± 4.3	•	•
23.4.86	5	12	50.0 ± 24.8	73.1 ± 6.2	9.9 ± 20.6	92.7 ± 2.3
30.4.86	2	6	72.6 ± 20.8	73.7 ± 6.0	5.6 ± 8.6	90.2 ± .6
6.5.86	3	9	55.7 ± 33.4	70.7 ± 5.4	•	•
Mean			68.2 ± 23.9	73.9 ± 4.8	4.4 ± 11.2	91.2 ± 1.6
Total		104	•	•	•	•

Table 2. Heart rate measurements in % of HR max for four competition matches (mean ± SD)

Date	Subjects	Measurements	% Time (medium int)	Heart Rate beats min^{-1}	% Time (high int)	Heart Rate beats min^{-1}
6.4.86	4	6	66.4 ± 12.0	77.2 ± 1.0	30.7 ± 12.8	91.1 ± 0.7
20.4.86	3	3	73.9 ± 6.6	76.7 ± 2.7	16.1 ± 3.4	90.4 ± 0.5
4.5.86	3	4	63.6 ± 4.7	75.9 ± 3.6	24.8 ± 4.0	91.7 ± 0.7
14.5.86	4	5	63.9 ± 13.9	77.4 ± 2.1	28.3 ± 14.8	92.1 ± 1.4
Mean			66.3 ± 11.2	76.9 ± 2.5	26.3 ± 12.1	91.4 ± 1.1
Total		18	•	•	•	•

Table 3. Lactate values during and after training (mM) (mean ± SD)

Date	Number of measurements	Lactate during training (mM)	Number of measurements	Lactate after training (mM)
11.2.86	●	● ●	●	
17.2.86	●	● ●	●	
24.2.86	●	● ●	●	
6.3.86	●	● ●	●	
24.3.86	●	● ●	●	
9.4.86	4	3.91 ± 1.70	4	1.92 ± 1.22
16.4.86	1	3.63 ± 0 ●	●	
23.4.86	3	4.70 ± 1.30	3	2.20 ± 0.96
30.4.86	6	2.49 ± 1.48	3	1.56 ± 0.23
6.5.86	2	2.38 ± 1.03	2	1.83 ± 0.29
Mean	●	3.32 ± 1.35	●	1.88 ± 0.75
Total	16	●	12	●

Table 4. Lactate values (mean ± SD) during and after the competitive matches (mM)

Date	No. of lactate measurement after 1st half	Lactate after 1st half	No. of lactate measurement post-match	Lactate post match
6.4.86	2	5.0 ± 2.0	4	4.0 ± 1.6
20.4.86	2	5.9 ± 0.1	2	3.2 ± 1.1
4.5.86	2	6.0 ± 1.8	3	5.7 ± 1.0
14.5.86	3	4.1 ± 1.1	4	3.0 ± 0.6
Mean	●	5.1 ± 1.6	●	3.9 ± 1.6
Total	9	●	13	●

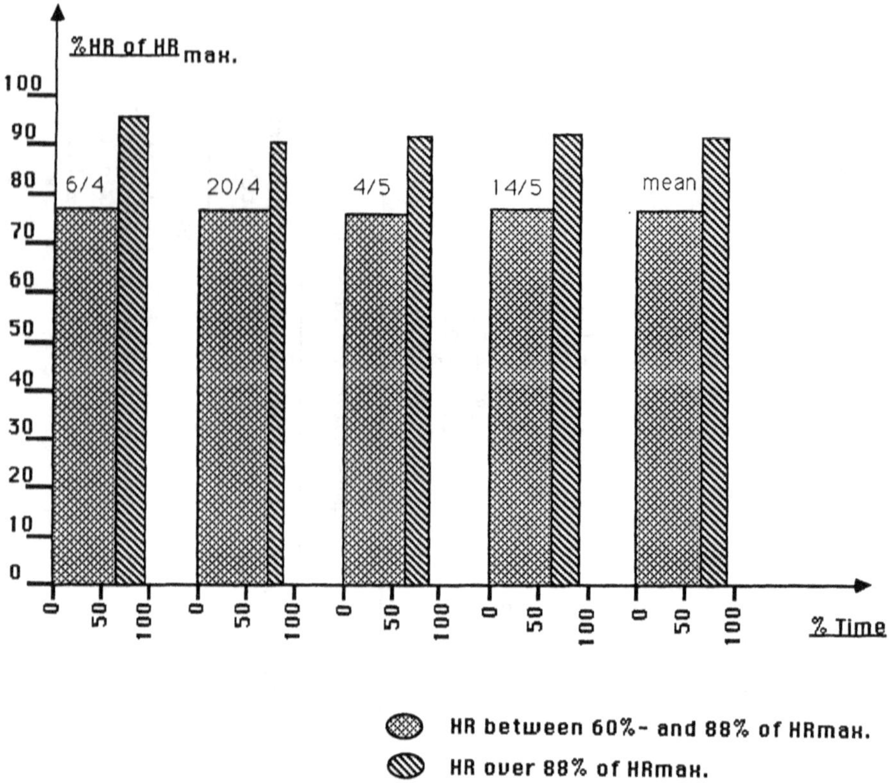

Figure 2. Heart rate (% HRmax) as a function of the time (% of match time) in which the players have been in the medium and high intervals during competition

measurable and comparable with the corresponding load of a competitive match. It is recognized that training in the coordination of movements and the training of the anaerobic and aerobic capacities are optimized through functional training, (Von Hollmann et al., 1978).

In this research the technical and tactical aspects were trained functionally. The training consisted of minor practice games with a limited number of players and limited size of playing ground.

As seen from Fig. 1 and Table 1 the differences between the various training sessions are considerable. In one case training was performed in the high interval area for 15% of the time, while in other cases the players never reached this level of exercise intensity. This shows that the training stimuli do not have a systmatic structure and do not necessarily involve regular bouts of 'high' intensity exercise.

The most important difference between match-play and training is the duration the players are in the 'high' intensity zone. During matches the players are in the high interval area for 26% of the time, which is significantly ($P < 0.0005$) longer than during training where the high interval represented 4% of the time. Therefore, it can be presumed that by increasing training intensity to the level of matches the effect of training on technical and tactical aspects would increase.

It is possible to exercise very hard in short bouts (with equivalent rest periods) for a long time without special use of anaerobic processes which lead to high lactate concentrations (Åstrand and Rodahl, 1977, p.399-401). Our results showed mean values of 2.7 mM in training and 4.4 mM in competition (See table 3 & 4). These correspond with results of other investigations (Von Hollman et al., 1978; Von Hollmann et al., 1981; Carli et al., 1986 and Poulsen et al., 1981). Although a few investigators have reported higher (6-10 mM) lactate values (Ekblom, 1986), our results suggest that anaerobic endurance training is not a particularly important consideration for soccer players. In the light of our results it may be that imperfect fitness in soccer players is due to the fact that the demands which a player must fulfil in the match situation have not been practised under sufficiently realistic conditions during training.

The competition match itself is a very valuable training stimulus for the individual player. The number of matches a player can participate in, is also a function of his training. Many foreign teams play about 70 competitive matches per year whereas Danish teams play approximately 40. These do not give the Danish players the same training value as many foreign players obtain.

References

Åstrand, P.O. and Rodahl, K. (1977) Textbook of Work Physiology. New York: McGraw-Hill.

Carli, G., Bonifazi, M., Lodi, L., Lupo, C., Martelli, G. and Viti, A. (1986) Hormonal and metabolic effects following a football match. Int. J. Sports Med., 7, 36-38.

Ekblom, B. (1986) Applied physiology of soccer. Sports Med., 3 50-60.

Poulsen, R., Hansen, P., Norgaard, L. (1981) En fodbold-fysiologisk undersogelse. Odense Universiteit, Unpublished report.

Von Hollmann, W., Liesen, H., Mader, A., Heck, H., Rost, R., Dufaux, B., Schurch, P., Lagerstrom, D. and Fohrenbach, R. (1981) Zur Hochst - und Dauerleistungsfahigkeit der Deutschen Fussball-Spitzenspieler. Deutche Zeitschrift fur Sportmedizin, 2, 113-120.

Von Hollman, W., Rost, R., Liesen, H., Mader, A. (1978). Physiologischinternistische Aspekte zum Fussballsport. Deutsche Zeitscrift fur Sportmedizin, 1, 29; 2,60.

Von Schmid, P., Dickhuth, H. H., Lehmann, M., Huber, G., Berg, A., Keul, J. (1983) Labordiagnostische Ergebnisse von Fussball- und Handballspielern. Deutche Zeitschrift fur Sportmedizin, 12, 365-375.

PHYSIOLOGICAL STRAIN IN 4-A-SIDE SOCCER

D. MacLaren, K. Davids, M. Isokawa*, S. Mellor and T. Reilly
Department of Sport and Recreation Studies, Liverpool Polytechnic, Byrom Street, Liverpool L3 3AF, England.
*Department of Physical Education, Tokyo Metropolitan University, Tokyo, Japan.

Introduction

The popularity of small-sided soccer, as represented by 4-, 5- or 6-a-side games, has paralleled the development of sports centres in the United Kingdom. Indeed on Merseyside the popularity of this form of soccer has further manifested itself in many successfully organised tournaments and leagues; nationally the game has progressed to a highly sponsored, televised 6-a-side tournament in which top professional teams participate. Furthermore, most soccer clubs use small-sided games as an integral part of their training and fitness schedules.

Despite the frequency of participation in small-sided soccer, there has been no investigation of the physiological strain imposed by playing such games. It was the intention of this study to monitor physiological strain incurred in playing 4-a-side soccer during:- (i) two legs of a cup final, and (ii) recreational matches.

Method

Three male outfield players from one team in the final of the Liverpool Polytechnic 4-a-side tournament volunteered for the study, having been informed of its details. A blood sample, from an antecubital vein, was taken before and immediately after the two-legs of the final; a similar procedure was used before and after a recreational match using the same subjects. The plasma was separated, removed and frozen for later analysis of adrenaline, noradrenaline, lactate, glucose and non-esterified fatty acids (NEFA). The plasma catecholamines were determined by 'high performance' liquid chromatography after clean-up and extraction on cation-exchange resin (Frayn and Maycock, 1983); the lactate and glucose were measured by an enzymatic photometric method using a Boehringer (UK) kit and the NEFA by a kit from Wako (Alpha Laboratories, U.K.).

One of the outfield players had his heart rate telemetred throughout the three matches. He had previously performed both a $\dot{V}O_2max$ assessment using a continuous incremental protocol to volitional exhaustion on a motorized treadmill and on a separate occasion, five 5 min sub-maximal runs on the treadmill during which time heart rate (HR) and $\dot{V}O_2$ were monitored. From these observations a regression line relating HR and $\dot{V}O_2$ was established.

Three further recreational matches were analysed during which three additional subjects, who previously had their $\dot{V}O_2max$ and HR-$\dot{V}O_2$ relationship determined, had their HR continuously monitored. Finger prick blood samples were taken before and after the matches, and deproteinized in cold 2.5% perchloric acid for later analysis of lactate concentration.

Results of the plasma hormones and metabolites were examined using Mann-Whitney tests to establish if there were significant variations from pre-match to post-match. Significant variations between the matches were similarly examined.

Results

Mean values for the plasma catecholamines, lactate, glucose and NEFA are presented in Table 1. Significant pre- to post-match differences were apparent for lactate concentrations for all matches and for glucose during the two legs of the final ($P < 0.05$). They represented an approximate increase of 30% and 56% respectively. In a recreational context there was no significant difference in lactate levels pre- or post-match between the three competitive players (4.5mM) and the three recreational players (4.9mM). No significant differences were apparent from pre- to post-match for plasma NEFA, although a 25% mean increase in concentration was observed.

Adrenaline levels were significantly higher prior to the first leg of the final than before the second ($P < 0.05$) into which the team carried a 7-1 goal lead. The values for the 2nd leg and the recreational match were not significantly different. This difference was not found in noradrenaline. Post-exercise values were 40% and 103% greater than pre-exercise concentrations for adrenaline and noradrenaline respectively.

The HR and estimated $\dot{V}O_2$ results are presented in Table 2. The values for the two legs of the final are for one subject only, whereas the recreation match values are for four subjects. The HR was sampled once every 3s, approximately. The $\dot{V}O_2$ data were calculated from individual HR-$\dot{V}O_2$ regression lines and were then expressed as a percentage of $\dot{V}O_2max$. A mean HR value of 172 beats min^{-1} was obtained irrespective of the match studied and this represented a $\dot{V}O_2$ of 3.95 l min^{-1}, corresponding to a work intensity of 82% $\dot{V}O_2max$. The mean energy expenditure of 79.4kJ min^{-1} was calculated from the mean estimated $\dot{V}O_2$ value.

Discussion

The range of post-match lactate values (range 3.1-7.3 mM) indicated that 4-a-side soccer appears to rely upon a significant contribution of its energy from glycogenolysis and glycolysis. Indeed such values are higher than those reported by Carli et al. (1986) for Italian semi-professional soccer players during an 11-a-side match but lower than those of by Ekblom (1986). Examination of the estimated energy expenditure data indicated that the 4-a-side soccer players were

Table 1. Mean values and ranges for the plasma concentrations of adrenaline, noradrenaline, lactate, glucose and NEFA

		Adrenaline (nM)	Noradrenaline (nM)	Lactate (mM)	Glucose (mM)	NEFA (mM)
Final (n=3)	Before	0.75(0.27-1.12)	2.44(1.64-3.40)	1.40(1.2-1.7)	5.50(4.77-6.60)	0.59(0.51-0.63)
(1st Leg)	After	1.16(0.33-1.74)	6.59(2.69-10.5)	[a]5.87(3.7-7.3)	[a]8.65(6.60-10.25)	0.77(0.63-0.98)
Final (n=3)	Before	0.37(0.16-0.60)	2.54(1.91-2.92)	1.40(1.2-1.6)	5.25(4.75-6.23)	0.59(0.45-0.81)
(2nd Leg)	After	0.41(0.24-0.63)	3.53(2.72-5.40)	[a]5.50(3.5-6.8)	[a]8.23(6.50-9.17)	0.76(0.5-1.03)
Recreational	Before	0.23(0.15-0.22)	2.15(1.55-2.70)	1.23(1.0-1.5)	5.03(5.0-5.10)	0.58(0.5-0.62)
(n=3)	After	0.28(0.18-0.35)	2.89(2.32-4.00)	[a]4.50(3.1-5.5)	7.67(5.15-9.10)	0.70(0.6-0.84)

[a]indicates $P < 0.05$

Table 2. Mean values for heart rate, estimated $\dot{V}O_2$ and % $\dot{V}O_2max$ during the three matches

	Heart Rate (beats min^{-1})		$\dot{V}O_2$(1 min^{-1})		%$\dot{V}O_2max$	
	1st Half	2nd Half	1st Half	2nd Half	1st Half	2nd Half
Final (1st Leg) (n=1)	174±10	171±11	4.0	3.87	84	81
Final (2nd Leg) (n=1)	172±8	172±8	3.9	3.9	82	82
Recreational (n=4)	171±17	172±20	3.95 (3.84-4.05)	3.99 (3.85-4.13)	80 (74-86)	81 (79-82)

working at an intensity of approximately 82% $\dot{V}O_2max$. This relatively high exercise intensity would support the contention that 'anaerobic' metabolism was high and thus resulted in significant elevation of lactate. Certainly the 4 mM threshold (V_{OBLA}) was exceeded in most cases.

Reference to research by Reilly and Ball (1984) would equate the mean post-recreation match lactate value of 4.5 mM and the mean post-final match values (5.87 and 5.50 mM for the two legs) to constantly dribbling the ball at 12.5 km h^{-1}, and greater than 14km h^{-1} respectively. However, it is appreciated that although the ball possession time is likely to be greater than during 11-a-side matches, there will be a significant proportion of time spent without the ball. This time spent without the ball is likely to involve significant periods of sprinting.

The observed elevated post-match plasma glucose concentrations may have arisen either as a consequence of haemoconcentration or enhanced liver glycogenolysis resulting from increased noradrenaline secretion. Since post-match noradrenaline levels were also elevated, the latter is a possibility. The small, but non-significant, rises in NEFA concentration were probably a result of haemoconcentration, since it is well established that lactic acid is an inhibitor of lipolysis.

The catecholamine response to the match conditions was most noticeable during the 1st leg of the final where an elevated pre-match adrenaline concentration (0.75 nM) was similar to that obtained prior to a "thrill" ride in a leisure park by Reilly et al. (1985), although the noradrenaline levels were higher in the present study. This reflects the anxiety placed on the players in anticipation of the matches, the level being greatest prior to the first competitive encounter. The post-match increases in catecholamine response were also greatest after the first match, representing a 55% and 170% increase in adrenaline and noradrenaline respectively; this implies that the stress and level of activity during this match was greater than in the other two matches. An increased level of activity would be reflected by an increase in post-match lactate values. Although the post-match concentrations of catecholamines and lactate were higher after the first match, they were not significantly different from the other two matches.

This similarity in exercise intensity was further reflected by the HR data, where mean values approximating 172 beats min^{-1} were found for all match conditions: qualitative differences in work-rate patterns betweeen the competitive and recreational matches might be discernible with motion analysis as employed by Reilly and Thomas (1976). The HR values observed were higher than those reported by Seliger (1968), Van Gool et al. (1983), and Reilly (1986). The latter two authors examined 11-a-side soccer, whilst the first named author used a 10 min match during which a 'Douglas bag' was carried by the players.

In conclusion, the metabolic demand required in playing 4-a-side soccer, particularly competitive matches, has an important implication for its use either as a training method for 11-a-side teams or as a recreational activity in its own right. The high aerobic and anaerobic requirements of the game (above that which is normally encountered during 11-a-side soccer) should mean that it would be effective as a general fitness training regimen.

References

Carli, G., Bonifazi, M., Lodi, L., Lupo, C., Martelli, G. and Viti, A. (1986) Hormonal and metabolic effects following a football match. Int. J. Sports Med., 7, 36-38.

Ekblom, B. (1986) Applied physiology of soccer. Sports Med., 3, 50-60.

Frayn, K. and Maycock, P. (1983) Sample preparation with ion-exchange resin before liquid-chromatographic determination of plasma catecholamines. Clin. Chim., 29, 1426-1428.

Reilly, T. (1986) The biological demands of elite soccer play. Proceedings of the XXIII FIMS World Congress of Sports Medicine (Brisbane).

Reilly, T. and Ball, D. (1984) The net physiological cost of dribbling a soccer ball. Res. Quart. Exerc. Sport, 55, 267-271.

Reilly, T. and Thomas, V. (1976) A motion analysis of work-rate in different positional roles in professional football match-play. J. Human Mov't. Stud., 2, 87-97.

Reilly, T., Lees, A., MacLaren, D. and Sanderson, F.H. (1985) Thrill and anxiety in adventure leisure parks. In: Contemporary Ergonomics: Proceedings of the Ergonomics Society's Annual Conference (edited by D.J. Oborne) pp210-214, London: Taylor and Francis.

Seliger, V. (1968) Energy metabolism in selected physical exercises, Int. Z. Angew, Physiol., 41, 231-240.

Van Gool, D., Van Gerven, D. and Boutmans, J. (1983) Heart rate telemetry during a soccer game: a new methodology. J. Sports Sci., 1, 154.

IS 'LACTIC ACID TOLERANCE' AN IMPORTANT COMPONENT OF FITNESS FOR SOCCER?

D. McA. Tumilty, A.G. Hahn, R.D. Telford and R.A. Smith
Australian Institute of Sport, P.O. Box 176, Belconnen, A.C.T., 2616, Australia.

Introduction

While significant involvement of the aerobic energy system in soccer is generally accepted, there are conflicting views on the relative importance of the two anaerobic energy systems, particularly on the extent of anaerobic glycolysis. Significant involvement of this energy pathway could indicate the need for training 'lactate tolerance'.

Previous studies have used two methods to assess involvement of the anaerobic energy systems-measurement of blood lactate levels in the game and observation of game activities. Cochrane and Pyke (1976), for example, found blood lactate levels of 1 - 2 mM in two players of the 1975 Australian national squad, samples being taken at half-time and full-time of a strenuous practice match. In contrast, Ekblom (1986) has frequently observed individual peak values above 12 mM during Swedish league games; he reported mean values for the team at half-time and full-time, ranging from 4 - 9.5 mM. Teams in the higher divisions showed the higher lactate levels.

In several studies, players have been observed during games and the time taken or the distance covered in performance of activities of different intensities were determined. Mayhew and Wenger (1985), observing North American Soccer league players, found that the ratio of time spent in high intensity:low intensity activities was 1:7. High intensity activity was defined as striding plus sprinting, and had a mean duration of 4.4 s. The authors concluded that the alactic system 'was probably the anaerobic system of primary importance'.

Withers et al. (1982) observed a number of players in the Australian Soccer League. From their data, the overall time ratio of high intensity:low intensity activities can be calculated at 1:14, with the mean duration of a high intensity activity being 3.7 s. They concluded that most of the energy for the high intensity work is probably supplied by the phosphagens.

Reilly and Thomas (1976) conducted extensive observations on the players from an English First Division team. Though results were reported only in terms of distances not times, and no inferences were drawn as to the source of anaerobic energy, the time ratio of high intensity activity can be estimated at 1:11. This lies between the values obtained by Mayhew (1:7) and Withers (1:14). The present study attempted to resolve the apparent contradiction between the results of these observational studies and Ekblom's (1986) measurements of blood lactate concentrations.

Method

The subjects (n=16) were junior soccer players (aged 16-19 years) of national standard. Selected physical and physiological characteristics are shown in Table 1. The figures are similar to those obtained on soccer groups tested elsewhere (Kirkendall, 1985).

Table 1. AIS junior soccer players - fitness measures

	Mean	S.D.
Skinfold sum (mm) (sum of 8 sites)	53.1	7.1
$\dot{V}O_2$ max (ml $kg^{-1}min^{-1}$)	58.9	3.4
Vertical jump (cm)	51.6	6.5
Sit and reach (cm)	+13.3	6.0
Knee extension (Nm) at 1.04 rad s^{-1}(Cybex)	233	34

Testing was conducted in two sessions on successive evenings. In the first session all players performed two repetitions of an agility test (Draper and Lancaster, 1985). After 5 min rest, they completed 6 sets, each of 3 maximal 20 m sprints. A 60 s rest was allowed between sets, while within sets the players sprinted every 20 s. Sprints were timed by a computerised electronic light gate system. After each set an ear-lobe arterial capillary blood sample was collected for determination of lactate concentration by an Analox LM3 analyser.

In addition, calf venous blood samples were drawn from half the players (n=8) immediately before and after the sprints. These were analysed for lactate by the Analox autoanalyser and for pH and bicarbonate by a Radiometer Acid-Base Analyser ABL-30.

The second session was centred around a full length game against a local team. Eight subjects (not the same 8 as on the previous night) had calf venous blood samples drawn immediately before warm-up and after the game for lactate, pH and bicarbonate determination.

Ten members of the team also performed 3 electronically timed maximal 20 m sprints within 15 min of the end of the game and (for eight players) after blood had been drawn.

Results

Tables 2 to 5 give the results of the two testing sessions. Statistical analysis was based on Student's t-test, for either correlated or independent samples as appropriate. The probability level for significance was set at 0.05.

Table 2. Calf venous blood sample: before (pre) and after (post) the sprints

n = 8	Lactate mM		pH		HCO_3 mM	
	pre	post	pre	post	pre	post
Mean	3.5	6.8[a]	7.257	7.183[a]	21.0	15.0
S.D.	0.8	1.6	0.024	0.060	1.0	2.9

a indicates significantly different ($P < 0.05$) from pre-game value

Due to technical difficulties, blood lactate readings were not obtained from all subjects after each set of sprints. Therefore the number of players for whom results are available varies from one sprint set to another, and the figures in Table 3 can be used only as an indication of the trend.

Table 3. Ear-lobe lactate after each sprint set

	Lactate level (mM)		
Time	Sample size	Mean	(± SD)
After set 1	9	5.0	± 1.4
" " 2	13	6.8	± 1.8
" " 3	12	7.8	± 2.1
" " 4	11	8.4	± 1.9
" " 5	8	8.9	± 1.5
" " 6	9	9.7	± 2.3

Table 4. Calf venous blood sample, pre-game and post-game

n = 8	Lactate mM		pH		HCO_3 mM	
	pre	post	pre	post	pre	post
Mean	1.0	2.4	7.281	7.335	22.1	21.8
S.D.	0.2	2.0	0.059	0.043	2.6	1.1

Mean (±SD) values for lactate, blood pH and HCO_3 before the game but after warm-up (pre) and after the game (post) are given in Table 4. None of the differences between pre- and post-game samples were significant.

Table 5. Comparisons (mean ±SD) of 20 m sprint times(s) : n = 10

	Fastest	Slowest
Session 1 (18 sprints)	3.036 ± 0.108	3.258[a] ± 0.116
Session 2 (3 post-game sprints)	Fastest 3.090[a] ± 0.129	

a means significantly different from the fastest time.

Discussion

The times, distances and intensities used in the sprint test are compared in Table 6 with values obtained from the observational studies on games. The proportion of distance spent sprinting all-out was much greater in the present study than would normally occur in a game. However, the time ratio of high intensity (sprinting plus fast running) to low intensity activities found in games (1:7, 1:11, 1:14) is quite similar to that used in the sprint test (1:9). The latter, lasting 10 min, may be regarded as reasonably representative of a vigorous portion of the game, especially as recovery intervals were of very low intensity.

Table 6. Times and distances at different intensities

Study	Comments	Distance(m) High intensity	Total	Time(s) High int.	Low int.	Ratio
Present	during test	378 (44%)	850*	56	502	1:9
	90 min game equivalent	3619	8226	542	4858	
Mayhew and Wenger	-	-	-	-	-	1:7
Reilly and Thomas	cruise	1810 (20.5%)	-	-		
	sprint	974 (11.2%)				1:35+(e)
	combined	2784 (31.7%)	8680			1:11+(e)
Withers et al.	striding	1506 (13.1%)				
	sprinting	666 (5.8%)				1:51(e)
	combined	2172 (18.8%)	11527			1:14
				(from mean times of high:low intensity work intervals)		

* Distance allows for recovery and returns to start
\+ Assumes speeds comparable to present study and that of Withers et al.
e indicates estimate.

The sprint test was structured to enable the rate of blood lactate accumulation to be determined. Table 3 indicates an early and progressive build up. A surprising finding was the pre-sprint mean venous lactate level of 3.5 mM (Table 2). The most likely explanation is that subjects had performed an agility test comprising 2 x 25 m sprints about 5 min before the initial blood sample was taken. The finding supports the claim by Jacobs et al. (1983) that anaerobic glycolysis begins a very short time after commencement of high intensity exercise. It also suggests that significant anaerobic glycolysis could be expected in a game.

Bicarbonate and pH were measured to gain a better idea of the demands placed on acid-base buffering mechanisms, since measurement of lactate alone is an uncertain indicator (Brooks, 1986). Pre- and post-sprint comparisons indicated that there was substantial hydrogen ion production and that buffering mechanisms had been considerably taxed (Table 2). The mean post-sprint ear-lobe lactates (9.7 mM; Table 3) were somewhat higher than the calf venous values (6.8 mM; Table 2). This may reflect the fact that ear-lobe and venous samples were not collected from precisely the same subjects, but could also be due to the flow of blood in the calf not being directly from the deep to the superficial veins (Williams and Warwick, 1980).

During the sprint test, there was a significant increase in the mean time taken to run 20 m (3.936 s to 3.258 s). The present findings indicate this may be due to intramuscular accumulation of hydrogen ions rather than to progressive phosphagen depletion as has been suggested (Dawson et al., 1984).

In contrast to the results of the first session, the game produced no signficant change in venous lactate, pH or bicarbonate. One possible reason is that the game was not of sufficiently high tempo to involve anaerobic glycolysis significantly. Ekblom (1986) did find that lactate levels were dependent on the standard of play, and the opponents of the AIS team in the game studied were of moderate ability.

Another possibility is that the players were able to effectively metabolise lactate and quickly correct temporary acid-base disturbances, enabling them to rapidly return to normal levels of lactate, pH and bicarbonate, even after intense efforts. However, at least two studies have indicated that after very high intensity efforts restoration of plasma bicarbonate concentration can take 30 min or more (Costill et al., 1984; Katz et al., 1984), though in these studies the exercise bouts were more severe than would be typical of a soccer game.

In conclusion the role of anaerobic glycolysis in soccer remains unclear, and hence there is also uncertainty concerning the need to develop a 'lactic tolerance' capacity. It cannot be assumed that anaerobic glycolysis has no role simply because sprints are usually brief. There is still a need to determine how fast and frequent soccer 'sprints' really are. The tempo of the game may be the crucial factor.

References

Brooks, G. (1986) The lactate shuttle during exercise and recovery. Med. Sci.Sports Exerc., 18, 360-368.

Cochrane, C. and Pyke, F. (1976) Physiological Assessment of the Australian Soccer Squad. Austr. J. Health, Phys. Ed. Recr., 73, 21-25.

Costill, D.L., Verstappen, F., Kuipers, H., Janssen, E. and Fink, W. (1984) Acid-base balance during repeated bouts of exercise: Influence of HCO_3 . Int. J. Sports Med., 5, 228-231.

Dawson, B., Ackland, T., Roberts, C. (1984) A new fitness test for team and individual sports. Sports Coach, 8, 12-44.

Draper, J.A. and Lancaster, M.G. (1985) The 505 Test: a test for agility in the horizontal plane. Austr. J. Sci. Med. Sport, 17, 15-18.

Ekblom, B. (1986) Applied physiology of soccer. Sports Med., 3, 50-60.

Jacobs, I., Tesch, P.A., Bar-Or, O., Karlsson, J. and Dotan, R. (1983) Lactate in human skeletal muscle after 10 and 30s of supramaximal exercise. J. Appl. Physiol. Respir., Environ. Exerc. Physiol., 55, 365-367.
Katz, A., Costill, D.L., King, D.S., Hargreaves, M. and Fink, W.J. (1984) Maximal exercise tolerance after induced alkalosis. Int. J. Sports Med., 5, 107-110.
Kirkendall, D.T. (1985) The applied sport science of soccer. Physician Sportsmed., 13, 53-59.
Mayhew, S.R. and Wenger, H.A. (1985) Time-motion analysis of professional soccer. J. Human Mov't. Stud., 11, 49-52.
Reilly, T. and Thomas, V. (1976) A motion analysis of work-rate in different positional roles in professional football match-play. J. Human Mov't. Stud., 2, 87-97.
Williams, P.L. and Warwick, R. (eds) (1980) Gray's Anatomy 36th Edit., pp. 757-759. Edinburgh: Churchill Livingstone.
Withers, R.T., Maricic, Z., Wasilewski, S. and Kelly, L. (1982) Match analyses of Australian professional soccer players. J. Human Mov't. Stud., 8, 159-176.

THE EFFECTS OF TRAINING AND MATCH-PLAY UPON MAXIMAL AEROBIC PERFORMANCE: A CASE STUDY

M.J. McKenna, E.R. Sandstrom and M.H.D. Chennells
Physiology Department, University of Melbourne, Parkville, Victoria, 3052, Australia.

Introduction

Professional football players follow heavy training and playing schedules. Australian Rules footballers may play up to two games and train five sessions, per week. Prior physical exercise, such as heavy endurance running on successive days, has been shown to be associated with an impairment of maximal aerobic work time and oxygen consumption (Costill et al., 1971). It was decided to investigate the effect of training for, and playing Australian Rules football, on the maximal aerobic, and hence, endurance performance of a single player. A case study design was chosen to overcome difficulties in obtaining professional footballers for serial tests during the season.

Methods

Repeated measures (n=20) of maximal oxygen uptake ($\dot{V}O_2$ max) were conducted on a single player, competing in the Victoria Football League. Physical characteristics of the player were:- age 23.0 years; height, 172.0 cm and weight, 74.0 (±0.7) kg. The $\dot{V}O_2$ max tests were conducted on a treadmill on consecutive days, with every attempt made to include full weekly testing. All tests were conducted prior to the training that day, at approximately 0830 hours, with the exception of the match day (Saturday) test which was conducted post-game at approximately 1800 hours. No tests were conducted on the morning of match days. During the course of the serial testing (some 4 months), the player participated in normal football training and competition.

Training was classified by i) duration, as short (up to 1.0 hour), moderate (1.0 to 1.5 hours), long (greater than 1.5 hours); and ii) intensity, as light - easy jogging, stretching, light ball games; moderate - the above as a warm-up, skill drills, some tackling exercises, interval runs (3/4 to full pace over 60-400m); and high - the above warm-up, skill and tackling drills, competitive drills including match practice, intervals of short (20-60m) sprints. The player's typical training and match schedule is shown in Table 1.

Table 1. Typical training and match schedule

Day:	Thursday	Friday	Saturday	Sunday	Monday	Tuesday	Wednesday
Duration:	Short	Rest	Competition	Short	Moderate	Long	Rest
Intensity:	High		Match	Light	Moderate	High	
Time(h):	1700		1400	0900	1700	1700	

Ventilatory gas analysis was conducted using a Jaeger Ergopneumotest (Jaeger, West Germany) with a Hewlett Packard 9815a programmable calculator. The gas analysers and the pneumotachograph were calibrated prior to each test. A fast incremental protocol was used for the $\dot{V}O_2$ max test, with speed, then gradient increased every 30s, until the subject was unable to maintain the running speed at the highest gradient reached. The highest $\dot{V}O_2$ attained was defined as the $\dot{V}O_2$ max.

For the purposes of statistical analysis the data from Saturday (n=2) and Sunday (n=1), were combined. The mean daily variation in $\dot{V}O_2$ max and other variables was then calculated using the following groups: Friday (n=5), Thursday, Saturday plus Sunday, Monday, Tuesday and Wednesday (all n=3).

Data were grouped according to the previous day's activity level, as well as the proximity of the test to the game. Data collected from tests conducted up to 24 hours after high intensity, long duration exercise (Saturday, Sunday and Wednesday), were combined and defined as 'heavy exercise'. The two tests conducted prior to the game (Thursday and Friday) were combined and defined as 'pre-game'. Tests conducted several days after the game and following low - moderate intensity and duration training on the previous day (Monday and Tuesday), were combined and defined as 'moderate exercise'.

The Kruskal-Wallis one-way analysis of variance by ranks test was applied to the data. If the variation was found to be significant at alpha 0.05, the Mann Whitney U test was applied to test for significance between particular groups.

Results

A significant variation of the daily $\dot{V}O_2$ max was seen (Figure 1, $P < 0.05$). The $\dot{V}O_2$ max values for each of Thursday, Friday, Monday and Tuesday were greater than the Saturday plus Sunday values (all $P < 0.05$).The $\dot{V}O_2$ max values for both Thursday and Tuesday were also greater than the Wednesday $\dot{V}O_2$ max value (all $P < 0.05$). No significant variation was seen in the daily maximal values of $\dot{V}E$, $\dot{V}CO_2$ or respiratory exchange ratio (R) (Table 2). From the $\dot{V}O_2$ max test, the only other peak measure to vary signficantly was 'work time' (WT), ($P < 0.05$, Figure 1). The WT for each of the Thursday, Friday and Tuesday tests was greater than the Saturday plus Sunday values, with the Thursday value also greater than that on Monday and Wednesday (all $P < 0.05$).

For the grouped data (Figure 2), significant variations were seen in each of $\dot{V}O_2$ max, WT and $\dot{V}CO_2$ (all $P < 0.01$). The pre-game $\dot{V}O_2$, $\dot{V}CO_2$ and WT were all greater than their respective post-heavy values (all $P < 0.005$). The post-moderate exercise $\dot{V}CO_2$, WT, (both

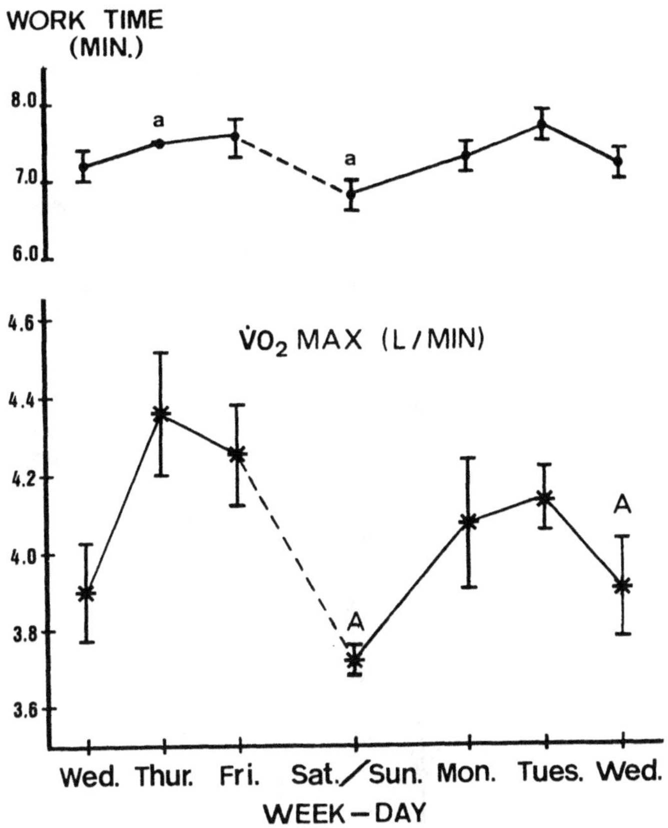

Figure 1. Variation of the mean daily maximal values of $\dot{V}O_2$ ($1\ min^{-1}$) and work time (min)

a Thur.,Fri.,Tues.> Sat./Sun. $P < 0.05$
Thur. > Mon., Wed. $P < 0.05$

A Thur.,Fri.,Mon.,Tues. > Sat./Sun. $P < 0.05$
Thur.,Tues. > Wed $P < 0.05$

Table 2. Mean (±SD) daily maximal values of $\dot{V}E$, $\dot{V}CO_2$ and R

Day:	Wednesday	Thursday	Friday	Saturday+Sunday	Monday	Tuesday
$\dot{V}E$ ($1\ min^{-1}$)	150.5	156.5	155.3	134.9	153.2	154.9
	±4.1	±3.2	±8.0	±6.0	±9.0	±8.0
$\dot{V}CO_2$ ($1\ min^{-1}$)	4.62	5.05	5.03	4.01	4.83	4.90
	±0.27	±0.22	±0.22	±0.28	±0.32	±0.22
R	1.20	1.16	1.21	1.08	1.19	1.19
	±0.04	±0.02	±0.05	±0.06	±0.05	±0.03

P < 0.05) and $\dot{V}O_2$ (P < 0.01) were greater than their respective post-heavy exercise values.

Body weight and maximal heart rate did not vary significantly, for either daily or grouped data.

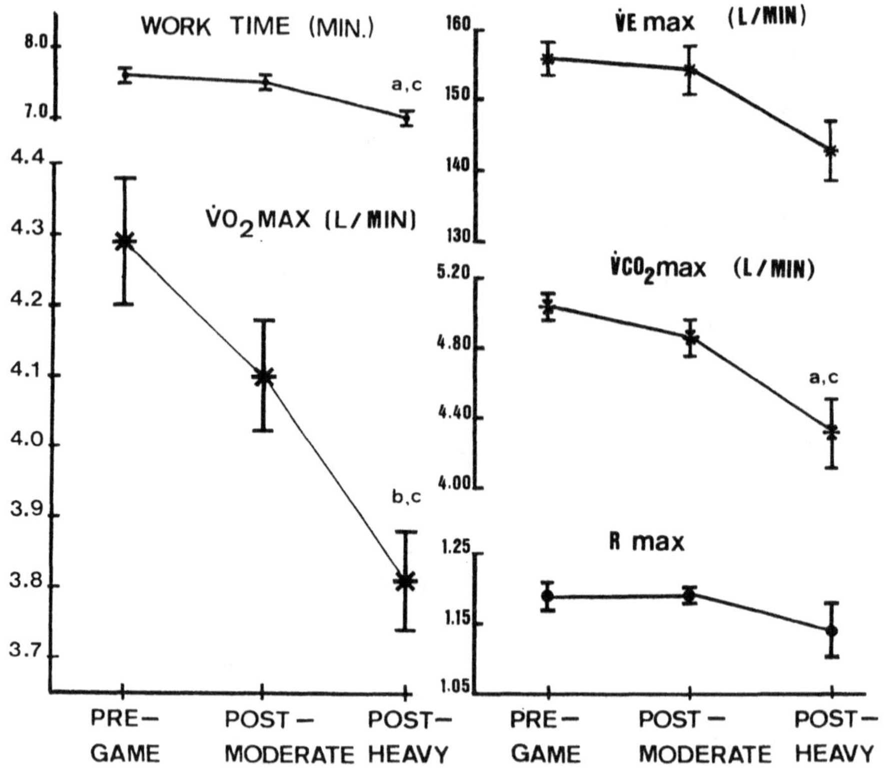

Figure 2. Variation of the mean grouped maximal values of $\dot{V}O_2$ (l min^{-1}), work time (min), $\dot{V}_E$ (l min^{-1}), $\dot{V}CO_2$ (l min^{-1}) and R

a	Post-Moderate	Post-Heavy	P < 0.05
b	Post-Moderate	Post-Heavy	P < 0.01
c	Pre-Game	Post-Heavy	P < 0.005

Discussion

The $\dot{V}O_2$ max of the player was found to be significantly reduced following both training and playing Australian Rules football. This reduction in endurance performance may limit the player's physical performance in subsequent training sessions, or more importantly, in a game.

Despite the similar coefficient of variation for $\dot{V}O_2$ max to that previously reported (Katch et al., 1982), the variation seen is not accounted for by a simple biological variation, but clearly reflects an exercise-related fluctuation in maximal work performance. This is shown by the strong association between the $\dot{V}O_2$ max and the player's activity level, on the previous day, as well as for the grouped data (Figures 1 and 2).

The reduction in $\dot{V}O_2$ max and WT after both training and playing Australian Rules football is consistent with reductions reported following prolonged exercise (Costill et al., 1971; Linnarsson and Eklund, 1982). The reduction observed in endurance performance in the current study, may be related to muscle glycogen depletion. Studies reporting a marked depletion in muscle glycogen have also found a reduction in maximal working capacity, expressed either through a decreased $\dot{V}O_2$ max (Costill et al., 1971) and/or through a decreased peak work load, or working time (Heigenhauser et al., 1983). Similarly, significant reductions have also been found in maximal $\dot{V}E$ and R (Linnarsson and Eklund, 1982; Heigenhauser et al., 1983), and $\dot{V}CO_2$ (Heigenhauser et al., 1983). The absence of a reduction in peak heart rate in the current study, despite the large decrease in work time, is consistent with previous studies (Costill et al., 1971; Heigenhauser et al., 1983). This suggests that the limitation to maximal aerobic performance seen in this study was due to peripheral, rather than central factors.

Several studies have reported the importance of muscle glycogen stores in soccer (Saltin, 1973; Currie et al., 1981; Jacobs et al., 1982). Consequently, a high carbohydrate diet is recommended for soccer players, to ensure optimal repletion of glycogen lost during the game (Jacobs et al., 1982). Maximal aerobic performance was markedly reduced following training and a game for Australian Rules football players. It is then likely that the player's physical performance during training and a game would be impaired. If it can be assumed that the reduced $\dot{V}O_2$ max was due to muscle glycogen depletion, a high carbohydrate intake may prevent fatigue from a match or training from adversely effecting subsequent performance.

References

Costill, D.L., Sparks, K., Gregor, R. and Turner, C., (1971) Muscle glycogen utilization during exhaustive running. J. Appl. Physiol., 31, 353-356.

Currie, D., Bonen, A., Belcastro, A.N., Kirby, R.L., Sopper, M. and Richards, A.R. (1981) Glycogen utilization and circulatory substrate responses during match play soccer and soccer training sessions (Abstract). Int. J. Sports Med., 2, 271.

Heigenhauser, G.J.F., Sutton, J.R. and Jones, N.L. (1983) Effect of glycogen depletion on the ventilatory response to exercise. J. Appl. Physiol. Respirat. Environ. Exerc. Physiol., 54, 470-474.

Jacobs, I., Westlin, N., Karlsson, J., Rasumusson, M. and Houghton, B. (1982) Muscle glycogen and diet in elite soccer players. Eur. J. Appl. Physiol., 48, 297-302.

Katch, V.L., Sady, S.S. and Freedson, P. (1982) Biological variability in maximal aerobic power. Med. Sci. Sports Exerc., 14, 21-25.

Linnarsson, D. and Eklund, B. (1982) Effect of long term skiing on maximal and submaximal exercise performance. In: Exercise and.Sport Biology (edited by P.V. Komi) pp. 185-190. Champaign, Illinois: Human Kinetics Publishers.
Saltin, B. (1973) Metabolic fundamentals in exercise. Med. Sci. Sports, 5, 137-146.

Part IV

Physiology of football training

SUCCESSFUL FORMULAE FOR FITNESS TRAINING

Peter Apor
Hungarian University of Physical Education, Alkotas, u.44, Budapest, and Children's Health Institute at Szabadsaghegy, Martonhegyi u.6., Budapest, Hungary.

Introduction

Soccer is among the most popular sports in the world, with well managed World Championships and international competitions and with great financial interest in many rich and developing countries. To play soccer does not need extreme stature or very rare physiological abilities. Playing it brings joy. One disadvantage is that subjects over 40-50 years of age are not recommended to play soccer competitively because of the risk of injuries and cardiovascular events.

Review of the Physiology of Soccer

Motion analysis of the game

Excellent studies have reported on the locomotion of players during games (Reilly and Thomas, 1976; Nettleton and Briggs, 1980; Withers et al., 1982; Ekblom, 1986). The reported distance covered by a player was 1.6 - 5.5 km or 5-10 km in a game (Wade, 1962; Zelenka et al., 1967) in the 1960's, while in the 70's and 80's the distance per game apparently rose to 9-11 km. To what extent this difference was due to methodologies is impossible to ascertain. About 8-18 per cent of the total distance covered is done at a high running speed. The high intensity of the whole game represents around 80% of the aerobic capacity. Blood lactic acid level rises to 7-8 mM but higher peaks are likely in spite of the experience that the 10-25 m maximal runs recur interspersed with 30-90s slow runs or walks.

The metabolic load

The oxygen demand increases above the level evoked by a simple run if any technical task involves participation of additional muscle groups, increases in intrapulmonary pressure and so on. Dribbling was found to increase the energy consumption by 5.2 kJ min^{-1} (1.24 $kcal.min^{-1}$) in the running speed range of 9-13.5 km h^{-1} (Reilly and Ball, 1984) and the perceived exertion (Borg scale) reflected higher stress when the ball has to be dribbled. Higher stride frequency and extra movements for kicking the ball explain the higher energy consumption. Aerobic efficiency during dribbling could characterise playing technique: technical superiority may be reflected in a smaller energy demand when running and dribbling with the ball.

Running sideways or backwards also increases the oxygen demand of locomotion compared to the 'normal' run (Reilly and Bowen, 1984).

Glycogen depletion in games can be as high as 84% of the total pool (Agnevik, 1970, cited by Kirkendall, 1985). Two games a week involves the possibility of an incomplete restoration of the muscle glycogen level from game to game (Jacobs et al., 1982).

Anthropometry and physiological capacities of players

Somatotype of top Hungarian soccer players is characterised by the 2.1: 5.1: 2.3 according to Heath-Carter parameters, which means that they belong to the balanced mesomorph category with only a few exceptions (Farmosi, 1986). The endomorphy of the players was found to be close to the value for sprinters, while in ectomorphy they resembled field hockey players (Toriola et al., 1985).

No special stature or somatic disposition is a pre-requisite for playing well in soccer (Kirkendall, 1985). Nevertheless specific statures may be exploited for tactical purposes, tall players for receiving free kicks or corners close to the opponent's goal.

Leg force of the players exceeds the 'average'. Knee extension torque was related to success in the game, according to Oberg et al. (1986). Like sprinters in track and field athletics, their knee flexion torque is relatively better developed than normal: the ratio between the knee flexor and extensor torque was 48, 61 and 75% at isometric, 0.52 rad s^{-1} (30° s^{-1}), and 3.14 rad s^{-1} (180° s^{-1}) angular velocity, while values of the controls were 42, 56 and 61%, respectively. Strength of the flexors seems to be crucial in the pathology of injuries (Burkett, 1970; Campbell and Glenn, 1982).

Height of the vertical jump (49-56 cm, Kirkendall, 1985) is similar to most other ball game players but it is inferior to that observed in volleyball players. Jumping performance throughout a minute was similar in the top and in the collegiate soccers teams.

Alactacid power of soccer players as determined by the Margaria test was high (169-181 kgm s^{-1}) in a study reported by Fox and Mathews (1979). These figures compare with 172 ($\pm$26) kgm s^{-1} reported by Maud and Shultz (1986) for 109 males regularly participating in vigorous physical activity.

Flexibility (maximal ankle excursion) of soccer players is usually worse than in the control subjects (Ekstrand, 1982; Oberg et al., 1984). This may be a consequence of the lack of proper stretching regimens.

Aerobic capacity is typically 15-20% better than the control values. Figures reported include 56-62 ml kg^{-1} min^{-1} (Raven et al., 1976), 58 in team (Jacobs et al., 1982), 61.2 (Hoette et al., 1986), 60-65 in the top American, Swedish and German teams (Ekblom, 1986). Caru et al. (1970) registered only 42-50 ml kg^{-1} min^{-1} in 14-18 year old players.

During a 9 week training period the aerobic capacity of boys 12 years of age was not changed from the 50 ml kg^{-1} min^{-1} value, nor was the knee extension force improved. Nevertheless, the oxygen consumption of a sub-maximal run was decreased (Berg et al., 1985). In another study the aerobic endurance characterised by the 12 min run-walk was surprisingly high as early as the 10-12 years age-group: about 2500 m was performed in the test time (Rigler and Orosz, 1986).

Hungarian Studies

From the early seventies a series of 'diagnostic' tests were performed with the participation of various Hungarian soccer teams. These cover aerobic capacity, lactacid capacity, anaerobic power and force, and muscle characteristics. Observations have been made on growing as well as adult players and some longitudinal studies have been performed.

Aerobic capacity measures
Maximal oxygen uptake of the best teams was always above 60 ml kg^{-1} min^{-1} while teams in the lower positions in the first League usually had lower values (Table 1). The rank-order of the aerobic capacity has been reflected in the actual position of the teams in the first division championship (Ekes et al., 1974):

Table 1. The relation between mean $\dot{V}O_2max$ and finishing position in the league in the top Hungarian clubs

	Relative aerobic capacity $\dot{V}O_2max$ (ml kg^{-1} min^{-1})	Position in the championship
Ujpesti Dózsa	66.6	1st
FTC	64.3	2nd
Vasas SC	63.3	3rd
Honvéd SE	58.1	5th

The aerobic capacity of soccer players has been measured in cross-sectional studies in 1973-73, in 1977 and in 1984. Data are presented in the Tables, 2, 3, 4 and 5. The members of the junior National Team have their aerobic power above 70 ml kg^{-1} min^{-1}, while players of the regional championship (Testnev. Foisk.) reached only a moderate value below 60 ml kg^{-1} min^{-1}.

A representative study on the players of one of the best clubs (FTC) revealed that the average $\dot{V}O_2max$(ml kg^{-1} min^{-1}) had not increased between 11-12 and 17 years of age, while the 12 min test performance approximated the 3000 m (Table 3) reported by Orosz (1979). A few years later the youth team (15-16 years of age) of the same club showed an average $\dot{V}O_2max$ of 66 ml kg^{-1} min^{-1} (Table 5).

We cannot expect that this difference reflects the aerobic ability of Hungarian soccer but it seems reasonable that by 18 years of age the players usually have a rather considerable - above 60 ml kg^{-1} min^{-1}-level of aerobic power. Some of the experiences point to the possibility that the older players and/or teams have the poorer performances and during the competitive season the aerobic capacity decreases due to improper maintenance of training.

Lactacid capacity
Lactacid test scores (Apor et al., 1972) of various sports groups are listed in Table 5. The highest run time (70-76 s) was measured in international level 400-1500 m track and field athletes. Soccer players are closer to the non-specifically trained control group

Table 2. Anthropometric and physiological parameters (mean ± SD) of 1st division soccer players in Hungary. The exercise for obtaining maximal responses was done on a treadmill

TEAMS	n	Age (years)	Weight (kg)	Height (cm)
Ujp.D.	10	22.9 ± 3.0	70.5 ± 4.0	176.5 ± 5.4
Honved	14	21.6 ± 6.4	73.5 ± 6.3	177.6 ± 4.3
SBTC	12	24.5 ± 3.0	73.1 ± 4.3	178.8 ± 4.8
Csep.I	18	26.0 ± 3.6	74.1 ± 5.2	178.2 ± 5.4
Csep.II	10	23.8 ± 2.9	75.1 ± 2.9	178.1 ± 3.6
Csep.Jun		18.0 ± 0.7	66.4 ± 6.8	175.1 ± 5.3

	$\dot{V}O_2max$ (ml min^{-1})	$\dot{V}O_2max$ (ml kg^{-1})	O_2pulse (ml beat^{-1})	$\dot{V}Emax$ (l min^{-1})
Ujp.D.	4545 ± 413	66.6 ± 3.8	24.5 ± 2.6	141.2 ± 7.0
Honved	4795 ± 754	65.4 ± 9.3	25.2 ± 4.7	125.2 ± 17.8
SBTC	4500 ± 300	62.4 ± 4.4	24.7 ± 1.8	130.1 ± 11.7
Csep.I	4249 ± 382	57.1 ± 7.4	24.2 ± 3.6	130.0 ± 17.2
Csep.II	4498 ± 414	59.9 ± 3.9	23.2 ± 2.9	145.7 ± 12.4
Csep.Jun	4035 ± 448	61.1 ± 8.4	21.0 ± 2.6	142.7 ± 17.7

	Vital capacity, ml (BTPS)	FEV_1/VC(%)
Ujp.D.	5790 ± 419	89.5 ± 7.5
Honv.	5900 ± 372	90.4 ± 7.2
SBTC	5360 ± 530	89.8 ± 10.0
Csep.I.	5430 ± 699	89.7 ± 8.6
Csep.Jun.	5140 ± 644	91.8 ± 7.6

Table 3. Physiological parameters of youth soccer teams (mean ± SD)

Team	n	Age	Body weight	$\dot{V}E$ max(ℓ min^{-1}) ml $kg^{-1}min^{-1}$)	$\dot{V}O_2max$	O_2pulse (ml beat)	WC_{170}/kg
National team	8	17.4 ± 0.31	68.6 ± 8.7	149.3 ± 17.4	73.9 ± 10.8	24.5 ± 2.43	4.218
FTC junior	10	18.2 ± 0.83	68.7 ± 6.7	142.0 ± 23.4	63.6 ± 8.0	23.4 ± 4.03	3.129
FTC youth	13	16.0 ± 0.21	67.8 ± 5.5	146.8 ± 21.2	63.2 ± 8.1	20.6 ± 5.10	
Csepel,jun.	13	18.0 ± 0.74	66.5 ± 6.9	142.7 ± 17.8	61.2 ± 8.5	21.0 ± 2.60	
Vasas,jun.	6	17.2 ± 0.98	70.8 ± 6.0	118.8 ± 22.9	55.0 ± 6.4	22.0 ± 5.82	3.107
Testnev.Foiskola	41	15.2 ± 1.64	57.5 ± 9.7	120.6 ± 25.0	56.2 ± 4.2	16.3 ± 3.03	2.617

Table 4. Cross sectional study of the soccer players of the top club, Hungary

Age, years	12 min test (m) mean	n	$\dot{V}O_2max$ (ml kg^{-1} min^{-1}) mean	n	Oxygen pulse/kg (ml $beat^{-1}$) mean	PWC_{170}/kg mean
11-12	2585 ± 18	127	56.0 ± 1.97	16	29 ± 0.01	3.16 ± 0.12
13	2595 ± 21	113	57.8 ± 2.3	15	30 ± 0.01	1.80 ± 0.12
14	2793 ± 17	156	51.4 ± 1.8	21	24 ± 0.02	- -
15	2800 ± 24	78	56.0 ± 1.2	31	26 ± 0.01	2.41 ± 0.20
16	2938 ± 15	140	58.6 ± 1.2	37	29 ± 0.01	2.70 ± 0.10
17	3021 ± 18	141	56.9 ± 1.3	33	28 ± 0.01	2.49 ± 0.10
18	2924 ± 52	12				

Table 5. Youth (15-16 years) champion soccer team, n = 17

	mean	SE
$\frac{\dot{V}O_2 (ml)}{W\ kg^{-1}}$ at 100 W	0.2805	0.0129
$\dot{V}O_2$(ml) at 12 km h^{-1}	245.6	6.5
$\dot{V}E$ max (l min^{-1})	125.9	4.60
$\dot{V}O_2max$ (ml kg^{-1} min^{-1})	66.5	2.27
Vastus lateralis		
Slow twitch fibres (%)	48.6	3.3
ST area μm^2	4007	419
FT area μm^2	4300	483
ATPase iμ.g^{-1} w.w.	9.61	0.894
Citrate synthetase iμ.g^{-1}w.w.	7.43	0.804
Aldolase iμ g^{-1} w.w.	33.08	1.413
Gastrocnemius		
Slow twitch fibres (%)	55.8	4.44
ST area (μm^2	2848	295
FT area ($\mu\ m^2$)	3770	415
ATPase (iμ g^{-1} w.w.)	9.55	0.62
Citrate synthetase (iμ g^{-1} w.w.)	11.56	1.478
Aldolase (iμ g^{-1} w.w.)	31.09	3.278
Vertical jumps without and with added weights		
Max. Voluntary		
Knee Extension, N:	241	87
Max. power (W)	1499	70
Max. power per kg	24.77	0.73
Force at Pmax per kg	10.92	0.746
a/F_o	0.3214	0.0816

Table 6. Lactacid (LA) test parameters (15 km h^{-1}, 20% slope, until exhaustion): values are mean ± SD

GROUP	N	LA run time (s)	LA max. power kgm s^{-1}	LA total power (kgm)
Modern	10	49.3 ± 9.9	56.5 ± 3.6	2960 ± 882
Pentathlon	11	40.5 ± 8.3	55.9 ± 3.6	2232 ± 358
Distance runners	13	49.5 ±12.2	52.1 ± 4.4	2523 ± 617
Soldiers, 21 years of age	22	25.4 ± 7.6	56.6 ± 7.2	1491 ± 427
Rowers,female	10	27.3 ± 6.3	27.0 ± 7.4	1280 ± 363
Soccer team, champion	14	36.0 ± 5.1	53.5 ± 5.8	2115 ± 203
Soccer team, second	14	31.1 ± 7.2	58.2 ± 6.2	1801 ± 429

(soldiers). Even after the 12 min run the blood acidosis was not too high (Tables 7 and 8). An improvement in the 12 min run score after two weeks 'grounding' training can be explained by improved motivation, marked with the higher acidosis (Table 7).

Table 7. 12 min runs, two weeks apart (53 1st League soccer players) : values are mean ± SD

	Jan. 8	Jan. 22
Distance	2952 ± 174	3121 ± 139
Art. cap. blood pH.	7.245 ± 0.0726	7.207 ± 0.059
Base excess	-10.66 ± 4.76	-12.07 ± 3.22

Low pH values were measured after the repetition (10 × 30 m) run but not during a 'special soccer test' which consisted of a slalom run with the ball (dribbling), passing and kicking. Thus it involved mainly technical tasks of moderate running speeds (Table 8).

In the 20 × 30 m run (Table 9) running speed was only 5-15 percent slower than that of the best 10 x 30 m. The 5 times 20 x 30 m run evoked a high, near maximum heart rate but the effect on blood acidosis was rather small. No sign of apparent fatigue was seen in the run scores or in the physiological measures during this test.

In recent years 15 × 30 m run test has been preferred with 10 s pauses between the runs (Orosz et al., 1983). Mean score of a First division team was 4.90 s at the end of the summer season and it was

Table 8. Blood pH in different tasks : values are mean (± SD)

TEAM	10 x 30 metres pH	Mean time(s)	n	'Special soccer test' pH	n	12 min run (m) pH		n
Csepel	7.05 ± 0.06	4.48	10	7.23 ± 0.04	19	7.15 ± 0.04	3316	16
Egyetert.	7.07 ± 0.05	4.55	6	7.22 ± 0.04	6	7.18 ± 0.02	3094	6
MTK	7.08 ± 0.05	4.48	20	7.16 ± 0.04	19	7.13 ±30.05	3230	18
Honved	7.10 ± 0.04	4.39	6	7.23 ± 0.02	18			
Ujpest	7.13 ± 0.06	4.41	6	7.23 ± 0.05	6	7.15 ± 0.06	3118	6
Vasas	7.19 ± 0.06	4.37	8	7.22 ± 0.07	10	7.16 ± 0.06	3194	6
Spart.	7.22 ± 0.03	4.71	6					
FTC	7.26 ± 0.08	4.43	6					

Table 9. 5 times 20 x 30 m run, soccer players.
(Start at each 20th s, 5 min pause among the 5 series)

Subjects	First	Second	Third	Fourth	Fifth	10 x 30 m separately
	time(s)		20 x 30 run			
Eg.	4.68	4.86	4.51	4.90	4.46	4.20
Ko.	4.79	4.70	4.46	4.76	4.37	4.17
We.	4.68	4.73	4.53	4.57	4.49	4.22
He.	4.60	4.49	4.63	4.74	4.61	4.27
	HR max					
Eg.	170	174	188	169	176	183
Ko.	180	178	182	178	182	182
We.	182	185	182	181	190	188
He.	159	188	185	176	187	186
	HR 5 min rest					
Eg.	670	-	650	-	640	660
Ko		700		680	620	650
We.	680		660		580	630
He.		590		610	630	610
	blood pH					
Eg.	7.27		7.30		7.27	7.12
Ko.		7.41		7.40	7.39	7.09
We.	7.36		7.38		7.39	7.15
He.		7.30		7.36	7.38	7.18

HR max: heart rate calculated from the first 6 s after the run
HR 5 min rest: sum of the heart rates measured at the beginning of the minutes of the recovery
Blood pH from the arterialised capillary blood, taken in the 3rd min of recovery

4.59 s after the 'grounding' training period. Decrease of the running speed during the 15 repetitions is not influenced by the age or by the trained state. These factors change only the intercept: all the 'fatigue lines' run parallel.

Alactacid anaerobic power

The anaerobic power (Margaria test, Table 10) of the soccer players was in the same range as of the other ball game players. Values are about 15-30% higher than that of the control group or of the long-distance runners. No seasonal or long-term follow up is available from our laboratory.

Table 10. Anaerobic alactacid power and vertical velocity (Margaria-test)

Group	kgm s^{-1}	m s^{-1}
Soccer team, 1st League	125 ± 11	1.51 ± 0.09
Soccer team, 3rd League	116 ± 7	1.68 ± 0.09
Handball team, 1st League	129 ± 10	1.67 ± 0.07
Soldiers, 21 years of age	102 ± 15	1.42 ± 0.14
Long distance runners	100 ± 11	1.48 ± 0.15
Ski runners	105 ± 10	1.48 ± 0.11
Girl students, 20 years of age	64 ± 11	1.15 ± 0.10

Force and muscle biopsy parameters of young soccer players

The best age-group team was tested in 1984 in our laboratory Players (age 15.8 ± 0.31 years) had 4-7 years training experience in soccer, few of them in track and field. They trained 3-4 times a week and played at least one game per week.

A steady state 100 bicycle exercise preceded the maximal treadmill run (Jaeger treadmill and Pneumotest). The players also performed several double-legged vertical jumps on a force platform (Tihanyi et al., 1983; Bosco et al., 1983) without and with 10, 20, 30 kg excess weight and bar on their shoulder. Force-velocity power curves were calculated from the mass and flight time values. A needle biopsy sample was taken from the gastrocnemius lateralis and vastus lateralis muscles for histochemical fibre typing (Fekete and Apor, 1981) and for enzyme activity analysis of the homogenate (ATPase, citrate dehydrogenase and aldolase, Boros-Hatfaludy et al., 1986). The volume of the lower leg and thigh was measured by the water-displacement method. Results are summarised in Table 5 referred to earlier.

In 1977 the team in the same position (16.6 ± 0.8 years of age) had a maximal ventilation of 133.6 (±22.07) l min^{-1}, a relative aerobic capacity of 61.0 (± 7.9) ml kg^{-1} min^{-1} and an oxygen pulse of 30.6 (± 3.7) ml $beat^{-1}$ kg^{-1}. It seems that the team of 1984 was marginally superior in aerobic power to its counterpart of seven years before.

The muscle composition of these young players was about average.

No or only modest fibre hypertrophy was observed. Enzyme activity values were inferior to those of the adult top sportsmen in Hungary (Quang, 1986), as were the force and power of the lower extremity in the jump tests.

Among the significant correlations it is worth mentioning the highly significant correlation between leg force and power, as well as between the aerobic capacity and the leg force and power, as well as between the aerobic capacity and the leg force. This may be partly accounted for by an effect of body weight. The larger the slow and fast fibres of the gastrocnemius muscle, the higher were the power and the force at the maximal power output. Highly significant correlations also existed between the leg volume and the fibre area data. One can say that a larger fibre area in the gastrocnemius coincides with a larger lower-extremity volume and with higher knee extension force and maximal power, in vertical jumps. Fibre parameters of the vastus lateralis failed to show similar significant correlations.

The area of the slow fibres in a muscle correlates well with the area of the fast fibres. The correlations between the fibre-type percentage and the area-values of the two muscles were lower but still significant.

Enzyme activities of the homogenate showed the 'expected' positive and negative connections with the fibre type percentage and with some force-power indices. There were negative correlations between the citrate synthase activity and FT area and between the aldolase activity and the per cent slow fibres. A positive correlation was found between ATPase activity and the maximal power.

In our case the less favourable aerobic efficiency (high oxygen uptake during the 100 W bicyling) coincided with smaller leg volume, with smaller fibre area, smaller leg power and force.

These data suggest that the 16 year old Hungarian soccer players have a medium aerobic capacity, while their muscle characteristics and muscle performance are not developed appreciably. The physiological test performances stand still around this age (Table 3) this is explained by a lack of proper training. Probably only the very devoted, 'talented' players develop further in being selected for the good adult teams.

Orosz and his co-workers (1983) followed the players who had been tested in 1976, six years before. They tried to establish which test could best forecast the 'talented' individuals. Fifteen tests were performed on the players in 1976 (part of which was performed on the treadmill, see Table 2):-

i) 15 × 30 m dash, with 10 s pauses between them
ii) 12 min run
iii) 30 m slalom run
iv) 30 m slalom run with ball
v) 30 m run
vi-x) Body dimensions, Lean body mass, Lower leg girth
xi) Size of the visual field
xii) Peripheral colour recognition
xiii) Visual critical fusion frequency
xiv) Simple reaction time
xv) Disjunctive peripheral reaction time (green-red)

Those who gave up playing soccer (79 subjects) were slow in the 15 times 30 m and in the slalom run with the ball. Players who were good in the repeated speed test and in technical skill were also excellent in the critical fusion frequency and in the speed of the peripheral colour recognition task. The size of the visual field was also larger in the 28 players who found their ways to the First division than in the 54, 'medium quality' players.

The score of the 12 min run did not separate the 3 groups. Neither was anthropometry informative from this point of view.

Conclusions

Soccer players' profiles have an aerobic power, muscle fibre and enzyme activity characteristics - particularly the key aerobic and key anaerobic enzymes - that suggest a moderately trained status. They have to be good at repeated short runs (high 'repetitive speed endurance'), they obviously have to be skilled with the ball. These abilities coincide with large visual field and quick response for movements in the peripheral (colour) visual field.

They do not need exceptional lactacid capacity, but they have to have a high alactacid power. Repeated involvement of high anaerobic power in very quick motions, combined with large visual field and quick-witted perception of the game situation is the measurable basis of good results (Apor and Pavlik, 1986).

To meet these requirements players should train their aerobic power to 3200-3000 m 12 min run score (above 65 ml kg^{-1} min^{-1} $\dot{V}O_2max$); they have to develop a musculature similar to sprinters in explosive power. Short but frequently repeated sprints are needed, interspersed with stretching and technical exercises because quick recovery is required in the short pauses between the maximal loads without lactic acid accumulation. The so-called 'mini-interval' exercise regimen is suggested for soccer players: 4-6 s maximal speed runs with maximally explosive starts and 20-30 s pauses (with stretching or ball exercises or jogging in this interval) seem to be a good 'sports specific' training practice.

Muscles, ligaments and ankles require very careful strength and soft tissue maintenance during the season (stretching, massage, baths, electrotherapy and so on) and proper healing of the lesions. Special dietary regimens are needed for the proper restoration of muscle glycogen after training and competition. Care must be taken in maintaining the basic physiological performance capacity, with regard to aerobic power, muscle power and muscle elasticity during the whole season.

References

Apor, P. and Pavlik, G. (1986) (Fitness of ball game players, their stress in training and games) In: Istvanfi, pp.58-82.

Apor, P., Szabo-Wahlstab, S., Miklos, M. (1972) Zusammen-hange zwischen einigen aeroben und anaeroben Parametern. In: Hansen, G., Mellerowicz, H. (Herausg.): 3. International Seminar fur Ergometrie, Berlin, Inst. f. Leistungsmedizin, pp.17-23.

Berg, K.E., La Voie, J.C. and Latin, R.W. (1985) Physiological training effects of playing youth soccer. Med. Sci. Sports Exerc. 17, 656-660.

Boros-Hatfaludy, S., Fekete, Gy., Apor, P. (1986) Metabolic enzyme activity patterns in muscle biopsy samples in different athletes. Eur. J. Appl. Physiol., 55, 334-338.

Bosco, C., Komi, P.V., Tihanyi, J., Fekete, Gy. and Apor, P. (1983) Mechanical power test and fibre composition of human leg extensor muscles. Eur. J. Appl. Physiol., 51, 129-134.

Burkett, L.S. (1970) Causative factors in hamstring strains. Med. Sci. Sport, 2, 39-42.

Campbell, D.E. and Glenn, W. (1982) Rehabilitation of knee flexor and knee extensor muscle strength in patients with meniscuctomies, ligamentous repair and chondromalacia. Phys. Ther., 62, 10-15.

Caru, B.L., LeCoultre, L., Aghemo, P. and Pinera Limas F. (1970) Maximal aerobic and anaerobic muscular power in football players. J. Sports Med., 10, 100-103.

Ekblom, B. (1986) Applied Physiology of soccer. Sports Med., 3, 50-60.

Ekes, E., Antony, B. and Malomsoki, J. (1974) (Maximal O_2 uptake of top soccer players. In Hungarian). Testnev. Sporteu. Szemle, 15, 265-269.

Ekstrand, J. (1982) Soccer injuries and their prevention. Linköping University, Sweden.

Farmosi, I. (1986) (Anthropometry in ball game players. (In Hungarian) In: Istvanfi, pp.27-57.

Fekete Gy. and Apor, P. (1981) Data on muscle fiber conversion and fibre splitting in man. Acta Physiol. Hung., 57, 163-7.

Fox, E.L. and Matthews, D.K. (1979) Physiological Basis of Physical Education and Athletics. Philadelphia: W.B. Saunders.

Hoette, C.A., Clark, B.A. and Wolff, G.A. (1985) Cardiac function and physical response of 146 professional football players to graded treadmill exercise stress. J. Sports Med., 26, 34-42.

Istvánfi Cs., (1986) Training of ball game players. (In Hungarian). Sport, Budapest.

Jacobs, I., Wrestlin, N., Karlsson, J. (1982) Muscle glycogen and diet in elite soccer players. Eur. J. Appl. Physiol, 48, 297-302.

Kirkendall, D.T. (1985) The applied sport science of soccer. Physician Sportsmed., 13, 53-59.

Maud, P.J. and Shultz, B.B. (1986) Relationship between and normative data for, three measures of anaerobic power In: Kinanthropometry III (edited by T. Reilly, J. Watkins and J. Borms) pp. 284-289. London: E and F.N. Spon Ltd.

Nettleton, B. and Briggs, C.A. (1980) The development of specific function tests as a measure of performance. J. Sports Med. Phys. Fit., 20, 47-54.
Oberg, B., Ekstrand, J. and Möller, M. (1984) Muscle strength and flexibility in different positions of soccer players. Int. J. Sp. Med., 5, 213-216.
Oberg, B., Möller, M., Gillquist, J. and , Ekstrand, J. (1986) Isokinetic torque levels for knee extensors and flexors in soccer players. Int. J. Sports Med., 7, 50-53.
Orosz, P. (1979) (Somatic development of young soccer players. In Hungarian) Doctoral dissertation, Testnev., Föisk., Budapest.
Orosz, P. (1983) A study on the repetitive speed-endurance in soccer players. (In Hungarian) Testnev. Föisk. Közl. No. I, 115-124.
Orosz, P., Fábian Gy., Pilvein, M. (1983) Data on talent selection and realization in soccer players. (In Hungarian) Testnev. Föisk.Közl. No. III, 71-110.
Quang, P. (1986) (Muscle characteristics and performance in man. In Hungarian) Ph.D. dissertation, Testnev. Föisk. Budapest.
Raven, P.B., Gettman, G.H., Pollock, M.L. and Cooper, K.H. (1976) A physiological evaluation of professional soccer players. Brit. J. Sports Med., 10, 209-16.
Reilly, T. and Ball, D. (1984) The net physiological cost of dribbling a soccer ball. Res. Quart. Exerc. Sport, 55, 267-271.
Reilly, T. and Bowen, T. (1984) Exertional cost of changes in directional modes of running. Percept. Motor Skills, 58, 49-50.
Reilly, T. and Thomas, V. (1976) A motion analysis of work-rate in different positional roles in professional football match-play. J. Hum. Mov't. Stud., 2, 87-97.
Rigler, E. and Orosz, P. (1986) Role and developing of conditional abilities in sport-game players. (In Hungarian) In Istvanfi, 1986.
Tihanyi, J., Apor, P. and Fekete, Gy. (1983) Zusammenhang zwischen ausgewahlten Absprungsmerkmalen und der Faserzusammensetzung der Oberschenkel und Wadenmuskulatur. Leistungs-sport, 13, 49-58.
Toriola, A.L., Salokun, S.O. and Mathur, D.N. (1985) Somatotype characteristics of male sprinters, basketball, soccer and field hockey players. Int. J. Sports Med., 6, 344-346.
Wade, A. (1962) The training of young soccer players. Med. Sport, 3, 1245-1251.
Withers, R.T., Maricic, Z., Wasilewski, S. and Kelly, L. (1982) Match analysis of Australian professional soccer players. J. Human Mov't. Stud., 8, 159-176.
Zelenka, V., Seliger, V. and Ondrej, O. (1967) Specific function testing in young players. J. Sports Med., Phys. Fit., 7, 143-147.

STRENGTH TRAINING AND KICK PERFORMANCE IN SOCCER PLAYERS

E. De Proft, J. Cabri, W. Dufour and J.P. Clarys
Department of Experimental Anatomy and Physical Education, Free University of Brussels, Laarbeeklaan 103, 1090 Brussels, Belgium.

Introduction

Although it has been extensively demonstrated that strength training improves performance and that strength characteristics are probably sport specific, there is little literature available concerning strength training of soccer players and its influence on their performance. Oberg et al. (1986) and Cabri et al. (1987) found significant differences in strength between soccer players and non-soccer players. Moreover, Oberg and co-workers (1986) could even demonstrate differences between high and lower level soccer players. Both studies agree that soccer players are generally stronger than non-soccer players and that soccer players have better fast-speed strength capabilities. It has also been confirmed that soccer players have a better kick performance than non-soccer players and that kick performance and concentric strength of the knee extensors and eccentric strength of the knee flexors are significantly correlated. In addition, concentric strength of the hip flexors and eccentric strength of the hip extensors are also significantly correlated with kick performance.

It is reasonable, therefore, to suppose that training the strength of the leg muscles might be of benefit to soccer players. Consequently, the aim of the present study was focussed on the influence of strength training on performance in soccer kicking.

Methods and Materials

The methods used in this study have been described extensively by Cabri et al. (1987).

Subjects

A total of 22 male soccer players, divided into adult soccer players (ASP) and young soccer players (YSP) and 20 male non-soccer players (NSP) were included in the experimental design (Table 1).

Strength training

Eleven soccer players (ASP: n=6; YSP: n=5) were asked to participate in a strength training programme, consisting of multiple repetitions at 80% of the maximal voluntary effort of different leg muscles, in addition to the normal soccer training. The programme lasted for one

Table 1. Anthropometric data of the subjects. Values are mean (±SD)

	N	age (yrs)	height (cm)	weight (kg)
Adult soccer players (ASP)	11	20.0±1.1	176.6±4.8	73.4 ± 8.8
Young soccer players (YSP)	11	15.5±0.7	170.0±4.3	60.5 ± 7.1
Non-soccer players (NSP)	10	23.0±1.5	178.1±4.0	70.7 ±11.1

full soccer season, twice a week, each session lasting for half an hour.

Measurements
Kick performance was measured on the soccer field. All subjects were asked to perform a maximal kick.

Isokinetic strength of knee flexors and extensors, and hip flexors and extensors, was measured by means of an isokinetic dynamometer (KIN-COM, Chattex Corp., TN) at a constant speed of 3.65 rad s^{-1}, during concentric and eccentric work.

Additionally, three functional performance tests were carried out for measuring explosive power. These were the vertical jump, the standing long jump and the triple jump on one leg. The tests described were performed at three different occasions:- before, in the middle and at the end of the training period.

The data, i.e. best kick performance, peak force of the different isokinetic strength tests, best trial of the functional performance measurements and linear velocities, were statistically handled by means of the Student t-test in order to evaluate any progress in strength and/or kick performance during and at the end of the training period. Pearson Product Moment correlation coefficients between kick performance and the different strength measurements were calculated to analyze the relations between kick performance and strength. In both tests, a probability value of 0.05 was taken to indicate significance.

Results

Comparing strength before and after the training period (Figure 1 and 2), the strength training group of the soccer players (both ASP and YSP) showed a significant increase not only in concentric and eccentric strength, but also in kick performance. Apparently, the strength training programme had a greater influence on eccentric strength development, for the strength increase seems to be higher than in concentric work. After strength training, the soccer players demonstrated an increase in eccentric strength of the knee flexors by 77% (10% for the non-strength training group) and an increase in concentric strength of the knee extensors by 25% (2% for the non-strength training group). Concentric strength of the hip flexors and eccentric strength of the hip extensors increased respectively by 15% and 35% (5 and 10% without strength training). The non-strength

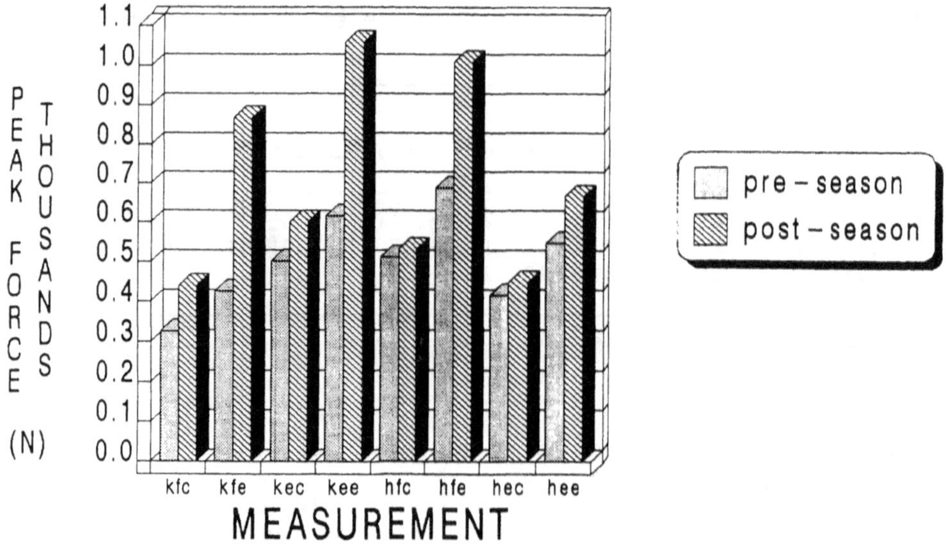

Figure 1. Isokinetic strength of the soccer players: strength training group, before and after the training period (one soccer season).
kfc: Knee Flexion Concentric
kfe: Knee Flexion Eccentric
kec: Knee Extension Concentric
kee: Knee Extension Eccentric
hfc: Hip Flexion Concentric
hfe: Hip Flexion Eccentric
hec: Hip Extension Concentric
hee: Hip Extension Eccentric

training group, however, did not show an increase in kick performance (Fig. 3).

The age ranges tested did not seem to significantly influence the results. Both the ASP and YSP groups showed the same tendencies already mentioned.

The correlations between strength and kick performance improved only in the strength training group. At the end of the training period, the correlation between kick performance and (i) concentric strength of the knee extensors (KEC) and (ii) eccentric strength of the knee flexors improved dramatically, by 15 and 20% respectively (Table 2), whereas the non-strength training group did not demonstrate an improvement of these relationships.

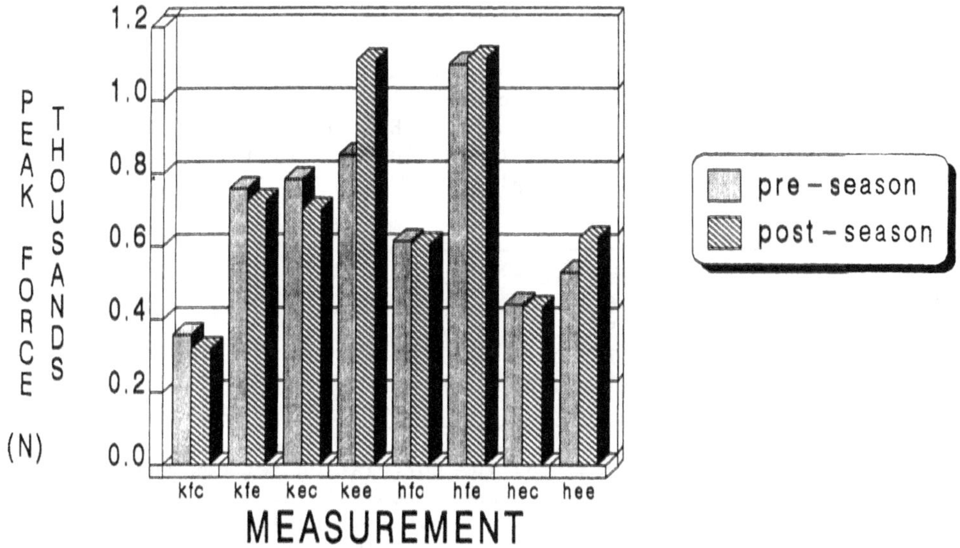

Figure 2. Isokinetic strength of the soccer players: non-strength training group, before and after the training period (one soccer season).
kfc: Knee Flexion Concentric
kfe: Knee Flexion Eccentric
kec: Knee Extension Concentric
kee: Knee Extension Eccentric
hfc: Hip Flexion Concentric
hfe: Hip Flexion Eccentric
hec: Hip Extension Concentric
hee: Hip Extension Eccentric

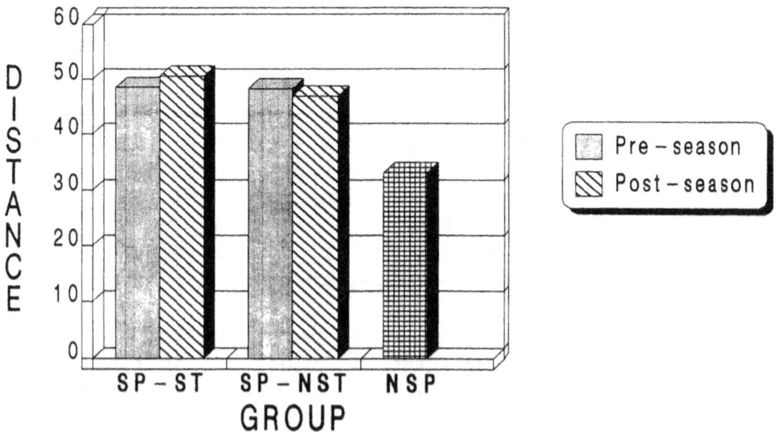

Figure 3. Kick performance of the soccer players - strength training group (SP-ST), the soccer players - non strength training group (SP-NST) and of the non-soccer players (NSP).

Table 2. Correlations between kick performance and isokinetic strength of the hip flexors concentrically (HFC), hip extensors eccentrically (HEE), knee extensors concentrically (KEG) and knee flexors eccentrically (KFE). Pre- and post-season (Pre - Post) and increase of these relations (Incr) are given

		Pre	Post	Incr.
Kick performance	HFC	.60	.85	+ 40
Kick performance	HEE	.56	.91	+ 65
Kick performance	KEC	.74	.85	+ 15
Kick performance	KFE	.77	.92	+ 20

In adolescent soccer players, the correlation between the kick performance and functional performance tests (i.e. the vertical jump) increased from r = 0.62 to 0.75. However, in adult soccer players, the relationship was significantly high only at the end of the training period ($r = 0.69$; $P < 0.05$).

Discussion

The results demonstrate the importance of incorporating strength training in a normal soccer training programme in order to increase not only strength but also (kick) performance. Previous investigations have also demonstrated this (Prins, 1978: Stevens, 1980; Kanehisa and Miyashita, 1983). Oberg et al. (1985) found a significant increase in strength in soccer players who in addition to their normal soccer training performed a 4-week strength training programme. It can be stated that the normal soccer training will increase strength, but that an individual strength training programme added to the soccer training will result in higher strength levels, better kick performance and better functional performances.

It is also demonstrated by the increase in the strength-kick performance correlations, that, given a certain level of technique, strength training will enhance the soccer players' performance. Moreover, it has been shown that soccer players have greater fast speed capabilities compared to non-soccer players (Oberg et al., 1986; Cabri et al., 1987), which is an important skill in high class soccer. Technical skill still remains an important determinant of the soccer kick. Although young soccer players have generally less strength than adult non-soccer players, their kick performance is far better.

It must be added that muscle strength is an important quality in athletes in order to reduce the risk of injury and in rehabilitation after injury (Sapega and Nicholas, 1981). During rehabilitation of soccer players, after knee injury for example, it is of great importance to pay special attention, not only to the knee extensors, but to the knee flexors as well, for it has been confirmed that the latter muscle group demonstrates great activity in the last phase of the soccer kick (De Proft et al., 1987). Moreover, eccentric strength of the hamstrings shows an even higher relation with kick performance than does the quadriceps muscle group and their response to strength training is also greater.

In conclusion, it can be stated that in soccer, strength training improves kick performance due to an increase in strength. Nevertheless developing technical skill (or neuromotor control) is still a predominant factor in the soccer kick and in kick performance.

References

Cabri, J. De Proft, E., Dufour, W. and Clarys, J.P. (1987) The relation between muscular strength and kick performance Paper presented at the First World Congress of Science and Football, Liverpool (U.K.), April, 1987.

De Proft, E., Cabri, J., Bollens, E., Dufour, W. and Clarys, J.P. (1987) Muscle activity in the soccer kick. Paper presented at the First World Congress of Science and Football, Liverpool (U.K.), April, 1987.

Kanehisa, H. and Miyashita, M. (1983) Specificity of velocity in strength training. Eur. J. Appl. Physiol., 52, 104-106.

Oberg, B., Moller, M., Ekstrand, J. and Gillquist, J. (1985) Exercises for knee flexors and extensors in uninjured soccer players: effects of two different programs. Int. J. Sports Med., 6, 151-154.

Oberg, B., Moller, M. Gillquist, J. and Ekstrand, J. (1986) Isokinetic torque levels in soccer players, Int. J. Sports Med., 7 50-53.

Prins, J.H. (1978) Histological changes in human skeletal muscle with isokinetic strength training at two distinct limb speeds. Dissertation Abstract International, 39(A), 4123.

Sapega, A. and Nicholas, J. (1981) The clinical usage of musculo-skeletal profiling orthopaedic sports medicine, Physician Sportsmed., 9, 80-81.

Stevens, R. (1980) Isokinetic vs isotonic training in the development of lower body strength and power. Scholastic Coach, 49, 74-76.

MORPHOLOGICAL AND METABOLIC ALTERATIONS IN SOCCER PLAYERS WITH DETRAINING AND RETRAINING AND THEIR RELATION TO PERFORMANCE

Jens Bangsbo and Masao Mizuno
August Krogh Institute, University of Copenhagen,
Universitetsparken 13, Copenhagen, Denmark.

Introduction

Successful soccer performance in each player is not only dependent upon technical, tactical and mental insight, but also upon the capablity to release the energy required during play. The type of physical activity demanded in soccer is classified as high intensity, intermittent exercise. Thus, both anaerobic and aerobic processes are required for energy liberation in individual players. Determinations of blood lactate concentrations during a match indicate that anaerobic energy yield plays an important role (Ekblom, 1986). Maximal aerobic work capacity expressed as maximal oxygen uptake ($\dot{V}O_2max$), is fairly high in elite soccer players (Ekblom, 1986) and during a game the relative contribution of aerobic process has been reported to account for 70 - 80% of maximal capacity (Reilly, 1979; Ekblom, 1986).

It has been well demonstrated that following endurance training, a marked adaptation occurs in the oxygen transport system and in the capacity of oxidative metabolism within skeletal muscles (Blomqvist and Saltin, 1983; Saltin and Gollnick, 1983). Cessation of the training causes a rapid decline in mitochondrial enzyme activities, while the effect on $\dot{V}O_2max$ and capillary supply in skeletal muscles is more moderate (Henriksson and Reitman, 1977: Houston et al., 1979: Coyle et al., 1984). In soccer players the effects of training and detraining on cardiovascular and metabolic characteristics have been studied (Fardy, 1969; Reilly and Thomas, 1977), but no information is available at the cellular level.

The present study, therefore, was undertaken to describe the effects of detraining and retraining, during the period where the competitive soccer season was interrupted for 7 weeks, on running performance, $\dot{V}O_2max$, skeletal muscle morphology and mitochondrial enzyme activities in semi-professional soccer players.

Methods

Subjects

Four semi-professional soccer players belonging to one of the top-class teams in Denmark, including one goal keeper (F.J.), were studied (Table 1). The subjects were informed about possible risks involved in this study before they gave their verbal consent to participate. All of the subjects had played for more than 13 years and had been regular players for at least 3 years.

General protocol

The subjects were studied at the end of the first half of the competition season (control), after 3 weeks of detraining and just before the beginning of the second half of the competition season following 4 weeks of retraining (Fig.1).

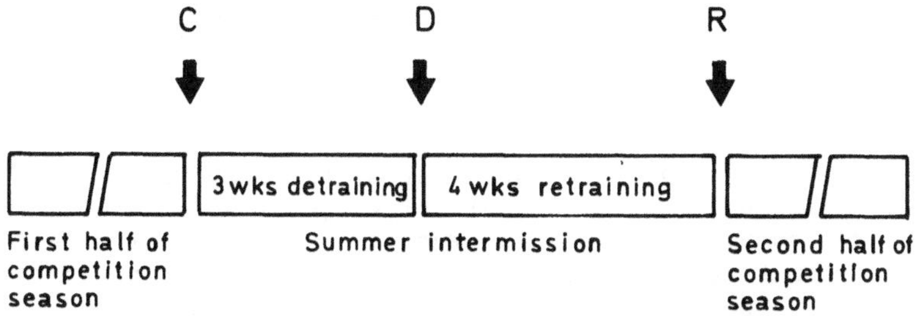

Figure 1. A schematic ilustration of the protocol employed in the present study indicating the control experiment (C), the experiment following detraining (D) and after retraining (R)

During the detraining period there was no soccer played at all, but the subjects were allowed to take part in other physical activities such as tennis, running and swimming. All physical activities were registered in the last month of the first half of the season, in the detraining period and in the retraining period by the players. From these records, training activity in the detraining period was estimated to be about 10% of the pre-detraining period level, while the level at the last week of the retraining period was 20% higher than before the detraining period.

Table 1. Physical characteristics of the subjects

	Age (yr)	Height (cm)	Weight (kg)	Maximal oxygen uptake (ml kg^{-1} min^{-1})	Maximal heart rate (beats min^{-1})
TC	23	174	69.2	57.9	194
CG	23	182	69.7	75.2	195
FJ	22	173	68.2	59.1	186
KT	24	185	67.8	72.7	196
Mean	23	179	68.7	66.2	193

Treadmill test

Running on a motor driven treadmill was used for determination of VO2max according to the protocol described by Saltin and Astrand (1967), where constant speed and step inclinations were employed.

Since the same procedure for measuring $\dot{V}O_{2max}$ was used in each experiment, treadmill running time to exhaustion was employed for evaluating short-term running performance.

Expiratory gas was collected in Douglas bags and the volume was measured on a Tissot spirometer. Oxygen and carbon dioxide concentrations were determined with paramagnetic O_2 (Servomex) and infrared CO_2 (Beckman LB-II) analysers, respectively. These analyzers were regularly calibrated during the day with a known concentration of gas determined by the Scholander technique. Maximal heart rate during treadmill running was recorded by precardial electrodes.

Field test

The field test specifically established for soccer players (Carlsson et al., 1983), which consists of sidestepping, jumping, turning around, backwards running and forwards running (4 times 540m), was performed for evaluating field running performance one day after the treadmill running experiments. As soon as the subject completed the test, blood samples were obtained from the finger-tip and lactate concentrations were determined spectrophotometrically (Lowry and Passonneau, 1972).

Muscle biopsies

Sampling

Muscle biopsies were taken from the lateral head of the right m. gastrocnemius by the percutaneous needle technique (Bergström, 1962). Muscle tissue was immediately dissected into two parts. One piece for enzyme analysis was frozen in liquid nitrogen. The remaining piece was mounted in embedding medium (O.C.T. Compound, Miels Tissue Tek) for histochemical analysis and frozen isopentane at its freezing point cooled with liquid nitrogen. The samples were thereafter stored in a freezer at -80°C until analyses were performed.

Enzyme activities

The muscle samples for determinations of mitochondrial enzyme activities were freeze dried in a thermoelectric freeze-dryer for 48 hours at -50°C and a pressure of 0.01 torr. Each sample was replaced and dissected under a microscope to remove blood, fat and connective tissue in a room where the temperatture (20°C) and humidity (less than 30%) were controlled. The dissected fibre fragments were homogenised at 1:400 dilution in an ice-chilled 0.3M phosphate buffer adjusted to pH 7.7 and containing 0.5 mg ml^{-1} of bovine serum albumin. Citrate synthase (CS) and 3-hydroxyacyl co-enzyme A dehydrogenase (HAD) activities were determined on the basis of the principle described by Lowry and Passonneau (1972) using a fluorimetric method of NAD-NADP coupled reactions as described by Essén-Gustavsson and Henriksson (1984). Enzyme activities were measured at 25°C and expressed as $\mu mol\ min^{-1}$ g dry weight $(wt)^{-1}$.

Histochemistry
Serial transverse sections 10 µm thick were cut, using a microtome at -20°C, and stained for myofibrillar ATPase reaction of pH of 9.4 (Padykula and Herman, 1955). Applying preincubations at different pH values (Brooke and Kaiser, 1970), the fibres were classified as slow twitch (ST) and fast twitch (FT) including sub-groups of FT fibres (FTa and FTb) under microscopy. The relative occurrence of fibre types was determined from a mean of 272 (range 202-334) fibres in each biopsy. The fibres identified as FTb (1.8-8.9%) were not included in further analyses.

Capillaries were visualised using the amylase-PAS method (Andersen, 1975). The number of capillaries per fibre and found around each fibre type as well as fibre cross-sectional areas were determined.

Statistics
Values are expresed as means with a range. Comparison between related observations were performed by the Friedman two-way analysis of variance (Siegel, 1956).

Results

Maximal oxygen uptake ($\dot{V}O_2max$) and performance (Fig. 2)
The control value for $\dot{V}O_2max$ was 4.4 (range 4.0-4.7) l min^{-1} and no significant changes was observed after detraining and retraining. However, there was a tendency for an increase following retraining, since 3 out of 4 subjects had a higher value than the control. Both short-term running and field running performance were impaired by 4% following detraining ($P < 0.01$) but were improved to the similar level after retraining ($P < 0.01$). The field running performance was even better than the control level ($P < 0.01$). The value for blood lactate concentration determined after the end of field tests was 5.7 (4.9-6.5)mM and was unchanged following detraining, while a 17% increase was observed after retraining ($P < 0.05$).

Mitochondrial enzyme activities (Fig.3)
The control values for CS and HAD activities were 45.8 (43.2-48.9) and 52.2 (46.9-57.8) µmol min^{-1} g dry $wt.^{-1}$, respectively. Following detraining HAD activity decreased by 27% ($P < 0.01$) and increased after retraining, but was still 12% lower than the control level ($P < 0.01$). A similar tendency was observed in CS activity, since 3 out of 4 subjects showed identical changes following detraining and retraining.

An additional determination was performed on two of the subjects and both enzyme activities appeared to be lowered already one week after detraining started (48.2 to 39.9 for CS and 52.0 to 35.2 µmol min^{-1} g dry $wt.^{-1}$ for HAD as the mean value of two subjects, TC and CG).

Muscle morphology
The relative occurrence of ST, FTa and FTb fibres determined in m. gastrocnemius before detraining was 55.9 (48.0 - 63.6), 39.8 (33 - 46.5) and 4.4 (3.0 - 5.5) %, respectively, and remained unchanged

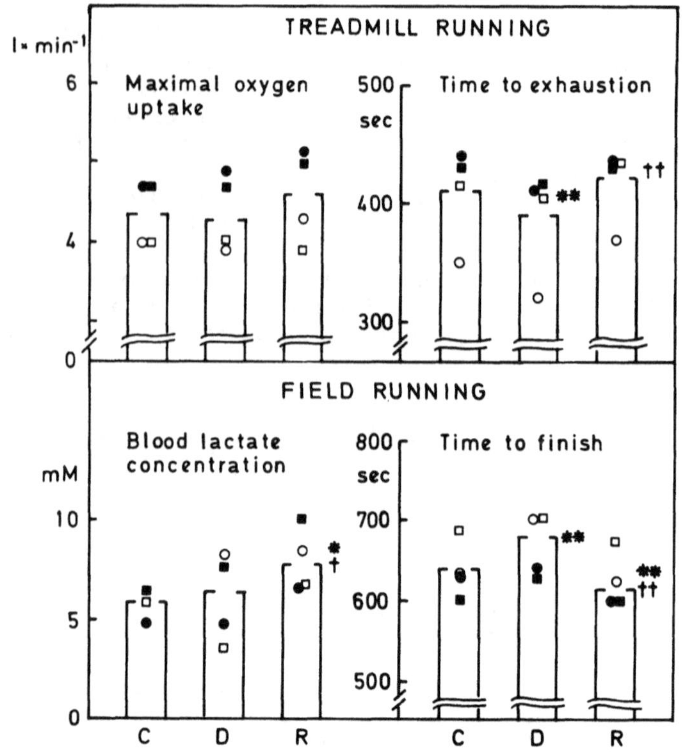

Figure 2. Maximal oxygen uptake and performance time determined in treadmill running as well as blood lactate concentration and performance time determined in field running obtained from the control experiment (C), the experiment following detraining (D) and after retraining (R). An individual mark corresponds to each subject (O = TC, ● = CG, □ = FJ (goalkeeper), ■ = KT). Field running test in the control experiment was performed in only 3 subjects. A significant difference compared with a control value (*. $P < 0.05$; **, $P < 0.01$) and a significant difference between D and R (+, $P < 0.05$; ++, $P < 0.01$) is marked.

through the period of time that this study was carried out. The mean fibre cross sectional area decreased by 7% following detraining ($P < 0.01$) and returned to the initial level after retraining. This was primarily due to the change in FTa fibre area (Table 2).

Although no change was detected in the number of capillaries per fibre, the number of capillaries found around ST fibres was decreased following detraining ($P < 0.01$) and increased after retraining compared with the control values ($P < 0.01$). The FTa fibres showed no change following detraining or after retraining (Table 3).

Table 2. Mean fibre cross-sectional area determined in biopsies from m.gastrocnemius obtained before detraining as a control (C), following detraining (D), and after retraining (R)

	Mean fibre area (μm^2)			Mean fibre type area (μm^2) ST fibres			FTa fibres		
	C	D	R	C	D	R	C	D	R
TC	6452	5550	5565	4974	5391	5341	6917	5722	6774
CG	4860	4787	5523	4985	5157	5249	5260	5020	6160
FJ	4920	4528	4408	4825	4669	4730	6343	5219	5923
KT	4649	4607	4652	5173	5035	4852	5569	5150	5692
Mean	5220	4868^{a}	5037^{+}	4989	5063	5043	6022	5278^{b}	6137^{++}

A significant difference compared with the control value is marked (^{a}, $P < 0.05$; ^{b}, $P < 0.01$).
A significant difference between the values determined after detraining and after retraining is marked ($^{+}$, $P < 0.05$; $^{++}$, $P < 0.01$).

Table 3. Capillary supply determined in biopsies from m.gastrocnemius obtained before detraining as a control (C), following detraining (D) and after retraining (R)

	No. of capillaries per fibre			No. of capillaries found around fibre types ST fibres			FTa fibres		
	C	D	R	C	D	R	C	D	R
TC	2.4	2.3	2.2	5.9	5.5	6.0	5.9	5.8	5.8
CG	2.4	2.5	2.8	6.4	6.1	6.6	5.4	5.9	6.1
FJ	2.5	2.4	2.4	6.2	6.1	7.0	7.3	6.0	6.4
KT	2.2	2.1	2.1	5.5	5.3	5.9	5.5	6.1	5.4
Mean	2.4	2.3	2.4	6.0	5.8^{b}	6.4^{++}6.0	6.0	6.0	

A significant difference compared from the control values is marked (^{a}, $P < 0.05$; ^{b}, $P < 0.01$)
A significant difference between the values determined after detraining and after retraining is marked ($^{+}$, $P < 0.05$; $^{++}$, $P < 0.01$).

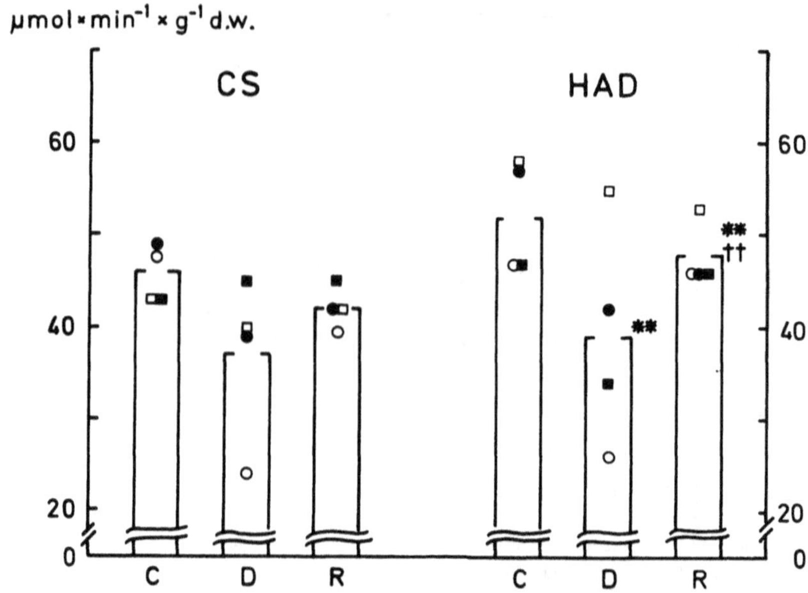

Figure 3. Citrate synthase (CS) and 3-hydroxyacyl co-enzyme A dehydrogenase (HAD) activity determined in biopsies from m. gastrocnemius. For symbols see Fig. 2 legend

Discussion

The mean $\dot{V}O_2max$ for the present elite soccer players was at the same level as reported for other players in elite teams (Ekblom, 1986). Morphological characteristics and mitochondrial enzyme activities in the present players are more similar to those seen in athletes involved in endurance events than strength trained individuals and non-elite socer players. Furthermore, training for soccer appears to cause a marked adaptation in oxidative potential within skeletal muscle (Table 4).

Running performance of the players was evaluated by a field test with movements relevant to soccer (Carlson et al., 1983), which is closely related to distance covered during a game (Ekblom, personal communication). The running performance in the control experiment was slightly lower than found in Swedish elite soccer players (Carlson et al., 1983). The cessation of soccer training for 3 weeks caused a marked decrease in running performance, but the control level was reached and even passed during 4 weeks retraining. Time to exhaustion on the maximal test showed the same tendency. Thus, the

Table 4. Morphological characteristics and mitochondrial enzyme activities determined in biopsies from m. gastrocnemius (G) and m. vastus lateralis (V) from non-athletes and individuals involved in different types of sport events

		Fibre type distribution (%)			Mean fibre area ($10^2.\mu m^2$)		No. of capillaries per fibre	Citrate synthase ($\mu mol.min^{-1}.g$ dry wt.$^{-1}$)	3-hydroacyl co-enzyme A dehydrogenase	References
		ST	FT a	FT b	ST	FT				
Non-athletes	G	51	49		43	47	1.5	-	-	Andersen and Kroese (1978)
	V	38	40	22	46	49	2.1	36	38	Andersen and Henrikson (1977) Saltin and Gollnick (1983)
Weight-lifters	V	41	59		66	110	2.1	-	-	Tesch et al. (1984)
Middle-distance runners	G	65	33	2	53	72	2.8	65	58	Okkels (1987)
Cross-country skiers	G	63	36	1	50	53	2.7	83	52	Mizuno et al. (1987)
Non-elite soccer players	V	42	41	18	50	65	1.9	-	-	Unpublished observation
Elite soccer players	V	40	60		55	70	-	-	-	Jacobs et al. (1982)
	G	56	40	4	50	60	2.4	46	52	Present study

ability for rather short-term high intensity exercise was impaired with detraining, but was at least re-established with relatively intensive retraining. In these periods no alterations were found in $\dot{V}O_2$max. It has previously been mentioned that $\dot{V}O_2$max is related to distance covered per game (Reilly, 1986). However, the present results albeit on a small sample, indicate that the work-rate during a match is not necessarily determined by the $\dot{V}O_2$max.

As seen in earlier studies (Houston et al., 1979; Coyle et al., 1984) detraining had a considerable, rapid negative effect on oxidative enzyme activities. In addition, measurements performed on two of the subjects showed that approximately half of the total reduction in the enzyme activities took place during the first week of detraining. Raising the oxidative enzyme activity with retraining is a slower process (Henrikson and Reitman, 1977; Houston et al., 1979). This was also seen in the present study, where mitochondrial enzyme level was increased after retraining, but the level was still lower than at the control experiment, although running performance was higher. It has been suggested that the mitochondrial enzyme activities in the exercising muscles may be an important factor in long-term performance (Gollnick and Saltin, 1982), so the change in enzyme activities may indicate that the endurance of the players was impaired at the start of the second half of the season when compared with the end of the first half.

Practical implications

For at least two reasons the level of physical activity has to be reasonably high in a detraining period, if the subsequent retraining period before competition is relatively short. First, the players can spend more time on other aspects of training, e.g. technical and tactical training. Second, it can ensure that the mitochondrial enzymatic activity of the players is as high as before detraining. Moreover, it is necessary to have a high level of physical training during the season, if the ability to perform short-term high intensity exercise after a pretraining period is going to be maintained

References

Andersen, P. (1975) Capillary density in skeletal muscle of man. Acta Physiol. Scand., 95, 203-205.

Andersen, P. and Henrikson, J. (1977) Capillary supply of the quadriceps femoris muscle of man: Adaptive response to exercise. J. Physiol. (Lond.), 270, 677-690.

Andersen, P. and Kroese, A.J. (1978) Capillary supply in soleus and gastrocnemius muscles of man. Pflugers Arch., 375, 245-249.

Bergström, J. (1962) Muscle electrolytes in man determined by neutron activation analysis on needle biopsy specimens. A study on normal subjects, kidney patients, and patients with chronic diarrhoea. Scand. J.Clin. Lab. Invest., 14, Suppl. 68.

Blomqvist, C.G. and Saltin, B. (1983) Cardiovascular adaptations to physical training. Ann. Rev. Physiol., 45, 169-189.

Brooke, M.H., and Kaiser, K.K. 1970) Three "myosin adenosine triphosphatase" systems. The nature of their pH lability and sulfhydryl dependence. J. Histochem. Cytochem., 18, 670-672.

Carlsson, C., Davidsson, T., Karlsson, H. and Wengrud, A, (1983) Löptestmodell for Fotbollskondition. Stockholm: Gymnastik- och Idrottshögskolan.
Coyle, E.F., Martin, W.H., Sinacore, D.R., Joyner, M.J., Hagberg, J.M. and Holloszy, J.O. (1984) Time course of loss of adaptations after stopping prolonged intense endurance training. J. Appl. Physiol., 57, 1857-1864.
Ekblom, B. (1986) Applied physiology of soccer. Sports Med., 3, 50-60.
Essén-Gustavsson, B. and Henriksson, J. (1984) Enzyme levels in pools of microdissected human muscle fibres of identified type. Adaptive response to exercise. Acta Physiol. Scand., 120, 505-515.
Fardy, P.S. (1969) Effects of soccer training and detraining upon selected cardiac and metabolic measures. Res. Quart., 40, 502-508.
Gollnick, P.D. and Saltin, B. (1982) Significance of skeletal oxidative enzyme enhancement with endurance training. Clin. Physiol., 2, 1-12.
Henriksson, J. and Reitman, J.S. (1977) Time course of changes in human skeletal muscle succinate dehydrogenase and cytochrome oxidase activities and maximal oxygen uptake with physical activity and inactivity. Acta Physiol. Scand., 99, 91-97.
Houston, M.E., Bentzen, H., and Larsen, H. (1979) Inter-relationships between skeletal muscle adaptations and performance as studied by detraining and retraining. Acta Physiol. Scand., 105, 163-170.
Jacobs, I. Westlin, N., Karlsson, J. and Rasmusson, M. (1982) Muscle glycogen and diet in elite soccer players. Eur. J. Appl. Physiol., 48, 297-302.
Lowry, O.H. and Passonneau, J.V. (1972) A Flexible System of Enzymatic Analysis, New York: Academic Press.
Mizuno, M., Juel, C., Rasmussen, T., Mygind, E., Scibye, B., Rasmussen, B. and Saltin, B. (1987) Limb skeletal muscle adaptation in well-trained athletes following training at altitude. Submitted for publication.
Okkels, T. (1987) Muscle morphology, metabolic potential and performance changes in middle distance runners after training with two levels of intense running. Int. J. Sports Med., in press.
Padykula, H.A. and Herman, E. (1955) The specificity of the histochemical method for adenosine triphosphatase. J. Histochem.Cytochem., 3, 170-195.
Reilly, T. (1979) Sports Fitness and Sport Injuries, London: Faber and Faber.
Reilly, T. (1986) Fundamental studies on soccer. Sportswissenschaft und Sportspraxis, 57, 114-120.
Reilly, T. and Thomas, V. (1977) Effects of a programme of pre-season training on the fitness of soccer players. J. Sports Med. Phys. Fit., 17, 401-411.
Saltin, B. and Åstrand, P.O. (1967) Maximal oxygen uptake in athletes. J. Appl. Physiol., 23, 353-358.
Saltin, B., and Gollnick, P.D. (1983) Skeletal muscle adaptability: Significance for metabolism and performance. In: Handbook ofPhysiology - Skeletal muscle (edited by L.D. Peacher and R.H. Adrian), pp. 555-631, Bethesda: Am. Physiol. Soc.
Siegel, S. (1956) Non-parametric Statistics for the Behavioural

Sciences. New York: McGraw-Hill.
Tesch, P.A., Thorsson, A., and Kaiser, P. (1984) Muscle capillary supply and fibre characteristics in weight and power lifters. J. Appl. Physiol., 56, 35-38.

EFFECTS OF 6 WEEKS PRE-SEASONAL TRAINING ON PHYSICAL FITNESS AMONG SOCCER PLAYERS

C. Islegen and N. Akgün
Sports Medicine Division, Ege University Medical Faculty, Bornova, Izmir, Turkey.

Introduction

Factors that determine physical fitness for soccer include aerobic capacity, anaerobic power, strength, speed, flexibility, agility, balance and coordination (Raven et al., 1976; Comucci, 1980). In order to be successful during the season, these factors must be elevated to high levels during the pre-season period by suitable training methods. This study examined the effects of pre-season training in Turkish footballers by measuring the aerobic capacity, maximal alactacid anaerobic power (MAAP), strength, flexibility and some skinfold thicknesses at the beginning and at the end of a six-week pre-season training period and comparing the results.

Material and Method

Subjects

Players (n=17) of a soccer team from the Third Division League in Turkey acted as subjects. Their mean (±SD) values were 24.5(± 3.1) years, 175(±6.8) cm, 69.9(±5.3) kg for age, height and weight respectively.

Procedure

Two indices of the aerobic capacity were used. The first was the 'Physical Working Capacity' determined as the subject's work-rate at a heart rate of 170 beats min^{-1} (PWC_{170}), on a Monark mechanically braked cycle ergometer. The other index was the $\dot{V}O_2$ max estimated from the heart rate values obtained during the sub-maximal loading on the same device (Åstrand and Rhyming, 1954).

A stair-run test (Margaria et al., 1966)was performed for the determination of MAAP. A 'Standing Vertical Jump' test was used for determining explosive power.

Left and right hand grip strength was measured with a 'Handgrip Dynamometer'. The 'Back and Leg Dynamometer' was used for measurement of both back and leg strength.

The 'Sit and Reach' test was used for determining flexibility of the lower back and posterior thigh muscles (Leighton, 1955).

Measurements were first done at the end of the seven week inactive period, or closed season. All these measurements were repeated after a six-week training period.

Training Programme

During the first three weeks the players performed low intensity runs (designed to be below the aerobic-anaerobic threshold) 5 days a week and 30-40 min every day. During the second 3 weeks, again for 5 days a week and 30-40 min every day, the intensity of the run was increased from time to time to force the aerobic-anaerobic threshold. This training programme was composed of 3-4x10 min runs, static and dynamic stretching exercises, technical exercises with the ball and 10-30 m sprints (Liesen, 1983).

Strength exercises were performed with extra weights two days a week. First the maximum lifting capacity of different muscle groups for each of the players was determined. Exercises were started with 40% of these maximal values. These weights were increased 10% every week. During the last two weeks muscular coordination exercises were performed with 70-85% of the maximal weights (Ehlenz and Grosser, 1983).

Results and Discussion

The pretraining (T_1) and post-training (T_2) results were compared with paired t-tests (Table 1). After the six week training period, the aerobic capacity (PWC_{170} and estimated $\dot{V}O_2max$), MAAP, explosive muscular power, muscular strength, flexibility had all improved significantly ($P < 0.01$). There was a small increase in the weight ($P < 0.05$) and a small decrease in the abdominal skinfold (P 0.05) at the end of the training period.

The increase in estimated $\dot{V}O_2max$ was from 42.35 (± 4.6) to 50.75 (± 379) ml kg^{-1} min^{-1} and the PWC_{170} increased from 2.38 (± 0.22) to 2.99 (± 0.22) W kg^{-1} min^{-1}. These changes represented improvements of 19.4 and 25.6% respectively. The MAAP was also increased from 156.4 (± 14.2) to 169.6 (± 18.0) kgm s^{-1}. There were average improvements of 3 cm in flexibility and 3.06 cm in the vertical jump.

There are not many comparative studies on soccer players at the pre-season stage and during the season. Reilly and Thomas (1977) observed no significant changes in weight, skinfold values, muscular power and strength measurements on 31 soccer players after a six-week pre-season training period. In this study, muscular strength and power were not changed because no specific exercises had been done for their improvement. However, Reilly and Thomas did report significant increases of 26.2% in the Harvard Index in their subjects. Losada (1980), Fardy (1969) and Vos (1980) have also found somewhat significant increases in $\dot{V}O_2max$ after a training period compared with values observed at the beginning of seasonal activity.

Improvement in cardio-respiratory function tests due to pre-season training is closely related to whether or not the player had done any exercises during the off-season to keep his aerobic capacity at a desirable level. Players who start the season with a low level of aerobic capacity because of detraining in the off-season, show a greater percentage change with the subsequent training. Whatever the state of fitness at the start of training the change in the $\dot{V}O_2max$ due to pre-season training is limited by physiological, metabolic and genetic factors to 25-50% according to various authors (Åstrand and Rodahl, 1977; Hollman et al., 1981).

Table 1. Pre- and post-training values of subjects (mean ± standard deviation)

Variable	Pre-training results	Post-training results
Height (cm)	175 ± 6.2	175 ± 6.2
Weight (kg)	70.0 ± 5.3	71.0 ± 4.8a
Skinfold		
Subscapula (mm)	10.9 ± 2.5	11.1 ± 2.5
Triceps (mm)	7.2 ± 1.4	7.2 ± 1.5
Suprailiac (mm)	7.2 ± 1.4	11.2 ± 4.1
Abdomen (mm)	12.8 ± 5.0	11.8 ± 4.3a
Thigh (mm)	9.9 ± 3.1	9.7 ± 3.0
Cardiorespiratory function tests		
Indirect $\dot{V}O_2$($l\ min^{-1}$)	2.953 ± 0.316	3.582 ± 0.294b
Indirect $\dot{V}O_2$($ml\ kg^{-1}\ min^{-1}$	42.35 ± 4.61	50.75 ± 3.79b
PWC_{170} (W)	166.5 ± 16.0	212.7 ± 17.8b
Muscular Power		
MAAP (kgm s^{-1})	156.4 ± 14.2	169.6 ± 18.0b
Vertical jump (cm)	54.6 ± 5.8	57.7 ± 4.8b
Strength		
Grip right hand (kg)	54.3 ± 6.2	57.2 ± 6.7b
Grip left hand (kg)	52.2 ± 6.4	55.6 ± 6.8b
Back (kg)	140.7 ± 2.3	165.4 ± 31.9b
Leg (kg)	128.9 ± 21.8	140.0 ± 22.8b
Flexibility		
Sit and Reach test (cm)	8.15 ± 8.09	11.07 ± 6.35b

a Significant at 0.05 level
b Significant at 0.01 level

It is concluded that the six weeks training programme did improve major physical fitness factors in soccer players. These changes were considered to be the results of starting the programme with low level physical fitness while the values for muscular strength reflected the absence of any specific strength training stimulus.

References

Åstrand, P.O. and Rodahl, K. (1977) Textbook of Work Physiology. New York: McGraw Hill.

Åstrand, P.O. and Ryhming, I. (1954) A nomogram for calculation of aerobic capacity (physical fitness) from pulse rate during submaximal work. J. Appl.Physiol., 7, 218.

Comucci, N. (1980) Evaluation of the soccer players' physical attributes. In: Proceedings of International Congress on Sports Medicine Applied to Football (edited by L. Vecchiet) pp.668-669. Roma: D. Guanella.

Ehlenz, H. and Grosser, M. (1983) Kraft-Training, Munchen: BLV Verlegspesellschof 1.

Fardy, P.S. (1969) Effects of soccer training and detraining upon selected cardiac and metabolic measures. Res. Quart., 40, 502-508.

Hollman, V., Liesen, H., Mader, A., Heck, H., Rost, R., Dufaux, B., Schurch, P., Lagerstrom,D. and Fohrenbach, R. (1981) Zur hochst und dauer-leistungs fahigkeit der Deutschen Fussboyyspitzen spieler. Dtsch. Zschr. für Sports Med., 5, 113-120.

Liesen, H. (1983) Aerobic-anaerobic threshold values of Turkey National soccer team. Communication to the 'Seminar for Football Trainers', (Izmir, Turkey).

Losada, A. (1980) Clinical and instrumental profile of the cardio-circulatory system of a football player. In: Proceedings of International Congress on Sports Medicine Applied to Football (edited by L.Vecchiet) pp. 103-112. Roma: D. Guanella.

Margaria, R., Aghemo, I. and Rouelli, E. (1966) Measurement of muscular power (anaerobic) in man. J. Appl. Physiol., 21, 1662-1664.

Raven, P.B., Gettman, L.R. Pollock, M.L. and Cooper, K.H. (1976) A physiological evaluation of professional soccer players. Brit. J. Sports Med., 10, 209-216.

Reilly, T. and Thomas, V. (1977) Effect of a programme of pre-season training on the fitness of soccer players. J. Sports Med. Phys. Fit., 17, 401-412.

Vos, J.A. (1979) Physiological comparison between Dutch soccer players and other teamsport men. In: Proceedings of International Congress on Sports Medicine Applied to Football (edited by L. Vecchiet) pp. 695-701. Roma: D. Guanella.

A PERIODIZED TOTAL CONDITIONING PROGRAMME FOR AUSTRALIAN RULES FOOTBALL

C.J. Jones : Footscray Institute of Technology, Ballaret Road, Footscray, PO Box 64, Victoria, Australia 3011. and Carlton Football Club, Melbourne, Australia.
S. Laussen : Melbourne Football Club, Melbourne, Australia.

Introduction

Australian Rules Football is a collision sport played by two teams of 18 players on a large oval field, each game comprising four quarters of 25 min playing time each. The rules of play provide for a game of continuous activity. Physical conditioning for Australian Rules Football has traditionally centred on the development of the player's aerobic capacity through endurance running (Smith, 1983). Little emphasis has been placed on other facets of physical conditioning (Taggert, 1982). In addition it has been the convention to commence pre-season training in the January following a competitive season which lasted from April to September of the previous year (Taggert, 1982). This results in the loss of practice time which might be better devoted to skill acquisition and enhancement (Taggert, 1982).

The traditional regimen is inconsistent with the current requirements of elite sports performance. Hahn et al. (1979) and Douge (1982) provided data which characterise the patterns of running required for participation in the sport. Australian Rules Football players are required to produce repeated bursts of high intensity activity interspersed with short recovery periods, a pattern similar to the demands of other field sports such as soccer.

Lindholm (1979) suggested that the coach may be viewed as a teacher and as such must practice sound educational principles. Cratty (1985) cited evidence of the success of 'athlete driven' methodology in athletic conditioning and participation. In the light of the inadequacies in the conditioning process, an 'athlete driven' model for the development of a scientifically based conditioning programme for Australian Rules Football was initiated in October 1981.

Method

All of the players registered with the Fitzroy Football Club for the 1981 season participated in a two-part procedure. The first required the completion of a Physical Conditioning Game-Requirement questionnaire : the second called for a 15 min follow-up interview. This was completed during October 1981. The results indicated a great (87% of questionnaire responses) concern of the players with a perceived lack of the upper body strength needed for successful participation at elite level. The athletes also expressed a need for a running programme more representative of the demands of the game.

A working party of five player representatives and two Physical Education Advisers examined the responses. They established the following protocol for training and monitoring:-

(i) Pre-season training would commence during the first week of November to allow a minimum of 6 weeks of conditioning prior to the Christmas vacation.

(ii) Two measures of upper body strength were chosen for use, a 1-Repetition Maximum bench press test (1RMBP) and a Body Weight bench press Repetition Maximum test (BWBM).

(iii) One hundred 100 m sprints would be completed by all players as a test of endurance prior to the Christmas vacation.

(iv) Varied pace running drills would be developed and used in an attempt to simulate game running stress during training.

Results and Discussion

Hahn (1979) reported players running distance as great as 10 km in a game of Australian Rules Football. Since the tempo and demands of the game appears to be increasing, it is reasonable to expect that players now cover distances in excess of this amount. The original 100 x 100 m test was an attempt to connect the time frame of game participation, 100 min, and the pattern of intermittent running inherent in the game.

Table 1. 100 x 100 m sprints

Year	n	Time frame (s)	Run time (s)
1981	54	60	18
1982	52	50	18
1983	47	50	17
1984	49	50	16.5

As illustrated in Table 1 the time between the start of each 100 m run, the time frame, and the speed of each run, were used to manipulate the intensity of the test on subsequent trials. The validity of the test for the players was confirmed by concurrent evaluation using an endurance running test for which external normative data were available. In this example the 12 min run was the comparative item.

Table 2. 12-minute endurance run

Year	n	Distance (s)	Range (s)
1981	43	3097	2700-3400
1982	58	3228	2930-3585
1983	41	3335	2940-3700
1984			No data

Test intensity was manipulated following evaluation of the questionnaire/interview process for each season by the Working Party. The training item central to running training was a varied pace drill. This drill was made up of four 75 m runs, four 75 m recovery jogs and eight 40 m sprints arranged in a continuous circuit. A 40 m sprint followed each 75 m effort. The time allowed for each run segment was self-selected by training groups as consistent with perceptions of game intensity. In practice the recovery jogs were completed in 45 s, the 75 m runs in 17 s and the 40 m sprints in 7 s. The maximum time completed by all players as a training group was 60 min in February 1983. In addition, telemetry of individual players showed heart rates were maintained in a training zone 70-85% of a heart rate maximum of 200 beats min^{-1}. It has been suggested that this range is consistent with training stimuli for improvement in cardiovascular function (Pyke 1980).

Table 3. 40 metre sprint

Year	n	Mean (s)	Range (s)
1981	28	5.78	5.67-6.34
1982	49	5.56	5.11-6.33
1983	34	5.37	5.14-6.08
1984	52	5.29	4.82-5.78

As previously indicated, the players' concern with the need to be stronger was at variance with the traditional emphasis in training. The strength training programme which was instituted exercised all of the major joints and muscle groups, and was consistent with accepted strength training practices. The players were expected to complete a minimum of three strength training sessions per week.

Table 4. 1-Repetition Maximum bench press

Year	n	Mean (kg)	Range (kg)
1981	20	75	50.0-122.7
1982		No data	
1983	43	89.3	54.5-136.4
1984	35	91.2	54.5-150.0

Each week contained one high volume, one medium volume and one "low volume high intensity" unit. A card system was used both as a recording tool and as a motivational device. Testing on the criteria occurred at six-week intervals throughout the year. A periodised adaptation of the programme was introduced for the 1983 season in accordance with the model proposed by Stone et al. (1982). In Table 4 it can be seen that 1-RMBP scores improved for each year, from a low of 75 kg in 1981 to 91.2 kg in 1984. Table 5 shows the data for BWBM; although there is no pattern of continuous improvement across the time period, it is noteworthy that in 1981, 50% of the players were unable to bench press their own body weight, whilst in 1984 only 4% could not achieve at least one repetition at this load.

Table 5. Body Weight bench press Repetition Maximum (BWBM)

Year	n	Mean (rep)	Range (rep)
1981	21	4.0	0-14
1982	42	7.7	0-21
1983	43	6.4	0-23
1984	50	6.1	0-27

The Working Party was instrumental in creating several other conditioning drills simulating game conditions. Two more of these are particularly relevant here. The first was a sequence of 40 m sprints designed to simulate the maximal running component of the game. The design format was similar to that used in the repetition 100 m test, i.e. a new sprint was begun every 20 s with each sprint to be completed in 7 s. The sprints were completed in blocks of 10 with a 2 min rest between sets. Table 3 shows a progressive reduction of the team's average 40 m sprint time over the training period. A game skill combat-running circuit was also designed to simulate the contesting segment of the game and thus to further enhance the game-specific conditioning of the athletes.

Conclusion

'Athlete-centred' methodology appears to be effective in promoting desirable changes in the conditioning of athletes playing Australian Rules Football at an elite level. This report describes an attempt to use athletes in the design and development of their own conditioning programmes. The evaluative tests and an improvement in game performance both suggest success was achieved. In particular sports specific conditioning drills were created from active consultation with the participants. Evaluation against normative data indicated improvement in physical performance parameters, thereby supporting the practices that had been introduced.

References

Cratty, B.J. (1985) Psychological Preparation and Athletic Excellence. New York: Mouvement Publications.

Douge, B. (1982) Testing in Australian Rules Football. Austr. Sports Coach, 6, 29-37.

Hahn, A., Taylor, N., Hunt, B., Woodhouse, T. and Shultz, G. (1979) Physiological relationships between training activities and match play in Australian Rule Football rovers. Aust. Sports Coach, 3, 3-8.

Lindholm, K. (1979) Coaching as teaching: seeking balance. Phi Delta Kappan, June.

Pyke, F.S. (1980) Physiology of training. In Towards Better Coaching (edited by F.S. Pyke). AGPS; Canberra.

Smith, R. (1983) Organising the training year for team sports. Austr. Sports Coach, 7, 6-13.
Stone, M.H., O'Bryant, H., Garhammer, J. and Rozenek, R. (1982) A theoretical model of strength training. Nat. Strength Condit. Ass. J., 4, 36-39.
Taggert, A. (1982) Australian football, pre-season training: a behavioural approach. Austr. Sports Coach, 6, 46-49.

EFFECT OF RECOVERY DURATION ON PERFORMANCE DURING MULTIPLE TREADMILL SPRINTS

D.J. Holmyard, M.E.Cheetham, H.K.A. Lakomy and C. Williams
Department of Physical Education and Sports Science,
University of Technology, Loughborough, Leics. LE11 3TU, England.

Introduction

Power output during multiple cycle ergometer sprinting is impaired when the recovery duration between bouts is short (30s) (Wootton and Williams, 1983). The ability to reproduce short bursts of maximal running exercise is of great importance in the 'multiple sprint' sports such as rugby, soccer and hockey. Until recently there has been no acceptable method for examining sprint running in the laboratory. A non-motorized treadmill has been modified for this purpose (Lakomy, 1984) and this has allowed the laboratory examination of both sprint running performance and of the metabolic responses to sprinting (Cheetham et al., 1984, 1986). The purpose of this study was to examine the influence of recovery duration and the preceding number of exercise bouts on the power output during sprint running.

Method

Subjects

Ten Rugby Union backs (University 1st XV; one scrum-half, two fly-halfs, three centres, two wing three-quarters and two fullbacks) whose mean (±SD) height, weight and age were 178.3±4.2cm, 77.5±4.8kg and 20.1±0.7 yrs respectively, volunteered to participate in the study. Subjects were highly motivated and were familiarised with treadmill sprinting in the week prior to the study. They agreed not to take part in training or match-play on the days before each of two treadmill running tests.

Equipment

A non-motorized treadmill was used for the sprint tests as this allowed the subjects to run at unrestricted speeds and to change speed as they fatigued. The modifications made to the non-motorized treadmill have been previously described by Lakomy (1984). Briefly, the treadmill was interfaced to a microcomputer which allowed the continuous monitoring of the horizontally applied force by means of a force transducer mounted on the rear cross-bar of the treadmill and the continuous monitoring of belt speed by means of a small generator mounted on the treadmill's front axle. External power output during the test was determined from the instantaneous product of the horizontally applied force and the treadmill belt speed.

Protocol

The two treadmill running tests consisted of ten 6 s sprints either with a 30 s recovery (30sR) or a 60 s recovery (60sR) between each sprint. The two tests were completed on separate days approximately 3 days apart and the order of tests was randomized between subjects. Five minutes before both tests two 30s sub-maximal runs were performed on the non-motorized treadmill at 10 and 12 km h^{-1}, which served both as a warm-up and to re-accustom the subjects to experimental procedures. The subjects then completed the first sprint, and all subsequent sprints, from a jogging start at 8 km h^{-1}.The subjects were asked to run as fast as possible from the start of both tests and were verbally encouraged throughout. Heart rate was recorded throughout the test and during 5 min of passive recovery by the interfacing of a heart rate monitor to a microcomputer.

Blood sampling and treatment

Capillary blood samples were taken in duplicate on both testing occasions at 4 min after the warm-up and at 1 and 5 min after the sprint test. The samples were deproteinized, frozen at -20°C and analyzed at a later date for blood lactate and glucose concentrations as described by Maughan (1982).

Terminology

Throughout this study 'peak power output' refers to the highest 1 s value of power attained during each 6 s sprint, whilst 'mean power output' refers to the average power output for the 6 s period. 'End power output' refers to the value of power in the last second of each sprint. 'Distance run' refers to the distance through which the subjects turned the treadmill belt during each sprint.

Statistical analysis

A two-way analysis of variance and Tukey test were used to examine differences in power output between the 30sR and 60sR tests and between the individual sprints during each test. A pooled t-test was used to examine differences between the post-exercise metabolite concentrations with the two recovery intervals. Results are presented as mean ± SD.

Results

Peak power output

The peak, mean and end power outputs during each sprint with the 30sR and 60sR intervals are shown in Table 1, whilst the differences in the power profiles between sprint 1 and sprint 10 for the two recovery intervals are shown in Fig.1. With the 30sR interval a 13.2% decrease in peak power output occurred between sprints 1 and 10. When the individual sprints were examined it was only during sprints 9 ($P < 0.01$) and 10 ($P < 0.05$) that peak power output was statistically lower than during sprints 1 and 2. During the test with the 60sR interval peak power output was well maintained with

Table 1. Peak, mean and end power output (watts) during ten 6 s sprints with either a 30 s or 60 s recovery interval (mean ± SD)

	1	2	3	4	5	6	7	8	9	10
Peak power										
60s	800	839	806	870	811	788	835	789	783	776
	±66	±92	±94	±86	±85	±41	±100	±87	±72	±69
30s	815	820	800	771	746	752	732	710	679	707
	±134	±107	±117	±114	±98	±91	±75	±46	±73	±68
Mean power										
60s	701	724	709	703	701	686	692	670	675	672
	±63	±66	±71	±55	±74	±52	±67	±70	±66	±67
30s	716	712	666	659	626	616[a]	596[b]	579[b]	565[b]	563[b]
	±118	±76	±97	±89	±69	±77	±63	±50	±72	±53
End power										
60s	675	679	680	567	612	519	618	570	555	599
	±68	±63	±83	±90	±110	±97	±111	±115	±116	±106
30s	713	635	617	548	568	495	471*	510	461	483
	±107	±84	±111	±86	±74	±126	±104	±102	±90	±75

significant difference between 30s and 60s recovery intervals
[a] $P < 0.05$, [b] $P < 0.01$

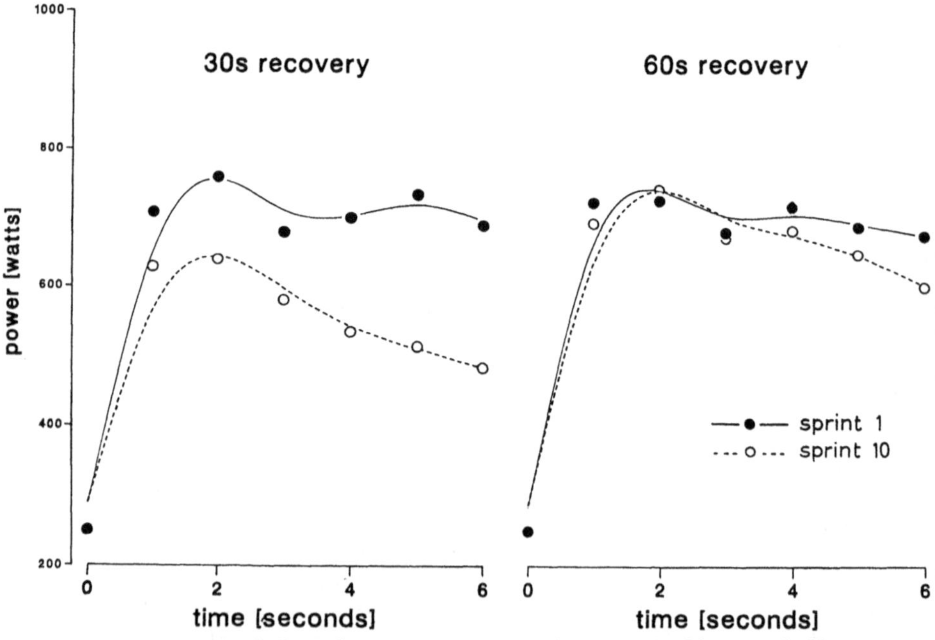

Figure 1. Power profiles for sprints 1 and 10 with 30 s and 60 s recovery intervals. Curves are formally fitted using a least squares model

only a 3.0% ($P > 0.05$) decrease from sprints 1-10. There were no differences in peak power output between corresponding sprints with the two recovery intervals, but over all 10 sprints the peak power output was highest during the 60sR interval test ($P < 0.05$).

Mean power output

Mean power output during each sprint with the 30sR and 60sR intervals is shown in Fig.2. With the 30sR a 21.4% decrease in mean power output occurred betwen sprints 1 and 10 and the mean power output during sprints 5-10 was less than that during sprints 1 and 2 ($P < 0.01$). During the 60sR interval test, mean power output was well maintained with only a 4.2% ($P > 0.05$) decrease from sprint 1 to 10. Sprints 6-10 with the 30sR interval all had a lower mean power output than the corresponding sprint with the 60sR interval ($P < 0.05$ sprint 6, $P < 0.01$ sprints 7-10). Those individuals achieving the highest peak power output during sprint 1 also had the largest decreases in mean power output between sprints 1 and 10 for 30sR ($r = 0.75$, $P < 0.05$). No such relationship was found for the 60s recovery interval.

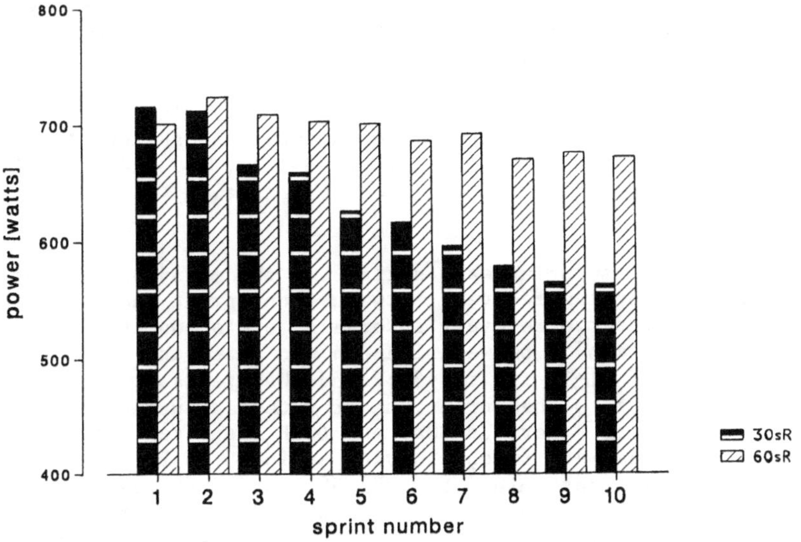

Figure 2. Mean power output during each sprint with 30 s and 60 s recovery intervals. (SD are omitted for clarity and are shown in Table 1).

End power output

During the test with the 30sR interval end power was decreased by 32.2% between sprints 1-10 and end power during sprints 6-10 was lower than that during sprints 1 and 2 ($P < 0.05$). When the recovery interval was 60s the end power output was better maintained, decreasing by 11.3% ($P > 0.05$) between sprints 1 and 10. When all 10 sprints were considered together, end power output was lower for the 30sR interval ($P < 0.05$), but because of the large inter-individual variations in end power output when corresponding sprints were compared, only for sprint 7 was there a statistically significant difference ($P < 0.01$) between the 30sR and 60sR interval test.

Distance run

The subjects moved the treadmill approximately 38m during all sprints with the 60sR interval. This distance is less than would be run outside, because the subjects were working against the resistance of the treadmill belt. When the recovery interval was 30s there was a 6.5% decrease in distance run between sprints 1 and 10 from 38.2±3.4m to 35.7±1.8m. The distance run in sprints 9 and 10 was less than that in sprint 1 ($P < 0.05$) and distance run in sprints 7-10 was less than that during sprint 2 ($P < 0.01$).

Blood lactate and blood glucose concentrations

The blood lactate and blood glucose concentrations following the warm-up and at 1 and 5 min after treadmill sprinting are shown in Fig.3. The warm-up caused only a small increase in blood lactate concentration as a result of the ten 6s sprints after both tests. At 1 min post-exercise blood lactate was increased to 17.83±2.06 mM and 17.52±2.29 mM for the 30s and 60s recovery intervals respectively. However, at 5 min post-exercise blood lactate was lower for the 60sR interval (17.73±2.01 vs 15.82±2.11, $P < 0.01$).

Blood glucose concentration after the warm-up was similar before the 30sR and 60sR tests (4.49±0.43 vs 4.45±0.36.) After exercise blood glucose concentration was higher after the 30sR test thanthe 60sR test at both 1 min (6.99±1.07 vs 6.25±1.11, $P < 0.05$) and 5 min (6.96±1.28 vs 5.96±1.08, $P < 0.01$) post-exercise.

Heart rate

The peak heart rates during each sprint and the mean heart rates before the test, during recovery between each sprint and after the entire test for the two recovery intervals, are shown in Fig.4. Heart rate (beats min^{-1}) between 1 and 4 min after the warm-up averaged 92±11 and 91±10 for the 30sR and 60sR tests. Standing on the treadmill prior to the sprint, heart rate was increased to 131±21 and 137±15 beats min^{-1} for the 30sR and 60sR tests respectively. The highest heart rates were reached during sprint 5 in both tests (188±18 and 180±14 beats min^{-1} for the 30sR and 60sR respectively). Heart rate during the recovery interval between each sprint was approximately 10 beats min^{-1} lower than the peak value during the sprint for both recovery protocols. Heart rate was decreased during recovery from 182±12 (30sR) and 172±11 (60sR) during sprint 10 to 116±11 and 115±10 beats min^{-1} respectively at 5 min post-exercise. Whilst there was a tendency for heart rate to be higher both during exercise and during recovery in the 30sR test compared to the 60sR test, there were no statistically significant differences in heart rate between the two recovery protocols ($P > 0.05$).

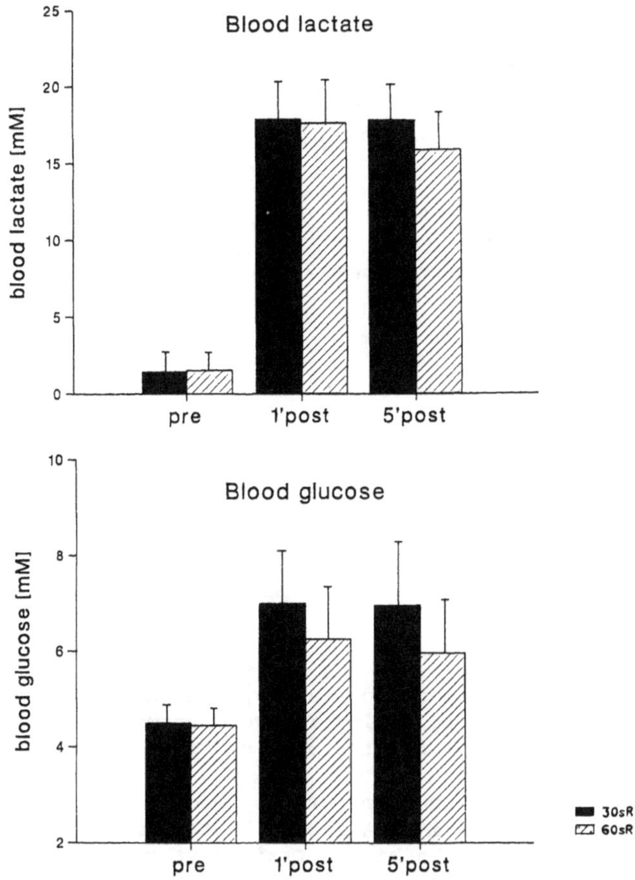

Figure 3. Blood lactate and blood glucose concentrations post warm-up (pre) and at 1 and 5 minutes after treadmill sprinting

Discussion

Mean power output during the 6s sprints in this study was higher than the mean power output recorded previously for male subjects during 30s of treadmill sprinting. This is not surprising as decreases in power output of approximately 50% occur during 30s of treadmill sprinting (Cheetham and Williams, 1985). However, power output during 6s treadmill sprinting was lower than that achieved during 6s of sprint cycling exercise (Boobis et al., 1982). This is probably because the resistive load is optimized in sprint cycling to give the highest power output (Dotan and Bar-Or, 1983), whereas in treadmill sprinting the resistance of the treadmill belt is fixed. The 13.2% and 21.4% decreases in peak and mean power output respectively between sprints 1 and 10 with the 30s recovery are of a similar magnitude to the 17.9% and 20.5% decreases found after only half the

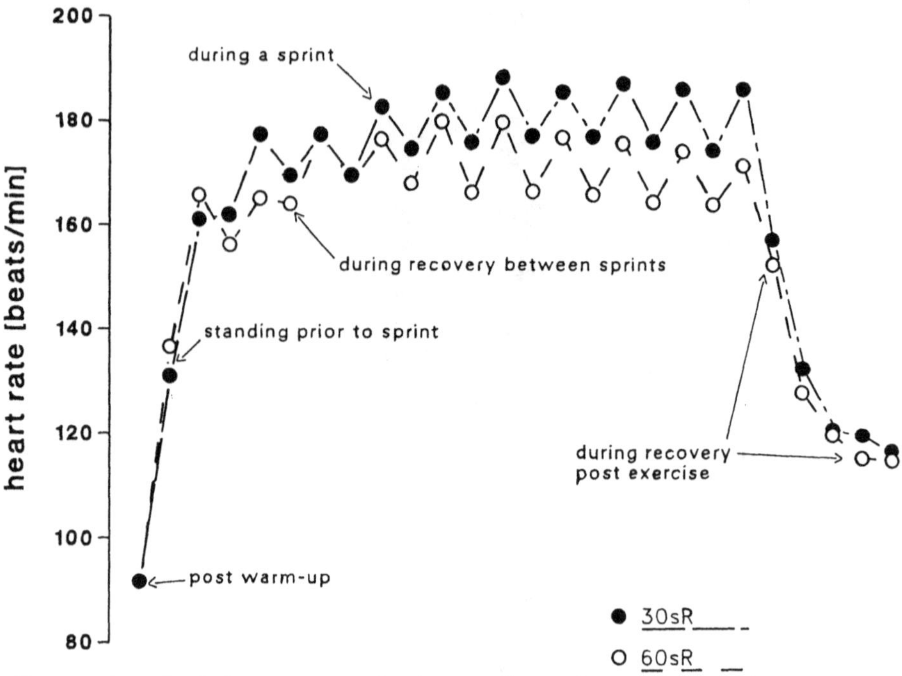

Figure 4. Peak heart rate during each sprint and mean heart rate before the test, during recovery between sprints and after the entire test for the 30 s and 60 s recovery intervals

number (5) of 6s cycle ergometer sprints (Wootton and Williams, 1983). Mean power output may have been better maintained in the present study because of the highly trained status of the subjects. Alternatively, power output during sprint running may be affected to a lesser degree by local fatigue of a particular muscle group than power output during sprint cycling. It is of interest that with the 30sR interval, power output was reduced by 21.4% between sprints 1 and 10, whilst the distance run was reduced by only 6.5%. It is possible that the smaller decrease in distance run is due, in part, to a modification of running style as fatigue develops during the test, but it is clear that as power is a derivative of both force and speed the major change with fatigue was a decrease in force exerted. A decrease in distance covered of 3m in 40m will have a marked influence on peformance in the game, but the effect of fatigue may be greater and less easily observed in those situations where power is also required, such as in tackling in rugby and soccer. The stressful nature of this exercise is indicated by the marked exercise-induced increase in blood lactate concentration, which indicates that anaerobic glycolysis is significantly contributing to the supply of energy during this type of exercise. It has been shown that during one 6s cycle ergometer sprint phosphocreatine (PCr) was decreased by 35%, adenosine-triphosphate (ATP) by 9% and glycogen by 14%, whilst muscle lactate was increased from 9 to 29 mM kg^{-1} dry wt (Boobis et al., 1982). If these rates of energy utilization were to continue in multiple sprint exercise it is clear that fatigue could result from both a reduction in energy supply and from acidosis in the muscle cell. In this study power output was relatively well maintained with the 60sR compared to the 30sR. This difference in recovery interval will have at least two effects. The longer 60s recovery will allow a greater resynthesis of PCr (Harris et al., 1976) and will also give more time for the translocation of hydrogen ions (H^+) from the muscle cell to the circulation. It is thought that H^+ causes fatigue either by inhibiting energy provision from anaerobic glycolysis through inhibiting the activity of phosphofructokinase (PFK) or by affecting the contractile mechanism itself (Hermansen, 1981). Therefore, the 60s recovery would allow greater energy provision from PCr and from anaerobic glycolysis. In addition, because of the increased H^+ and lactate efflux between sprints in the 60sR test, it is possible that muscle lactate concentration was lower in the last few sprints of the 60sR test than during the 30sR test. This suggestion is supported by the lower blood lactate concentration found at 5 min post-exercise after the 60sR test in this study. Thus, the inhibition of contractile activity by acidosis would be less in the later sprints of the 60sR test. However, an additional finding in this study is that with both the 30sR and 60sR intervals peak power output was better maintained than mean power ouput and the greatest changes with fatigue were in the ability to maintain power output throughout the 6s, as indicated by the large decreases in end power output. If acidosis was inhibiting the contractile mechanism, then peak and mean power output would be equally affected. As peak power was better maintained, this would suggest that the problem might be one of energy supply or that the site of fatigue lies outside the muscle cell. As it is likely that inhibition of PFK will be overcome by positive modulators of glycolysis during exercise, it is possible that to prevent glycogen depletion, glycolysis is inhibited elsewhere in the pathway such as at the phosphorylase reaction as suggested by McCartney et al. (1986).

In summary, this study has shown that performance during brief duration multiple treadmill sprints is affected both by the recovery interval and by the preceding number of sprints. With the 30s recovery only 5 sprints could be performed before fatigue reduced mean power output, whereas with the 60s recoveory the power output was maintained throughout the test. The larger decrements in performance with the 30s recovery interval may be due to an incomplete resynthesis of PCr and also to greater acidosis, because of the limited time for translocation of H^+ from muscle to blood.

References

Boobis, L.H., Williams, C. and Wootton, S.A. (1982) Human muscle metabolism during brief maximal exercise. J. Physiol., 338, 21-22P.

Cheetham, M.E., Boobis, L.H., Brooks, S. and Williams, C. (1986) Human muscle metabolism during treadmill sprinting. J. Appl. Physiol., 61, 54-60.

Cheetham, M.E. and Williams, C. (1985) Blood pH and blood lactate concentration following maximal treadmill sprinting in man. J. Physiol. Lond., 361, 79P.
Cheetham, M.E., Williams, C. and Lakomy, H.K.A. (1985) A laboratory sprint running test: metabolic responses of sprint and endurance trained athletes. Brit. J. Sports Med., 19, 81-84.
Dotan, R. and Bar-Or, O. (1983) Load optimization for the Wingate Anaerobic Test. Eur. J. Appl. Physiol., 51, 409-417.
Harris, R.C., Edwards, R.H.T., Hultman, E., Nordesjo, L.O., Nylind, A. and Sahlin, K. (1976) The time course of phosphorylcreatine resynthesis during recovery of the quadriceps muscle in man. Pflugers Arch., 367, 137-142.
Hermansen, L. (1981) Effect of metabolic changes on force generation in skeletal muscle during maximal exercise. In: Human Muscle Fatigue: Physiological Mechanisms. (Ciba Foundation Symposium 82) pp. 75-88. London: Pitman Medical.
Lakomy, H.K.A. (1984) An ergometer for measuring the power generated during sprinting. J. Physiol., 354, 33P.
Maughan, R.J. (1982) A simple, rapid method for the determination of glucose, lactate, pyruvate, alanine, 3-hydroxybutyrate and acetoacetate on a single 20 µl blood sample. Clin. Chim. Acta, 122, 231-240.
McCartney, N., Spriet, L.L., Heigenhauser, G.J.F., Kowalchuk, J.M., Sutton, J.R. and Jones, N.L. (1986) Muscle power and metabolism in maximal intermittent exercise. J. Appl. Physiol., 60,1164-1169.
Wootton, S.A. and Williams, C. (1983) The influence of recovery duration on repeated maximal sprints. In: Biochemistry of Exercise. Int. Series on Sports Sciences (edited by H.G. Knuttgen, J.A. Vogel and J.R. Poortmans) pp.234-238, Vol. 13. Champaign, Il: Human Kinetics.

Part V

Fitness test profiles of footballers

BIOLOGICAL PERFORMANCE OF GERMAN SOCCER PLAYERS (PROFESSIONALS AND JUNIORS) TESTED BY SPECIAL ERGOMETRY AND TREADMILL METHODS

P.E. Nowacki, D.Y. Cai, C. Buhl and U.Krümmelbein
Institute of Sports Medicine Justus-Liebig-University Giessen
Kugelberg 62, 6300 Giessen, West Germany.

Introduction

The standard method of determining the physical and cardiorespiratory performance capacities of subjects is bicycle ergometry. Similar to the bicycle ergometer test described by Nowacki (1975) and Nowacki and Schäfer (1984) in which subjects are stressed with work loads proportional to body weight, is a method set up to correlate work load and body weight on the treadmill by changing its speed and slope Nowacki (1983). Furthermore Nowacki and Cai (1986) presented a work load test on the treadmill especially designed to consider the mode of stress of soccer players during training and match-play. Despite the large number of soccer players all over the world, one still has to agree with Bachl and Prokop (1977) that research dealing with performance capacity of professional soccer players is lacking. For the purpose of a detailed investigation several football teams of both amateur and professional leagues have been tested on a bicycle ergometer. The teams included players of the German 1974 World Championship team, the national team players nominated for the 1982 World Championship, and the most successful 1981 German Youth team (European and World Champions). Subsequently, in addition to the bicycle ergometer tests, two selected teams were further subjected to the special treadmill test and the field test.

Methods

Subjects

Following extensive medical and orthopaedic examination (including ECG at rest, lung function, fat determination) soccer players of the 1974 and 1982 German national teams (mean age: 26.6 ± 3.2 years and 25.5 ± 3.1 years respectively), of the A-Youth National team of 1981 (mean age: 17.9 ± 0.3 years), and players of several other teams were tested. The players nominated for the 1982 World Championship trials were tested in 1981.

Bicycle ergometry

Soccer players were uniformly tested on a bicycle ergometer to the point of exhaustion in a sitting position with incremental work rates (1 W kg^{-1} body weight). According to the diagram shown in Fig. 1 it is possible to distinguish between trained and untrained subjects,

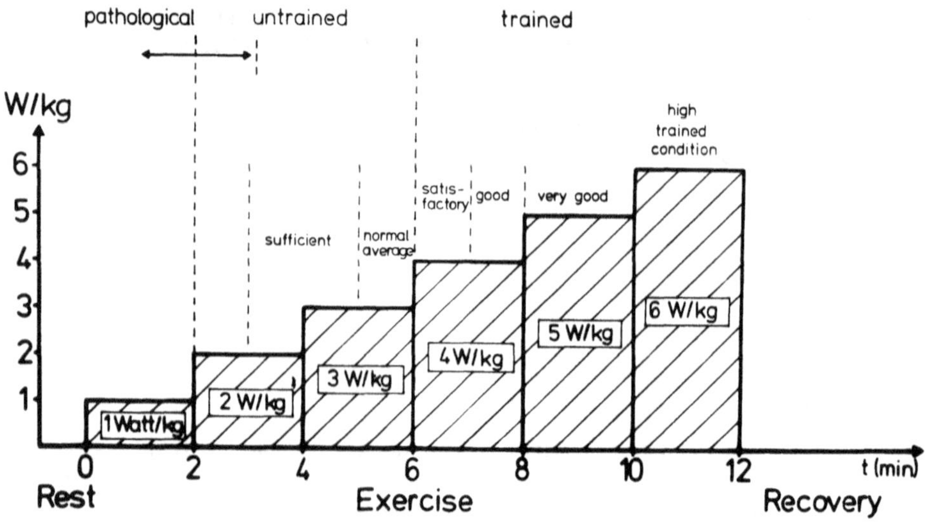

Figure 1. Criteria for evaluation of physical performance capacity following exhaustive bicycle ergometry

and to evaluate their physical performance capacity. The 'Ergotest' electrically braked universal ergometer (E. Jaeger, Wuerzburg, FRG) was used. The physical performance capacity was defined as the total work load ($wmin^{-1}$) attained on the bicycle ergometer

Treadmill
For the first 15 min of the treadmill exercise (illustrated in Fig. 2 and Fig. 3) speed was kept at 9 km h^{-1}, and was then raised to 12 km h^{-1}. Within the first 3 min a slope was set at 0%. The following time was then subdivided into 4 min periods, each period starting with a slope elevated by 2% compared to the preceding one. After 1 min this slope was raised by 4% for another minute, and was then decreased by 2% in the third minute. In the first half of every fourth minute the exercise was interrupted, and blood samples were taken from earlobes to determine lactate concentration: in the second half the work load was adjusted to that of the third minute. By this method the physical performance capacity of subjects can be assessed as follows: reaching just the third 4-min period (speed 9km h^{-1}, slope 10-14%) subjects are considered as satisfactorily trained, entering the fourth 4-min period (speed 12 km h^{-1}, slope 10-14%) subjects can be characterized as well trained, and working longer than 20 min (speed 12 km h^{-1}, slope 15%) on the treadmill, subjects are deemed to be very well trained. The treadmill "Laufergotest" (E.Jaeger, Wuerzburg, (FRG)) was employed.

The heart rate was registered electrocardiographicaly using the tri-recorder 'Cardiomat' (Hellige, Freiburg im Breisgau, FRG) and simultaneously controlled on the screen of single channel oscilloscope made by the same company. Respiratory and metabolic data were continuously registered in an open system, with a pneumotachograph and the complete set of measuring instruments for

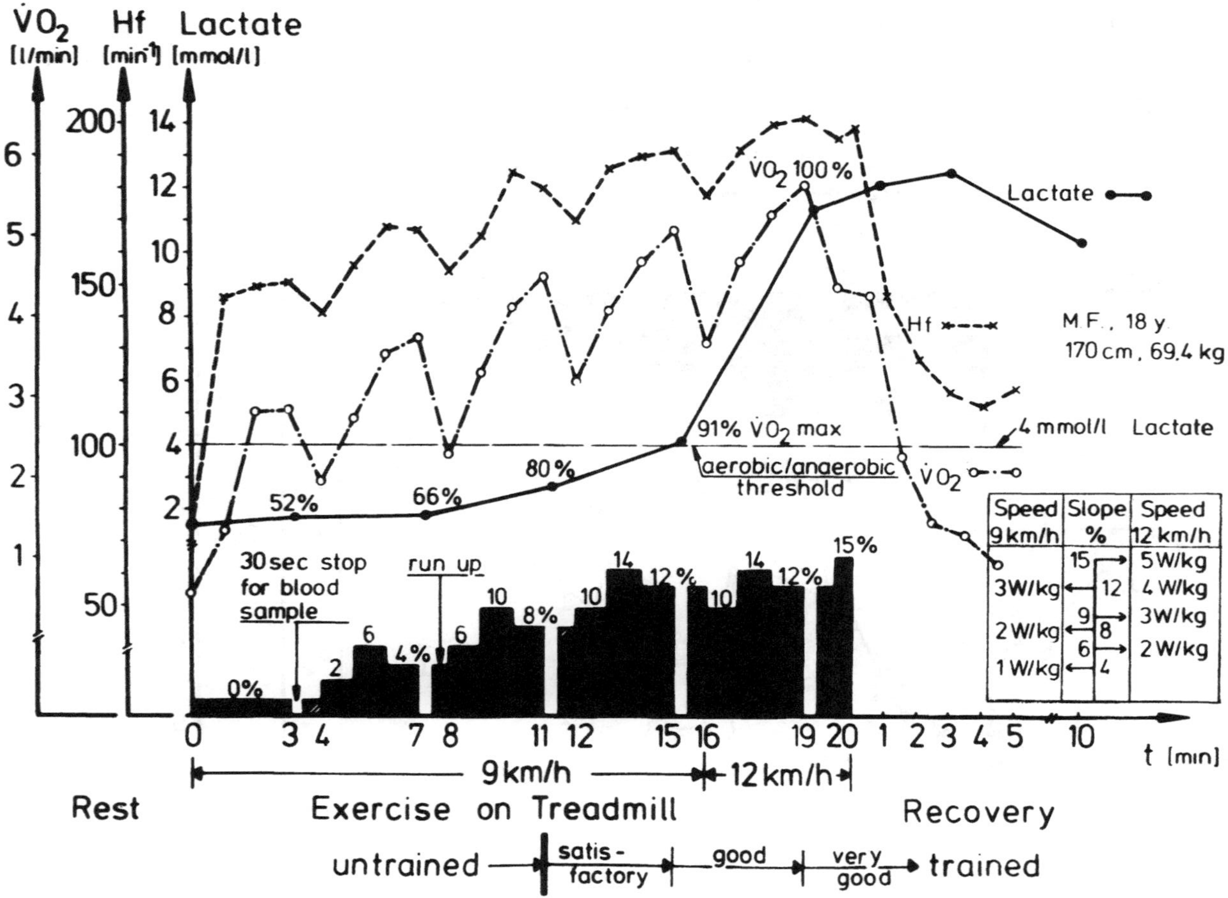

Figure 2. Special treadmill test for football players (soccer) designed by Nowacki, Krümmelbein, Giessen, (FRG), and Cai, Shanghai (PR China)

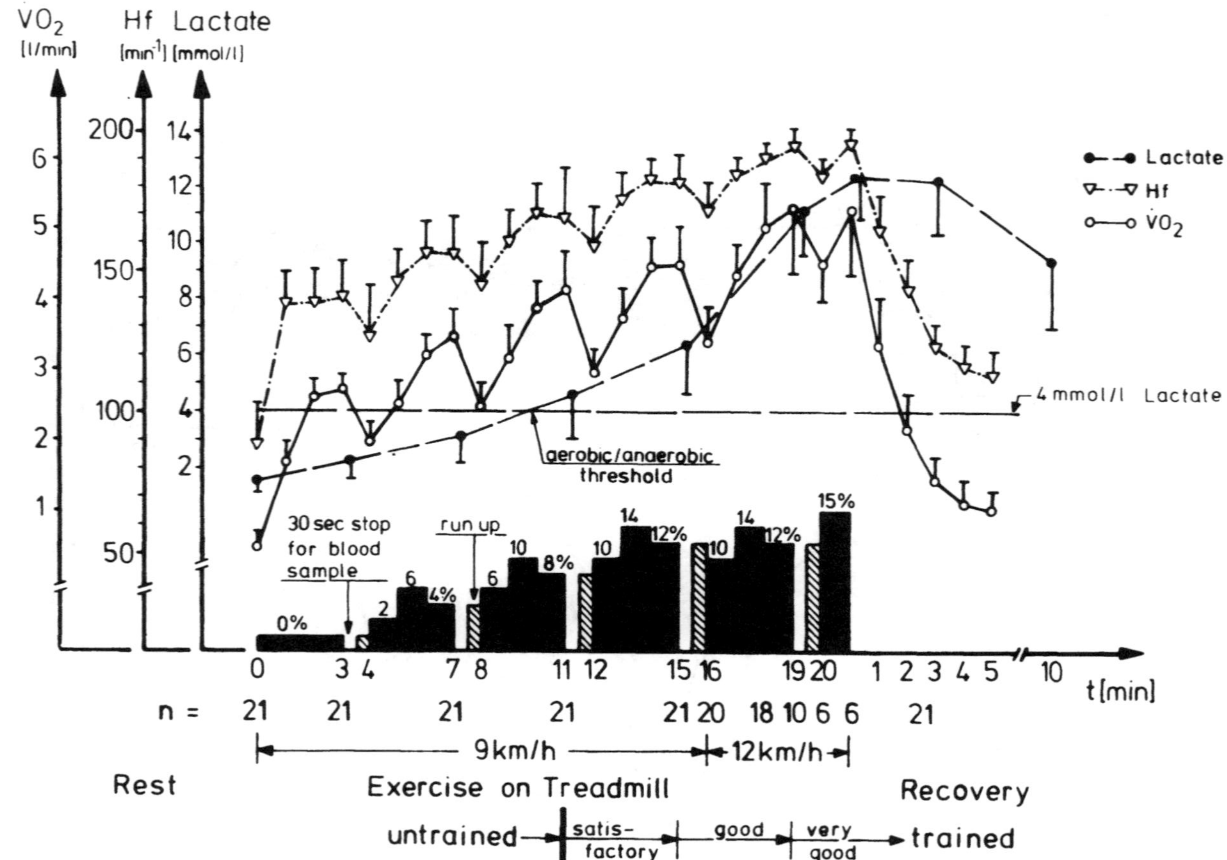

Figure 3. Reaction of the heartbeat frequency and of the oxygen uptake in combination with the lactic acid production of selected players of the A-Youth Team of the Giessen Football Club (VfB) during and following the special treadmill test for football players

cardiorespiratory diagnoses of E. Jaeger, (Wuerzburg, FRG); the data were run through a computer allowing immediate documentation. Analysis of blood lactate concentration was performed by the enzymatic method with a fixed wave length spectrophotometer (Eppendorf Company, Hamburg, FRG).

Field test

After a 3 min warm-up phase, subjects had to carry out a series of special runs which were repeated till exhaustion. The series consists of five different elements: slalom-running (40 s), heading 30 s), running back and forth with the ball (20 s),sprinting without the ball (20 s), and running diagonally to fixed marks (45 s). Between each element there was a 5 s interval, except between the sprinting and diagonal running where a 10 s period was allowed. After the warm-up phase and at the end of each series a 1 min interval was employed (30 s for blood sampling from earlobes to determine lactate concentrations, and palpation of pulse rate and another 30 s for running back to the starting point). From one series to the following either the running distance or the frequency of heading was further extended without changing the times given for each element.

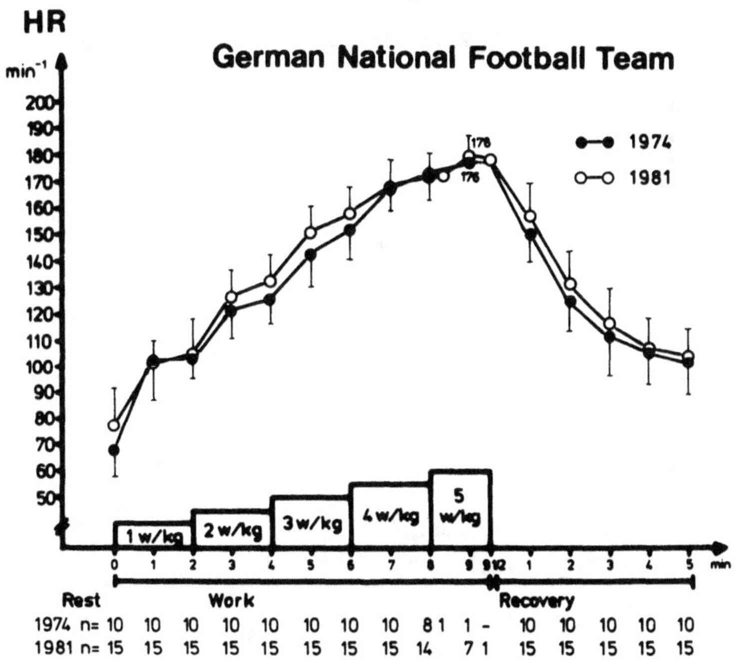

Figure 4. Reaction of the heartbeat frequency of the 1974 World Football Champion and the first runner-up in the 1982 World Championship, the Federal Republic of Germany, during and following exhaustive bicycle-ergometry

Results and Discussion

The physical performance capacity of the players of the 1974 and 1982 German national teams has increased significantly ($P<0.01$) from 1480 ± 221 in 1974 to 1727 ± 197 $wmin^{-1}$ in 1982. According to the criteria for evaluation of the physical performance capacity, in 1974 only one player of the German national team (P. Breitner) could be tested for 1 min at 5 W kg^{-1} but in 1981 seven players of the 1982 German team worked for 1 min at 5 W kg^{-1}, and another one (K.H. Foerster) lasted 1.5 min at the same work level. The captain of the 1982 side (K.H. Rummenige) achieved the highest work total, 1 min at 5 W kg^{-1} corresponding to 400 W.

The cardiac responses of the 1974 and 1982 German national teams were almost identical (Fig. 4) with a maximum heart rate (HR) of 173 (± 7) and 176(± 8) beats min^{-1} respectively. Although these values are fairly low, the players had worked to full capacity, assessed objectively as well as subjectively. Other authors (Schleusing (1965); Bachl and Prokop, (1977)) obtained equally low values when applying exhaustive bicycle ergometry.

Cardiorespiratory performance capacity of the 1974 and 1982 German national soccer teams is shown in the curves representing relative oxygen uptake and oxygen pulse (Fig. 5 and 6). The progression of

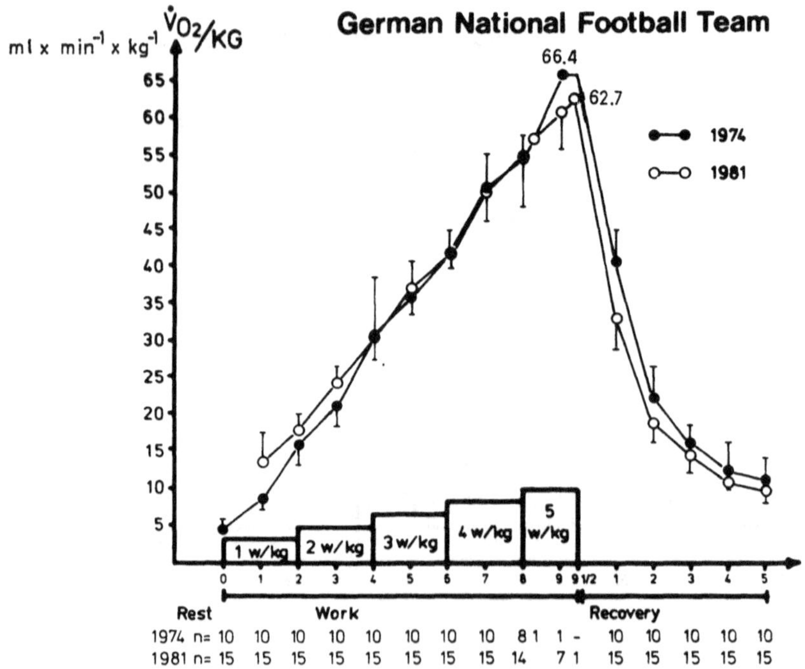

Figure 5. Reaction of the relative oxygen uptake of the 1974 World Football Champion and the first runner-up in the 1982 World Championship, the Federal Republic of Germany, during and following exhaustive bicycle-ergometry

both curves is almost identical at the sub-maximum levels which underlines the high quality of the method of evaluation as well. The somewhat higher values in relative oxygen uptake (ml kg^{-1} min^{-1}) and in oxygen pulse ($\dot{V}O_2$/ HR) in 1981, after the first minute of work, are due to methodological circumstances. In 1974, values at rest were still registered when 'sitting still', whereas in 1981 exercise commenced at 1 W kg^{-1} after a 1-2 min 'period of no-load running'.

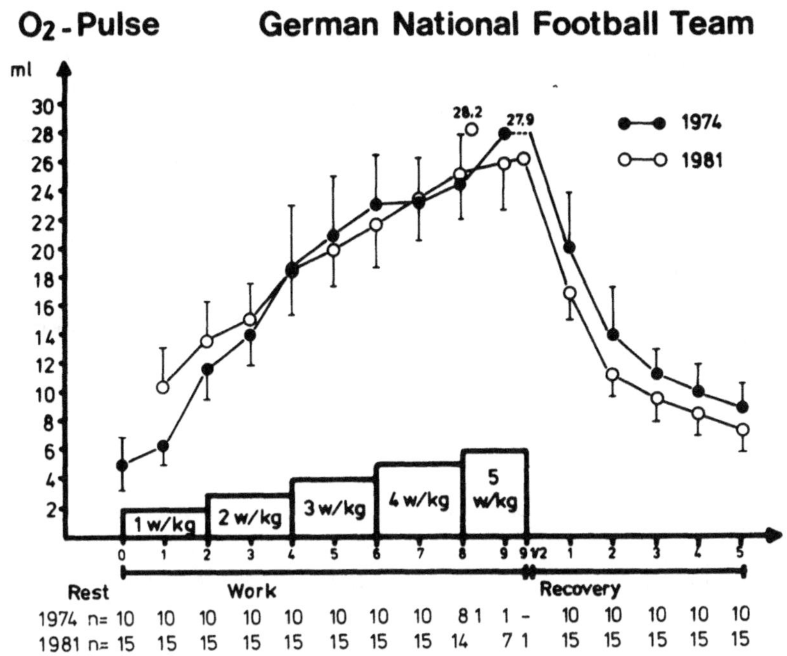

Figure 6. Reaction of the oxygen pulse of the 1974 World Football Champion and the first runner-up of the 1982 World Championship, the Federal Republic of Germany, during and following exhaustive bicycle-ergometry

The modern day game of soccer has produced the 'offensive defence' player. Playing in such a way taxes the physical fitness of these players. In 1974, P. Breitner, left defence, very successfully demonstrated the possibilities of such a way of playing during the World Championship tournament. The biological performance data on this player ($\dot{V}O_2$ max = 66.4 ml kg^{-1} min^{-1}) showed that, at the time, he surpassed the rest of the German team by a substantial margin. It is none the less amazing that when tested for the 1982 World Championship P. Breitner, at that time playing as a central defender, showed an aerobic capacity ($\dot{V}O_2$ max) of 60.7 ml kg^{-1} min^{-1}, which is still above average. A comparison between the maximum biological performance data of the German national teams of 1974 and 1982, and the data of successful German professional and amateur teams (FC Kaiserslautern, Eintracht Frankfurt, Oli.-Bürstadt) revealed that the

Table 1. Maximum relative oxygen uptake and maximum oxygen pulse of several soccer teams tested by Nowacki and coworkers in comparison with values of football players tested by other authors

Authors	Team	n	Mean age (years)	$\dot{V}O_2$ max ($ml\ kg^{-1}\ min^{-1}$)	Maximal O2 pulse ($ml\ beat^{-1}$)	Test mode
Present authors	Third Division Hessen League TSV Battenberg	10	24.3 ± 4.2	69.2 ± 7.8	29.1 ± 2.4	Special tread mill test for footballers
Present authors	A-Youth Hessen League VfB Giessen team	21	16.9 ± 0.7	68.8 ± 7.5	26.1 ± 3.9	Special tread mill test for footballers
Hollmann et al.(1981)	German 1978 National Team	17	26.5 ± 3.8	62.0 ± 4.5	----	Treadmill test
Nowacki and de Castro (1984)	Hessen League VfB Giessen team	17	24.2 ± 5.2	59.8 ± 7.1	23.9 ± 3.0	Treadmill test in relation to body weight
Nowacki and de Castro (1984)	German team 1981/82 World Championship, second place.	15	25.5 ± 3.1	59.5 ± 5.4	26.7 ± 5.4	Bicycle-ergometry
Dickhut et al (1981)	First German National League	14	25.0 ± 3.5	58.4	---- .	Treadmill test
Nowacki and de Castro (1984)	A-Youth National team Europe and World Champion 1981	16	17.9 ± 0.3	58.3 ± 6.9	21.9 +2.5	Bicycle ergometry
Bachl and Prokop (1977)	Austrian National Team 1975	9	24.9 ± 3.5	58.3 ± 4.3	22.7 ± 2.1	Treadmill test in relation to body weight
Nowacki and de Castro (1984)	Schoolboys National Team 1975	16	15.2 ± 0.2	56.7 ± 7.2	19. ± 2.6	Bicycle ergometry
Hollmann et al.(1981)	German 1978 National Team (goal keepers)	4	29.5 ± 3.4	56.2 ± 1.2	----	Treadmill test
Nowacki and de Castro (1984)	German Amateur Champion 1978 Oli.Büstadt	15	26.4 ± 3.8	56.0 ± 5.2	23.0 ± 2.4	Bicycle ergometry
Nowacki et al.(1984a)	First German National League (Bundesliga) Eintracht Frankfurt 1982	14	25.7 ± 5.6	55.9 ± 4.7	23.4 ± 2.1	Bicycle ergometry
Dickhut et al.(1981)	Second German National League	11	25.9 ± 4.±	54.8	----	Bicycle ergometry
Nowacki et al.(1984b)	German National Team World Champion 1974	10	26.6 ± 3.2	54.5 ± 6.8	25.3 ± 3.6	Bicycle ergometry

Nowacki et al.(1984b)	Hessen League VfB Giessen Team	13	24.7 ± 3.3	53.3 ± 9.7	21.0 ± 4.2	Bicycle ergometry
Nowacki et al.(1984a)	First German National League (Bundesliga) 1.FC Kaisers-lautern	20	25.8 ± 3.5	52.7 ± 7.2	22.9 ± 2.5	Bicycle ergometry
Schnabel et al.(1981)	Second German National Liga	17	24.3 ± 4.2	52.1 ± 4.3	23.6 ± 2.3	Treadmill test
Nowacki and de Castro (1984a)	A-Youth Hessen Team 1979	17	16.8 ± 0.2	50.9 ± 7.5	18.9 ± 2.0	Bicycle ergometry
Schnabel et al.(1981)	Amateur Team Regional (Landesauswahl)	13	23.0 ± 2.6	50.0 ±5.7	24.± 1.4	Treadmill
Schnabel et al.(1981)	DFB Youth National Team	17	17.9 ± 0.5	48.7 ± 5.7	20.7 ± 2.4	Treadmill test
Nowacki and de Castro (1984)	C-Youth National Team	23	14.2 ± 0.2	48.4 ± 3.7	15.7 ± 1.6	Bicycle ergometry
Schnabel et al.(1981)	C-Youth Regional (Landesauswahl)	20	14.7 ± 1.0	48.1 ± 4.0	17.4 ± 2.8	Treadmill test
Nowacki and de Castro (1984)	C-Youth Team Londorf-Kessel-1979	12	13.6 ± 0.6	47.8 ± 9.9	11.2 ± 2.3	Bicycle ergometry
Nowacki and de Castro (1984)	B-Youth National Team 1982		17.3 ± 0.2	47.7 ± 4.7	17.9 ± 2.2	Bicycle ergometry
Nowacki and de Castro (1984a)	A-Youth Hessen Team 1974	10	17.3 ± 0.5	46.0 ± 6.8	17.5 ± 2.1	Bicycle ergometry
Nowacki and de Castro (1984)	B-Youth TSG Leihgestern 1979	11	16.0 ± 0.8	45.1 ± 4.4	15.4 ± 2.1	Bicycle ergometry

latter showed results that were only slightly lower than the professionals (Table 1). The same is true for the world's most successful 1981 German Youth team (European and World Champions), which achieved on average a maximum oxygen uptake of 58.3 (± 6.9)ml kg^{-1} min^{-1}. All junior players were members of National League clubs and therefore had already experienced professional training conditions.

Bachl and Prokop (1977) had the same results when comparing Austrian football teams, ranging from minor leagues to First and Second National Leagues and up to the national team. The teams in the higher leagues, displaying almost equal or only slightly superior biological performance data compared to the minor league teams were successful apparently due to better technique and a more economical manner of play, especially during the final phase of a football game.

The comparatively high lactic acid production after the exhaustive test on the bicycle ergometer points towards a well developed anaerobic capacity in soccer players (Fig. 7). On the other hand, players who achieved lower lactate values on the same power output may still have 'reserves'. This assumption might possibly be tested through comparative field studies of football players in training and competition.

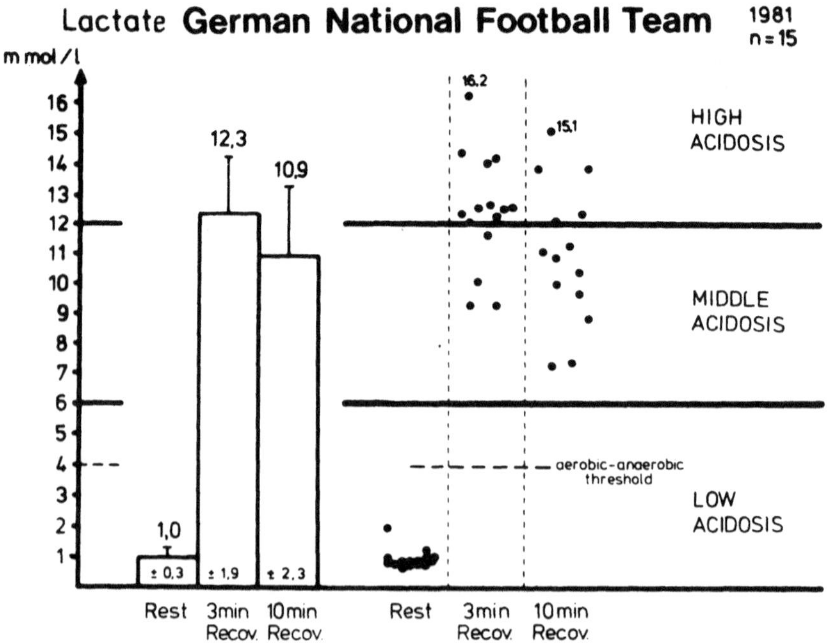

Figure 7. Lactic acid production of the players nominated for the 1982 German National World Championship soccer team at rest and following exhaustive bicycle-ergometry

Oxygen uptake, lactate concentrations, and heart rate data of one player of the A-Youth team of the VfB-Giessen Football Club obtained using the special treadmill test are used as illustration of results in Fig. 2. In the nineteenth minute a heart rate of 202 beats min^{-1} was measured, and the oxygen uptake reached its maximum value of 5.579 l min^{-1} (referred to as 100%). At the beginning of each 4 min period oxygen uptake was measured to be at 52%, 66%, 80% and 91% (periods 1-4). At the end of each 4 min period (exactly between 3 and 3.5 min of each period) lactate concentrations were found to be 1.9, 1.95, 2.3, 4.1 and 11.7 mM respectively.

Similar results were observed in the 21 selected players of the same team. The heart rate reached maximum values of 196 (± 4) beats min^{-1} and the maximum oxygen uptake was measured at 5.28 (+ 0.92) min^{-1} (Fig. 3).

The regular change of work rate caused the increase in the amount of oxygen needed by the muscles, because the cardiorespiratory system and muscles must adapt their function from time to time to suit the change in the work rate. Therefore, the actual work rate in this special test is a little higher than that usually noted in standard tests. However, this special test can be recommended to measure the physical capacity of those subjects, such as ball players, who engage in irregular work bouts. In these kinds of sports the work load changes in an irregular fashion throughout the whole game.

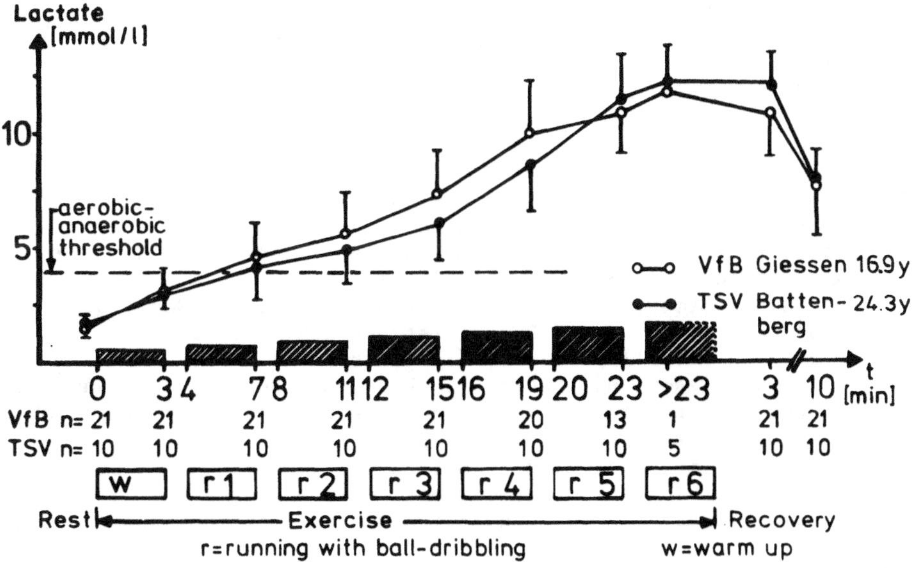

Figure 8. Reaction of the lactic acid production of selected players of the A-Youth Team of the Giessen Football Club (VfB) and the Third Division Battenberg Amateur Club (TSV) at rest, during the following special field test.

Fig. 8 illustrates the progressive rise of lactate concentrations in selected soccer players (n = 21, and n = 10, respectively) of the A-Youth Team of the Giessen Football Club (VfB) and the Third Division Battenberg Amateur Club (TSV) stressed under field test conditions. Already within the first series of the five different forms of runs, the lactate levels of both teams passed the so-called 'aerobic-anaerobic' threshold to reach the maximum values of 10.8 (± 1.9)mM (VfB), and of 12.0 (± 1.4)mM (TSV) (3rd min of recovery). In comparison to the special treadmill test, where the 'aerobic-anaerobic' threshold was surpassed after 15 min, blood lactate concentratins of football players stressed in the field test passed this threshold before 7 min. Heading and sprinting seem to be possible explanations for this phenomenon. Whether field tests can substitute for laboratory investigations is a matter for further investigation. Comparison with other data reports can establish that the cardiorespiratory performance capacity of soccer players has reached a higher stage of development than can be observed in other kinds of ball-game sports. Nowacki (1971) reported a maximum oxygen uptake of 52.5 (± 7.8)ml kg^{-1} min^{-1} when applying the same testing method to the 1978 World Champion handball team (FRG Team), 49.4 (± 7.9)ml kg min^{-1} when testing a National League ice hockey team, and 48.7 (± 6.5)ml kg^{-1} min^{-1} when testing the 1982 German volleyball champions, USC Giessen. A further increase in the aerobic capacity of soccer players up to the level of top rowers (70 ml kg^{-1} min^{-1}) or even to the level of cross-country skiers (85-90 ml kg^{-1} min^{-1}) is hardly necessary since such an extreme development in endurance capacity is likely to lead to deficiencies in other areas, such as speed and technique.

References

Bachl, N. and Prokop, L. (1977) Wie gut trainiert sind österreichische Fussballer? Leistungsdiagnostische Standortbestimmung aus der Sicht des Sportphysiologen. Österr. J. Sportmed., 7, 3-10.

Dickhut, H.H., Simon, G., Bachl., N., Lehmann, M., and Keul, J. (1981) Zur Höchst - und Dauerleistungsfähigkeit von Bundesligafussballspielern. Leistungssport, 11, 148-152.

Hollmann, W., Liesen, H., Mader, A., Heck, H., Rost, R., Dufaux, B., Schürch, P., Lagerström, D., and Föhrenbach, R.(1981) Zur Höchst- und Dauerleistungsfähigkeit der deutschen Fussball-Spitzenspieler. Dtsch. Z. Sportmed., 32, 113-120.

Nowacki, P.E. (1971) Die Spiroergometrie im neuen Untersuchungssystem für den Spitzensport. Leistungssport, 2, 37-51.

Nowacki, P.E. (1975) Möglichkeiten der medizinischen Leistungsdiagnostik In: DSB: Bundesausschuss Leistungssport. Information zum Training. Medizinische Betreuung des Leistungssportlers in Training und Wettkampf Beiheft zu Leistungssport, 3, 77-119.

Nowacki, P.E.(1983) Zur Standardisierung der Laufbandspiroergometrie. In: H. Mellerowicz and I.W. Franz, (Editors): Standardisierung, Kalibrierung und Methodik in der Ergometrie. Perimed-Verlag, Erlangen, 259-278.

Nowacki, P.E. and Cai, D.Y.(1986) A new protocol for ergometric treadmill tests. In: Abstracts: The XXIII FIMS World Congress of Sports Medicine Brisbane, Australia, 20-28 Sept., (edited by V Kippers. A.W. Parker, and N.C. Wilson) p.201.

Nowacki, P.E. and de Castro, P.(1984) Development of the Biological Performance of German National Football Teams (FRG, Juniors and Professionals) In: Current Topics in Sports Medicine. Proceedings of the World Congress of Sports Medicine, Vienna 1982 (edited by N. Bachl, L. Prokop and R. Suckert) pp. 560-575, Wien, München, Baltimore: Urban and Schwarzenberg-Verlag.

Nowacki, P.E. and Schäfer, D.(1984) Die physical working capacity (PWC_{170}) bei körpergewichtsbezogener Ausbelastung auf dem Fahrradergometer und ihre Bedeutung als Leistungsparameter in Abhängigkeit von Alter, Geschlecht und Sportart. Therapiewoche, 34, 3835-3853.

Nowacki, P.E., Hafermann, P. and Psiorz, J.(1984) Sportmedizinisches Leistungsprofil einer Bundesliga-Fussballmannschaft. Therapiewoche, 34, 3893-3903.

Nowacki, P.E., Hafermann, P. and Psiorz, J.H. (1984) Entwicklung des biologischen Leistungsprofils der Deutschen Fussballmannschaften, 1974-1982. In: Stellenwert der Sportmedizin in Medizin und Sportmedizin 2. Symposium der Sektion "Sportmedizinische Forschung und Lehre an den Hochschen" des Deutschen Sportärztebundes (Deutsche Gesellschaft für Sportmedizin e.V.) Tübingen, 5-8, Mai 1983 (edited by D. Jeschke) pp. 596-603, Berlin, Heidelberg, New York, Tokyo: Springer-Verlag.

Schleusing, G. (1965) Trainingsanpassungserscheinungen von Herz und Kreislauf bei Fussball - und Handballspielern im Vergleich zu anderen Sportarten, Medizin und Sport, 5, 101-104 .

Schnabel, A., Kindermann, W. and Schmitt W.M. (1981) Aerobe Kapazität von Fussballspielern unterschiedlicher Spielstärke. Dtsch. Z. Sportmed., 32, 120-127.

DEFINITION OF THE PHYSIOLOGICAL PROFILE OF THE SOCCER PLAYER

M. Faina, C. Gallozzi, S. Lupo, R. Colli, R. Sassi,* C. Marini,
Institute of Sports Science, Department of Physiology and Biomechanics, Italian Olympic Committee, Via dei Campi Sportivi 46, Rome 00197, Italy.
*Lazio Sports Association.

Introduction

Soccer is a sport where all too often attention is focussed almost exclusively on technical and tactical aspects to the relative neglect of physiological factors. Organic function as a component of fitness surely plays a major role in sports performance and, in this respect, the physical conditioning of players should no longer be reported as a minor factor.

Soccer, like many other team sports, features a sequence of stages involving anaerobic demands as well as others involving aerobic demands. Indeed such an alternation has given rise to some confusion concerning many aspects related to performance. for example the type of 'endurance' needed for the game. Endurance in soccer is sometime interpreted as depending, fundamentally, on anaerobic performance capabilities (that is, the capability of repeating the effort which is always at high intensity). Alternatively, the type of endurance required for the game is regarded as that typically involving 'long duration' exercise, having merely aerobic characteristics and a training methodology where great importance is attached to workloads which are uniform and not too intense.

The data relating to maximal aerobic power of soccer players ($\dot{V}O_2max$) reported in the literature (Berg et al., 1985; Caru et al., 1980; Ekblom, 1986; Luhtanen, 1980: Rost and HolLmann, 1983) generally indicate values ranging from 55 to 60 ml $kg^{-1}min^{-1}$. On the other hand, there are few data available (Luhtanen, 1980) concerning fast contraction characteristics of the leg extensor muscles (explosive strength), these being an indication of the qualities of muscular elasticity in the major muscular group involved in the game. It should be remembered that in the counter-movement vertical jump test (Bosco, 1985), the jump effectiveness (height) depends on the explosive strength of the subject, and his coordination capabilities in addition to his muscle elasticity.

The alactacid anaerobic power of players determined using the stair run test of Margaria et al. (1966) and examined by both Luhtanen (1980) and Smaros (1980), reached fairly good levels. Furthermore, the study carried out by Oberg et al. (1984) on the dynamic strength of quadriceps muscles of soccer players are of interest. This study, which employed an isokinetic dynamometer, showed that in top level soccer players, the ratio between the strength developed at a higher speed of contraction (4.19 rad s^{-1}) and that developed at a lower speed (1.05 rad s^{-1}) was better than that observed in players at a lower level.

Therefore, according to the reports reviewed, it would seem that top players have a fast muscle contraction capability, a good anaerobic power and an above average level aerobic power.

To evaluate the demands of play, the easiest detectable parameters during a match are blood lactate and heart rate (HR). In a Swedish study (Ekblom, 1986) the HR was observed during a soccer match and while it showed an intermittent trend, it tended to stay on at a relatively high level. In this connection, it should be pointed out that play and recovery periods in soccer are generally short: this explains the intermittent trend of the HR and the high to medium levels of work intensity recorded.

Moreover, Ekblom (1986) noted a significantly higher blood lactate in A-Division matches compared to matches played in lower divisions. This suggests that one qualifying factor for soccer players is not so much the quantity of work performed (total distance covered) as the intensity with which it is carried out.

In the Department of Physiology and Biomechanics of the Institute of Sports Science (Rome), soccer has been studied for some time by following a working schedule which includes, eventually, the application of training methodologies, the aim of which is to develop specific functional capabilities. In order to outline the working schedule, an analysis of the physiological characteristics of the player and play itself was first established.

Material and Methods

Altogether 17 amateur (age 22 ± 4.1 years, height cm 178.5 ± 5.9cm, weight 72.1 ± 8 kg) and 27 professional (age 26 ± 4.8 years, height 177.2 ± 4.5 years, weight 74. 4 ± 5.8 years) soccer players, were examined. Furthermore a top level athlete (considered by the press in the last World Cup as one of the world's best players) has been evaluated to point out his physical characteristics compared to the average values of those of the amateur and professional groups. They were subjected to treadmill ergometry, a series of jump tests and measurement of isometric leg strength.

The following tests were included:

i) Treadmill test : (6 amateurs, 27 professionals and 1 top level) to detect the maximum aerobic power; the running speed on the level-treadmill (Laufergotest, Jaeger) was increased by 2 km h^{-1} every 2 min to exhaustion. During the test the heart rate (HR) was recorded and respiratory gases were analyzed by means of an automatic system (Dataspir, Jaeger).

ii) Jump test: (17 amateurs, 17 professionals and 1 top level) the test was performed by using a conductance board connected to an electronic clock (Ergo jump; Bosco, 1985), which enabled the measurement of the contact and flight time of one or more consecutive jumps.
The test involves the measurement of the displacement of the centre of gravity of the athlete in three different jump attempts. These are:

a) Squat jump (SJ): vertical jump from a squatting position with hands placed on hips; this performance is carried out by using mainly the contractile components of the leg extensor muscles;

b)Counter-movement jump (CMJ): the vertical jump is preceded by a counter movement at the bottom (stretch-shortening muscle cycle); during this performance the contractile, elastic and coordination components contribute to a succesful jump. From the CMJ-SJ ratio the elasticity coefficient is thus obtained, this being the percentage increase of the jumping capability caused by the intervention of elastic energy;

c) Drop jump (DJ): vertical jump following a fall from a bench of variable height (40-60 cm); in this instance, the performance is mainly subject to the elastic reactive component of the muscle groups.

iii) Ergo jump 15 s: (17 amateurs, 17 professionals and 1 top level) the test consists of a series of counter movement jumps without any interruption for 15 s; the average height reached when jumping, the work and power output were calculated. The test is an indication of the power of the athlete's alactacid anaerobic mechanism, this being expressed in relation to body weight (W kg^{-1}).

iv) Leg extensor strength: (6 amateurs, 17 professionals and 1 top level) an electronic isometric dynamometer (MK7; Dal Monte, 1987) was used; the parameter is indicated as maximal strength relative to body weight (N kg^{-1}).

In order to indirectly evaluate the energy used during competition, a filmed analysis of play and recovery periods in a set of matches played during the 1986 world championships was eventually performed.

Results

The amateur soccer players examined on average showed a maximum oxygen uptake of 64.1 (± 7.2) ml kg^{-1} min^{-1}. In the professionals the mean value was 58.94 (± 6.13) ml kg^{-1} min. This difference did not reach statistical significance ($0.05 < P < 0.10$). Analysis amounting to the positional roles showed that the aerobic power was highest in midfield players (61.18 ± 7.85), then defenders (58.95 ± 5.61) and, finally, forward players (5.41 ± 3.85). Statistically, these latter differences were not significant ($P > 0.10$). The VO_2max of the top level player was 63.2 ml kg^{-1} min^{-1}.

Table 1. Muscle power characteristics in the amateur and and professional players (mean ± SD) and 1 top level player

Squat jump (cm)	34.2 ± 4.0	40.4 ± 5.2	35
CMJ (cm)	36.9 ± 4.8	43.5 ± 4.9	48
Drop Jump (cm)	33.7 ± 4.4	42.2 ± 6.5	35
CMJ-SJ ratio(%)	7.87	7.6	34
Ergo 15 (W kg^{-1})	24.1 ± 3.6	25.1 ± 2.5	25.2

The muscular power values measured in amateurs, professionals and 1 top level are presented in Table 1. Statistically, all the differences between the two groups proved to be highly significant ($P < 0.005$), except the elasticity (CMJ - SJ Ratio) and alactacid anaerobic power (Ergo 15s) parameters.

The relative strength ratio measured in amateurs was 43.36 (±4.61) N kg^{-1} whereas in professionals the mean value was 40.61(±3.43), N kg^{-1}. This difference was without any statistical significance ($P > 0.10$). The relative strength of the top level player was 48.66 N kg^{-1}.

In the filmed analysis of play periods in matches played during the world championships, it was observed (Fig.1) that 51% of the actions lasted 20 s or less. Very few actions lasted more than 60 s. In addition, it is most interesting to note that recovery periods, although these refer to the whole team and not to individual players, are even shorter than the duration of the actions themselves.

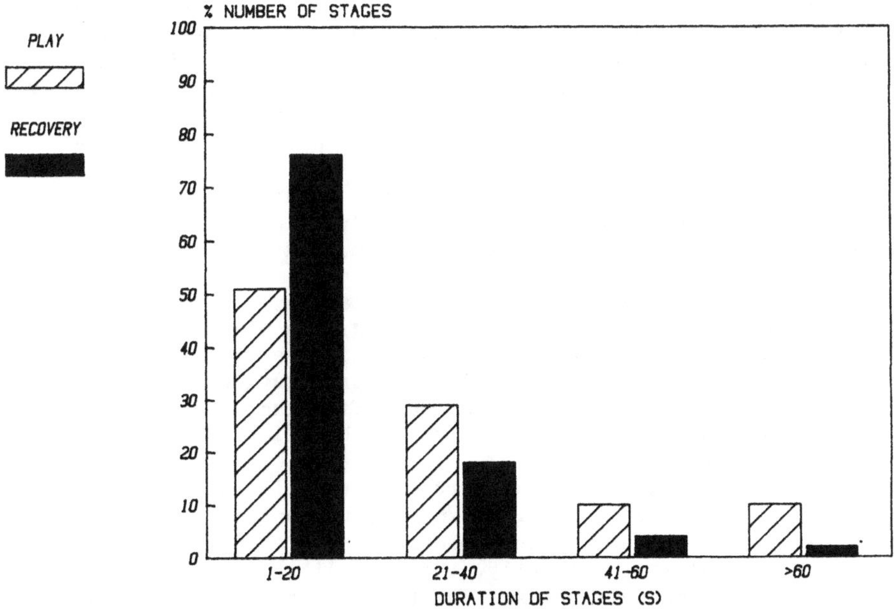

Figure 1. Play and recovery stages in professional soccer. The hatched columns represent the percentage of playing actions. The black columns represent the percentage of recovery stages. The playing and recovery stages are divided by their time of duration

Discussion

The soccer players examined in this study both amateurs as well as professionals, had aerobic power values slightly higher than those of sprinters (52 ml kg^{-1} min^{-1}) (Bosco, 1985) and slightly lower than the average of 366 athletes (61.8 ml kg^{-1} min^{-1}) evaulated in 1986 in our Institute. The population of these athletes was formed in a thorough heterogenous fashion from team games athletes, long distance runners and sprinters, of average and top level abilities.

Differences were more marked when comparison was made between the footballers' aerobic power and the one of long distance athletes who had higher values (85 ml kg^{-1} min^{-1}) (Åstrand and Rodahl, 1970). The comparison with the sedentary group gave lower values (44 ml kg^{-1} min^{-1}).

It is interesting to note that amateur soccer players had a higher aerobic power than professionals. It was also noted, in confirmation of the widespread idea of 'global play', that there were not any significant differences among the various positional roles, even though midfield players showed a higher aerobic power than the players. The top level player showed an aerobic power about the average of professional players.

The explosive muscular power of soccer players, both amateurs and professionals, was found to be slightly lower than that of typical power-performance athletes (32 W kg^{-1}), yet clearly higher than that of endurance athletes (23 W kg^{-1}) (Bosco, 1985). The values measured in the professionals was clearly better than those measured in amateurs. It seems that professionals have a greater explosive muscular power and this parameter, as opposed to aerobic power, seems to discriminate between the playing levels. This is in agreement with findings of Oberg et al. (1984) for dynamic strength. The alactacid anaerobic power followed the same pattern although in this case it was not statistically discriminating.

The strength test showed that soccer players, both amateurs and professionals, are not particularly strong. As yet, we are unable to state whether this is a correct physiological profile of the soccer player or whether it is due to a lack of preparation in this respect. Nevertheless it could be indicative that the top level soccer player had a coefficient of strength ratio (RS) higher than the other players.

The overall observations, supported by the literature, underlines the image of the soccer player as an athlete endowed with great qualities of muscular power and able to supply energy through anaerobic metabolism. Generally, these qualities are followed by an average level of aerobic power. The top soccer player in this study showed an aerobic power not particularly high, a good alactacid anaerobic power, a satisfactory value of strength ratio. Finally, he exhibited excellent explosive strength in the leg muscles, associated with an elasticity and coordination coefficient which were just as good.

Results suggest that the physiological preparation for soccer must be structured in such a way as to enable the player to develop and then to keep intact, during the season, these fundamental muscular qualities rather than provide him with a guarantee to sustain medium to low intensity exercise for a long time.

The recommendations for soccer arising from this research are as follows:

i) it is necessary to have and develop a good (possibly excellent) power and capability of fast muscular activation;

ii) aerobic power is not necessarily a factor limiting the performance nor should a higher value be a crucial criticism in the selection of talent; however, it is important that it be adequately developed through a proper modulation of training loads;

iii) endurance training must be aimed at developing a prompt recovery during competition of muscular function;

iv) in order to develop soccer specific endurance, the application of training methodologies that include administration of intense and repeated loads is appropriate:

v) long duration and low to medium intensity endurance training should be avoided, as this does not stimulate the fundamental qualities required for the game.

References

Åstrand, P.O. and Rodhal, K. (1970) Textbook of Work Physiology. New York: McGraw Hill.

Berg, K.E., La Voie, J.C. and Latin, R.W. (1985) Physiological training effects of playing youth soccer. Med. Sci. Sports and Exerc., 17, 656-660.

Bosco, C. (1985) Elasticita e forza esplosiva negli sport di potenza. Roma, Sss.

Caru, B., Le Coultre, L., Aerhema, P., and Pinera Limas, F. (1970) Maximal aerobic and anaerobic muscular power in football players. J. Sports Med. and Phys. Fit., 10, 100-103.

Dal Monte A. (1983) La Valutazione Funzionale dell'Atleta' Firenze: Sansoni.

Ekblom, B. (1986) Applied physiology of soccer. Sports Med., 3, 1, 50-60.

Luhtanen, P., (1980) A longitudinal physiological, technical and tactical evaluation of football. In: Proceedings First International Congress on Sports Medicine Applied to Football. Rome: Don Guanella.

Lupo, S. and Dal Monte, A. (1987) Primi risultati ottenuticon il nuovo dinamometzo isometrics MK7 nella velutazione delle forza negli etlets (in press).

Margaria, R., Aghemo, P. and Rovelli, E. (1966) Measurement of muscular power (anaerobic) in man. J. Appl. Physiol., 21, 1662-1664

Oberg, B., Gillquist, J., Moller, M. and Ekstrand, J. (1984) Isokinetic torque levels for knee extensors and knee flexors in soccer players. Int. J. Sports Med., 5, 50-53.

Rost, R. and Hollmann, W. (1983) Athlete's heart, a review of its historical assessments and new aspects. Int. J. Sports Med., 147-165

Smaros, G. (1980) Energy usage during football matches. In: First International Congress of Sports Medicine Applied to Football. Rome: Don Guanella.

PRE-SEASON FITNESS PROFILES OF PROFESSIONAL SOCCER PLAYERS

J.E. White, T.M. Emery, J.E. Kane, R. Groves and A.B. Risman
Department of Human and Environmental Sciences, West London Institute of Higher Education, Borough Road, Isleworth, Middlesex TW7 5DU, England.

Introduction

The sport of soccer has not been studied extensively by sports scientists although reviews of the various demands of the game have been documented (Reilly, 1979; Kirkendall, 1985; Ekblom, 1986; Reilly, 1986). Furthermore, with the exception of longitudinal studies during the competitive season (Thomas and Reilly, 1979; Reilly and Thomas, 1980) and the influence of pre-season training upon fitness levels in soccer players (Reilly and Thomas, 1977a), little attention has been devoted to the fitness status of professional soccer players during the period between competitive seasons of play. Notwithstanding the difficulties of assessing sports-related fitness in general and soccer fitness in particular (Reilly and Thomas, 1977b), this study attempted to determine a profile of pre-season fitness in professional soccer players using selected variables relevant to the fitness demands of the competitive season.

Methods

Seventeen professional soccer players constituting the first team squad of a prestigous First Division club were included in the study which was conducted two or three weeks prior to the start of the English Football League season. The descriptive data of the subjects are outlined in Table 1.

A series of fitness related evaluations was undertaken following habituation to the exercise laboratory and the procedures for assessment. Body composition estimates were determined from the sum of four skinfold measures (Durnin and Womersley, 1974), body mass index from the ratio weight/height^2 (Garrow, 1983) and physique from somatotype ratings (Heath and Carter, 1967). Physical performance measures included:- explosive leg strength calculated from vertical jump and reach scores using the Lewis nomogram (Mathews and Fox, 1976), absolute and relative power using the Margaria-Kalamen stair run test (Margaria et al., 1966; Kalamen, 1968) and agility using the Illinois agility run test (Cureton, 1970).

Physiological measures included the determination of maximal aerobic and anaerobic work indices during continuous, incremental exercise to voluntary exhaustion on a bicycle ergometer. Following a

Table 1. Characteristics of the first team squad of professional soccer players (n = 17)

Variables	Mean	±	SE
Age (Yrs)	23.3	±	0.9
Height (cms)	180.4	±	1.7
Weight (kg)	76.7	±	1.5
Body Mass Index (W/Ht^2)	23.6	±	0.4
Body Fat Estimate (%)	19.3	±	0.6
Endomorphy	2.6	±	0.2
Mesomorphy	4.2	±	0.2
Ectomorphy	2.7	±	0.2

standardised 5 min warm-up exercise at 2.0 kp and 60 rev min^{-1}, subjects performed 2 min work increments of 0.5 kp at the same pedalling frequency until standardised maximal aerobic power criteria had been achieved (B.A.S.S., 1986). Cardiorespiratory measures were obtained using standardised ECG and automated expired air analysis (Contronic 200 MGA - mass spectrometer), and earlobe mixed arteriovenous blood samples were taken, for subsequent determination of lactate using an enzymatic method (Analox LM2). All assessments were made during the period of pre-season training approximately two to three weeks prior to the start of the regular competitive season. Training schedules were monitored during this same period for a representative one week duration.

Results

Body composition measures revealed elevated estimates of percent body fat along with body mass index scores. Somatotype ratings indicated relatively low endomorphy and ectomorphy with moderate mesomorphy levels (Table 1).

Cardiorespiratory and blood lactate responses to graded, incremental exercise are presented in Figure 1. Linear trends observed in heart rate and oxygen consumption were matched by a curvilinear blood lactate response to incremental increases in work load. Peak heart rate, oxygen consumption and lactate values were observed following an average of 15 min of exercise which corresponded to an average work load of 5.75 kp (Table 2). The lactate "threshold" value of 4.0 mM was achieved after 9.5 min exercise and corresponded to approximately 87% maximal heart rate and 77% maximal oxygen consumption values.

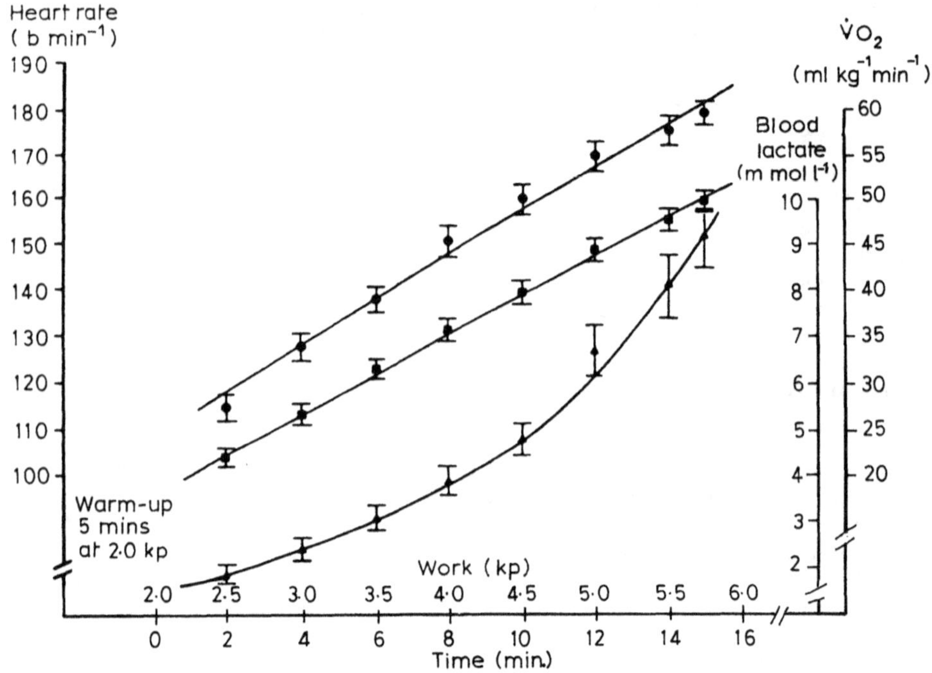

Figure 1. Heart rate, $\dot{V}O_2$ and blood lactate responses to a graded incremental exercise test

Table 2. Cardiorespiratory and anaerobic capacities of the first team squad of professional soccer players N = 17)

Variables	Mean	±	SE
Heart rate max (beats min^{-1})	179.2	±	2.4
$\dot{V}O_2max$ (ml kg^{-1} min^{-1})	49.6	±	1.2
Time to exhaustion (min)	15.0	±	0.5
Maximal work load (kp)	5.75	±	0.13
Time to 4 mM La (min)	9.5	±	0.75
Blood La at exhaustion (mM)	9.10	±	0.64
Heart rate (beats min^{-1})	155.5	±	3.3
% HRmax at 4 mM La.	86.9%	±	1.8%
$\dot{V}O_2$ (ml kg^{-1} min^{-1}) at 4 mM La	37.5	±	1.2
%$\dot{V}O_2$max at 4mM La	77.1%	±	3.3%

Physical performance measures are presented in Table 3. Explosive leg strength, determined from vertical jump height together with anaerobic power, derived from the stair run test, showed moderate levels, whilst agility run times were unexceptional.

Table 3. Performance characteristics of the first team squad of professional soccer players (N = 17)

Variables	Mean	±	SE
Explosive leg strength ($kgm\ s^{-1}$)	131.8	±	3.3
Vertical jump height (cm)	59.8	±	1.3
Anaerobic power ($kgm\ s^{-1}$)	204.8	±	4.5
(Stair run) ($kgm\ kg^{-1}\ s^{-1}$)	2.6	±	0.1
Agility run (s) (Illinois test)	16.4	±	0.1

Table 4. Pattern of pre-season training schedule of the first team squad of professional soccer players

Days	Game-Related Training (min)	Fitness/Conditioning (min)
Monday	75.00	115.00
Tuesday	85.00	65.00
Wednesday	Recreational Activities (Golf)	
Thursday	90.00	105.00
Friday	Game Preparations	
Saturday	Game Day	
Sunday	Free Day	
Totals (min) (535.00 min 8h 55min)	250.00 (4h 10min)	285.00 (4h 45min)
Proportions (%)	46.7%	53.3%

Analysis of the weekly training schedules utilised during the pre-season training period revealed that an average player's training was concentrated into three days per week. It consisted of approximately three hours per day, with one recreational day and one day devoted to the competitive game (Table 4). The distribution of training activities indicated that the time devoted specifically to 'fitness related' and 'game related' training practices was approximately 53% and 47% respectively.

Discussion

Anthropometric results indicated that this particular group of professional soccer players was not readily distinguished by general physique characteristics. Body mass index (23.5) was within the normal limits (Garrow, 1983) but located toward the upper end of the normal range (20-25). Although caution should be exerted in interpretation of B.M.I. in athletic populations with elevated muscle mass, the mesomorphic ratings of this particular group show they were outside this category. The estimated percentage of body fat (19.3%) was considerably higher than that reported by Reilly (1979) in other studies which document a range of 10-16% even though players with comparable height and weights were investigated. Notwithstanding the recent criticism of the use of skinfold measures in the estimation of body fat (Clarys, 1987), the sum of four skinfold sites measured (29.8 mm) would indicate excess superficial adipose tissue stores.

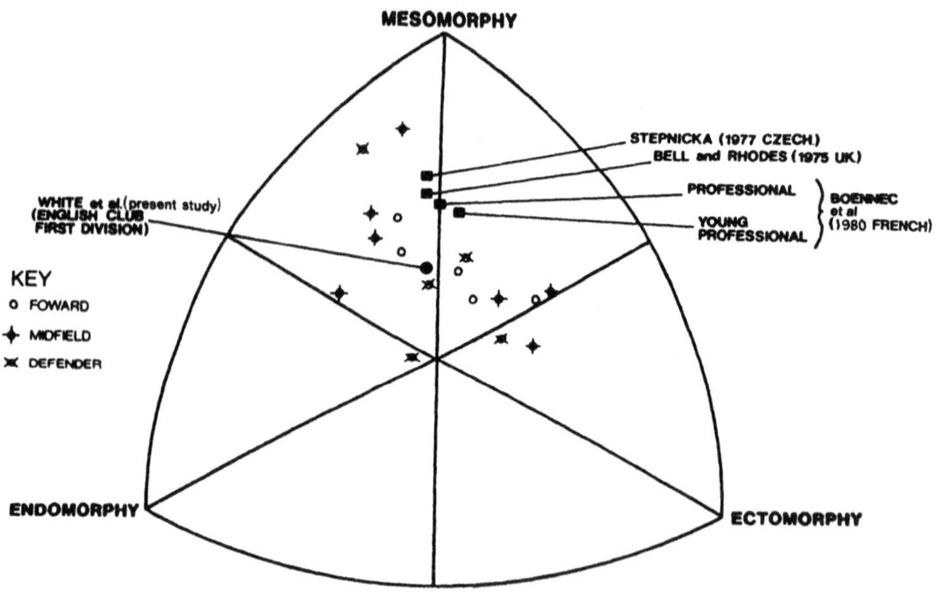

Figure 2. Somatotype of professional soccer players

The somatotype distribution of the group as well as individual players is presented in Figure 2, and comparisons with other studies of professional soccer players is readily apparent. While the somatotype of English College players has been reported to vary around 3:5:2.5 (Bell and Rhodes, 1975), the present group with a somatotype of 2.6:4.2:2.7, showed lower mesomorphy estimates than those in other studies, and, both as a group as well as individually, deviate considerably from the somatochart area associated with European professional soccer players (Boennec et al., 1980; Stepnicka, 1977). Furthermore, there was no readily discernable clustering of players into somatoplot distributions associated with positional roles of forwards, midfield players and defenders and only the goalkeeper was identified as an 'outlier.'

Physiological responses to exercise showed comparable levels of maximal heart rates to those reported by Reilly (1979) in other studies, although the mean maximal oxygen uptake value of 49.6 ml kg^{-1} min^{-1} was considerably below the range 56-66 ml kg^{-1} min^{-1} reported in various groups of professional soccer players (Reilly, 1979). Indeed the expected levels among top class international players of 60-65 ml kg^{-1} min^{-1}, with some individuals above 70 ml kg^{-1} min^{-1} (Ekblom, 1986), were not apparent even though several players among the squad had considerable international experience. Moreover, even allowing for expected lower $\dot{V}O_2max$ levels due to the use of a cycle ergometer protocol rather than a treadmill, the present values are similar to those obtained in non-specifically trained males of similar age using identical exercise protocols.

Blood lactate changes indicated that the 4.0 mM 'threshold' level (Heck et al. 1985) occurred during relatively low levels of cardio-respiratory demand corresponding to approximately 87% HR max and 77% $\dot{V}O2max$ at around 70% of the maximum work load. Peak lactates of 9.1 mM at 15 min were considerably below those reported during laboratory exercise tests involving treadmill running in elite soccer players who averaged 14.2 ± 2.1 mM (Ekblom, 1986). Furthermore, since reported values during competitive games often exceed 12.0 mM (Ekblom, 1986) with corresponding oxygen uptake levels averaging 80% VO2max during play, it would appear that both aerobic power and anaerobic tolerance of the subjects in the present study were somewhat limited.

Physical performance measures indicated vertical jump scores (59 ± 1.3 cm) comparable to those reported by Reilly and Thomas (1977) and Thomas and Reilly (1979) in English First Division players who achieved scores of 58.0 ± 1.1 cm and 55.5 ± 1.2 cm, with similar explosive leg strength values since body weights were closely matched. Anaerobic power derived from stair run times showed similar levels of absolute power (204.8 ± 4.5 kgm s^{-1}) compared with those obtained by Kalamen (1968) in track sprinters (201.8 ± 4.5 kgm s^{-1}) but considerably lower than professional American Football players (240-271 kgm s^{-1}). Even so, relative power scores (2.60 ± 0.1 kgm kg^{-1} s^{-1}) were significantly higher than those reported by Withers (1977) in young players (1.65 kgm kg^{-1} s^{-1}). Agility run times, however, were slower than those observed in U.S.A. professional soccer players (15.5 ± 0.14 s) reported by Cureton (1970) and in unpublished work on English Football League First Division players (15.3 ± 0.20 s) by Davies (1982).

Summary

It was concluded that in this sample of professional soccer players, body composition and physique characteristics were comparable with other groups of games players. Furthermore, physiological indices of performance indicated relatively low aerobic and anaerobic capacities, which were accompanied by unexceptional performance capabilities compared with other games playing groups. The training schedules utilised suggested a 'minimal' approach to preparation and the problems of detraining and/or loss of specific fitness during the 'off season' represents a potential limitation to optimal performance in professional soccer players.

References

Bell, W. and Rhodes, G. (1975) The morphological characteristics of the association football player. Brit. J. Sports Med., 9, 196-200.

Boennec, P.M., Prevot, M. and Ginet, J. (1980) Somatotype desportif de haut niveau, resultats dans huit disciplines differentes. Medicine du Sport, 54, 45-54.

British Association of Sports Sciences (1986) Position statement on the physiological assessment of the elite athlete. (edited by T.Hale, A. Hardman, P. Jakeman, C. Sharp and E. Winter).

Clarys, J.P. (1987) The skin-fold - myth and reality. J. Sports Sci., 5 (in press).

Cureton, T.K. (1970) Illinois agility run. In: Physical Fitness Workbook for Adults. Champaign, Illinois: Stipes Publishing Co.,

Davies, B. (1982) Observations on an English League first division football club performance abilities (Unpublished report: University of Salford).

Durnin, J.V.G.A. and Womersley, J. (1974) Body fast assessed from total body density and its estimation from skinfold thickness.Brit. J. Nutr., 32, 77-97.

Ekblom, B., (1986) Applied physiology of soccer. Sports Med.,3, 50-60.

Garrow, J.S. (1983) Indices of adiposity. Nutrition Abstracts and Rev. Clin. Nutr., 8, 697-708.

Heath, B. and Carter, J. (1967) A modified somatotype method.Amer. J. Phys. Anthrop., 27, 54-74.

Heck, H., Mader, A., Hess, G., Mucke, S., Muller, R. and Hollman, W. (1985) Justification of the 4 mmol/l lactate threshold. Int. J. Sports Med., 6, 117-130.

Kalaman, J. (1968) Measurement of maximum muscular power in man. Unpublished doctoral dissertation, Ohio State University.

Kirkendal, D.T. (1985) Applied sports science of soccer.Physician Sportsmed., 13, 53-59.

Margaria, R., Aghemo, P. and Rovelli, E. (1966) Measurement of muscular power (anaerobic) in man. J. Appl. Physiol., 21, 1662-1662-1664.

Mathews, D.K. and Fox, E.L. (1976) The Physiological Basis of Physical Education and Athletics. London: W.B. Saunders Co.

Reilly, T., (1979) What Research Tells the Coach about Soccer. Washington, D.C. American Alliance for Health, Physical Education, Recreation and Dance.

Reilly, T., (1986) Fundamental studies on soccer. In: Sportspielforschung: diagnose prognose (edited by H. Kasler and R. Andreson). pp114-120. Hamburg: Verlag Ingrid Czwalina.

Reilly, T. and Thomas, V. (1977a) Effects of a programme of pre-season training on the fitness of soccer players. J. Sports Med.Phys. Fit., 17, 401-402.

Reilly, T., and Thomas, V. (1977b) Applications of multivariate

analysis to the fitness assessment of soccer players. Brit.J. Sports Med., 4, 183-184.
Reilly, T. and Thomas, V. (1980) The stability of fitness factorsover a season of professional soccer as indicated by serial factor analyses. In: Kinanthropometry II (edited by M. Ostyn, G. Beunen, J. Simons). pp245-257. Baltimore, University Park Press.
Stepnicka, J. (1977). Somatotypes of Czechoslovak athletes. In: Growth and Development (edited by O. Eiben). Physique Symposia Biology Hungary, 20, 357-264.
Thomas, V. and Reilly, T. (1979) Fitness assessment of EnglishLeague soccer players through the competitive season. Brit.J. Sports Med., 13, 103-109.

MAXIMAL ANAEROBIC POWER OF INDIAN SOCCER PLAYERS ACCORDING TO PLAYING POSITION

J.L. Bhanot
Research Centre in Physical Education and Sports,
Department of Human Biology
Punjabi University, Patiala-147002, India.

Introduction

Different sports require different levels of anaerobic power. Anaerobic power has been shown to be especially important in certain field positions in hockey (Bhanot and Sidhu, 1982). However, its contribution in the game of football, which like hockey is considered to be an endurance event (Saltin and Åstrand, 1967; Bhanot and Sidhu, 1981), has not been fully explained. The present study aimed to find out whether a relationship exists between the maximal anaerobic power of football players and their playing positions.

Materials and Methods

The study was conducted on 84 soccer players at Netaji Subash National Institute of Sports, Patiala. They included 8 goalkeepers, 26 backs, 13 half-backs and 37 forwards. Maximal vertical velocity was determined by the technique used by Margaria et al. (1966) and Bhanot and Sidhu (1981). The mechanical work output, described as anaerobic power by Margaria et al. (1966), was estimated from maximal vertical velocity and body weight.

The present day team formation in the game of soccer in India is 4-2-4. This refers to the field positions of 4 back or defenders (2 central, one on each side), 2 half-backs or midfield players (one on the right and one on the left) and 4 forward, outside right, inside-right, inside left and outside left. Differences between positions were examined with multiple 't' tests.

Results

In body weight, the backs were found to be the heaviest, followed by goalkeepers, half-backs and forwards (Table 1). The goalkeepers were not significantly different from the backs or half-backs, but they were significantly heavier than the forwards ($P < 0.05$).

The centre backs were heavier, faster and possessed better anaerobic power than wing backs. The differences were significant only in the case of anaerobic power ($P < 0.05$).

Table 1. Means (±SD) for body weight, vertical velocity and anaerobic power in goalkeepers, backs, half-backs and forwards

Field Position	N	Body weight (kg)	Vertical velocity ($m\ s^{-1}$)	Anaerobic power (W)
Goal	8	62.46 ± 5.53	1.976 ± 0.21	1210 ± 161
Backs	26	65.20 ± 6.54	1.714 ± 0.19	1096 ± 150
Half-backs	13	60.80 ± 6.78	1.748 ± 0.20	1042 ± 90
Forwards	37	58.29 ± 5.12	1.821 ± 0.15	1040 ± 109

Discussion

From the observations, it is clear that at certain field positions, the players are heavier in body weight, faster in vertical velocity and possess better anaerobic power than in others. These positional differences could be attributed to the game's tactical roles like defending, passing or feeding, and attacking. Depending upon the field position and the requirement at a particular moment, a player utilizes the required energy either through aerobic or anaerobic mechanisms for handling the game situation successfully.

The goalkeeper is under constant threat from the opposing forward line in that he may be tested at any moment with little warning. He needs good anticipation and quick body movements. This may be the reason that in the present sample the goalkeepers possessed the best vertical velocity and anaerobic power values. Among football players, the goalkeepers have been reported to be fastest in reaction times for both hand and foot (Bhanot, 1986). Their lower body weight than the backs might be helpful in diving, to catch or clear the football quickly on the ground or in the air, depending upon the game situation.

Though the backs were the slowest in vertical velocity, their body weight allows them to have anaerobic power values better than half-backs and forwards and next only to goalkeepers. This high level of anaerobic power might help the backs in winning the ball and clearing it successfully, or in joining with their forwards when on the attack. Quick reaction times and good anaerobic power enable the backs to tackle the forwards more successfully (Bhanot, 1986). Their high body weight may be due to increased muscle mass which might be an advantage in kicking the ball.

The midfielders or half-back line and the forwards possessed almost equal vertical velocity and anaerobic power values. The reason may be that in the game, though the half-line players function mainly as feeders and providers for the forwards, they also play an attacking role periodically and so their vertical velocity and anaerobic power profiles are similar to those of forwards. The half-line and forward-line players in soccer have been shown to be equal in reaction times of hand and foot (Bhanot, 1986). The lower anaerobic power in half-backs and forwards compared to backs and goalkeepers may be because they derive relatively more energy aerobically during the game and might be expected to have the higher aerobic power values.

It was observed that the centre backs had better anaerobic power results than the wing backs. With a 4-2-4 formation, the centre backs function predominantly as defenders, while the wing backs function both as defenders and feeders. Consequently they possess anaerobic power profiles more like the half-backs.

From the findings, it is clear that soccer players do vary in anaerobic power profiles according to their field positions. These positional differences may reflect differential demands on anaerobic energy sources during play. The relative importance of anaerobic power in training for soccer should take into consideration the field position of the player.

Acknowledgements

The author wishes to thank Mr. Amarjit Singh Bains, Mr. Gurcharan Singh and Mr. H.R. Arora for their assistance in the preparation of the manuscript.

References

Bhanot, J.L. and Sidhu, L.S. (1981) Maximal anaerobic power in national level Indian players. Brit. J. Sports Med., 15, 265-268.

Bhanot, J.L. and Sidhu, L.S. (1982) Maximal anaerobic power in national hockey players. Brit. J. Sports Med. 17, 34-39.

Bhanot, J.L. (1986) Reaction time and different field positions in football players. In: Proc. of Second International Sports Science Conference (edited by C.K.Giam and K.C. Teh) pp 191-197. Singapore: Singapore Sports Council.

Margaria, R., Aghemo, P. and Rovelli, E. (1966) Measurement of muscular power (anaerobic) in man. J. Appl. Physiol., 21, 1662-1664.

Saltin, B. and Åstrand, P.O. (1967) Maximal oxygen uptake in athletes. J. Appl. Physiol., 23, 353-358.

PHYSIOLOGICAL CHARACTERISTICS OF 12-YEAR-OLD SOCCER PLAYERS

W. Bell Department of Physical Education and Human Movement Studies, South Glamorgan Institute of Higher Education, Cyncoed, Cardiff, CF2 6XD.

Introduction

There is, generally, an increasing volume of knowledge slowly accumulating about the relation between physical activity and the growing child, some of which has been obtained from children who compete in specific sporting activities. There is, however, surprisingly little information concerning the physiological characteristics of children who participate competitively in Soccer, despite the game being a popular and widespread recreational and competitive sport. The present study, therefore, seeks to provide details of some fundamental physiological characteristics of the young competitive soccer player.

Methods

Subjects of the study consisted of 18 boys of mean age 12.3 years who formed part of a much larger group of children who had been studied longitudinally throughout adolescence. Selection was made on the grounds that the subjects' first choice of competitive sport was soccer. All the boys played competitively for their school teams and for teams outside school. Many had obtained representative schoolboy honours. Each boy was assigned to his preferred playing position. The sample then consisted of 2 goalkeepers, 7 defenders, 4 midfield players and 5 strikers.

Anthropometric measurements were taken according to the recommendations of Weiner and Lourie (1981). Stature was measured to the nearest 0.1 cm using a stadiometer with the subject being stretched upwards to the fullest extent. Body mass was taken on a beam balance to the nearest 50 g.

Body density was determined by hydrostatic weighing. Each subject was seated in water heated to 30°C. A forced maximal exhalation was made before underwater weight was recorded. Repeated trials were taken until a plateau had been attained, the mean value of these measurements being used as the final underwater weight. A correction was made for residual volume using the closed-circuit nitrogen dilution technique. Duplicate measurements were taken and the mean value used. Total body fat (TBF) was calculated from body density using the equation derived for children by Lohman, Boileau and Slaughter (1984). Fat-free mass (FFM) was obtained by the subtraction of TBF from total body mass.

Maximal aerobic power ($\dot{V}O_2$ max) was assessed from sub-maximal work tests with a correction being made for underestimation (Davies, Barnes and Godfrey, 1972). Subjects were exercised on a Monark bicycle ergometer. Ventilation was measured using a dry gas meter (Parkinson and Cowan) fitted to the input side of a three-way respiratory valve. The output from the valve was connected to a mixing chamber from which a continuous sample of expired air was directed to O_2 and CO_2 gas analysers (Beckman). Both instruments were calibrated before each experiment with determined gas mixtures. Cardiac frequency was monitored using an ECG. A discontinuous series of increasing work loads was used, each lasting 6 min. Ventilation was recorded over the last 2 min of exercise; cardiac frequency, O_2 and CO_2 fractions were obtained during the last 30 s of exercise.

The age at which peak velocity in height occurs is one of a number of indicators which can be used to identify maturational status. Since these subjects were part of a larger group of children which had been studied longitudinally over a 4 or 5 year period, height had been measured annually until it was ascertained that the peak velocity in height (PHV) had been attained for each child. The PHV and the age at which it occurred were determined using third-degree polynomials (Largo et al., 1978). The adolescent period was scanned at three-monthly intervals with the largest observed value being used as the estimate of PHV. The age at which PHV occurred was obtained from these same measurements.

Results

Descriptive statistics for all variables according to playing position are given in Table 1. Stature was found to be greatest in goalkeepers (156 cm). Strikers (152 cm) were slightly taller than defenders (148 cm) with midfield players (148 cm) being similar in size to defenders.

Strikers had the greatest body mass: there was about a 1 kg difference between strikers (40 kg) and goalkeepers (39 kg) and between goalkeepers and defenders (38 kg). Midfield players, at around 35 kg, were noticeably lighter than the other positions.

Using analysis of variance the differences between the various playing positions in either height or weight were non-significant ($P<0.05$). The mean overall height of all players was 150 cm which is at about the 60th centile for British children; the mean overall weight was 38 kg which is around the 50th centile (Tanner and Whitehouse, 1976).

Of the outfield players, defenders and strikers had similar relative amounts of TBF (14%), with midfield players having slightly less (11%). Only one goalkeeper was available for measurement (9%). None of the differences in body fat between playing positions was significant ($P<0.05$).

The $\dot{V}O_2$ max was expressed in absolute terms ($l\ min^{-1}$) and also relative to three aspects of body size - body weight, FFM and height. There was not a great deal of difference in the absolute levels of $\dot{V}O_2$ max between the playing positions ($P<0.05$). Midfield players and strikers had values of 2.2 $l\ min^{-1}$, defenders and

Table 1. Mean values (±SD) for body size, body composition and aerobic power ($\dot{V}O_2$ max)

	GK (n=2)	Defenders (n=7)	Midfield (n=4)	Strikers (n=5)	All positions (n=18)
Stature (cm)	155.7 3.0	147.6 4.8	148.2 3.4	152.0 6.8	149.8 5.5
Body mass (kg)	38.6 5.4	37.5 4.6	35.3 2.7	39.8 2.8	37.8 3.9
TBF (%)	8.8	13.5 4.1	10.5 3.0	13.8 6.1	12.73 4.53
$\dot{V}O_2$ max (l min^{-1})	1.97 0.01	2.04 0.25	2.15 0.10	2.22 0.21	2.11 0.21
$\dot{V}O_2$ max(ml kg^{-1} BM min^{-1}	51.4 7.0	55.1 6.4	61.1 3.4	55.9 4.8	56.23 5.80
$\dot{V}O_2$ max(ml kg^{-1} FFM min^{-1})	58.8 4.2	63.0 4.7	66.8 5.5	65.1 6.1	64.0 5.4
$\dot{V}O_2$ max(l m^2 min^{-1})	0.81 0.03	0.93 0.08	0.98 0.07	0.96 0.10	0.94 0.09
Age at PHV (years)	14.3 1.3	14.9 0.7	14.1 0.7	13.8 1.0	14.3 0.9

goalkeepers 2.0 l min^{-1}. There was greater variation in values when $\dot{V}O_2$ max was calculated relative to body size. In all the relative expressions of $\dot{V}O_2$ max midfield players had the largest values, followed by strikers, defenders and finally goalkeepers. However, like all the other dimensions observed so far the differences were not large enough to be significant ($P<0.05$).

Age at PHV varied from 13.8 years in strikers to 14.9 years in defenders ($P<0.05$). The overall mean value was 14.3 years.

Because of a lack of significance between the various playing positions in any of the variables measured, the measurements for all positions in each variable were pooled. The mean descriptive statistics determined from the pooled values are included in Table 1.

Discussion

Although the differences in stature and body mass were not significantly different between playing positions it seems likely that they reflected, to some extent, the positional requirements of the game at a junior level. Goalkeepers are usually the tallest and heaviest of players, with midfield players being the shortest and lightest. Defenders and strikers usually fall midway between these two types.

Defenders and strikers had much the same proportion of their body weight as fat (14%); midfield players were seen to have smaller amounts (11%). These values are at a reasonable level for boys of this age. At 12 years of age most boys are probably close to the take-off point of adolescence. During this period most boys tend to lose fat, so that it is very likely that these levels will be reduced over the next few years. The mean overall value for TBF was 13%. For 11 year old players Vrijens and Van Cauter (1985) found a value of 18%. The results for body size and body composition in the present group of young players are thus similar in their positional arrangement to those obtained in young adult players (Bell and Rhodes, 1975; Bell, 1983).

Absolute levels of $\dot{V}O_2$ max varied between 1.97 l min^{-1} for goalkeepers and 2.22 l min^{-1} for strikers. The variation between playing positions was indeed quite small. The average $\dot{V}O_2$ max for all players was 2.1 l min^{-1}. This value is at the 50th centile for $\dot{V}O_2$ max standards (Cameron et al., 1980).

Expressed relative to body mass the mean $\dot{V}O_2$ max value was 56 ml kg^{-1} min^{-1}. Values were lowest for goalkeepers (51 ml kg^{-1} min^{-1}) and highest for midfield players (61 ml kg^{-1} min^{-1}). The values for defenders and strikers (55 ml kg^{-1} min^{-1}) fell midway between those two positions. Although the differences between positions were not significant, these figures would seem to indicate that the positional requirements of children resemble those of adults. In an organised and disciplined team, even at a junior level, there will be a tendency to have some measure of positional responsibility. Caru et al. (1970) have reported a value of 52 ml kg^{-1} min^{-1} for 14 year old Italian players. Professional soccer players are seen to have higher relative mean values ranging from 58 ml kg^{-1} min^{-1} (Raven et al., 1970) to 67 ml kg^{-1} min^{-1} (Ekblom, 1986).

The $\dot{V}O_2$ max expressed on the basis of FFM displayed the same relationship between positions as did $\dot{V}O_2$ max related to body mass. Values ranged from 59 ml $kg^{-1}min^{-1}$ to 67 ml kg^{-1} min^{-1}, the overall mean being 64 ml kg^{-1} min^{-1}.

It is appropriate during growth to express $\dot{V}O_2$ max in relation to height since it provides a more stable standard for comparative purposes. The use of height in this way has some practical importance, for example in considering the influence of training on children, where it may be necessary to exclude the effect of growth. On the basis of height 2 midfield players again demonstrated a larger $\dot{V}O_2$ max value (0.98 l m^2 min^{-1}) than either strikers (0.96 l m^2 min^{-1}) or defenders (0.93 l m^2 min^{-1}). All outfield players had larger values than goalkeepers(0.81 l m^2 min^{-1}).

Age at PHV occurred earliest in strikers (13.8 years) and latest in defenders (14.9 years). For midfield players and strikers the ages at PHV were 14.1 and 14.3 years respectively. Differences were not significant and the mean of all positions was 14.3 years. This compares with a value of 14.1 years for boys in the United Kingdom (Tanner at el., 1966). Thus players are seen to be of average maturational status.

In conclusion the present study has shown that 12 year old Soccer players are slightly above average in height, and have average values for weight, aerobic capacity and maturational status. Oxygen uptake values were inclined to reflect positional requirements. Whether this is a desirable trend or not will depend upon the philosophical view taken about the development of young players. Total body fat values were all at a reasonable level. At 12 years of age, therefore, Soccer players can be regarded as being a fairly homogeneous group of young athletes.

References

Bell, W. (1983) Homogeneity of body composition in Association Football players. In: Proceedings Sport and Science (edited by D.A. Brodie, J. Burnie, R.G. Eston, F. Sanderson and J.J. Thornhill), F2, 1-7. School of Physical Education and Recreation, University of Liverpool: Society of Sports Science Conference.

Bell, W. and Rhodes, G. (1975) The morphological characteristics of the Association Football player. Brit. J. Sports Med., 9, 196-200.

Cameron, M., Mirwald, R.L., and Bailey, D.A. (1980) Standards for the assessment of normal and absolute maximal aerobic power. In Kinanthropometry II, (edited by M. Ostyn, G. Beunen and J. Simons), pp 349-359. Baltimore: University Park Press.

Caru B., Le Coultre, L., Aghemo, P., and Pinera-Limas, F. (1979) Maximal aerobic and anaerobic power in football players. J. Sports Med. Phys. Fit., 10, 100-103.

Davies, C.T.M., Barnes, C., and Godfrey, S. (1972) Body composition and maximal performance in children. Human Biol., 44, 195-214.

Largo, R.H., Gasser, T., Prader, A., Stuetzle, W., and Huber, P.J. (1978) Analysis of the adolescent growth sport using smoothing spline function. Ann. Human Biol., 5, 421-434.

Lohman, T.G., Boileau, R.A., and Slaughter, M.H. (1984) Body composition in children and youth. In: Advances in Paediatric Sport Sciences Vol I, Biological Sciences (edited by R.A. Boileau). Champaign, Illinois: Human Kinetics Publs.

Raven, P.B., Gettman, L.R.,Pollock, M.L., and Cooper, K.H. (1976) A physiological evaluation of professional soccer players. Brit. J. Sports Med., 10, 209-216.

Tanner, J.M., and Whitehouse, R.H. (1976) Clinical longitudinal standards for height, weight, height velocity, weight velocity and the stages of puberty. Arch. Dis. Child., 51,3, 170-179.

Tanner, J.M., and Whitehouse, R.H. and Takaishi, M. (1966) Standard from birth to maturity for height, weight, height velocity and weight velocity: British children, 1966. Arch. Dis. Child., 454-471: 613-635.

Vrijens, J., and Van Cauter, C. (1985) Physical performance and specific skills in young soccer players. In: Children and Exercise XI, (edited by R.A. Binkhorst, H.C.G. Kemper and W.H.M. Saris), pp. 285-292, Champaign, Illinois: Human Kinetic Publ.

Weiner, J.S. and Lourie, J.A. (1981) Practical Human Biology. London: Academic Press.

ISOKINETIC MUSCLE STRENGTH OF SOCCER PLAYERS

Haruhiko Togari, Jiro Ohashi and Tetsuro Ohgushi*
Department of Sports Sciences, University of Tokyo, 3-8-1 Komaba, Meguro-ku, Tokyo 153, Japan.
*Colleges of Arts and Sciences, Sophia University, Japan.

Introduction

Leg muscle strength is an important factor in playing soccer. It is clear from Asami and Togari's (1968) report that there is a close correlation between the knee extension strength and ball speed. Recently the isokinetic principle has been used to evaluate dynamic strength in many branches of sports sciences. Muscle strength of soccer players has been studied by a number of techniques. Isokinetic data have been reported by Öberg et al. (1984), Poulmedis (1985), and Kirkendall (1985).

The purpose of this study is not only to measure the dynamic muscle strength of leading Japanese soccer players, analysing their typical profiles, but also to discuss and compare various levels of technical ability. Additionally, differences between regular players and substitutes, and between the different playing positions were examined.

Methods

Altogether 181 persons were examined, consisting of 20 Japan national team members, 86 Japan Soccer League (JSL) players (37 regulars and 49 substitutes), 40 candidates for the Universiade national team and 35 candidates for the national youth team. Cybex II (Lumex Co., New York) apparatus was used to measure the leg extension power at the velocity levels of 1.05, 2.09, 3.14, 4.19 and 5.24 rad s^{-1}. The subjects sat in an experimental chair which permits the knee joints to extend from 90 degrees to 180 degrees. The range of motion was 90 degrees, starting at 90 degrees of flexion and proceeding to full extension. The highest peak torque was recorded during three isokinetic contractions at each of the five velocities.

Results

Table 1 shows the mean and standard deviation values of peak isokinetic muscle strength. In extensor muscle torque the value of 1.05 rad s^{-1} was the highest.

It was further observed that the more angular velocity increased the more isokinetic torque decreased. With regard to various technical levels, the national team and the JSL players tended to be

Table 1. Mean and standard deviation values of isokinetic muscle strength and the mean and standard strength on technical levels

	Height (cm)	Weight (kg)	Age (years)	1.05 rad s^{-1} (Nm)	2.09 rad s^{-1} (Nm)	3.14 rad s^{-1} (Nm)	4.19 rad s^{-1} (Nm)	5.24 rad s^{-1} (Nm)
	175.3	69.7	24.2	254.4	201.8	157.4	123.2	101.2
Japan national	5.79	5.03	2.48	52.41	36.83	24.35	17.09	16.53
	20	20	20	20	20	20	20	20
	174.2	69.8	25.6	245.0	202.6	161.8	133.1	102.4
Japan Soccer League	4.91	5.00	3.01	44.99	33.78	21.91	21.04	17.48
	37	37	37	37	27	37	27	37
	176.1	68.9	20.5	230.0	170.8	148.6	107.1	94.7
Universiade national	4.18	4.53	1.00	30.08	26.04	24.44	20.53	13.67
	40	40	40	40	16	40	16	40
	175.5	67.9	17.5	237.2	180.7	146.4	116.3	96.5
Youth national	5.61	5.44	0.71	33.11	41.92	21.76	24.42	16.14
	35	35	35	35	12	35	12	35

Table 2. Mean and standard deviation values of isokinetic muscle strength for different playing positions

	Height	Weight	Peak torque (Nm)			Peak torque/Weight (Nm kg^{-1})		
			1.05	3.14	5.24	1.05	3.14	5.24
	(cm)	(kg)	(rad s^{-1})	(rad s^{-1}	(rad s^{-1})	(rad s^{-1})	(rad s^{-1})	(rad s^{-1})
	180.0	73.8	255.1	154.4	101.4	3.59	2.15	1.39
Goalkeeper	2.79	3.12	41.12	26.98	17.59	0.52	0.32	0.22
	20	20	20	20	20	20	20	20
	176.0	69.3	237.6	150.0	97.5	3.38	2.16	1.42
Defender	4.61	5.23	42.67	25.54	16.51	0.54	0.34	0.25
	54	54	53	54	54	54	54	54
	172.9	66.5	232.0	149.8	95.6	3.52	2.25	1.44
Midfielder	4.59	4.63	36.52	23.12	14.89	0.54	0.30	0.22
	41	41	41	41	41	41	41	41
	173.9	67.8	228.6	153.3	96.8	3.41	2.28	1.43
Forward	4.85	5.29	49.83	26.84	18.26	0.64	0.34	0.25
	61	61	61	61	61	61	61	61

stronger than the candidates for the national youth team and for the Universiade team at all velocity levels, even though the difference was not statistically significant ($P > 0.05$).

Fig. 1 shows that regular players were slightly stronger than substitutes. However the differences observed between these groups were non-significant ($P > 0.05$).

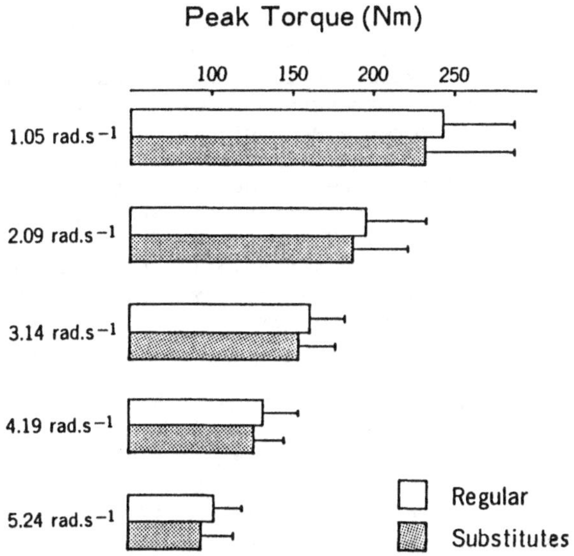

Figure 1. Isokinetic muscle strength of Japan Soccer League players

Table 2 shows the means (±SD) for absolute and relative values of isokinetic muscle strength according to the four playing positions. Relative values were obtained by dividing the strength by body weight ($Nm\ kg^{-1}$).

On the whole goalkeepers were superior at the lowest velocity level, and they were significantly stronger than forwards at 1.05 rad s^{-1} ($P < 0.05$). At 3.14 rad s^{-1} and 5.24 rad s^{-1}, however, there was only a small difference between goalkeepers and field players. When positional features were reviewed, superiority at 1.05 rad s^{-1} was recognised in the order of defenders, midfielders and forwards, but at 3.14 rad s^{-1} there was almost no observable difference.

Discussion

The members of the Japan national team and JSL players were found to be rather stronger at all velocity levels than the other groups. When compared with other studies, the data at 3.14 rad s^{-1} were similar to those of the members of the US national team (Ekblom, 1986) and were higher than values of Swedish players (Oberg et al., 1984) and Greek elite soccer players (Poulmedis, 1985).

In this study the differences between various technical levels were not statistically significant. The reason for this is possibly that the leg extension movement used in this study resembles the kicking motion in a game and that the principal muscles involved in both movements are practically the same. This muscle group is usually well trained in the case of a soccer specialist; therefore, the quadriceps are highly trained in these players.

In their study, Togari et al. (1979) analysed the difference in physique and physical fitness between regular players and substitutes in the Japanese Soccer League. According to the report, regular players were significantly superior to others in many items of measurement including muscle strength. However, with regard to leg extension strength the difference was not distinctive. In other words, for leg extension strength, it seems that it is not possible to find any significant difference in soccer players because they have attained a certain level of trainability whether they are regular players or substitutes. The results of regular players, who always showed good performance at all velocities, indicate that successful soccer players have better leg extension strength than others who have been trained in the game for a long time. This agrees with the results of other researchers reviewed by Ekblom (1986).

Oberg et al. (1984) studied the isokinetic muscle strength of Swedish soccer players. They reported the superiority of goalkeepers, which was attributable to genetic factors such as muscle fibre type, neuromuscular patterns, and also to the effects of training. This may be so, but it may also be true that it was simply the better physique of goalkeepers which affected the performance. From the results obtained by using Nm cm^2 body surface in the report of Oberg and co-workers and Nm kg^{-1} in this study, the difference between goalkeepers and outfielders was non-significant. This leads to the following explanation. Since goalkeepers have better physiques than others, the absolute value is markedly superior, but the muscle strength per unit cross-sectional area is not always greater in goalkeepers than in outfield players. This may indeed be accounted for by genetic factors such as muscle fibre composition. Acquired factors during training may also play an important role.

Among outfielders, defenders showed a slightly better performance than others. This might be the result of their better physique rather than due to a specific characteristic of that position.

The results obtained can be summarised as follows:

(i) The Japan national team and the JSL players were stronger than the candidates for the youth national team and for the Universiade team in muscle strength at all velocities.

(ii) Regular players were always stronger than substitutes in muscle strength at all velocities, though the difference was not statistically significant.

(iii) With regard to comparison between positions, goalkeepers and defenders showed the best performance at the low velocity, while at the middle and high velocities no significant differences were found between playing positions.

References

Asami, T. and Togari, J. (1968) Studies on the kicking abilities in soccer. Res. J. Phys. Educ., 12, 267-272.

Ekblom, B. (1986) Applied physiology of soccer. Sports Med., 3, 50-60.

Kirkendall, D.T. (1985) The applied sport science of soccer. Physician Sportsmed., 13, 53-59.

Öberg, B., Ekstrand, J., Möller, M. and Gillquist, J. (1984) Muscle strength and flexibility in different positions of soccer players. Int. J. Sport Med., 5, 213-216.

Poulmedis, P. (1985) Isokinetic maximal torque power of Greek elite soccer players. J. Orth. Sports Med. Sports Physical Therapy, 6, 293-295.

Togari, H., Asami, T., Adachi, N., Yamamoto, K., Sugiyama, S. and Ohashi, J. (1979) A study on physical fitness of the top soccer players in Japan. The Proceedings of the Department of Physical Education, College of General Education, University of Tokyo, 13, 33-42.

THE RELATION BETWEEN MUSCULAR STRENGTH AND KICK PERFORMANCE

J. Cabri, E DeProft, W. Dufour and J.P. Clarys
Department of Experimental Anatomy and Physical Education,
Free University of Brussels, Laarbeeklaan 103, 1090 Brussels,
Belgium.

Introduction

The relation between strength measurements (by means of a dynamometer) and performance is still a widely discussed topic in sports research. The relation between muscle strength and performance of the athlete 'in the field' is a subject of controversy, not only in biomechanics, but also in other research fields dealing with muscle power.

Nevertheless, some investigators have demonstrated positive correlations between the force, measured in the laboratory, and 'functional' or practical tests. Perrine and Edgerton (1975) found high correlations between isokinetic strength (at a speed of 6.29 rad s^{-1} and both the 50 m dash and the vertical jump (r = 0.63 and 0.93), and demonstrated improvements in performance after fast isokinetic leg thrust exercises. Prins (1978) also found these improvements in the vertical jump, but only when training was performed at a fast speed (2.26 rad s^{-1}), not at a slow speed (0.61 rad s^{-1}). Stevens (1980) recorded jump-height gains after 8 weeks of isokinetic training. He also demonstrated the superiority of isokinetics over weight training. Bosco et al. (1983) found high correlations between isokinetic movements and ballistic type of activities, and concluded that the motor unit activation pattern is velocity dependent. Kanehisha and Myashita (1983) also found a significant relation between peak force (measured at v = 3.65 rad s^{-1}) and the velocity of a 50 m sprint.

Among soccer practitioners, it is well known that soccer players demonstrate a better kick performance than non-soccer players, for technical skill is a dominant element in this matter. The angle of placing the foot at impact, the angle of launching the ball, and the angle between the trunk and the vertical axis discriminate soccer players from non-soccer players (De Proft et al., this conference).

In an attempt to establish isokinetic torque values, Oberg et al. (1986) found that concentric muscle strength of knee flexors and extensors is significantly higher in soccer than in non-soccer players. But the question whether performance and technical skill interfere with these differences measured in the laboratory still remains open. The present study therefore is focussed on the relation between strength of the leg muscles and kick performance in soccer players.

Methods

Subjects

Eleven high level soccer players (SP; mean age 20 years), and a control group of 10 adult non-soccer players (NSP; mean age 23 years, students in physical therapy) were used in the experimental design. The anthropometric characteristics are given in Table 1.

Table 1. Anthropometric data of the subjects. Values are mean (±SD)

	N	Age (yrs)	Height (cm)	Weight (kg)
Soccer players	11	20.0 ± 1.1	176.6 ± 4.8	73.4 ± 8.8
Non-soccer players (NSP)	11	23.0 ± 1.5	178.1 ± 4.0	70.7 ± 11.1

Experimental design

Strength measurements

Strength of both extensors and flexors at the knee joint and the hip joint was measured by means of an isokinetic dynamometer (KIN-COM, Chattex Corp., TN), at an angular velocity of 3.65 rad (210 degrees) s^{-1}, both during concentric and eccentric contractions. Independent studies have confirmed the reliability of the dynamometer in measuring angle, velocity and force within an error of 3% (Hart et al., 1985). Because of the high velocities of the limbs during a soccer kick, the highest speed was selected to measure strength. After an extensive warm up, the following strength measurements of the dominant leg were carried out:-

i) knee flexion - concentric and eccentric contraction (KFC and KFE);

iii) knee extension - concentric and eccentric contraction (KEC and KEE),
(the subjects were tested in a sitting position, the hip was fixed at 120 degrees of flexion, both trunk and thigh were fixed by means of straps, the shin pad was positioned 2 cm proximal to the internal malleolus);

iii) hip flexion - concentric and eccentric contracton (HFC and HFE);

iv) hip extension - concentric and eccentric contraction (HEC and HEE),
(the subjects were standing on one leg, the shin pad fixed at the level of the femoral condyles, and the subjects were asked to simulate a "normal" kick with maximal effort).

The rotational axis of the joints investigated was aligned with the shaft of the dynamometer.

Five trials were done for each test, and the best force value was used for statistical analysis. The rest period between each test was standardised to 3 min. All force values were corrected for influences of gravity.

Kick performance

In order to evaluate a sport specific performance task, kick performance, i.e. the ability to kick a soccer ball as far as possible using a standardised technique, was measured. The kick performance was defined as the distance from the start position to the place of impact of the ball on the ground. A take-off run of three paces was allowed to standardise the pre-kick movement. The best shot of three trials was registered for analysis. Cinematographic and light trace analysis of the movement was added to evaluate the kicking technique and to calculate the linear velocities of the lower limb segments.

Performance tests

Additionally, three performances tests were included to evaluate explosive power of the leg extensor muscles according to Letzelter (1983) and Clarke (1976):-

i) The Jump and Reach Test (J and R), or the vertical jump performance: from a semi-squatting position, the subject was asked to perform a vertical jump, with no allowance for a preparatory counter-movement (Bosco et al., 1983). The difference between the height of the subject (with his arm in the upright position) and the marked sign of the jump was then calculated.

ii) The Standing Long Jump (SLJ): from a standing position, the subject was asked to perform a jump in the horizontal direction, with no take-off run allowed. The distance between the start and the place of contact of the heel on the ground was then measured.

iii) The Triple Jump on the Left Leg (TJL) and Right Leg (TJR): from a standing position on either left or right leg, the subject was asked to perform three consecutive jumps. The distance between the start and last heel contact was measured.

From each of the performance tests, only the best trial (of three) was taken into consideration for analysis.

Peak forces, maximal kick performance, maximal jump performances and velocities at the different joints were statistically handled by means of Student t-tests and Pearson Product Moment correlation coefficients. A probability value of 0.05 or less was accepted at significant.

Results

Isokinetic strength

When isokinetic strength is considered, soccer players (SP) demonstrated significantly greater forces than non-soccer players (NSP) at both concentric and eccentric knee flexion, eccentric knee extension, concentric hip flexion and at both concentric and eccentric hip extensions (KFC, KFE, KEE, HFC, HEC, and HEE: see Figure 1). Although not significant, a similar tendency was found at the concentric knee extension and eccentric hip flexion (KEC, HFE).

Performance

The kick performance results indicated a significant difference between SP and the NSP group (Figure 2). As expected, the soccer players were able to kick the ball further than the non-soccer players.

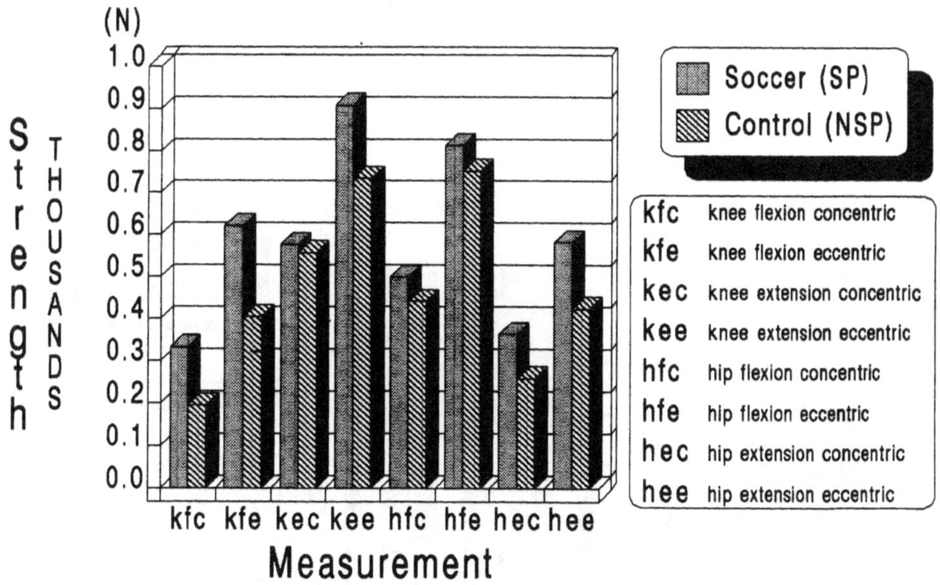

Figure 1. Isokinetic strength (peak force) of soccer players (SP) and non-soccer players (NSP) for the knee flexion concentric and eccentric (KFC and KFE), the knee extension concentric and eccentric (KEC and KEE), the hip flexion concentric and eccentric (HFC and HEE), and the hip extension concentric and eccentric (HEC and HEE).

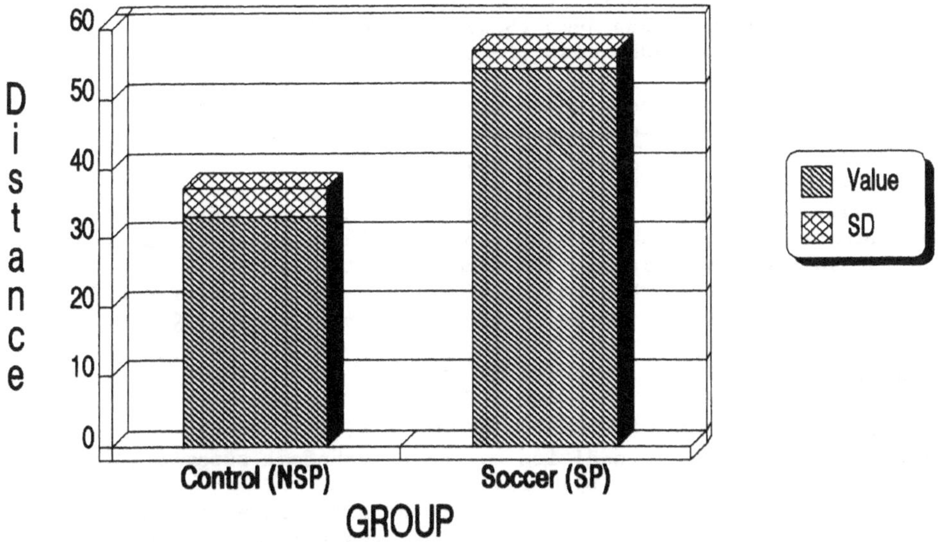

Figure 2. Kick performance of soccer and non-soccer players (control)

A significant difference between SP and NSP was found in both left and right triple jumps (TJL, TJR) (Figure 3). Neither the Jump and Reach test nor the Standing Long Jump was found to discriminate between the groups.

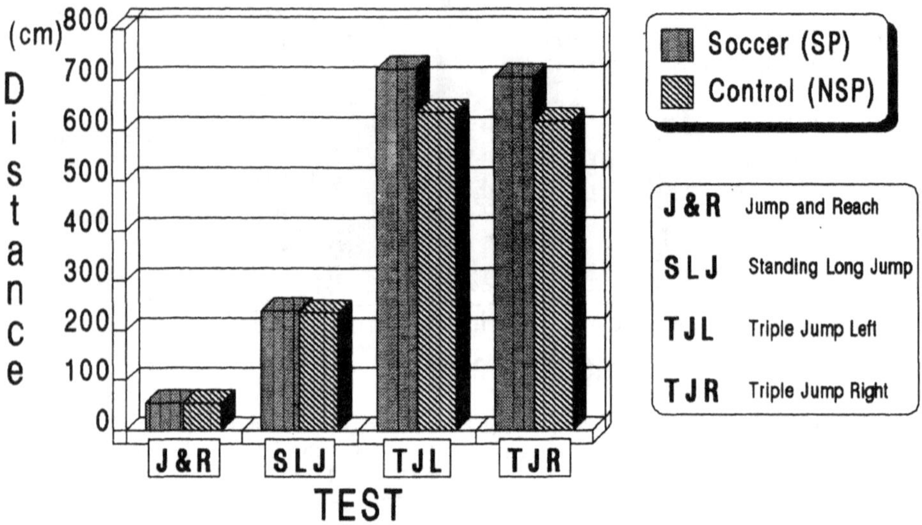

Figure 3. Functional performance tests of soccer and non-soccer players (control): the jump and reach test (J and R) the standing long jump (SLJ), and both triple jumps on one leg (TJL and TJR, resp. left and right leg)

Considering the linear velocities of hip, knee and ankle (Figure 4), all data were found to be higher in the SP group.

Correlations

The analysis of the inter-relationship between the different parameters measured is shown in Table 2. In the soccer players, kick performance was correlated significantly with KFE ($r = 0.77$), KEC($r = 0.74$) HFC ($r = 0.60$), HEE ($r = 0.56$), the J and R test ($r = 0.69$), and with the linear velocity of the ankle ($r = 0.64$) ($P \leqslant 0.05$).

Discussion

Our findings confirm the results of Oberg et al. (1986). In general soccer players are, in addition to their technical superiority, also stronger than non-soccer players.

However, we did not find a significant difference in concentric strength of the knee extensors, although the same trend can be demonstrated. Moreover, kick performance was greater in soccer players. This would imply that having greater muscular strength will result in a greater kick performance. The finding that kick

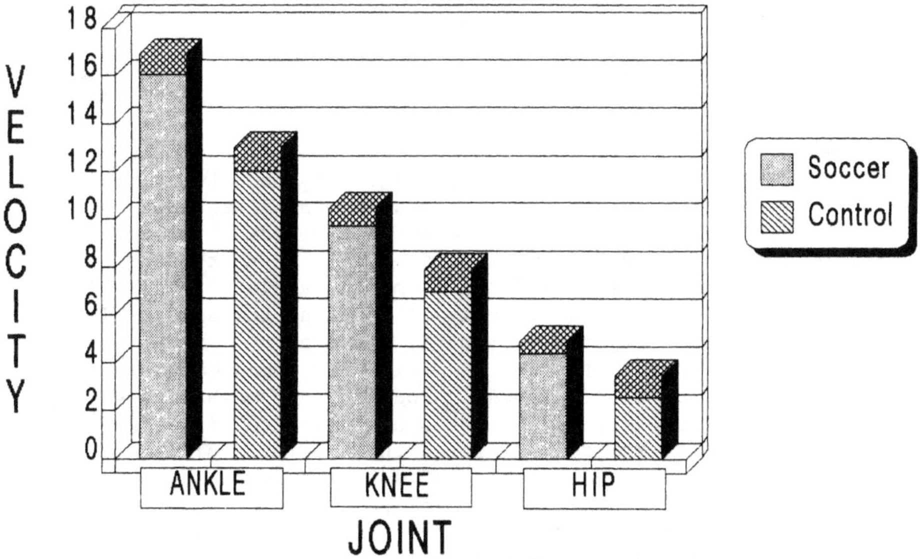

Figure 4. Linear velocities of the joints measured in soccer and non-soccer players (control) during a standardised soccer kick movement

Table 2. Pearson Product Moment correlation coefficients between kick performance coefficients between kick performance (KP) and: eccentric strength of knee flexors (KFE), concentric strength of knee extensors (KEC), concentric strength of hip flexors (HFC), eccentric strength of hip extensors (HEC), jump and reach test (J and R), and ankle linear velocity (ANV)

	KFE	KEC	HFC	HEE	J and R	ANV
KP	0.77	0.74	0.60	0.56	0.69	0.64
J and R	0.65	0.70	0.56	0.60	-	-

performance correlates significantly with concentric strength of the knee extensors and eccentric strength of the knee flexors, corroborates this statement.

In agreement with Oberg et al. (1986), we can state that the influence of specific soccer training can be responsible for the strength differences. It seems that soccer players demonstrate a greater kick performance, not only because of their technical skills, but also because of a more efficient use of their muscular system. The correlations with the kick performance suggest that greater eccentric (concentric) strength of the hamstrings (quadriceps) induces a better kick performance. This has proved to be an important factor in the kicking motion: at the end of the kick, EMG activity of the knee flexors is recorded due to co-activation at the end of the extension phase. Therefore, it is clear that eccentric strength of the hamstrings needs special attention when considering training aspects.

The greater fast-speed capabilities in soccer players indicate that this function is an important skill factor in soccer. This finding is confirmed by Oberg et al. (1986), and by our velocity measurements at the hip, knee and ankle. It seems that soccer players are able to generate more strength in a shorter period of time than non-soccer players, which results in higher limb segment velocities. This would improve the impulse moment at impact with the ball, resulting in a better kick performance. Both the angle between the trunk and the vertical and the launching angle of the ball are additional skill factors positively influencing the soccer kick, and differentiating soccer from non-soccer players.

The positive correlations between kick performance and isokinetic strength (at the level of the knee) confirm that measuring strength by means of an isokinetic dynamometer has practical implications. In addition, it can be stated that strength training could be effective in increasing the kick performance of soccer players.

A test rationale consisting of kick performance, eccentric strength of the knee flexors and concentric strength of the knee extensors, is proposed to evaluate skilled performance characteristics of soccer players. The relation between the strength tests described here might represent an interesting ratio to be evaluated more extensively.

References

Bosco, C., Mognoni, P. and Luthanen P. (1983) Relationship between isokinetic performance and ballistic movement. Eur. J. Appl. Physiol., 51, 357-364.

Clarke, H.H. (1976) Application of Measurement to Health and Physical Education. New Jersey: Prentice Hall Inc., 171-174.

De Proft, E., Cabri, J., Bollens, E., Dufour, W. and Clarys, J.P. (1987) Muscle activity in the soccer kick. Paper presented at the First World Congress of Science and Football, Liverpool (U.K.), April, 1987.

Hart, D., Miller, L. and Stauber, W. (1985) Effect of cooling on force oscillations during maximal voluntary eccentric exercise. Experimental Neurology, 90, 73-80.

Kanehisa, H. and Miyashita, M. (1983) Specificity of velocity in strength training. Eur. J. Appl. Physiol., 52, 104-106.

Letzelter, H.Z. (1983) Methoden und Inhalte der Krafttrainungs. Ahrensburg: Cruvalina, 318.

Oberg, B., Moller, M., Gillquist, J. and Ekstrand, J. (1986) Isokinetic torque levels in soccer players. Int. J. Sports Med., 7, 50-53.

Perrine, J.J., and Edgerton, V.R. (1975) Isokinetic anaerobic ergometry. (Abstr.) Med. Sci. Sports, 7, 78.

Prins, J.H. (1978) Histological changes in human skeletal muscle with isokinetic strength training at two distinct limb speeds. Dissertation Abstracts International, 39 (A), 4123.

Stevens, R. (1980) Isokinetic vs isotonic training in the development of lower body strength and power, Scholastic Coach, 49, 74-76.

A FITNESS PROFILE AND ANTHROPOMETRIC ANALYSIS OF FIRST AND SECOND CLASS RUGBY UNION PLAYERS

P. Rigg and T. Reilly
Liverpool Polytechnic, Department of Sport and Recreation Studies, Byrom Street, Liverpool L3 3AF., England.

Introduction

Rugby Union football is a team game, which is unique in many of its traditions, rules and mores. It is the major winter sport of Wales, New Zealand and South Africa and is currently played in forty countries worldwide.

The team incorporates two playing units - 8 forwards (ball winners), and 7 backs (ball carriers). A variety of profiles of body composition and fitness is apparent in both playing units, the reason for this heterogeneity being the diversity of playing skills required by the game itself.

Despite the game's worldwide popularity, there have been few comprehensive investigations of the anthropometric and physiological characteristics of elite Rugby Union players. Three main areas of examination are evident:-

(i) General fitness profiling, involving basic fitness tests such as vertical and broad jumps, sit-ups and press-ups.

(ii) Physiological profiling, including measurement of aerobic power, cardiovascular performance, and anaerobic power output.

(iii) Anthropometric profiling, incorporating somatotyping, measures of body composition, body proportions and basic measurements such as height and weight.

Integration of the afore-mentioned areas yields a multivariate approach towards profiling. This type of multi-factorial assessment of fitness has proved successful in evaluation of soccer players (Reilly and Thomas, 1977; 1980).

There are basic descriptive data on rugby players from the three main approaches towards fitness profiling. Maud (1983) produced a comprehensive report on the fitness and body parameters that described one amateur U.S.A. Rugby Union team. Fifteen subjects thus engaged in tests to assess anthropometry, flexibility, muscular endurance, aerobic and anaerobic power. Comparisons were made between forward and back line units: this work was later furthered by Maud and Shultz (1984), in assessing the 1982 U.S.A. national squad. They found significant differences between forward and back line players in anthropometric variables including height, weight, percent fat, lean body mass, but not in muscle strength, power or aerobic capacity. The small sample size in these studies restricted the inferences that can be made.

Vanderfield (1975) and Webb and Lander (1983) have undertaken general fitness assessment of Rugby players. Williams et al. (1973) and Bell (1980) have also supplied examples of baseline physiological profiling for this sport.

Anthropometry has been considered in some detail by Bell (1973, 1979, 1980). Bell's (1973) study involved second class players; he found that body shape was essentially uniform for forwards and backs, but that forwards had more body fat (19.5% against 12.2%), particularly in the areas of maximum contact, essentially the upper body.

Although the areas previously described have been explored, it is apparent that considerable gaps still remain in our knowledge about Rugby Union footballers. Notably, analysis of first class British players is very limited, as is research authenticating a discrimination between playing positions and between standards of play, factors which make Rugby Union so unique.

It is reasonable to assume that the various playing roles impose specific demands on players, so that fitness requirements will vary according to playing position. It is also likely that a higher level of fitness is called for the higher the standard of play. The aim of this study was twofold:-

(i) to determine whether any differences in fitness profiles exists between the five positional categories;

(ii) to examine differences in fitness profiles and body composition values between first and second class Rugby Union players.

Methods

The research involved the analysis of data on forty-eight 1st and 2nd Class Rugby Union players. The 1st class players were selected from Liverpool, Waterloo and Leicester Rugby Union Football Clubs' 1st team squads; the 2nd class players were recruited for the study from Liverpool Polytechnic R.U.F.C., 2nd and 3rd teams. The subjects were sub-divided into 5 positional categories as shown in Table 1.

Table 1. Positional categories and numbers of subjects tested

Category	Positions	Number of Subjects 1st Class	2nd Class
1. Front row	Prop, Hooker	5	5
2. Second row	Locks	4	3
3. Back row	No. 8, Flanker	5	5
4. Half-backs	Scrum half; Fly half	4	4
5. Backs	Wing, Centre, Full-back	6	7

All forty-eight subjects, performed a comprehensive battery of tests, during two periods of testing (except for the 1st class front row forwards). The first session involved four pairs of tests, undertaken at the respective Rugby clubs' premises. The second session was conducted in the laboratory at Liverpool Polytechnic. This session involved anthropometric data collection and tests of aerobic and anaerobic capacity. Standard procedures were adopted throughout the research; a brief summary of the protocols utilised in each test follows.

The performance tests comprising the first session incorporated muscle strength and endurance tests, leg power, suppleness, speed and agility. The procedures are briefly described:-

Muscle strength and endurance: (i) Floor push-ups; the push-up procedure was repeated once every two seconds. Scoring consisted of the maximum number of floor push-ups. (ii) Sit-ups; the maximum number of sit-ups was recorded. Counting was ceased if a pause was taken at the top or bottom of the action, the hands were unclasped, or the subjects pushed upwards from the elbows.

Leg power: (i) Vertical jump and (ii) Standing broad jump. The greatest of three attempts was recorded to the nearest cm (Adams et al., 1963).

Suppleness: (i) Dynamic flexibility according to Fleishman(1964) and (ii) Sit and reach test according to Wells and Dillon (1952).

Speed and agility: (i) 40 m sprint, was conducted from a standing start on a marked Rugby Union pitch. The faster of two attempts was recorded to the nearest 0.1s. (ii) Western Motor Ability run (W.M.A.) was conducted as described by Youanez (1976).

The second session carried out in the laboratory consisted of basic anthropometric measures, the Wingate Anerobic Test and the measurement of physical work capacity (PWC_{170}).

Anthropometry: (i) Body fat, was recorded at four sites (biceps, triceps, sub-scapular, supra-iliac), using Harpenden skinfold calipers. The percentage body fat was calculated according to the procedures of Durnin and Womersley (1974): (ii) Somatotype, using Heath and Carter's (1976) modified somatotype procedure.

The Wingate Anaerobic test was performed using the standard procedure of Dotan and Bar-Or (1983). Three values were recorded Peak Power, Mean Power and Peak Power/Body Weight.

The PWC_{170} test was performed according to the procedure described by Watson and O'Donovan (1976).

Results

The performance test profiles of the players are presented in Table 2. Results were examined for significance using analysis of variance and t-tests.

In the 1st Class players performance on the sit-ups and press-ups was poorest in the second row forwards and best in the backs (sit-ups) and front row (press-ups). This trend was not replicated among the 2nd Class group. The poorest jumping performances tended to be among the front-row forwards, although differences between the groups were non-significant ($P > 0.05$). In the sprint tests the backs and half-backs were the fastest, front row and second-row forwards the slowest. There were no clear trends in the flexibility data which discriminated between the playing positions for both levels of play.

The 1st Class front row players as a group had significantly higher values that their 2nd class counterparts in press-ups and sit and reach ($P < 0.05$): differences in the standing broad jump and vertical jump tests were not significant ($P > 0.05$). The back row players of the 1st Class Group were significantly different from those of 2nd Class standard in the sit and reach test and in the vertical jump ($P < 0.05$). The half-backs of the 1st Class sample were significantly better in press-ups and sit-ups that the 2nd Class half-backs ($P < 0.05$). The backs of 1st Class standard performed significantly better than did those of the 2nd Class group in these same two tests ($P < 0.01$). The faster performances of the 1st Class players in the sprint and agility runs did not reach significance ($P < 0.05$).

The laboratory based data are contained in Table 3 for both the 1st Class and 2nd Class players. The second row forwards were the tallest and heaviest, half-backs the smallest and lightest for both standards of play. At both levels of play the backs were the leanest: the highest percent body fat was found in front row forwards at 1st Class level and second row at 2nd Class. The overall mean somatotype of the players was 2.5; 5.0; 2.0. Differences between playing positions were non-significant ($P > 0.05$). The best performance on the Wingate Anaerobic tests were obtained by the back row players, but only among the top class group. When values were expressed relative to body weight, results for the backs approached those of the 1st Class back row players and were the highest among the 2nd Class players. On the aerobic test (PWC_{170}) the highest values were found in the back row players in the 1st Class group, no clear trend being discernible among the 2nd Class players.

Significant differences were observed for second row forwards between the two standards of play in height, weight, percent body fat, endomorphy and in the PWC_{170} test ($P < 0.05$). Differences between 1st and 2nd Class players were also found among the back row forwards in height, all three Wingate Anaerobic test variables and in PWC_{170} ($P < 0.05$). The 1st Class half-backs were higher than their counterparts at the lower level of play in mesomorphy ($P < 0.01$) while the 1st Class backs were significantly better than those in the 2nd Class group on the PWC_{170} test. The mean overall somatotype of the 1st Class players (2.5: 4.9: 1.7) was not significantly different from those at the lower level ($P > 0.05$).

Discussion

Results confirmed the existence of unique characteristics of Rugby Union players according to positional role and standard of play. Body size, indicated by height and weight, proved to be the most predictable source of variability between positions. The 1st Class, second row players, for example, were on average 24 cm taller and 24 kg heavier than the half-backs. The greatest homogeneity was seen in somatotype which differed little between the defined positional categories and the level of play. This duplicates earlier findings that differences between the main positional categories are distinguished by characteristics of body size rather than shape (Reilly and Hardiker, 1981).

Although the 1st Class front row players had generally better fitness profiles than those of the 2nd Class group, only the results

Table 2. Fitness performance profiles (mean ± SD) 1st and 2nd Class players

Test		Front row	Second row	Back row	Half-backs	Backs
Press-ups	1st Class	41.2 ± 8.6[a]	31.8 ± 18.6	38.4 ± 8.8	39.0 ± 3.2[a]	33.8 ± 3.9[b]
	2nd Class	26 ± 3.4	17.3 ± 3.1	42 ± 22.1	28.5 ± 6.6	24 ± 4.5
Sit-ups	1st Class	79.4 ± 50.1	63.3 ± 9.7	71.6 ± 22.2	87.5 ± 2.5[a]	95.7 ± 24.5[b]
	2nd Class	56.3 ± 2.9	55 ± 5	85.2 ± 75.4	51.8 ± 7	57.9 ± 17.1
Vertical Jump (cm)	1st Class	50 ± 7	52 ± 3[a]	53 ± 5[a]	55 ± 3	57 ± 2
	2nd Class	45 ± 4	52 ± 3	46 ± 5	51 ± 3	51 ± 7
Broad Jump (cm)	1st Class	2.12 ± 5[a]	2.24 ± 5	2.27 ± 23	2.4 ± 19	2.30 ± 20
	2nd Class	2.00 ± 92	2.25 ± 5	2.22 ± 13	2.3 ± 17	2.30 ± 17
40 m sprint (s)	1st Class	6.38 ± 0.5	6.28 ± 0.22	6.12 ± 0.2	5.82 ± 0.2	5.8 ± 0.4
	2nd Class	6.7 ± 0.2	6.5 ± 0.1	6.16 ± 0.2	6.0 ± 0.2	6.1 ± 0.2
W.M.A. (s)	1st Class	17.9 ± 0.7	18.5 ± 0.6	17.2 ± 0.7	17.0 ± 0.4	16.9 ± 0.8
	2nd Class	18.6 ± 6.9	18.8 ± 0.1	17.7 ± 0.6	17.3 ± 0.4	17.4 ± 0.9
Sit and Reach (cm)	1st Class	10.2 ± 4.7[a]	5.9 ± 4.3	11.7 ± 5.5[a]	4.3 ± 6.5	9.8 ± 4.8
	2nd Class	0.63 ± 7.5	8.2 ± 5.5	3.7 ± 4.3	5.8 ± 3	8.1 ± 4.6
Dynamic flexibility	1st Class	23.2 ± 5.5	20.8 ± 2.1	19.6 ± 5.6	23.2 ± 3.8	21.3 ± 4.3
	2nd Class	20.8 ± 1.7	16.0 ± 9.6	23.2 ± 0.8	21.3 ± 2.2	23.9 ± 2.8

a, indicates $P < 0.05$; b, $P < 0.01$

Table 3. Anthropometry, anaerobic and physical work capacities (mean values ± SD), 1st Class and 2nd Class players

Test		Front row	Second row	Back row	Half-backs	Backs
Height (cm)	1st Class	176.7 ± 3.7	196.7 ± 6.1[a]	184.8 ± 5.9[a]	172.8 ± 5.4	180.4 ± 4.8
	2nd Class	176.2 ± 2.7	185.3 ± 2.1	176.1 ± 4.1	172 ± 2.2	179.6 ± 4.6
Weight (kg)	1st Class	89.2 ± 3.7	100.8 ± 6.7[a]	86.5 ± 6.8	77.0 ± 5.8	80.2 ± 4.6
	2nd Class	80.0 ± 8.1	86.7 ± 8	80.9 ± 5.8	72.0 ± 8.9	77.3 ± 5.2
Body Fat (%)	1st Class	13.6 ± 2.1	11.1 ± 1.2[a]	11.5 ± 2.5	12.1 ± 1.2	10.4 ± 1.5
	2nd Class	12.4 ± 3.4	13.3 ± 1	12.3 ± 2.1	11.7 ± 1.3	11.0 ± 2.9
Peak Power(W)	1st Class	-	914 ± 46	1071.0 ± 108[a]	858.0 ± 32	888.0 ± 46
	2nd Class	937.0 ± 79	861.0 ± 84	878.0 ± 121	809.0 ± 47	941.0 ± 142
Mean Power (W)	1st Class	-	797.0 ± 70	903.0 ± 39[a]	618.0 ± 32	767.0 ± 68
	2nd Class	755.0 ± 103	699.0 ± 47	735.0 ± 118	674.0 ± 73	656.0 ± 237
Peak Power	1st Class	-	7.9 ± 1.1	10.6 ± 1.2[a]	8.0 ± 0.4[b]	9.68 ± 0.18
($W\ kg^{-1}$)	2nd Class	9.3 ± 1.3	8.2 ± 0.2	8.6 ± 0.9	9.4 ± 0.3	9.9 ± 1.4
PWC_{170} (W)	1st Class	210.0 ± 37	246.0 ± 22	258.0 ± 38[a]	204.0 ± 37	238.0 ± 61[a]
	2nd Class	210.0 ± 35	210.0 ± 9	186.0 ± 40	180.0 ± 11	174.0 ± 20

a, indicates $P < 0.05$; b, $P < 0.01$

for height, weight, endomorphy and mesomorphy proved to reach statistical significance. Although the highest values of percent body fat were noted in the front row players, the levels were still below the average for the general population. They were still below the 14.6% reported by Bell (1980) for rugby forwards and close to the 12.7% found by Williams et al (1973). The front row members were the least mobile of the players and this was reflected in their sprint times. Their superior performances in the press-ups reflect the role of the props in pushing against the opposing scrum.

Teams depend on their second row players for winning possession in the line-out. In this respect, height, leanness and jumping ability are beneficial. It seems that the second row players in the top class clubs gain advantage because of their height rather than anaerobic and jumping test performances. The best jumpers were the backs and half-backs at the 1st Class level, their performances being slightly better than those of English League professional soccer players (Thomas and Reilly, 1979).

The back row players, particularly at 1st Class level, demonstrated fitness profiles of all-round athletes. They were the fastest of the categories of forwards and were the most flexible in the sit and reach test. They were the best group on the aerobic capacity test and on the Wingate Anaerobic test. Their power outputs on the latter tests were appreciably better than those reported for well-trained sports science students on the same test (Parry-Billings et al., 1986), although the superiority is largely explained by differences in body weight. The high values on the PWC_{170} test fits in with their foraging role in loose-play.

The half-backs showed good results for sit-ups and press-ups and tended towards high mesomorphy values. Their good performances in the sprints supplemented their scores in the jump tests. These qualities would be important in order to neutralise the speed and anaerobic power of the 1st Class back row players. Overall the backs were the fastest group: this is compatible with their role of running with the ball.

The present study demonstrated differences between 1st and 2nd Class players and suggests differences in fitness requirements according to the level of Rugby Union played. A higher standard of fitness seems to be required at the more competitive level of play. Besides, body size and fitness profiles were shown to be specific to positional categories: this specificity was more strongly dictated by positional role in the 1st class compared to the 2nd class level of play. The analysis was insensitive to examining individual playing positions, for example, that of full-back among the backs or hooker among the front row. This required a considerably greater sample than was available but points to a direction that future research might take.

References

Adams, W.C., Haskell, W.L., Holtinger, W.L., Leight, R.D. and Penny, W.J. (1963) Foundations of Physical Activity. Champaign Ill: Stipes Publishing Company.

Bell, W. (1973) Anthropometry of the young adult college Rugby player

in Wales. Sport Bibliography, 7, 298-299.
Bell, W. (1979) Body compositions of Rugby Union football players. Brit. J. Sports Med., 13, 19-23.
Bell, W. (1980) Body composition and maximal aerobic power of Rugby Union forwards. J. Sports Med. Phys. Fit., 20, 447-451.
Dotan, R. and Bar-Or, O. (1983) Load optimization for the Wingate anerobic Test. Eur. J. Appl. Physiol. Occup. Physiol., 44, 737-743.
Durnin, J.V.G.A. and Womersley, J. (1974) Body fat assessed from total-body density and its estimation from skinfold thickness measurements on 481 men and women aged from 16 to 72 years. Brit. J. Nutr., 32, 169-179.
Fleishman, E.A. (1964) The Structure and Measurement of Physical Fitness. Englewood Cliffs, NJ: Prentice Hall.
Maud, P.J. (1983) Physiology and anthropometric parameters that describe a Rugby Union team, Brit. J. Sports Med., 17, 16-23.
Maud, P.J. and Shultz, B.B. (1984) The U.S. national rugby team: a physiological and anthropometrical assessment. Physician Sportsmed., 12, 86-99.
Parry-Billings, M., Reilly, T. and MacLaren, D. (1986) The measurement of anaerobic power and capacity: studies on the Wingate Anaerobic Test. Soc. Nat. Instit. Phys. Educ. Sports J., 9, 48-58.
Reilly, T. and Hardiker, R. (1981) Somatotype and injuries in adult student rugby. J. Sports Med. Fit. 21, 186-191.
Reilly, T. and Thomas, V. (1977) Application of multivariate analysis to the fitness assessment of soccer players. Brit. J. Sports Med., 11, 183-184.
Reilly, T. and Thomas, V. (1980) The stability of fitness factors over a season of professional soccer as indicated by serial factor analyses. In: Kinanthropometry II (edited by M. Ostyn, G. Beunen and J. Simons) pp.247-257. Baltimore: University Park Press.
Thomas, V. and Reilly, T. (1979) Fitness assessment of English League soccer players through the competitive season. Brit. J. Sports Med., 13, 103-109.
Vanderfield, D.G. (1975). Fitness testing of Rugby players. Austr. J. Sports Med., 14, 14-15.
Watson, A.W.S. and O'Donovan, D.J. (1976) The relationship of level of habitual activity to measures of leanness-fatness, physical working capacity, strength and motor ability in 17 and 18 year old males. J. Appl. Physiol., 36, 618-624.
Webb, D. and Lander, J. (1984) An economical fitness testing battery for high school and college Rugby teams. Sports Coach, 7, 44-46.
Wells, K. and Dillon, E. (1952) The sit and reach test - a test of back and leg flexibility. Res. Quart., 23, 115-118.
Williams, C., Reid, R.M., and Coutts, R. (1973) Observations on the aerobic power of university Rugby players and professional soccer players, Brit. J. Sports Med., 7, 390-391.
Youanez, M.S. (1976) Wester Motor Ability Tests. University of Western Ontario, London, Canada: Physical Fitness Research Laboratories.

AEROBIC AND ANAEROBIC POWER OF RUGBY FOOTBALL PLAYERS

Y. Ueno, E. Watai and K. Ishii
Nippon College of Physical Education,7-1-1, Fukazawa, Tokyo, Setagaya-ku, Tokyo, Japan.

Introduction

Several investigators have recently attempted to determine the maximal anaerobic power from different viewpoints (Katch 1974; Evans and Quinney 1981; Dotan and Bar-Or 1983; Simoneau et al., 1983: LaVioie et al., 1984: Patton et al., 1985). Attention has been devoted to establishing the best method of eliciting the maximal mechanical power output and to clarifying the energy patterns in such short-term, strenuous activities. The purpose of this study was to examine the relationship between maximal anaerobic and aerobic power of Rugby football players by measuring their maximal mechanical power outputs and their maximal oxygen intakes.

Methods

Subjects

Ninety-nine inter-college level (Japan) Rugby Union football players volunteered as subjects. They were classified broadly into three groups by their playing positions:- forward players (FW), half-back players (HB), three-quarters back players (TB).

Measurement of mechanical power output

An electrically braked bicycle ergometer (Combi Power Max V) was utilized to measure the mechanical power output. A load relative to body weight (0.1 kp kg^{-1}) was imposed on each subject for 7 s. The mechanical power outputs generated during the maximal pedalling bout were digitized by means of a microcomputer linked to the bicycle ergometer.

Measurement of maximal oxygen uptake

Maximal oxygen uptake ($\dot{V}O_2$ max) was determined with a progressive work test on a bicycle ergometer (Monark). Expired gas was collected by the Douglas bag method. The O_2 and CO_2 concentrations of the mixed expired gas were analyzed with the Sanei (1 H 21) gas monitor.

Statistical Procedure

A two-way analysis of variance (ANOVA) was employed to assess the differences between groups. The level of significance was set at the 0.05 level.

Results

The data are summarised in Table 1. Values are presented as mean with SD in parenthesis.

Table 1. Physical characteristics and $\dot{V}O_2$ max, $\dot{V}O_2$ max/body weight, peak power and peak power/body weight according to playing positions

Position	n	Height (cm)	Weight (kg)	(Aerobic) $\dot{V}O_2$max ($l\ min^{-1}$)	$\dot{V}O_2$max ($ml\ kg^{-1}\ min^{-1}$)	(Anaerobic) Peak power (W)	Peak power ($W\ kg^{-1}$)
Forward	44	176.5 (5.9)	80.6 (8.5)	4.37 (0.6)	54.7 (7.2)	1047.4 (119.2)	13.02 (1.0)
Half-back	17	168.5 (3.6)	66.3 (4.2)	3.70 (0.5)	55.8 (6.7)	907.7 (99.7)	13.68 (1.2)
Three-Quarters	38	171.9 (3.9)	69.5 (5.1)	3.77 (0.4)	54.5 (6.4)	948.3 (79.7)	13.66 (0.9)
Total	99	173.4 (5.7)	73.9 (9.0)	4.01 (0.6)	54.8 (6.8)	985.3 (116.4)	13.38 (1.1)

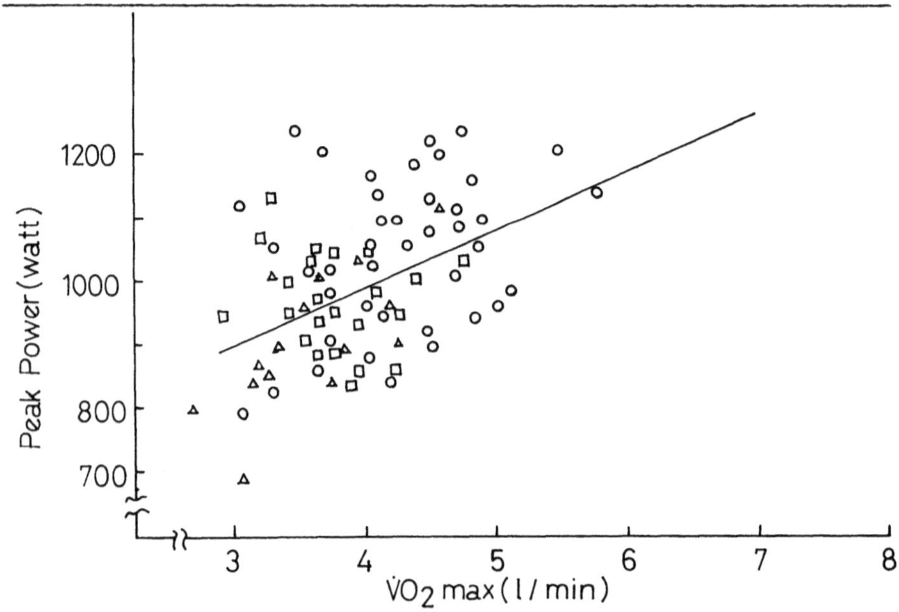

Figure 1. Relationship between $\dot{V}O_2$max($l\ min^{-1}$) and peak power(watt)

The $\dot{V}O_2$ max of forward (FW) players (4.37 $l\ min^{-1}$) was greater than that of the three-quarters (TB) group (3.77 $l\ min^{-1}$) or the half-back (HB) players (3.70 $l\ min^{-1}$). The differences between FW and TB and between FW and HB were significant ($P<0.001$). When the $\dot{V}O_2$ max was expressed relative to body weight, it was found to be higher in HB players (55.8 ml kg^{-1} min^{-1}) than in FW and TB players. However, the differences between the three groups were not significant. The greatest value of all peak power outputs was 1047.4 W in FW players. There were significant differences between FW and TB players and between FW and HB players ($P<0.001$). The mean power was closely associated with peak power ($r=0.987$, $P<0.001$). Therefore, peak power alone is employed as representative of anaerobic power in the Discussion section.

The $\dot{V}O_2$ max was closely related to peak power ($r=0.460$: $P<0.001$) (Fig.1). However, when values were corrected for body weight, the significant relation between peak power and $\dot{V}O_2$ max was not found.

Discussion

According to a previous study of the maximal aerobic power of Japanese elite athletes (Kuroda et al., 1973), the maximal oxygen uptakes of Rugby Football players were 3.99 l min^{-1} (52.1 ml kg^{-1} min^{-1}). The present results (4.01 l min^{-1}; 54.8ml kg^{-1} min^{-1}) agree closely with those of the previous study. Based on other findings the mean $\dot{V}O_2$ max obtained in this study coincided with that of wrestlers and weight-lifters (Saltin and Åstrand, 1967) and handball players, badminton players and sprinters (Hollman and Heck, 1971).

As for the anaerobic power outputs, the peak power of Rugby Football players was 985.4 W (13.4 W kg^{-1}), which was greater than that reported previously for college students (Katch and Weltman, 1979; Evans and Quinney, 1981; Crielaard and Pirnay, 1981; Dotan and Bar-Or, 1983; Nakamura et al., 1984). Particularly, it should be noted that the absolute peak power (1047.4 W) of FW players was greater than that of the sprinters studied by Crielaard and Pirnay (1981). As for the value relative to body weight, the peak power obtained in this study (13.35 W kg^{-1}) was greater than that of the middle and long-distance runners (10.63 and 10.51 W kg^{-1} but less than that of the sprinters (14.16 W kg^{-1}).

Several investigators have reported on the relationship between maximal aerobic and maximal anaerobic power (Katch and Weltman, 1979: Crielaard and Pirnay, 1981; Boulay et al., 1985). There are some contradictary findings on the relationship between them. Findings have varied from reports of a high, negative correlation between the two parameters to others that have reported no relationship. Results may be influenced by factors such as the difference in muscle fibre type (Komi et al., 1977; Bar-Or et al., 1980; Simoneau et al., 1985), the balance of pH (MacCartney et al., 1983) and the effects of enzyme activities (Gollnick et al., 1973; Taunton et al., 1981; Boobis et al., 1983) because different types of athletes were employed as subjects in those studies. Therefore, the specificities of these sports events appeared to affect the relationship between aerobic and anaerobic powers. The present study found that there was a positive, linear relationship between $\dot{V}O_2$ max and peak power ($Y=91.025x + 620.577$, $r=0.460$). The correlation could be explained by the common influence of body weight since $\dot{V}O_2$ max was not significantly associated with peak power when both variables were expressed per unit body mass. Besides, the FW players who possessed a large muscle volume had greater values in both parameters than HB players who had less muscle volume. This reinforces the view that the differences in body size accounted for the significant correlation between anaerobic power and aerobic power when values were expressed in absolute terms. Therefore, $\dot{V}O_2$ max/body weight of HB and TB players would tend to equal or exceed that of FW players when the influence of body weight is eliminated.

It seems that FW players had larger $\dot{V}O_2$ max ($1\ min^{-1}$) and peak power (W) because their body weights and muscle volumes were larger than the others. On the other hand, it is noted that HB players who had less body weight had larger $\dot{V}O_2$ max ($ml\ kg^{-1}$) and peak power ($W\ kg^{-1}$) than FW players. In relative terms the HB and TB players were better in both aerobic power and anaerobic power than FW players. This would allow the half-backs especially, to move around the field more effectively than FW players in the actual game.

References

Bar-Or, O., Dotan, R., Inbar, O., Rothstein, A., Karlsson, J. and Tesch, P. (1980) Anaerobic capacity and muscle fibre type distribution in man. Int. J. Sports Med., 1, 82-85

Boobis, L., Williams, C. and Wootton, S.A. (1983) Human muscle metabolism during brief maximal exercise. J. Physiol., 338, 21.

Boulay, M.R., Lortie, G., Simoneau, J.A., Hamel, P., Leblanc, C. and Bouchard, C. (1985) Specificity of aerobic and anaerobic work capacities and powers. Int. J. Sports Med., 6, 325-328.

Crielaard, J.M. and Pirnay, F. (1981) Anaerobic and aerobic power of top athletes. Eur. J. Appl. Physiol., 47, 295-300.

Dotan, A. and Bar-Or, O. (1983) Load optimization for the Wingate Anaerobic Test. Eur. J. Appl. Physiol., 51, 409-417.

Evans, T.A. and Quinney H.A. (1981) Determination of resistance settings for anaerobic power testing. Canad. J. Appl. Sport Sci., 6, 53-56.

Gollnick, P.D., Armstrong, R.B., Saltin, B., Saubert, C.W. Sembrowich, W.L. and Shephard, R.E. (1973) Effect of training on enzyme activity and fibre composition of human skeletal muscle. J. Appl. Physiol., 34, 107-111.

Hollman, W. and Heck, H. (1971) Herzleistungsfahigkeit und Sport. Arztliche Fortbildung, 1, 62-67.

Katch, V.L. (1974) Body weight, leg volume, leg weight and leg density as determiners of short duration work performance on the bicycle ergometer. Med. Sci. Sports, 6, 267-270.

Katch, V.L. and Weltman, A. (1979) Interrelationship between anaerobic power output, anaerobic capacity and aerobic power. Ergonomics, 22, 325-332.

Komi, P., Rusko, H., Vos, J. and Vihko, V. (1977) Anaerobic performance capacity in athletes. Acta Physiol. Scand., 100, 107-114.

Kuroda, Y., Itoh, S., Tsukagoshi, K., Amemiya, T. and Susuki, Y. (1973) Maximal oxygen uptake in Japanese top athletes. The 2nd Report in Sports Sciences of Japan Amateur Athletic Association (Tokyo).

LaVoie, N., Dallaire, J., Brayne, S. and Barrete, D. (1984) Anaerobic testing using the Wingate and Evans-Ouinney protocols with and without toe stirrups. Canad.J. Appl. Sport Sci., 9, 1-5.

MacCartney, N., Heigenhauser, G.F. and Jones, N.L. (1983) Effects of pH on maximal power output and fatigue during short-term dynamic exercise. J. Appl. Physiol., Respirat. Envir. Exerc. Physiol., 55, 225-229.

Nakamura, Y., Mutoh, Y., and Miyashita, M. (1984) A method of determining maximal anaerobic power using a bicycle ergometer. Japan J. Sports Sci., 3, 834-839.

Patton, J.F., Murphy, M.M. and Frederick, E.A. (1985) Maximal power outputs during the Wingate Anaerobic Test. Int. J. Sports Med., 6, 52-85.

Saltin, B. and Åstrand, P.O. (1967) Maximal oxygen uptake in athletes. J. Physiol., 23, 353-358.

Simoneau, J.A., Lortie, G., Boulay, M.R. and Bouchard, C., (1983) Tests of anaerobic alactacid and lactacid capacities: Description and reliability. Canad. J. Appl. Sport Sci., 8, 277-270.

Simoneau, J.A., G. Lortie., Boulayt, M.R., Marcotte, M., Thibault, M.C. and Bouchard, C. (1985) Human skeletal muscle fibre type alteration with high-intensity intermittent training. Eur. J. Appl. Physiol., 54, 250-253.

Taunton, J.E., Maron, H. and Wilkinson, J.G. (1981) Anaerobic Performance in Middle and Long Distance Runners. Canad. J. Appl. Sports Sci., 6, 109-113.

POWER OUTPUT OF RUGBY FORWARDS DURING MAXIMAL TREADMILL SPRINTING

M.E. Cheetham, R.J. Hazeldine, A. Robinson and C. Williams
Department of Physical Education and Sports Science, University of Technology, Loughborough, Leics. LE11 3TU, England.

Introduction

It has been said that sheer muscular power (strength applied at speed) is the basis of physical effort in rugby (Evans, 1973). Because of methodological problems the measurement of the maximal power of rugby footballers has been confined to tests of explosive or passive strength such as the Sargeant jump or hand grip test, whilst the determination of power output during running has been limited to treadmill and field tests which measure, or predict, maximal aerobic power ($\dot{V}O_2$max). During such tests body weight must be supported throughout the run so oxygen uptake is quite rightly expressed in relation to body weight, with the consequence that rugby forwards with their particularly high body weight have relatively low $\dot{V}O_2$max values compared to other groups (Bell, 1980; Williams et al., 1973). In Rugby Union football the power required to win the ball is to a large extent supplied by the heavy body weights of the forwards. Furthermore, it has been estimated that one third of the distance run by a rugby forward during an international game is covered at maximal pace with the remainder at approximately three quarter pace (Williams, 1976). Maximal sprinting activity requires a power output which is 2-3 times greater than the maximal aerobic power (Wootton, 1984). Therefore, it is of interest and of relevance to examine the power output of rugby forwards during maximal running activity and to express this power output both in absolute terms and in relation to body weight. Thus the purpose of the present study was to examine the power output of rugby forwards during maximal treadmill sprinting and to make comparisons with some previously collected data on rugby backs of the same playing standard.

Methods

Subjects

Ten student Rugby Union forwards (1st XV; two props, two second row, 5 flankers and one number 8) whose mean (±SD) height, age and weight were 1.85±0.06m, 20.7±0.6 yrs and 92.5+6.9 kg respectively, volunteered to participate in the study and to perform a maximal 30 s sprint on a non-motorized treadmill. These highly motivated subjects were familiarized with treadmill sprinting in the week prior to the study and agreed not to take part in training or match-play on the day before the treadmill running test.

Equipment

A non-motorized treadmill was used for the sprint test as this allowed the subjects to run at unrestricted speeds and to change speed as fatigue occurred. The modifications made to the non-motorized treadmill have been previously described (Lakomy, 1984). Briefly the treadmill was interfaced to a microcomputer which allowed the continuous monitoring of the horizontally applied force by means of a force transducer mounted on the rear cross-bar of the treadmill and the continuous monitoring of belt speed by means of a small generator mounted on the front axle of the treadmill. The instantaneous product of the horizontally applied force and treadmill belt speed was used to determine external power output during the test.

Protocol

Five minutes before the 30 s sprint, two 30 s sub-maximal runs were performed on the non-motorized treadmill at 10 and 12 km h^{-1} which served both as a warm-up and to re-accustom the subjects with experimental procedures. The 30 s sprint was commenced from a jogging start at 8km h^{-1}. The subjects were asked to run as fast as possible from the start of the test and were verbally encouraged throughout. Heart rate was recorded during the sprint and throughout 5 min of passive recovery.

Blood sampling and treatment

Capillary blood samples were taken in duplicate after the sub-maximal warm-up and at 5 min post-exercise. They were deproteinized, frozen at -20°C and analysed for blood lactate and glucose concentrations as described by Maughan (1982).

Terminology

Throughout this study 'peak power output' refers to the highest value of power attained during the test, whilst 'mean power output' refers to the average power output for the 30 s period. 'End power output' refers to the value of power in the last second of the sprint. 'Fatigue' refers to the decline in power output over the 30 s period of the test and is expressed as the difference between peak and end power output as a percentage of the peak power output. Results are presented as mean$\pm$SD.

Results

Power output

The power profile generated during the 30 s sprint is shown in Fig.1. Peak power output of 830$\pm$149W was reached between 2 s and 8 s into the test for all individuals. The power profile shows a slightly lower peak than this, because of inter-individual variations in the time taken to reach peak power output. After attainment of peak power output there was a continuous decline in power for the remainder of the sprint, resulting in an overall decrease of 48$\pm$11% throughout the time period of the test. Therefore, the mean power output of 579$\pm$49W was substantially lower than the peak value. When power output was expressed in relation to body weight the peak and mean power outputs were 8.96±1.32 W kg^{-1} and 6.28±0.54 W kg^{-1} respectively. Those forwards with the highest peak power, expressed in absolute terms or in relation to body weight, also experienced the greatest fatigue during the test ($r=0.82$, $P<0.01$).

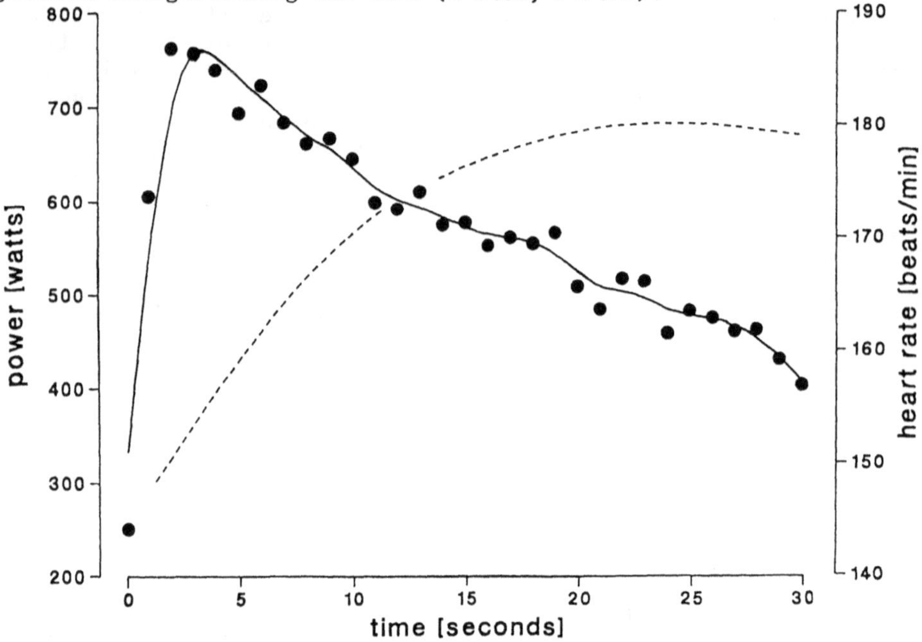

Figure 1. Power output and heart rate of rugby forwards during a 30 s treadmill sprint (n=10). Curves are formally fitted with a least squares method

Heart rate

Heart rate (beats min^{-1}) during the 30 s sprint is illustrated in Fig.1 and shows that whilst power output was declining heart rate was at first rapidly increased and averaged 150±12 and 170±20 beats min^{-1} between 0-5 and between 5-10 s into the sprint respectively. Thereafter, there was only a small increase in heart rate with an average value of 179±13 beats min^{-1} during the last 5 s of the test. After the sprint heart rate was decreased to 147±11 after 1 min recovery and to 106±10 beats min^{-1} at 5 min post-exercise.

Blood lactate and glucose concentrations

Blood lactate was increased from 1.77±0.47 mM to 14.38±2.11 mM and blood glucose from 4.66±0.39 mM to 5.45±0.62 mM as a result of the 30 s sprint. Those forwards with the highest peak power in relation to body weight also had the greatest increases in blood lactate and blood glucose concentrations ($r=0.72$, $P<0.05$ and $r=0.71$, $P<0.05$ respectively). The correlations between mean power wt^{-1} and the increase in blood lactate and blood glucose concentrations were much lower ($r=0.48$, $P>0.05$ and $r=0.19$, $P>0.05$ respectively).

Discussion

It is considered that power is required in rugby football for the making and breaking of tackles, explosive acceleration, snap shoves in the scrum and forcefully ripping in a maul (Williams, 1976). It wsuld be expected, therefore, that rugby forwards would have a relatively large power output. In the present study peak power output for the rugby forwards was the highest that has been recorded for male subjects performing this particular running test, including a group of rugby backs of a similar playing standard (Cheetham and Williams, 1984, 1985). The mean power output was lower than that for the previously tested rugby backs, because of the greater fatigue experienced by the forwards during the 30 s period of the test. Power output during treadmill sprinting has previously been shown to be related to body weight (Lakomy, 1984). Therefore, the higher absolute peak power output of the rugby forwards was due to their greater body weight (92.5±6.9 kg vs 79.5±6.73 kg). Whilst absolute power is important in any contact situation in the game, the rugby forward must also have the ability to transport this body weight at speed around the field. Therefore, power output in relation to body weight is probably a better predictor of running performance in the game. When the power output was expressed in relation to body weight the forwards had a markedly lower peak (8.96±1.32 W kg^{-1} vs 10.12±1.32 W kg^{-1}) and mean power output (6.28±0.54 W kg^{-1} vs 8.03±0.86 W kg^{-1}) than the rugby backs.

In this study those forwards with the highest peak power output in absolute terms, or in relation to body weight, also experienced the greatest fatigue during the test and had the largest increases in blood lactate concentration. Blood lactate concentration at 5 min post-exercise has been shown to be indicative of muscle lactate at the end of exercise for this particular running test (Cheetham et al., 1986). Therefore, it is possible that those individuals with the highest peak power output also had the greatest contribution from anaerobic glycolysis to energy supply during the test, but as a consequence suffered the greatest fatigue because of the ensuing acidosis in the muscle cell. However, the increase in blood lactate concentration for the forwards was substantially lower than that for the previously tested rugby backs (12.62±0.62 mM vs 16.52±1.23 mM), whereas fatigue was greater for the forwards. It is possible that as a result of training the backs have developed a higher buffering capacity allowing them to reduce the change in muscle pH for a given lactate concentration.

In summary this study has shown that the power output of rugby forwards during sprint running can be satisfactorily examined in the laboratory. Those forwards with the highest peak power output are likely to experience the greatest fatigue during a 30 s test. The absolute peak power output of rugby forwards was higher than that for rugby backs, but when the power was expressed in relation to body weight both peak and mean power output during treadmill sprinting was lower for the forwards than for the backs.

References

Bell, W. (1980) Body composition and maximal aerobic power of rugby union forwards. J. Sports Med. Phys. Fit., 20, 447-451.

Cheetham, M.E., Boobis, L.H., Brooks, S. and Williams C. (1986) Human muscle metabolism during sprinting. J. Appl. Physiol., 61, 54-60.

Cheetham, M.E. and Williams, C. (1984) Anaerobic power of male games players and endurance trained athletes. J.Sports Sci., 2, 197-198.

Cheetham, M.E. and Williams, C. (1985) Blood pH and blood lactate concentration after maximal treadmill sprinting. J. Physiol., 361, 79P.

Evans, E.G. (1973) Basic fitness testing of rugby football players. Brit. J. Sports Med., 7, 384-387.

Lakomy, H.K.A. (1984) An ergometer for measuring the power generated during sprinting. J.Physiol., 354, 33P.

Maughan, R.J. (1982) A simple rapid method for the determination of glucose, lactate, alanine, 3-hydroxybutyrate and acetoacetate on a single 20µl blood sample. Clin. Chim. Acta, 122, 231-240.

Williams, C., Reid, R.M. and Coutts, R. (1973) Observations on the aerobic power of university rugby players and professional soccer players. Brit. J. Sports Med., 7, 390-391.

Williams, R. (1976) Skilful Rugby. London: Souvenir Press Ltd.

Wootton, S.A. (1984) Influence of diet and training on the metabolic responses to maximal exercise in man. PhD thesis: Loughborough University of Technology.

Part VI

Medical and environmental aspects of football

ACHILLES TENDINITIS IN SOCCER

A.B. Stibbe,
Chief Medical Staff, A.F.C. Ajax, Middenweg 401, P.O.Box 41885,
1009DB, Amsterdam, The Netherlands.

Introduction

Soccer is the largest participation sport in Holland with about one million registered players, of which half are youths. Though acute injury is the main problem in soccer, overuse injuries are common among players. According to Ekstrand (1982) 30% of all soccer injuries are overuse injuries. Adductor tenosynovitis and Achilles tendinitis are the most common types. In this article Achilles tendinitis and all the measures to prevent this disabling condition are considered.

Though Achilles tendinitis is especially associated with runners, soccer players also frequently incur this condition. In the last five years the professional players of Ajax (Amsterdam) had three ruptures of the Achilles tendon, one of which was a total rupture, the other two partial. In two cases there was a history of Achilles tendinitis. Four percent of absences for medical reasons concerned Achilles tendinitis and six percent involved a rupture.

As great care is taken with these complaints, which means a direct reduction of training and games, there was no case of severe tendinitis with prolonged absence. Plaster therapy, injection therapy or surgical treatment were not necessary in any instance.

The Acute Rupture of the Achilles Tendon

Acute subcutaneous rupture is a typical sport injury with increasing incidence. Though it occurs characteristically in poorly conditioned individuals, it is not infrequently seen among professional soccer players.

Evaluation of an acute rupture is based solely on physical examination. Patients are unable to stand on tip-toe. Fresh cases are easily diagnosed from a visible and palpable gap in the tendon at the site of rupture. The squeeze test of Thompson in which pressure on the calf does not result in passive flexion of the foot is decisive. The therapy of choice in young active people is primary suture.

Tendinitis and rupture are not the only disabling conditions in and around the Achilles tendon (Table 1). In this respect bursitis and Sever's disease are also discussed.

Table 1. Achilles tendon pathology

Tendinitis
Rupture
Bursitis
Periosititis
Avulsion
Apophysitis (Sever's disease)

Achilles bursitis is an inflammation of the bursa between the Achilles tendon and the calcaneus. The soccer shoe, especially a new one, may irritate a prominence on the calcaneus, causing retrocalcaneal bursitis. Palpating the tendon with the thumb and index finger elicts tenderness anterior to the attachment of the tendon. X-rays may reveal a prominence on the calcaneus which in rare cases has to be removed. It is known as Haglund's exostose.

The conservative measures described for treating Achilles tendinitis are also used to treat retrocalcaneal bursitis. Local injections of steroid may be helpful, but care must be taken to avoid injection directly into the tendon.

Sever's disease or traction apophysitis of the heel is a harmless condition occurring only in children during the period of active growth of the calcaneal apophysis. As it is frequently seen in our young soccer players, it merits some comment.

It was formerly believed to be an example of osteochondritis, but it is now generally agreed that it is nothing more than a chronic strain at the attachment of the posterior apophysis. It may thus be regarded as analogous to Osgood-Schlatter's disease of the tibial tubercle. The child is usually between 8 and 13 years old. He complains of pain behind the heel and a slight limp may be noticed. On examination there is a tenderness over the lower posterior part of the tuberosity of the calcaneus. Radiography usually fails to show any alteration from the normal. In most cases treatment is not required, because the symptoms will eventually subside spontaneously.

Achilles Tendinitis

In general there are four types of Achilles tendinitis (Table 2). It is important to make this subdivision because each has its own measures and therapy.

Table 2. Achilles tendinitis

Tendinose (Achillodynie)
Tendinitis
Peritendinitis (Crepitans)
Insertion tendinopathy

The Achillodynie represents a local degeneration of Achilles tissue. On physical examination a tender nodule is found at about 3 - 5 cm proximal to the calcaneal insertion. It is always a sign of longer existing complaints.

The Achilles tendinitis shows an inflammatory reaction with swelling over a part of the tendon.

Achilles tendinitis crepitans is a condition in which the complete tendon is swollen and painful. When the swelling lasts for a longer period, you can hear a noise like walking in the snow, in plantar and dorsi-flexion.

Insertion tendinopathy refers to a painful condition at the attachment of the tendon on the calcaneus.

Aetiology

Achilles tendinitis may be caused, apart from too much training, by two training errors - running on hills and wearing shoes with rigid soles. Additional stress to the Achilles tendon occurs when the runner lands hard when running downhill and during toe-off in running uphill or against the resistance of an inflexible sole. A shoe with an inadequately padded heel wedge or a soft heel counter that does not stabilize the heel may also contribute to injury.

Biomechanical problems such as tibia vara, functional talipes equinus, tight hamstring and calf muscles, and a cavus foot are also associated with Achilles tendinitis. Heel or forefoot varus deformities cause the foot to land in an excessively supinated position and hyperpronate in midstance to compensate, which puts torque on the tendon. These repetitive stresses on the Achilles tendon at heel strike and toe-off, along with running on hills or uneven terrain, inflict small cumulative tears in the tendon that produce the inflammatory response seen clinically.

So the Achilles tendinitis usually is caused by mechanical overloading and wearing improper shoes. It is amplified by anatomical and biomechanical faults along with violence and in some cases disease (Table 3).

Table 3. Aetiology of Achilles tendinitis

Exogenous	Endogenous
Training errors	Anatomical disorders
Surface	Biomechanical disorders
Shoes	General disorders
Climate	
Type of activity	
Technique	
Warm-up	
Cool-down	
Trauma	

Aching pain or stiffness characterize Achilles tendinitis. The patient experiences a burning pain that appears first after a heavy training session, especially the next morning. Later it appears early during warming-up, becomes less severe during practice and then worsens after the training.

The pain may also appear when the patient gets out of bed in the morning but may then gradually subside during the day. When there is pain in the night or at rest there is very likely a rupture. It is important to make this subdivision because the therapy and prevention differ. The prognosis of stage one is excellent when the right measures are taken while stage four is poor, especially when the patient is injected with steroids.

It is important to ask about the circumstances that could have been the cause of the tendinitis (see exogenous aetiology).

Physical Examination

It is necesary to have a full examination including the lower back and feet. This reveals the anatomical and biomechanical disorders already referred to. Since 25% of all Achilles tendon ruptures are missed, it is best to have all patients tip-toe and perform the Thompson test when they have complaints of the lower leg.

Local examination reveals tenderness. This tenderness is usually 4-5 cm proximal to the insertion into the calcaneus, but which may also be diffused along the tendon. In severe cases crepitus, swelling and a tender nodule develop.

During physical examination, gentle palpation of the tendon as the ankle moves from plantar flexion to dorsiflexion can reveal crepitations - tendinitis crepitans. As has been mentioned the player may have one or more biomechanical problems - cavus foot, tight calf muscles and functional hyperpronation.

Diagnosis

As mentioned before, Achilles tendon pathology is a clinical diagnosis. Nevertheless it can be useful to have a lateral X-ray view made, especially in patients more than 30 years old. It can show a Haglund's exostose, a tendon calcification and diminishing of the triangle of Kager.

Therapy

Rest is the key-word in the treatment of all types of Achilles tendinitis. This can mean that the patient must reduce his mileage and avoid hills and banked roads. A heel lift inserted into the shoe is also effective in the way it helps relax the Achilles tendon at heel strike. A tape can also be useful. Trying to 'run through' may convert a mild injury into a severe one demanding total rest or immobilization.

When acute symptoms, especially swelling, are present anti-inflammatory measures are indicated. Ice-therapy is useful but it has to be used for at least 20 min. Physiotherapy in the form of curapuls is also beneficial. Oral medication can be helpful, but steroids are contra-indicated due to the risk of tendon rupture.

When the swelling persists for a longer period, an infiltration can develop. The therapy is different, especially in that improvement of the blood flow is essential. For that purpose ice can be applied, in this case 5 times a day for 5 min. Histamine-iontoforese will improve blood flow. Stretching exercises must be continued to prevent scar tissue and to maintain flexibility.

Sometimes nodule formation is the only sign of chronic overuse of the Achilles tendon. Again vasodilatation is important. This means ice-massage and radar therapy (microwave radiation) are all appropriate. Transverse friction, according to the method of Cyriax (Cyriax and Russell, 1980) will make the scar tissue flexible. Ultrasound therapy may help recalcitrant injuries.

Despite all these conservative measures and through the common delay in seeking proper treatment many cases become chronic and resistant to treatment. Compared with other inflammatory overuse injuries Achilles tendinitis causes patients to abandon their activities for a longer time. Surgery could be needed.

Tenolysis, in which the thickened paratenon is divided, can help. In more severe cases, in which a nodule is palpable, surgical exploration of the tendon is indicated. The degenerative material is excised and the remainder of the tendon sutured. In extreme cases the plantaris tendon is used to reinforce the repair.

Prevention

After this review of the Achilles tendon pathology, a note about prevention of the injury is added. This can be divided into primary, secondary and tertiary prevention.

To discuss primary prevention it is necessary to know about the aetiology of Achilles tendinitis (see aetiology). Some aspects can now be considered. A physical check-up will reveal anatomical and biomechanical disorders. In leg length difference a heel-lift can be very useful. If excessive pronation is present an orthotic device should be used. The cavus foot is a more difficult problem, but a heel wedge permanently inserted between the midsole and inner sole helps absorb the impact at heel strike.

One should know that soccer players are, in general, less flexible than other athletes and that there is a direct correlation between muscle tightness and strain. The present design of soccer training seems to promote muscle tightness. Thus, redesign of the warm-up with more emphasis on flexibility and the addition of a cool-down should help to reduce injuries.

Achilles tendinitis is especially caused by training errors, so professional advice on control of the performance is essential. It is more important to practice intensively than extensively. Avoid hills and banked roads when running. It is advisable also to vary running with swimming, rowing or cycling. Another exogenous cause is the running shoe, especially one with rigid soles. A shoe with an inadequately padded heel wedge or a soft heel counter that does not stabilize the heel may also contribute to injury.

Table 4. Primary Prevention

Screening	- Leg length difference	(Heel wedge)
	- Pes cavus with hyperpronation	(Orthotic device)
	- Tight calf muscles	(Stretching exercise)
Training	- Reduce mileage	
	- More intensive than extensive	
	- Swimming, Rowing, Cycling	
Surface	- No hills	
	- No banked roads	
Shoes	- Flexible sole	
	- Well moulded Achilles pad	
	- Heel wedge (> 15 mm)	
	- Rigid heel counter	
	- Heel lift	
Warm-up/ Cool-down	- Stretching exercises	

The soccer shoe, especially a new one with a rigid heel counter, can be responsible not only for bursitis but also for tendinitis. This tendinitis is called the 'external friction syndrome'.

Early recognition of symptoms of Achilles tendinitis is essential to prevent a severe injury (secondary prevention). An attempt to 'run through' may convert a mild injury into a severe one. It is important not only for the physician to be aware of the complaints and symptoms of tendinitis, but also for coaches, trainers and the player himself to be convinced to take measures whenever pain and/or stiffness occur in and around the Achilles tendon.

Finally tertiary prevention means adequate therapy and rehabilitation. The details have been provided earlier.

Prevention is not possible without a thorough knowledge of the aetiology, clinical condition and therapy of the injury. Prevention is only significant if we are convinced about the extent of the problems of sports injuries, not only for the health care but also for the success of a soccer team.

References

Cyriax, J. and Russell, G. (1980) Textbook of Orthopaedic Medicine. London: Bailliere Tindall.

Ekstrand, J. (1982) Soccer injuries and their prevention. Doctoral thesis, Linkoping University (Sweden).

MUSCLE CONTRACTURES OF SOCCER PLAYERS - RELATIONSHIP WITH KNEE COMPLAINTS AND THE EFFECT OF STRETCHING EXERCISES

M. Weber and J.U. Baumann
Orthopaedic Clinic, University of Basel, Kinesiology Laboratory, Felix Platter-Spital, CH-4055 Basel, Switzerland.

Introduction

Painful knee joints are common in soccer players and there is a variety of causes. This study is concerned with prevention of injuries and chronic overload of joint surfaces and ligaments. A reduction of muscle elasticity, combined with shortening - so-called muscle contractures - impairs the performance of the athlete. Muscle contractures lead to a reduction of the functional range of motion of the corresponding joints. Because muscles are arranged in functional chains, one contracted muscle interferes with the whole chain and thus with the total pattern of movement. Bi-articular muscles such as m. rectus femoris, the ischio-crural group and gastrocnemius are particularly prone to contracture. The reduction of the range of motion of one or several muscles leads to a concentration of stress within the joint structures. In addition, muscle contractures reduce the flexibility and adaptability of the player. It must be expected, that a reduced range of motion of muscles and joints increases the probability of an injury.

Testing for muscle contractures is simple. No expensive apparatus is needed. A careful examiner and a joint goniometer are all that is required to detect muscle contractures.

For prevention and treatment of muscle contractures, stretching exercises were recommended by Wiktorsson-Möller et al. (1983), Henricson et al. (1983) and many other authors. This study aims at evaluating their effect on soccer players and their knee disorders. Stretching exercises should particularly have a preventive effect on chronic overloading of the knee joint. At the same time they are expected to improve running speed, mobility and performance of the players. These aspects require long term follow-up examinations and could not be adequately evaluated in this work. Stretching exercises must be used cautiously because they can be harmful to persons with hypermobile joints and ligaments.

Such hypermobile athletes are rare; among soccer players. They were reported by Ekstrand and Gillquist (1982) to be regularly affected by contractures of the thigh and leg muscles. A need was felt to evaluate the knee complaints of soccer players in a series of soccer clubs. The benefits of stretching exercises performed regularly by more than half the players in this study were assessed systematically with specific reference to extensibility and mobility of two muscle groups in the thigh and the effect on knee complaints.

Material and Methods

Soccer players (n = 95) from 6 teams ranging from the first professional to the fourth amateur division of Northwestern Switzerland were studied. The players were distributed in 3 age groups:- 10-19 years (n=3), 3.2% of total; 20-29 years (n=78), 82.1% of total; 30-39 years (n=14), 14.7% of total.

There were small differences in age distribution among the clubs, showing a tendency towards a higher age in the clubs of the top divisions. The distribution of the body weights of the 95 players is shown in Table 1. The heavier players were clearly accumulated in the best placed clubs.

Table 1. Distribution of body weight and height of players (n=95). Values are given as a percent of the total

Body Weight	%	Height	%
50 - 59 kg	1.1	160 - 169 cm	5.3
60 - 69 kg	33.7	170 - 179 cm	48.3
70 - 79 kg	49.5	180 - 189 cm	45.3
80 - 89 kg	14.7	190 - 199 cm	1.1
90 - 99 kg	1.1		

Height distribution is included in Table 1. The mean standing height varied considerably among the clubs, but no clear relation between the mean height in each club and its playing performance was detected.

The training intensity in the 6 clubs varied between 5 times a week (32.6% of players) to twice weekly (48.4%). Altogether 78% of the footballers had been active players for 11-20 years. Stretching exercises had been performed 3 times a week or more frequently over a period of at least 3 months by 44.2% of the club members, twice weekly by 7.4%, less frequently by 15.8% and not at all by 32.6%. Players in the highest ranking clubs were found to be the most active.

Methods of Testing

A questionnaire was filled in by each athlete in presence of the first author, reporting on training activities, stretching exercises, knee injuries, as well as on previous and present knee related complaints.

Testing for contractures of the hamstring muscle group consisted in passive flexion of one hip joint to 30°, followed by passive flexion of the corresponding knee as far as possible. The deficit in knee extension to a neutral position was measured with a Protek goniometer. For this study, a hip flexion angle of only 30° was chosen instead of the commonly used 90° angle because this knee angulation is frequently reached in kicking activities. An extension deficit of the knee measuring 30° and more was defined as pathological, indicating a significant hamstring muscle contracture. This group contains the following individual muscles:- m. semimembranosus, m. semitendinosus, m. gracilis, m. biceps femoris. The m. rectus femoris was examined for contractual shortening by passive flexion of the knee joint with the hip joint extended to the neutral position. A knee flexion angle of 105° or less was considered as pathological, indicating a contracture of M. rectus femoris.

The results of the study were evaluated statistically by the χ^2-test. A probability value equal to less than 0.05 was taken to indicate significance.

Results and Discussion

History of knee pain

A history of knee pain was reported in 58.9% of all players: 15.8% had been treated for a meniscal injury, 13.4% for a tear of a cruciate ligament and 17.9% for damage to the collateral ligaments of the knee joints. The highest incidence of knee related complaints and of reported knee injuries was observed in the lowest ranking clubs. A history of knee complaints does not imply, however, that these symptoms persisted at the time of examination.

Relation between muscle shortening and stretching exercises

Table 4 shows the relationship between muscle shortening (contracture) and stretching exercises. Statistical evaluation by the χ^2-test shows a highly significant relation between reported stretching exercises and the measurements of muscle length $\chi^2 = 29.1$; $P = 0.005$).

The study clearly demonstrates, that stretching exercises as they were performed by the individuals examined are effective in maintaining or obtaining muscle length and extensibility within normal limits. In other words they can prevent or cure muscle contractures.

Table 2. Contingency table relating contracture and stretching exercise

	Stretching	No Stretching	Sum
Muscle shortening	11	26	37
No muscle shortening	50	8	58
Sum	61	34	95

Relation between knee pain and muscle shortening (contracture)

Among the 29 players with knee complaints on examination, 14 had muscle contractures. Among the 66 persons without knee pain, 23 had muscle contractures. Whilst muscle contractures were present in half the players with knee complaints, only about 1/3 of those free of knee pain had contractures. The difference in muscular shortening between individuals with and without knee complaints was not statistically significant by the χ^2-test. Inspite of this statistical result the percentage of players with simultaneous occurrence of knee complaints and muscle contractures was observed to be considerably higher than the percentage with knee complaints but without muscle contractures.

This finding was further corroborated by our special study on the group of players with long standing knee disorders (see later Section).

Relation between knee complaints and stretching exercises

On the day of examination, 30.5% of all players reported knee related complaints. Among the 64.2% of all players who had performed stretching exercises, 31.1% had knee complaints. Among the 35.8% of all players who did not use stretching, 10 (or 29.4%) complained about their knees.

Thus clearly no effect of stretching exercises on the knee complaints present in these players could be observed. This means, that our test subjects had knee complaints whose origin might have been partially connected with muscle shortening. Stretching exercises had no effect, however, in curing these disorders.

Evaluation of players with long term knee disorders

Of the 29 players with knee complaints on the day of examination, 20 had long term impairments of knee joint function. Of these 18 were evaluated in a special part of the study. In total 42 different pathological conditions due to injuries were found; 35% were related to the menisci, 25% to the cruciate ligaments and 30% to the collateral ligaments. A varus deformity at the knee, related to tibia vara, was noted in 17 of the 18 players; in all except one of these 18, m. rectus femoris was shortened by contracture. In 14 of the 18 examined players, there was a significant contracture of the hamstring muscle group in one or both legs with an extension deficit of the knee of 30-55° when the hip was placed at a right angle. Thus, muscle contractures of knee flexor and extensor muscles were present in the majority of the players whose knee joints showed signs of long standing damage.

It is our opinion that the observed findings regarding the correlation between simultaneous presence of knee complaints and muscle contractures are important for the planning of training activities. This is particularly so in view of the reported evidence concerning the effectiveness or stretching exercises for preventing or correcting the shortening of muscles into a state of contracture. Finally, it must be realised that all the subjects evaluated were active football players at the time of examination despite their knee complaints.

While many authors, for example Jenoure et al. (1984), Anderson (1980), Spring (1981) and Esnault (1986), claimed, that stretching exercises 'feel good' and that elastic muscles with a full range of motion are beneficial to the mobility and speed of the athletes, they are not a cure-all. Two thirds of the players with knee complaints were suffering from long standing knee disorders and all, but one, had a varus knee deformity. This indicates, that most of these knee joints had some degree of ligamentous instability. In the presence of knee instability, a moderate degree of muscle contractures would enhance stability and have a beneficial effect.

On the basis of this study it appears, that stretching exercises seem to play a useful part in the training programme of soccer players with intact, non-injured knee joints. In the presence of knee instability, however, muscle stretching exercises for the hamstring muscle group and m. rectus femoris should be used cautiously or not at all, depending on the individual case.

References

Anderson, B. (1980) Stretching: USA. Shelter Publication.

Ekstrand, J. and Gillquist, J. (1982) The frequency of muscle tightness and injuries in soccer players. Amer. J. Sports Med., 10, 75-78.

Esnault, M., Viel, E. and Harichaux, P. (1986) La pratique du stretching, our étirements myo-tendineux et aponéurotique, neurophysiologie, anatomie et méthodologie. Cinésiologie, 25, 137-146.

Henricson, A., Larsson, A., Olsson, E. and Westlin, N. (1983) The effect of stretching on the range ofmotion of the ankle joint in badminton players. J. Orthop. Sports Phys. Ther., 5, 74-77.

Jenoure, P., Feinstein, R. and Segesser, B. (1984) Refléxions au sujet du stretching. Med. Hyg., 42, 2417-2422.

Spring, H. (1981) Muskelfunktionsdiagnostik nach Janda. Schweiz. Z. Sportmed., 29, 143-146.

Wiktorsson-Möller, M., Oberg, B., Ekstrand, J. and Gillquist, J. (1983) Effects of warming up, massage and stretching on range of motion and muscle strength in the lower extremity. Amer. J. Sports Med., 11, 249-252.

FORTY YEARS OF HEAD AND CERVICAL SPINE FATALITIES IN AMERICAN FOOTBALL: 1945-1984

Frederick O. Mueller and Carl S. Blyth
University of North Carolina, 311 Woollen Gymnasium,
Chapel Hill, North Carolina 27514, U.S.A.

Introduction

The American Football Coaches Association began collecting football fatality data in 1931 and has continued for every year since with the exception of 1942. Football has benefitted from these surveys because the research results have been the basis for football rule changes and improvement in equipment.

The purpose of this research was to discuss the aetiology of football head and cervical spine fatalities that have occurred in the United States since 1945. Forty years of data collection, 1945-1984, detail the incidence of American football head and cervical spine fatalities. Upon establishing the incidence and aetiology of head and cervical spine fatalities from 1945-1984, the data were divided into ten-year spans of time and concentrated on the variables that have either increased or decreased fatalities. The paper concludes with a discussion of the major preventative measures that have been given credit for the reduction of head and cervical spine fatalities in the past ten years.

Data Collection

Data were collected on a national level from all organized football programmes through personal contact and questionnaires on each football fatality. Information collected included personal data on the injured player, equipment data, injury type and body part, and pertinent information on the exact circumstances of the accident. Fatalities that resulted from participation in the fundamentals of football are considered direct, while fatalities that were caused by systemic failure as a result of exertion during participation in a football activity are considered indirect. For the purpose of this report the data will use only direct fatality information.

Results

1945-1984

Each year from 1945-1984 has produced a head or cervical spine fatality in football. As illustrated in Table 1, there were 643 fatalities from 1945-1984. Head injuries accounted for 433 or 67.3

per cent, cervical spine injuries account for 111 or 17.3 percent and 99 or 15.4 percent were attributed to other injuries. Head and cervical spine fatalities combined were associated with 84.6 percent of the total.

Table 1. Football head and cervical spine fatalities 1945-1984

Body part	Frequency	Percent
Head	433	67.3
Cervical Spine	111	17.3
Other	99	15.4
Total	643	100

The type of injury associated with the majority of head fatalities was the sub-dural haematoma, numbering 337; skull fractures numbered 18. Almost all of the cervical spine fatalities were fractures, dislocations, or fracture-dislocations.

A majority of the head fatalities happened during participation in games (61.2 percent), and as shown in Table 2, 73.7 percent were to high school players. A majority of the cervical spine fatalities also happened in games, and 64.0 percent were to high school players. It should be pointed out that there are greater numbers of football players at the high school level than either the college or professional ranks.

Table 2. Football head and cervical spine fatalities 1945-1984 according to level of play

	Head		Cervical spine	
Level of Play	Frequency	Percent	Frequency	Percent
College	28	6.4	19	17.1
High School	319	73.7	71	64.0
Professional	13	3.0	12	10.8
Sandlot	73	16.9	9	8.1
Total	433	100.0	111	100.0

A majority of the players who died as a result of either a head or cervical spine injury were involved in tackling or being tackled.

1945-1954

In this decade improvement took place in the football helmet and the plastic-shelled helmet was first introduced. A single-bar face mask was introduced in the early 1950's. The fundamentals of football play an important role in injury prevention, and during this decade the techniques of blocking and tackling used the shoulder as the initial contact point. Player participation during this time averaged approximately 7 000 000 per year.

During this decade there were 87 head fatalities and 32 cervical spine fatalities in all levels of football (Table 3). Other injuries accounted for 34 fatalities. Head and cervical spine injuries were responsible for 77.7 percent of the fatalities from 1945-1954 and 18.5 percent of the fatalities from 1945-1984.

Table 3. Head and cervical spine fatalities: totals by decades

	Head		Cervical Spine	
Year	Frequency	Percent	Frequency	Percent
1945-1954	87	20.1	32	28.8
1955-1964	115	26.6	23	20.7
1965-1974	162	37.4	42	37.9
1975-1984	69	15.9	14	12.6
Total	433	100.0	111	100.0

As illustrated in Table 4, 67.8 percent of the head fatalities and 81 percent of the cervical spine fatalities took place in games. As mentioned earlier, a majority of the injured players, 57.1 percent, participated at the high school level (Table 5).

Sub-dural haematomae were related to 80.4 percent of the head fatalities. Fractures were shown to be the cause of 81.3 percent of the cervical spine fatalities.

To help prevent serious football injuries and fatalities, it is important to know the exact activity the individual was involved in at the time of the injury. Tackling and being tackled were responsible for 47.1 percent of the head fatalities and 71.9 percent of the cervical spine fatalities.

1955-1964

In the late 1950's the techniques of blocking and tackling used the shoulder as the main area of initial contact. Players were told to keep their heads up, aim at the opponent's mid section and, at the last second before contact, slide their head to one side and make contact with their shoulder. Toward the end of this period of time there was a move to make initial contact with the head. The football helmet continued to improve and the one-bar mask moved to the two-bar, and some players had full face masks to protect a fractured nose or other facial injury.

From 1955-1964 there were 115 head fatalities, 23 cervical spine fatalities, and 37 other fatalities. Head and cervical spine injuries were responsible for 78.9 percent of the fatalities during this decade and 21.5 percent of the fatalities from 1945-1984. There was an average of approximately 8 500 000 football participants during the decade from 1955-1964.

Table 4. Head and cervical spine fatalities by decades game vs practice

	1945-1954	1955-1964	1965-1974	1975-1984
Head				
Game	59	58	108	40
Practice	12	41	46	27
Unknown	16	16	8	2
Cervical Spine				
Game	26	16	30	10
Practice	1	5	10	4
Unknown	5	2	2	0

Fifty-one per cent of the head fatalities and 69.6 percent of the cervical spine injuries took place in games. A majority of the injured players, 69.6 percent, participated at the high school level. Seventy-seven percent of the cervical spine fatalities were fractures.

As was the case in the prior decade, tackling and being tackled were responsible for a major share of the fatalities. Forty-three percent of the head fatalities and 60.9 percent of the cervical spine injuries were due to tackling or being tackled.

The 1955-1964 data show an increase in the percentage of head fatalities when compared to the previous decade and a slight decrease in the percentage of cervical spine fatalities.

1965-1974

The period of 1965 to 1974 in football became well known for terms like spearing, butt blocking and tackling, face to the numbers and face to the chest. Tackling and blocking techniques involved placing the face of the tackler or blocker into the chest of the individual being tackled or blocked. The initial contact was now being made with the head. Players were wearing full face masks and felt well protected when striking with their head. It was also a time when cervical spine inuries were causing permanent disabilty to football participants.

The data starting in 1965 and ending in 1974 produced 162 head fatalities, 42 cervical spine fatalities, and 19 other fatalities. Head and cervical spine injuries were associated with 91.5 percent of the fatalities during this decade and 31.7 percent of the fatalities from 1945-1984. Both figures show a dramatic increase from the two previous decades. During the decade 1965-1974 participation figures ranged from a low of 11 000 000 to a high of 13 000 000.

Table 5. Head and cervical spine fatalities by decades:- level of play

	1945-1954	1955-1964	1965-1974	1975-1984
Head				
College	5	8	11	4
High School	52	82	127	58
Professional	9	3	1	0
Sandlot	21	22	23	7
Cervical Spine				
College	4	5	8	2
High School	16	14	30	11
Professional	9	2	1	0
Sandlot	3	2	3	1

Sixty-seven percent of the head fatalities and 71 percent of the cervical spine fatalities took place in games. A majority of the injured players, 77 percent, participated at the high school level. Seventy-two percent of the head fatalities were sub-dural haematomae, and 66.6 percent of the cervical spine fatalities were fractures.

The 1965-1974 data reveal a dramatic percentage increase in both head and cervical spine fatalities when compared to the previous two decades. The 1968 football season was also associated with 36 fatalities, the greatest number since 1931, and all were head and cervical spine fatalities.

1975-1984

Many important changes have been made in football during this ten year period and they have helped reduce the number of head and cervical spine fatalities. In 1976 a change in football rules made it illegal to butt block, face tackle, or spear. These terms involved using the frontal area or top of the helmet and/or the face mask to make initial contact with the opponent. The National Operating Committee on Standards for Athletic Equipment (NOCSAE) developed a safety standard for the football helmet that went into effect during the 1978 season for colleges and the 1980 season for high schools. From 1975 to 1984 there were 69 head fatalities, 14 cervical spine fatalities, and nine other fatalities. Head and cervical spine injuries were associated with 90.2 percent of the fatalities during this decade and 12.9 percent of the fatalities from 1945-1984.

Fifty-eight percent of the head fatalities and 71.4 percent of the cervical spine fatalities took place in games, and a majority of the injured players, 75 percent, participated at the high school level. Eighty-seven percent of the head fatalities were sub-dural haematomae, and 78.6 percent of the cervical spine fatalities were fractures.

Tackling and being tackled were again involved in a majority of the fatalities. These activities were associated with 52.2 percent of the head fatalities and 85.7 percent of the cervical spine fatalities.

Discussion and Recommendations

Head and cervical spine fatalities accounted for 84.6 percent of all football fatalities from 1945-1984, and the decade with the highest percentage was 1965-1974. There was a dramatic decrease in both numbers and percentages from 1975-1985. Chi-square analysis ($P < 0.05$) was used to demonstrate a significant increase or decrease in fatalities between the decades. There was a significant increase in both head and cervical spine fatalities between the decades 1955 through 1964 and 1965 through 1974 and a significant decrease between the latter period and the decade 1975-1984. Preventative measures given credit for the reducton of these fatalities have been the 1976 rules changes, the helmet standard, improved medical care and improved coaching techniques.

There has been a definite decline in the number of football head and cervical spine fatalities during the past ten years, 1975-1984. Suggestions for reducing head and neck fatalities are as follows:-

i) Mandatory medical examinations and medical history should be taken.

ii) A physician should be present at all games and practice sessions. If this is not possible, emergency measures must be provided.

iii) Athletes must be given proper conditioning exercises which will strengthen their necks so that participants will be able to hold their heads firmly erect when making contact.

iv) Coaches should drill the athletes in the proper execution of the fundamentals of football skills.

v) Coaches and officials should discourage the players from using their heads as battering rams when blocking and tackling.

vi) When a player has experienced or shown signs of head trauma (loss of consciousness, visual disturbance, headache, inability to walk correctly, obvious disorientation, memory loss), he should receive immediate medical attention and should not be allowed to return to practice or competition without permission from the proper medical authorities.

Acknowledgement:
This research was supported by the American Football Coaches Association, the National Collegiate Athletic Associations, and the University of North Carolina at Chapel Hill.

CAN SENIOR CITIZENS PLAY SOCCER SAFELY?

T. Kohno, N. O'Hata, H. Morita, T. Shirahata, S. Onodera and M. Sato
Division of Sports Medicine, Health Science Center, The Jikei University School of Medicine, 3-25-8 Nishishinbashi, Minato-ku, Tokyo, 105, Japan.

Introduction

The need for sports activity by senior citizens is widely recognised. In recent years sudden deaths during or after exercise have been reported. According to Tokutome (1986) coronary disease is the most frequent cause of these sudden deaths, while Murayama (1985) has argued that coronary disease is a background factor.

To prevent sudden deaths, a sports medical check-up is recommended. A medical check-up in sports medicine differs from a general check-up in an inactive situation by the addition of active loading, i.e. exercise testing. Its purpose is to determine the intensity of exercise which an individual can endure and to discover any latent diseases which might be exacerbated by exercise.

However, few senior citizens who do participate in sports have a sports medical check-up and so there are few data about the health and safety of senior citizens who exercise frequently (Murayama, 1984). This is especially important to those senior citizens who play soccer since it is a physical contact sport. Therefore, we gave sports medical check-ups to a group of senior citizens who have played soccer regularly over the past 45 years (since college). The major questions of interest were firstly, is it safe to continue to play soccer after reaching middle age? Secondly, what kind of restrictions should be suggested to those who want to continue to play soccer?

Method

Eleven male soccer players with an average age of 60.5 years participated in this study. All had regularly played soccer about 2 hours a week for about the last 40 years. All had been playing soccer at least since college.

Subjects first completed a medical history and took a medical check-up. Table 1 shows the items in the medical check i) physical examination; ii) urine examination; iii) blood chemistry examination; iv) X-ray examination; v) anthropometry - height, body weight, back muscle strength, agility, flexibility; vi) cardiopulmonary function (at rest).

Based upon examination of their medical history, their resting ECG and an individual medical consultation, subjects were cleared for participation in treadmill testing. The treadmill was chosen as a testing device because of the familiarity of the subjects with walking and running.

Table 1. Elements of the medical check-up given to subjects

General Status	
Urinalysis	Protein Sugar, Urobilinogen, Occult blood test, Sediment.
Complete Blood	WBC, RBC, Hb, Ht, MCV, MCH, MCHC, Platelet, E.S.R.
Blood Chemistry	GOT, GPT, LDH, ChE, TBi, DBi, IBi, ALP, LAP, UN, TC, γ-GTP, TP, Alb, A/G, Cl, Na, K, Ca, Fe, FBS, HDL-Cholesterol, Glycohaemoglobin-Al, UIBC, TIBC.
Serological Test	RA, ASLO, CRP, HBS-Ag, HBS-Ab, TPHA, Blood Type.
X-Ray Examination	Chest, Knee, Ankle, Foot, Lumbar Spine.
Anthropometry	Height, Body Weight, Sitting Height, Skinfolds.
Cardiorespiratory Function	Vital Capacity, Blood Pressure, ECG (at rest) Maximum Oxygen Consumption ($\dot{V}O_2max$), Maximum Ventilation, Exercise ECG.
Fundamental Motor Ability	Back Strength, Sidestep, Trunk Extension, Vertical Jump, Trunk Flexion, Grip Strength, Jumping Reaction Time.

Treadmill testing began at a 3% grade and a speed of 4 km h^{-1}. The grade was held constant throughout, and the speed was increased 0.6 km h^{-1} every minute. Exercise ECG's were recorded for each minute during and also immediately after testing. Blood pressure was measured pre- and post-exercise testing. During the treadmill test a physician monitored the ECG of the subject and stopped the test if any major abnormalities (as described by Doba and Hatano, 1986) occurred.

Maximum oxygen consumption ($\dot{V}O_2max$) was measured by an automatic metabolic measurement system (System-5, by AIC, Japan).

Results

Profiles

The physical profile of the sample group is shown in Table 2. This indicates that middle-aged and aged soccer players in our sample are one standard deviation above the national norms (Iizuka, 1985) for their age group in height and sitting height. The proportion of body fat in the sample group was 17.1%, which is lower than the normal 20.5%. In reaction time, vertical jump and sidestep, the sample group was more than one standard deviation above normals. In back strength they were only slightly better than normals. In terms of trunk flexion the sample group was just slightly inferior to normals.

The sample group's average $\dot{V}O_2max$ was clearly superior to normals (0.8 SD above normals). They were the same as normal in terms of ventilation.

Table 2. Profiling of subjects vs. Japanese norms

Item		Subjects Mean	Subjects SD	Japanese norms Mean	Japanese norms SD	Significance
Height	(cm)	167.1	3.29	158.4	6.2	b
Body weight	(kg)	64.2	6.19	55.2	8.77	
Sitting height	(cm)	91.4	2.99	85.6	4.2	a
Chest girth	(cm)	91.4	4.28	87.1	6.7	
Back strength	(kg)	113.2	19.4	101.2	19.7	
Side step	(number)	41.9	5.72	34.7	6.36	b
Trunk extension	(cm)	31.9	8.97	32.8	5.2	
Vertical jump	(cm)	43.0	7.02	32.8	5.2	b
Trunk flexion	(cm)	6.9	4.27	7.5	6.0	
Reaction time	(ms)	278.0	24.31	444.9	71.8	b
Grip strength (R)	(kg)	41.6	4.79	39.3	6.65	
Grip strength (L)	(kg)	38.5	6.0	*		
$\dot{V}O_2max$	ml kg^{-1} min^{-1}	38.5	9.23	28.0	5.21	b
$\dot{V}Emax$	(1 min^{-1})	103.2	21.17	105.7	18.9	

Notes: For Subjects N = 11.
* Grip strength: Japanese norms are only given for both hands averaged together.
a $P < 0.05$; b $P < 0.01$

ECG at rest, under load, and after exercise

Irregularities such as ST-T changes (which indicates ischaemic change) and arrhythmic changes were not found in resting ECG's. However, in exercise and post-exercise ECGs six out of the eleven subjects showed lowering of ST-T and/or arrhythmic changes. Five showed lowered ST-T and one had pre-ventricular contractions.

In one case, a 61 year old forward player, 5 min after loading began, ST lowering was observed at II, III, aVF, V5 and V6. His heart rate was 148 beats min^{-1}. In this example he recovered 8 min after loading stopped (See Figures 1a and 1b).

Including the above case, six players were given echocardiograms and no evidence of heart disease was found. In Table 3 the maximum heart rate during exercise and blood pressure before and after exercise are shown for each subject. None of the players had high blood pressure before exercise. There was no abnormal rise of blood pressure due to loading. The average maximum heart rate was 165 beats min^{-1} and was lower than the average figure of 171 beats min^{-1} for Japanese age-equivalents.

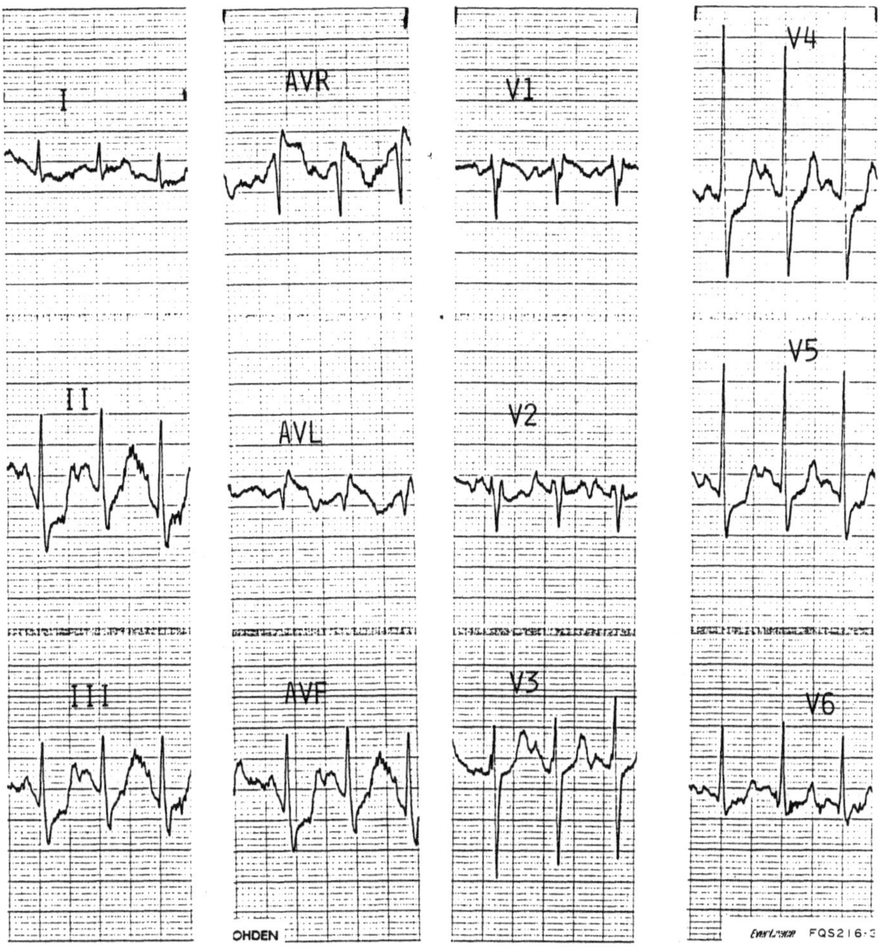

Figure 1a. The ECG 5 min after loading began

Discussion

In developing an exercise prescription, intensity, duration and frequency have to be taken into consideration. Our subjects, who graduated from college about forty years ago and who are now company executives, generally practice soccer once a week for two hours. Healthwise, it would be ideal for them to have moderate exercise five or six times a week; at least, they should exercise three times a week. Our subjects, however, maintained better physical strength than normal because of their single weekly soccer practice over the last forty years. This indicates that senior citizens can maintain their physical fitness if they have regular exercise such as two hours a week in addition to their daily routine.

Cardiac problems are one of the most serious concerns when senior

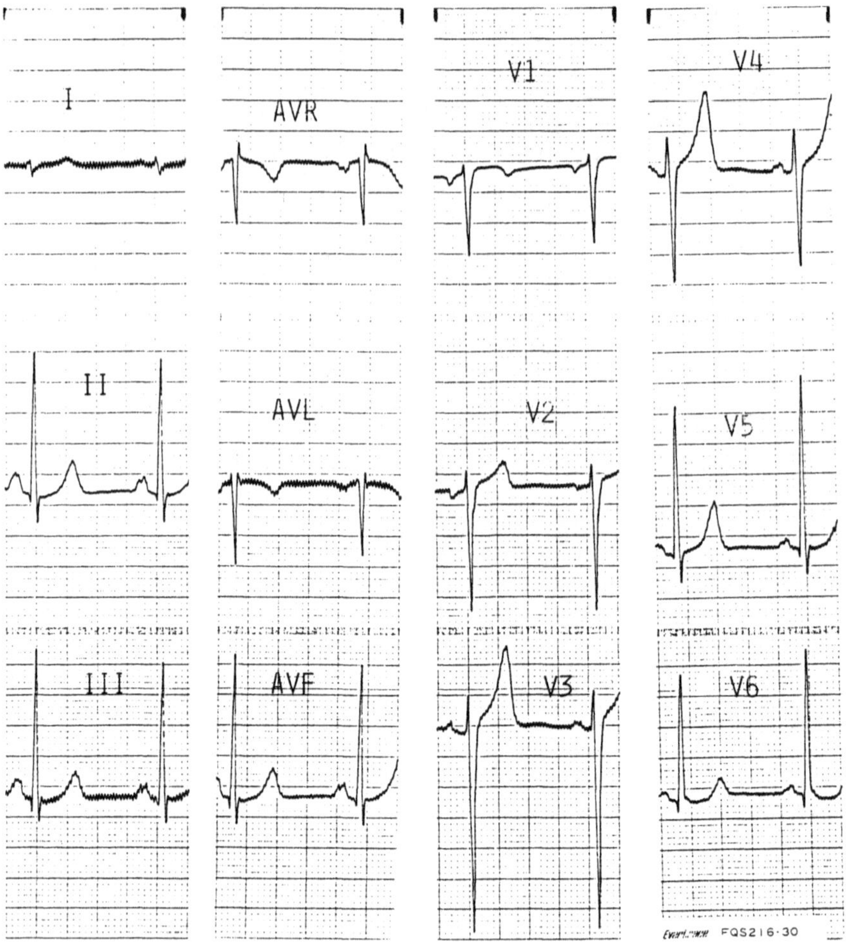

Figure 1b. The ECG 8 min after loading began

citizens practice sports. Murayama (1985) mentioned that coronary insufficiency is the main cause of sudden death whilst exercising. In order to examine cardiovascular problems, an exercise ECG is necessary. While our subjects were at rest, they did not show any indication of ischaemic changes (such as ST-T depression) or arrhythmia. During and after the exercise ECG test, six of them showed ST depression and arrhythmia: five of them showed ST depression and one, pre-ventricular contractions.

The case of the one who had pre-ventricular contraction, we decided, was not serious because the contraction did not take place repeatedly nor show R on T. The five who had ST depression did not have to take an angiography or cardiac scintigraphy because their echocardiograms ruled out any heart diseases, their ST depressions were between 1.5 mm and 2 mm, they had practiced soccer regularly,

Table 3. Subjects' heart functioning and the response to exercise testing

Subjects Initials	Age (yrs)	Maximum Heart Rate (beats min^{-1})	Blood Pressure Before Exercise (mmHg)	Blood Pressure After Testing (mmHg)
N.Y.	56	176	122/84	190/90
N.F.	59	167	140/70	200/70
M.H.	57	183	114/62	221/110
I.M.	60	154	121/82	195/75
I.S.	61	144	128/87	174/105
S.S.	67	171	140/94	174/78
O.M.	69	157	127/66	195/85
I.F.	59	180	153/85	205/95
O.Y.	57	163	120/80	160/80
N.K.	62	146	144/84	220/90
O.T.	59	169	120/80	130/60
Average	60.5	165	129/79	188/85

and the intensity of the exercise they had when the ST depressions appeared was the same as when they practice soccer.

When we considered Sakamoto's (1985) suggestion that those who show ST depression without any symptoms during exercise testing should check whether they have ischaemic heart disease or not, we decided that they should take the exercise ECG test every six months. Shephard (1986) suggested that those with ST depression and with no other cardiac symptoms are able to practice soccer as long as no further ST depression takes place. Following his suggestion, we advised our subjects to continue their soccer practice on the following conditions: i) When they play, they should pay attention to their heart rate. Considering ST depression and exercise intensity, it should not exceed 140 per minute; ii) They should warm-up for about 15 to 20 min so that their heart rates can gradually go up to 140 beats min^{-1}.

Although soccer players generally follow soccer's Seventeen Rules, for all older players in Japan, we support the following practices which are already used in Japanese senior citizen games. Play 20 min halves, use a small-sized ball, play on a grass or artificial grass field, substitute freely and only play opponents of the same age.

References

Doba, M. and Hatano, Y. (1986) Heart Disease and Exercise Tokyo: Asakura Publishing Co.

Iizuka, T. (1985) The Norms of Japanese Physical Fitness. Tokyo: Fumaido Publishing Co.

Murayama, M. (1985) Accidents in cardiovascular systems caused by sports and prevention. Public Health, 49, 257-262.

Sakamoto, S. (1985) Holter ECGs of senior citizens during jogging or a marathon race. J. Clin. Sports Med., 2, 533-563.Shephard, R. (1986) Physical training for the elderly. Clinics in Sportsmed., 5, 515-532.
Tokutome, S. (1986) Actuality of sudden death during exercise. Medical Progress, 137, 442-444.

IS HEADING THE BALL A DANGEROUS ACTIVITY?

M. Stewart Townend
Department of Mathematics, Statistics and Computing, Liverpool Polytechnic, Liverpool L3 3AF, England.

The Problem

The incidence of head injuries is a common cause for concern in various sports. In some sports, such as mountaineering, the risk of head injury can be reduced through the use of proper protective equipment. In other sports such as boxing, blows to the head are part of the fighter's permitted arsenal. In soccer heading a ball is a permitted tactic and constitutes a fundamental skill of the game.

Several authors, for example Atha et al. (1984) and Benedek and Villars (1974), have made a study of a punch to the head in boxing. Their results show that for a punch delivered by a heavyweight fighter impact forces to the opponent's head of the order of 6300 Newtons (N) with initial head accelerations of approximately 80 g (where g represents the acceleration due to gravity) occur. Some of the dangers of large forces to the head are that they may:-

(i) produce surface deformation - bruising, broken nose and so on, especially in boxing;

(ii) cause high head accelerations leading to high internal pressures and consequent brain damage.

According to Benedek and Villars (1974) fatalities can be anticipated for initial head accelerations of 200 g or more, while the value of 80 g reported above could be sufficient to cause unconsciousness. This latter value is a useful guide for comparisons. There are frequent reports in the soccer press about players who having been concussed (perhaps due to an accidental collision with another player) have played on with no recollection of events.

Since heading is a common action in soccer it is considered useful to develop a model with which to determine the magnitude of both the initial blow to the head and the initial acceleration of the head. Comparison of the values with those reported for boxing then enables the injury potential of the heading action to be assessed. This will provide an important contribution to the game of soccer given its popularity with young people.

The Assumptions

The collision between the head and the ball is modelled as an oblique impact between two rigid moving spheres. One represents the head, of

mass m_H kilogram (kg), and the other the ball of mass m_B kg.
For simplicity, and without loss of generality, the head is assumed to be moving horizontally immediately prior to the impact with a velocity of u metres per second (m s^{-1}) while the horizontal and vertical components of the ball's velocity are u_B and v_B m s^{-1} respectively.

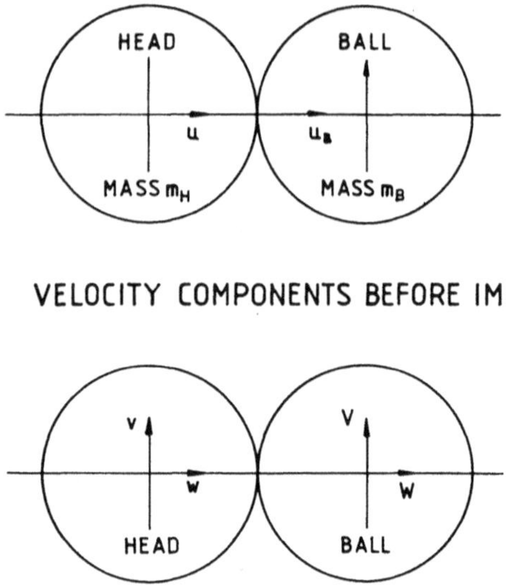

Figure 1. The velocity components of the head and ball before and after impact

It is acknowledged that in general prior to the impact the head is not the only part of the player's body which is moving and therefore that the value of m_H should be modified accordingly. This is not done in this analysis since the objective is to obtain a simple model which will readily give an estimate of the order of magnitude of the blow to the head rather than an absolute value. The assumption regarding the rigidity of the spheres is similarly defended.

The Model

Application of the principle of conservation of momentum along the line of centres at impact gives:-

$$m_H u + m_B u_B = m_H w + m_B W \qquad (1)$$

where w and W (m s^{-1}) represent the horizontal components of velocity of the head and ball respectively immediately after impact.

Newton's experimental law relating to collisions gives:-

$$W - w = - e(u_B - u), \qquad (2)$$

where e denotes the coefficient of restitution between the ball and the player's head.

If it is now assumed that the spheres are smooth (the likely presence of perspiration or sweat which will lubricate the surface and reduce friction between the head and the ball on the head makes this a reasonable assumption) and that the impulsive blow has no component perpendicular to the common normal at impact, then the components of velocity of the ball and the head, in this direction, are unaltered by the impact so that:-

$$v = 0 \quad \text{and} \quad V = v_B, \qquad (3)$$

where v and V (m s^{-1}) represent the vertical components of velocity of the head and ball respectively immediately after impact.

The speed of the head immediately after impact is given by:-

$$\sqrt{(v^2 + w^2)} = w, \text{ since } v = 0, \text{ where}$$

$$w = \frac{(m_H - em_B)u + m_B u_B(1 + e)}{m_H + m_B}, \qquad (4)$$

from equations (1) and (2).

The effect of a large force, denoted by F Newtons (N), acting for a short time Δt seconds (s) is assessed in terms of the impulse I, defined as:-

$$I = F.\Delta t. \qquad (5)$$

The impulse itself is determined by the change in momentum of the object caused by the application of the force. Thus the impulse I experienced by the head is given by:-

Impulse = Change in momentum of head

= Momentum of head after impact − Momentum of head before impact

i.e. $$I = m_H w - m_H u \qquad (6)$$

The magnitude of the impulsive force received by the head is thus obtained from equations (4), (5) and (6) as:-

$$F = \frac{m_B m_H}{m_B + m_H} \cdot \frac{(1 + e)}{\Delta t} \cdot | u_B - u | . \qquad (7)$$

Results

The following data were obtained from an analysis of high speed film of a demonstration of the heading action by a skilled college soccer player:-

i) horizontal velocity of player's head before impact; $u \sim 3 - 5 \text{ m s}^{-1}$
ii) horizontal velocity of ball before impact; $u_B \sim -10 \text{ m s}^{-1}$
iii) duration of head-ball contact, $\Delta t \sim 0.015$ s,

while the coefficient of restitution, e, was found experimentally to be of the order of 0.8.

The magnitude of the force experienced by the head is then given, in terms of the head mass m_H kg and the ball mass m_B kg as:-

$$F \simeq 1800 . \frac{m_B m_H}{m_B + m_H} .$$

The value of the coefficient 1800, which can be seen from equation (7) to depend on e, u_B, u and Δt is greater for elite soccer players and less for junior players but is generally found to be of the order 1500-2000.

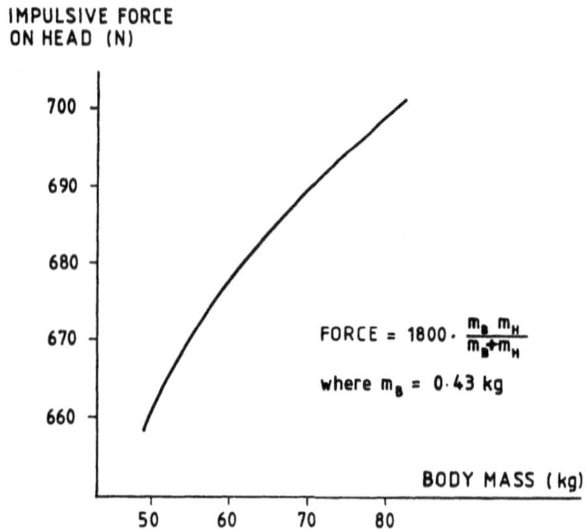

Figure 2. Graph of the magnitude of the impulsive force on the head, $|F|$, versus body mass of the player using a standard soccer ball of mass 0.43 kg

Analysis of Results

The impulse force $|F|$ is plotted as a function of the player's body mass in Fig. 2., it being assumed that the mass of the player's head is 0.05 x body mass and that the mass of the ball is 0.43 kg. The figure shows that the impulsive force to the head increases almost linearly with the mass of the player, for the range of body masses considered.

The initial acceleration of the head due to receiving the blow of magnitude $|F|$ is determined using Newton's second law of motion $|F| = m_H a$, where a denotes the acceleration of the head in metres per second per second (m s^{-2}). For the range of body masses and force magnitudes shown in Fig.2 the initial acceleration of the head is of the order of 20 g - 25 g, and is considerably less than that reported in boxing by Benedek and Villars (1974).

Figure 3 shows the almost linear variation of the impulsive force $|F|$ with the mass of the ball, for players of specific body masses. As expected, the use of a lighter ball reduces the impulsive blow to the head.

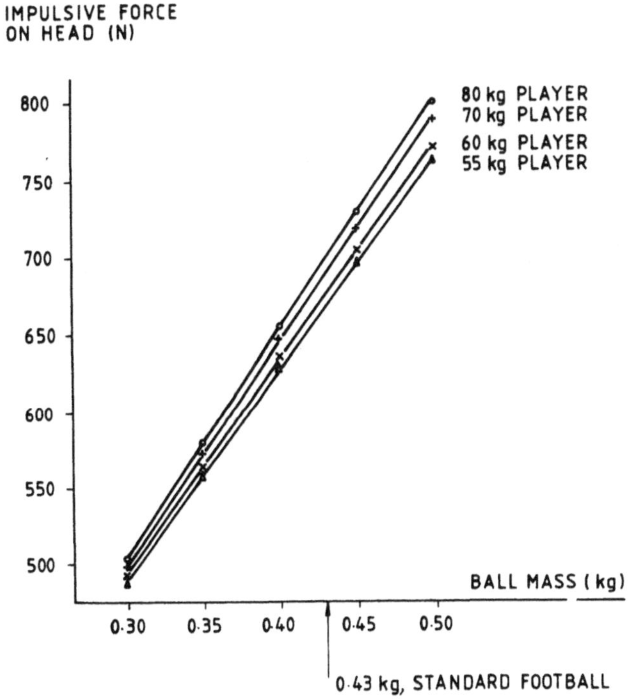

Figure 3 Graph showing the variation of the magnitude of the impulsive force on the head, $|F|$, with ball mass, m_B, for players of different weight

Table 1 shows that lightweight players experience a proportionately larger impulsive blow to the head than heavier players, for a specific set of values of the dynamic parameters e, u_B and u. There are therefore strong grounds for the practice of using lighter footballs with junior (and hence lighter) players.

Table 1. The variation of the impulsive force F on the head with body mass of the player (BW)

Mass of player (kg)	Impulsive force on head Newtons (N)	Bodyweights (BW)
55	669	1.24 BW
60	677	1.15 BW
70	689	1.00 BW

Conclusion

The model presented shows that the magnitude of the impulsive blow to the head due to the heading action in soccer is approximately one order of magnitude less than that reported in boxing. It is concluded that heading a football is not per se a dangerous activity.

Acknowledgements

The author wishes to thank Paul Charlish and David Williams of the Department of Sport and Recreation Studies at Liverpool Polytechnic for their help with data collection.

References

Atha, J., Yeadon, M.R., Sandover, J. and Parsons, K. (1984) Measuring the mechanical properties of a heavyweight's punch. J. Sports Sci., 2, 188-189.

Benedek, G.B. and Villars, F.M.H. (1974) Physics with Illustrative Examples from Medicine and Biology, Volume I, pp. 4-75. Reading, Mass.: Addison-Wesley.

QUANTIFICATION OF IMPACT ACCELERATIONS OF THE HEAD DURING THE HEADING OF A FOOTBALL

I. Burslem and A. Lees
Department of Sport and Recreation Studies, Liverpool Polytechnic, Byrom Street, Liverpool L3 3AF, England.

Introduction

The effect of repeated blows to the head is well documented in boxing. As early as 1928 Martland described the so-called punch drunk syndrome. Roberts (1969) investigated 224 former professional boxers and 17% showed chronic neurological damage attributable to boxing. Ross et al. (1983) showed that even boxers with a moderate number of bouts may suffer cerebral atrophy.

How much damage can occur after multiple headings of the ball during football was questioned by the 'Sunday Times' in 1974, and it advocated that scientific studies should be undertaken. Very little research has been undertaken into the skill of heading. Mawdsley (1978) undertook a biomechanical analysis of heading and highlighted the importance of timing. Tysvaer and Storli (1981) conducted a questionnaire study and found a low percentage of serious head injury but 16.4% of players complained of symptoms including headaches, dizziness and neck pains.

Holbourn (1943) showed that for blows of long duration the shear strains in the brain are proportional to the force magnitude. For short duration blows the injury is proportional to the change of velocity (i.e. acceleration). The changeover occurs somewhere in the region between 200-2 ms, with blows of less than 2 ms being of short duration. Plagenhoef (1971) showed that duration of impact of the ball on the head in soccer to be 23 ms while Schneider (1984) found duration of impact to be between 13-18 ms. Although these times lie in the changeover region it can be assumed that the blow tends to be of long duration, and that shear stresses in the brain and possible injury are related to the magnitude of the force action.
In terms of the rotational deceleration magnitudes which are likely to cause injury Holbourn (1943) found that magnitudes of 7500 rads s^{-2} could cause concussion in man. Stalnaker et al. (1977) obtained similar values of between 5450 and 8950 rads s^{-2} for impacts in which there was no external damage or visible brain injury in cadavers.

Method

One subject was used in this investigation. He was a male sports scientist who played soccer and was accustomed to the apparatus as he had taken part in a previous pilot study.

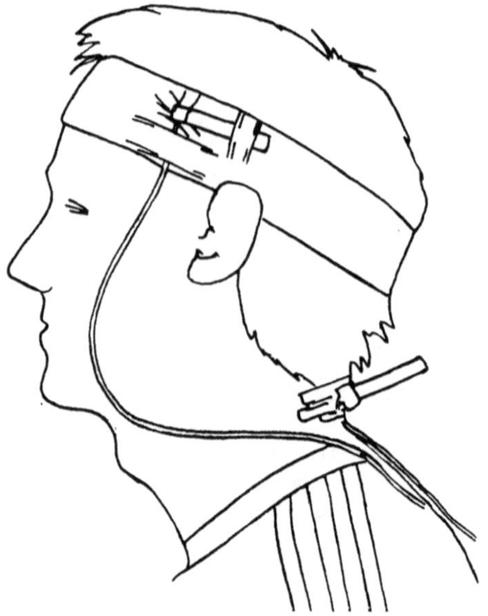

Figure 1. Attachment of the accelerometer to the subject

Two piezoceramic accelerometers were attached to the subject onto the back of the neck and another was securely attached to a headband with tape and positioned on the side of the head (Fig.1). The leads from the accelerometer were brought over the shoulder and taped in position. The signals from the accelerometer were recorded on an ultra-violet oscillograph. The camera used was a Locam 11 16mm high speed motion camera and was set at 400 frames per second. A synchronization unit was used to record a voltage pulse on the oscillograph and produce a light flash on the film. The flash was also the signal for the subejct to jump and head the thrown ball.

The rotational acceleration of the head (x) was found using the formula:-

$$x = (a_2\cos\emptyset_2 - a_1\cos\emptyset_1)/r$$

A description of the notation is given in Fig.2.

The values for a_1 and a_2 were read off directly from the accelerometer traces. The values for $\emptyset_1$ and $\emptyset_2$ were obtained from the cine film.

Two supplementary studies were undertaken. The first was to examine the characteristic accelerometer traces obtained with a group of six skilled subjects and four unskilled subjects. Characteristic traces are shown in Figs. 3 and 4. The second was undertaken to show the effect of impact on the general acceleration profiles of the movement. The subject was asked to jump and head an 'imaginary ball' and then it was repeated actually heading the ball. This resulted in two different traces being recorded.

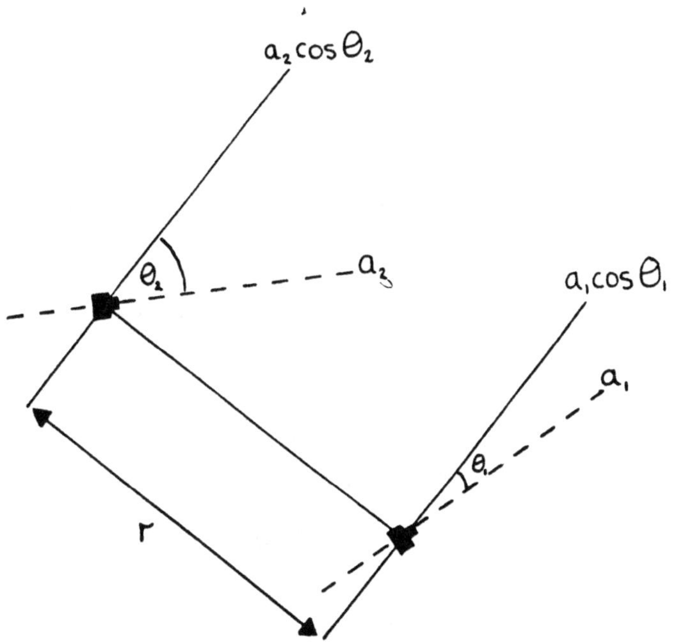

Figure 2. Notation used in calculating the rotational deceleration of the head

Results

The values for the rotational deceleration of the head caused by impact with the ball calculated from the equation above can be seen in Table 1. A typical accelerometer trace from which these results were obtained can be seen in Fig.3.

Table 1. Rotational deceleration of the head due to impact with the ball (rad s^{-2}). 1 subject, 5 trials

Frame	Trial 1B	Trial 1C	Trial 2A	Trial 2B	Trial 2C	Mean	
1	-73.4	-	-	-1.0	-108.8	-61.1	
3	-75.4	-106.2	-23.9	-15.9	-91.1	-62.5	
5	-67.1	-92.9	-53.9	-30.5	-50.4	-58.9	
7	-97.2	84.8	-62.9	-14.1	-81.3	-34.1	contact
9	-106.3	-209.9	-221.2	-173.6	-249.0	-192.0	
11	-261.3	102.5	-184.0	-136.2	-132.5	-122.3	
13	-257.4	-28.2	-6.4	+42.5	-127.0	-75.3	
15	+51.4	+80.2	+74.1	+232.8	+17.0	+91.1	
17	+38.6	+21.7	38.3	+132.3	+80.1	+62.2	
18	-	+57.1	+116.1	-	-	+86.6	

Negative sign indicates deceleration
Positive sign indicates acceleration

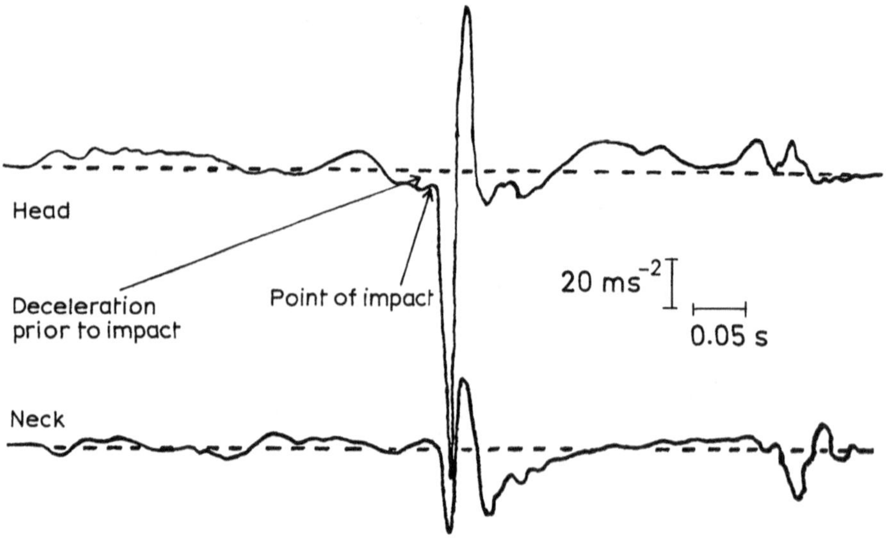

Figure 3. Accelerometer trace of skilled subject

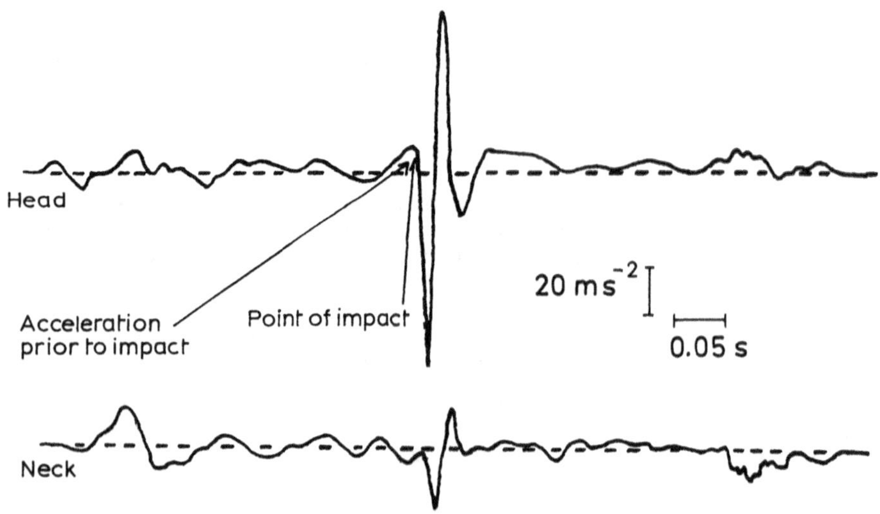

Figure 4. Accelerometer trace of unskilled subject

The point of impact is characterised by the sharp deceleration peak exhibited on both the head and neck traces. This was confirmed by (i) synchronisation of the film data to the accelerometer traces, and (ii) no sharp deceleration peak was found on the traces of a subject heading an imaginary ball.

Discussion

An analysis of the accelerometer traces shows three main phases - the take off, the characteristics at and around impact, and post-impact including the landing. Identification of these features was helped by comparison of accelerometer traces of the action with and without contact with the ball.

During take off and in preparation for the header, the head accelerometer shows a period of acceleration as the head and body rise in preparation for impact and then again as the subject is bringing his head forward for contact. Just before impact the head begins a period of deceleration; this is produced by rigidity of the head, neck and shoulders in an attempt to absorb the shock of impact. During this period the neck accelerometer tends to show acceleration, thus demonstrating the interaction of the head and neck in order to produce segment rigidity. These findings tend to support the comments of Mawdsley (1978) who stated 'The forward velocity of the head, relative to the trunk, must be reduced to almost zero to produce rigidity but the deceleration must not come so soon as to lose the forward velocity of the head altogether'.

The important phase of the movement, the impact, is characterised by a period of sharp deceleration as the ball contacts the head, then adapting to the presence of the ball this deceleration reduces until, as the ball is leaving and immediately afterwards, there is a period of acceleration. Too much significance should not be attached to this latter peak as it may well be an artefact resulting from the method of fixation of the accelerometer. After this short period of acceleration there is a longer period of deceleration as the head regains control of its motion.

Mawdesley (1978) found this latter period of deceleration following impact stating it was to 'prevent the head from snapping forward following the release of pressure after impact with the ball'. The duration of impact was calculated as being at 15 ms, agreeing with the previous values found by Plagenhoef (1971) and Schneider (1984). The landing is characterised by a series of oscillations as the smooth curve is interrupted by impact with the ground.

An important difference was found between the acceleration traces of skilled and non-skilled subjects. For skilled subjects prior to impact, the head consistently shows a period of deceleration; thus if the neck exhibits more of the whole body characteristics it can be said that the body is accelerating forwards, but the head is decelerating to produce rigidity ready for impact. This deceleration prior to impact is not found with any consistency in those traces of non-skilled subjects. So we can say that in the non-skilled subjects the head was not consistently set rigid ready for impact. This lack of rigidity would mean that the head could suffer more movement upon impact and consequently greater rotation than if it was set rigid.

This difference between skilled and non-skilled subjects highlights the importance of timing and its application to coaching. If there is apprehension in heading, as there might be when young children are learning, then it is likely that this apprehension would manifest itself in incorrect timing and the learning of a faulty technique. It would thus seem of paramount importance that children are taught to head the ball in the correct place on the forehead, not to be afraid of the contact and to watch the ball onto the head.

The values obtained for linear and rotational acceleration appear to be too low to cause any injury compared to the values reported by Holbourn (1943) and Stalnaker et al. (1977). However the values quoted in the literature are those related to the levels needed to produce concussion in individuals, and not with the injury effect resulting from many more minor blows to the head. It should also be remembered that the values reported here were obtained in the laboratory and it is reasonable to assume that higher values would be obtained in a game situation.

References

Holbourn, A.H.S. (1943) Mechanics of head injuries. Lancet, 11, 438-441.

Mawdesley, H.P. (1978) A biomechanical analysis of heading. Momentum, 3, 16-21.

Plagenhoef, S. (1971) Patterns of Human Motion, Englewood Cliffs, New Jersey: Prentice Hall,

Roberts, A.H. (1969) Brain Damage in Boxers. London: Pitman Medical Publishsing Co. Ltd.

Ross, R.J., Cole, M., Thompson, J.S. and Kim, K.H. (1983) Boxers' computed tomography E.E.G. and neurological evaluation. J. Amer. Med. Ass., 249, 211-213.

Schneider, K. (1984) Das Risko Einer Hirnverletzung Beim Fussball-Kopfstoss. Unfall-Heilkunde, 87, 40-42.

Stalnaker, R.L., Melvin, J.W., Nisholtz, G.S., Alem, N.M. and Benson, J.B. (1977) Head impact response. Society of Automative Engineers Transactions, 86, 3156-3170.

Tysvaer, A. and Storli, O. (1981) Association football injuries to the brain. A preliminary report. Brit. J. Sports Med., 15, 163-116.

JET LAG IN STUDENT RUGBY LEAGUE PLAYERS FOLLOWING A NEAR MAXIMAL TIME-ZONE SHIFT

T. Reilly and S. Mellor
Department of Sports and Recreation Studies, Liverpool Polytechnic, Byrom Street, Liverpool L3 3AF, England.

Introduction

Jet lag refers to the cluster of feelings that are associated with disruption of normal circadian rhythms. These rhythms refer to cyclical variations in biological functions that oscillate with a period of about 24 hours. They are either endogenous or exogenous in origin, the latter being the more adaptable when the environmental cues that determine the characteristics of the rhythm are altered.

Body temperature is a fundamental variable in circadian rhythmicity, its changes throughout a day conforming closely to a cosine wave. Many aspects of human performance are known to vary with time of day in close association with the body temperature curve. These include isometric strength, reaction time, movement time, co-ordination and agility, all of which are components of performance in rugby football. In crossing time zones the normal curve in body temperature is shifted in phase, taking about one day per time zone crossed to adapt to the new local time (Reilly, 1987).

Despite their close association with body temperature, circulatory and metabolic rhythms are partially independent: the curve in heart rate, for example, peaks earlier than that of oxygen uptake ($\dot{V}O_2$) whilst body temperature has its peak a little later in the evening (Reilly and Brooks, 1982). The rhythm in minute ventilation ($\dot{V}E$) is also relatively stronger than that of $\dot{V}O_2$. Consequently, not only may the main rhythms be shifted in phase but many may be temporarily controlled only loosely by their biological clocks. At this time while the rhythms are desynchronised and adapting to the new time zone at different rates, the rugby player may be disorientated and dispirited until the symptoms of jet-lag abate. Physiological rhythms affected include body temperature, the sleep-wake cycle, pulse rate, ventilation, blood pressure and renal function.

Loss of sleep may also be incurred in trans-world travellers. Circadian rhythms are known to persist under conditions of sleep deprivation. A study of indoor footballers playing for over 91 hours found that their work-rate varied throughout each day in cyclical fashion, peaking in the evening as body temperature reached its high point. A fall in activity from day to day represented an underlying 'fatigue' trend (Reilly and Walsh, 1981). In prolonged flight the desynchronisation of biological rhythms is distinct from the more basic fatigue associated with sleep loss and with travel per se.

This background is provided to adumbrate a particular difficulty to be faced by international rugby teams travelling from the British Isles to compete in Australia or New Zealand. The first Rugby Union World Championships in 1987 is an example of likely occurrence of early difficulties, as teams are prohibited by the international governing body from arriving at their competitive destinations well in advance of the first match. The organisation of the World Student Rugby League Championships in New Zealand in summer, 1986, provided an opportunity for monitoring the visiting British team to observe the severity of jet lag encountered and the rate at which adaptation occurred.

Methods

Subjects were members of the British team which competed in the Rugby League World Championships for students in summer 1986. Prior to departure for Australia and New Zealand, the subjects (n = 14) agreed to co-operate in a study of jet-lag and performance in the early stages of the tour. None of the subjects had experienced a near-maximal time-zone transition before.

The itinerary of the party was as follows. On August 14th the squad left Britain: the team arrived in Sydney on August 16th at 0730 hours local time, following a flight of 30 h duration and a time zone shift of 9 h. During the flight attempts were made to switch in advance to Australian time by changing watches to local Sydney time and adjusting the sleep-wake schedule accordingly. This strategy was to prove impractical on a flight with many stops and frequent meal breaks. Players were also prevented from sleeping before 2200 hours on the day of arrival. They had two 'friendly' matches in Australia within one week, prior to departure for New Zealand and a further 2 hours time-zone shift.

The severity of jet-lag was subjectively assessed using a 7-point scale, the highest value representing severe jet lag. This was administered in the morning (0800 hours) and evening (1800 hours) local time for four days, i.e. until the day before the first match of the tour. In this time the quality of sleep was rated on a subjective scale, rank 1-7, the higher value representing the better quality sleep. Muscular strength was measured also twice a day using a Takei Kigi-Kogyo grip dynamometer.

Obtaining reliable body temperature data from these subjects turned out to be impractical. It was possible for one of the investigators to follow essentially the same route one month later and employ a single-subject research design. Measurements were made of oral temperature as frequently as possible during each day using a clinical thermometer held sub-lingually for 5 min. Care was taken that influence of extraneous factors (exercise, meals, drink) was kept to a minimum. Generally 10 data points were obtained each day. These were examined by cosinor analysis to establish the acrophase (peak time) of oral temperature for each day. Measurements were also made of subjective ratings of jet-lag. Data were collected until three days after the subjective ratings were neutral throughout the whole day. Observations were repeated on the return journey from Christchurch involving one week on the Australian east coast.

Results

Rugby players

All 14 players participated in the 8 testing sessions on the 4 days after arrival in Australia. Comparisons between days and between times of day were formally made using multiple 't' tests.

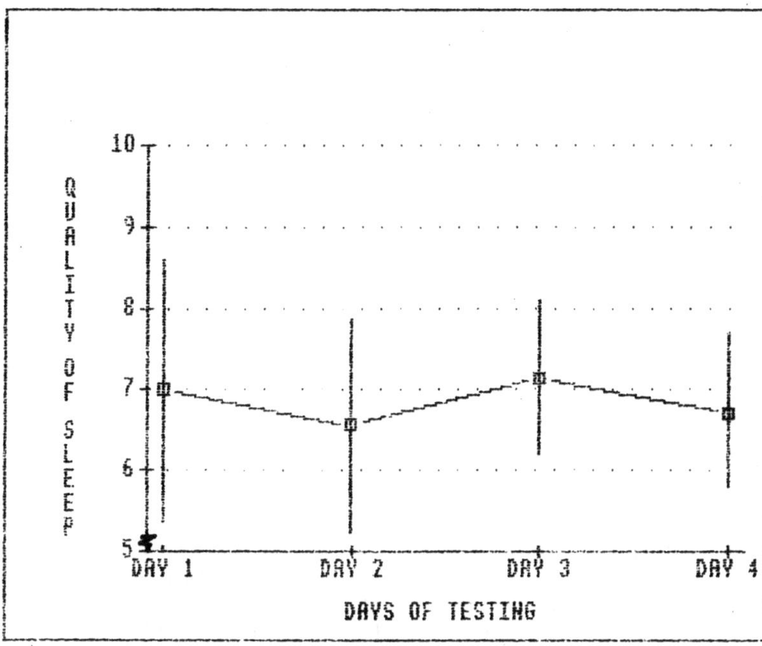

Figure 1. Subjective sleep ratings for players for the days after arrival in Australia

Results for sleep ratings are displayed in Figure 1. This indicates that the quality of sleep obtained was good on each of the nights. There were no significant differences in the ratings of sleep quality between any of the four nights ($P > 0.05$). None of the subjects found difficulty in sleeping.

The self-analysis of jet-lag is illustrated for the first four days in Australia in Figure 2. Jet-lag was perceived to be most severe on the second day of testing, that is the fifth day after leaving Britain. The symptoms of jet-lag were felt to be greater in the evening than in the morning for the first two days monitored ($P < 0.01$). Thereafter there were no significant differences between the times of day, although jet-lag was still present at the time that the last measurements were made.

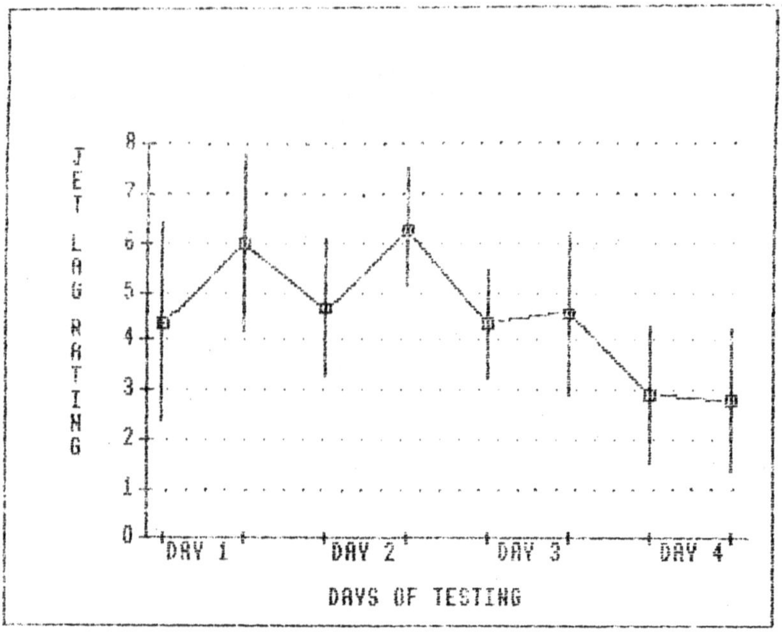

Figure 2. Ratings of jet-lag for four days after arrival in Australia

The grip strength data showed a progressive improvement in performance with each day of testing (Table 1). Day 1 represents the first day of testing, three days after leaving London. Morning values were significantly greater than the evening values on Day 1 ($P < 0.05$) and Day 2 ($P < 0.01$). No time of day effects were observed on the day after. By Day 4 of testing the diurnal trend was reversed, the mean grip strength in the evening being significantly greater than morning values ($P < 0.001$).

Table 1. Grip strength (kg) for four days after the day of arrival in Sydney from London. Morning and evening values are given as mean ± SD

	Morning	Evening
Day 1	49.1 ± 4.3	48.3 ± 4.5
Day 2	49.3 ± 4.5	48.5 ± 4.7
Day 3	49.1 ± 4.4	49.4 ± 4.6
Day 4	48.8 ± 4.3	50.4 ± 4.8

Single subject

The acrophase in oral temperature was determined for each day on the outward (eastward) and return (westward) legs of the trip. These values are shown in local time in Figures 3 and 4 respectively. Pre-flight observations showed that the peak in oral temperature consistently occurred at about 1730 hours. The initial data points after departure reflect overnight stays in Singapore (September 10) and Perth (September 11) before a further 2 hour phase-shift in flying to the east coast of Australia. The acrophase in oral temperature at this time was found about 0330 hours. The peak occurred earlier each day until it stabilised at about 1730 hours. This coincided with the disappearance of jet lag ten days after departing from London.

Eastward flight

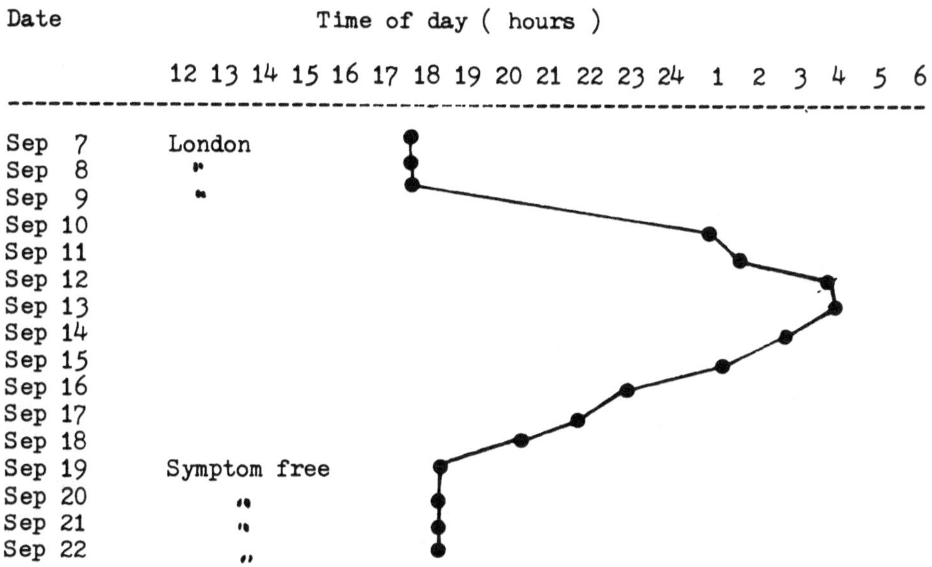

Figure 3. Acrophase of oral temperature given in local time : values are for the eastward flight

The return journey included a one-night stop-over in Singapore (October 9), the acrophase being shown as Sydney time since it occurred in-flight. The curve in oral temperature stabilised again at about 1730 hours, ten days after leaving Australia. Jet lag ratings were positive for a further two days.

Discussion

Observations on the Rugby League players indicated that none of them had difficulty in sleeping on the nights immediately after arrival at their destination in Australia. The first night's sleep was probably enhanced by the sleep loss incurred in-flight. Recommendations to

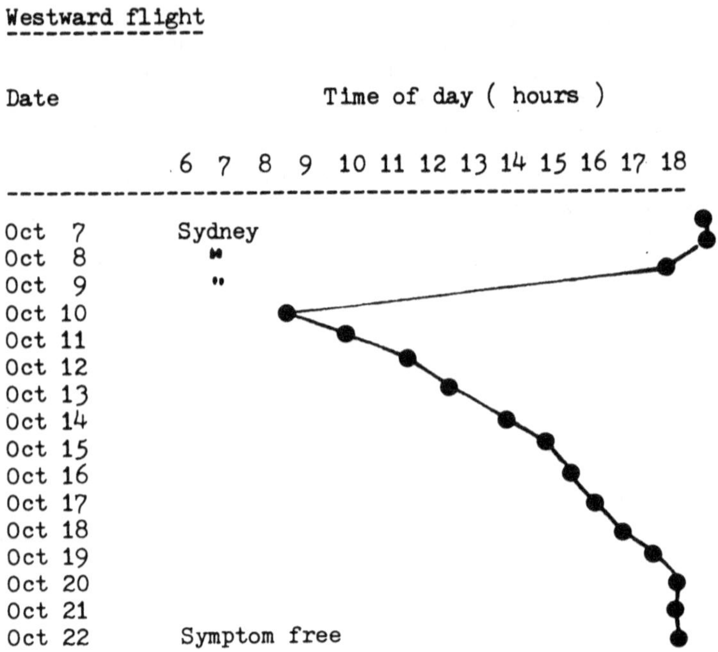

Figure 4. Acrophase of oral temperature in local time for the westward journey

subjects were to avoid anchoring their rhythms to the time-zone of departure by prolonged naps at the time they felt drowsiest during the flight. To what extent this strategy was implemented or effective in accelerating adaptation of rhythms to the new time-zone is indeterminable.

Jet lag symptoms at first were felt less acutely in the morning than in the evening. This is likely to be due partly to the refreshing effects of the preceding sleep which would decrease symptoms and partly to the prevailing arousal level. Arousal generally follows the curve in body temperature during the day (Colquhoun, 1971) and would be expected to peak early in the morning on the first days after arrival (Figure 3). This bias towards more severe evening symptoms tended to disappear as the acrophase in body temperature regressed to eventually stabilise at an evening peak time. The absence of a time of day effect after Day 3 is in accord with this reasoning.

Ratings of jet lag were still positive when measurements were terminated and so it was not established how long it took for subjects to become symptom-free. Extrapolation from the available data to neutral ratings suggests that zero values would be attained nine days after leaving London. This estimate is likely to contain error associated with individual differences.

Similar trends were evident in the grip strength data which at first were higher in the morning than in the evening. This is contrary to usual observations, as muscular strength is found to be greater in the evening than in the morning (Baxter and Reilly, 1983; Wilby et al., 1987). The present data reflect a desynchronisation of the rhythm in grip strength for the first three days of measurement. The re-adjustment of the rhythm to environmental cues is suggested by the reversal of the initial time of day effect on Day 4, six days after setting out from London. More data points per day are needed to establish when the normal circadian rhythm in grip stength was restored. The results do suggest that, at least for the first three days of measurement, the grip strength was adversely affected. They suggest also that training sessions might best be scheduled for the morning rather than the evening in the first couple of days after arrival, because of this impairment in muscular strength.

The single-subject data demonstrate that oral temperature provides a useful clue to the rate at which biological rhythms adapt to time-zone transitions. No specific attempts were made to hasten adaptation, e.g. altering sleep patterns before departure, dietary regimes as recommended by Ehret and Scanlon (1983), and so on. The observations vindicate the conventional guidelines of allowing one day to adapt for each time-zone crossed. Most authorities consider it easier to adapt to desynchronisation after westward compared to eastward flights (Minors and Waterhouse, 1981). This may not apply to near-maximal time-zone shifts, as present data indicated no apparent differences with the direction of travel.

In summary, this study found evidence of jet lag persisting for some days after a near-maximal time-zone shift. The severity of symptoms varied with time of day. During this time muscular strength of the Rugby League players was suppressed, although they were able to participate in daily training. Observations on oral temperature suggest that it is a good index to employ for monitoring the rate of adaptation to a new time zone and for predicting the disappearance of symptoms of jet-lag.

References

Baxter, C. and Reilly, T. (1983) Influence of time of day on all-out swimming. Brit. J. Sports Med., 17, 122-127.

Colquhoun, W.P. (1971) Biological Rhythms and Human Performance. New York: Academic Press.

Ehret, C.F. and Scanlon, L.W. (1983) Overcoming Jet-Lag. New York: Berkeley Publishing Corporation.

Minors, D.S. and Waterhouse, J.M. (1981) Circadian Rhythms and the Human. Bristol: John Wright.

Reilly, T. (1987) Circadian rhythms and exercise. In: Exercise: Benefits, Limits and Adaptations (edited by D. MacLeod, R.J. Maughan, M. Nimmo, T. Reilly and C. Williams) pp. 346-366. London: E. and F.N. Spon Ltd.

Reilly, T. and Brooks, G.A. (1982) Investigation of circadian rhythms in metabolic responses to exercise. Ergonomics, 25, 1083-1197.

Reilly, T. and Walsh, T.J. (1981) Physiological, psychological and performance measures during an endurance record for 5-a-side soccer play. Brit. J. Sports Med., 15, 122-128.

Wilby, J., Linge, K., Reilly, T. and Troup, J.D.G. (1987) Spinal shrinkage in females: circadian variation and the effects of circuit weight-training. Ergonomics, 30, 47-54.

PHYSIOLOGICAL RESPONSES TO ACUTE, MODERATE HYPOXIA IN ELITE SOCCER PLAYERS

Jens Bangsbo, Klaus Klausen, Thomas Bro-Rasmussen and Jan Larsen
August Krogh Institute, University of Copenhagen, 13 Universitelsparken, DK-2100 Copenhagen, Denmark.

Introduction

The ability to work at high intensity is markedly impeded when the oxygen pressure is reduced, e.g. corresponding to an altitude higher than 2000 m. Thus, the maximum oxygen uptake is decreased and ventilation and blood lactate concentration during severe, submaximal exercise are increased when subjects exercise at low pressure as in a pressure chamber (Hermansen and Saltin, 1966; Saltin, 1967; Bangsbo et al., 1987).

The Danish National soccer team qualified for the 1986 World Championship in Mexico, where most of the playing fields were situated at an altitude higher than 2000 m. Hence, the purpose of the present study was to evaluate the physiological responses of the players to moderately lowered oxygen pressure. Soccer is characterised as a high intensity, intermittent exercise (Ekblom, 1986). Thus the players' reaction to hypoxia was tested by means of an intermittent exercise test.

Materials and Methods

In the spring before the 1986 World Championship in Mexico, 21 players of the Danish National soccer team were tested. Their mean (range) age, weight and heights were 26(20-36) years; 77 (65-95) kg and 183 (167-194) cm, respectively. Five players including three goalkeepers were players from the Danish National League and the remainder were from different European clubs.

General protocol

Each player was allowed one day off work for the testing in the laboratory. The subjects arrived at the laboratory between 0800 and 1000 hours. For blood sampling a catheter was inserted into a vein on the back of the left hand. The subjects then went through a pre-test and after 10 min rest they completed an interval test at 760 mmHg (normoxia). Two hours later a reduced pre-test and the same interval test were performed at 565 mmHg (hypoxia) corresponding to an altitude of 2500 m above sea level (Fig. 1a). All tests were carried out on a Krogh cycle ergometer in a low pressure chamber (Elma, Sweden).

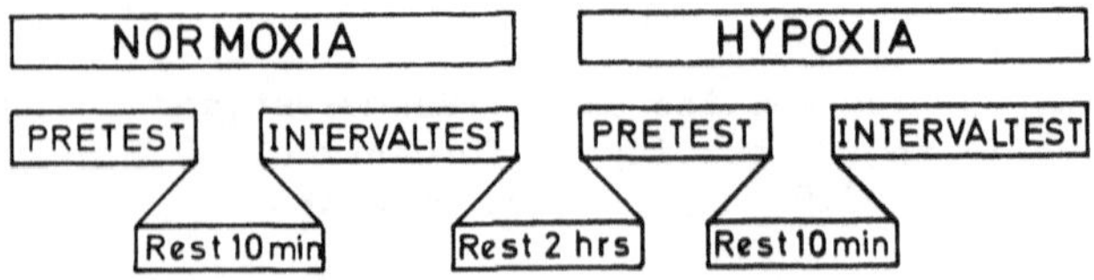

(a)

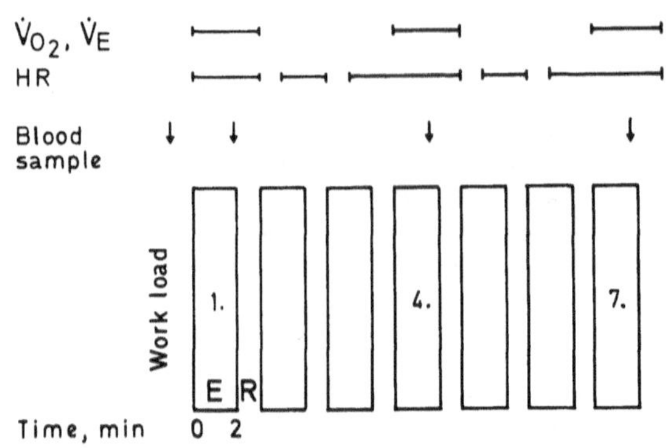

(b)

Figure 1. General protocol (a). Testing procedure during the interval test; E = 2 min exercise periods, R = rest time (b)

2.2 Testing procedures

Before the pre-test a blood sample was taken. The pre-test consisted of two 6 min periods with sub-maximal work loads (mean ± SDs 151.8 ± 25.3 and 244.0 ± 30.6 W), followed by a maximal test where the work load was continuously increased until exhaustion within 1-2 min. At the end of each of the two sub-maximal work loads heart rate (HR), oxygen uptake ($\dot{V}O_2$) and pulmonary ventilation ($\dot{V}E$) were measured. The aim of the brief maximal test was to determine the players' maximal HR and hence HR was registered continuously during the test. The maximal test was not performed in hypoxia.

Another blood sample was taken before the interval test. The interval test consisted of seven 2 min exercise periods. The results from the pre-test were used to determine a work load (mean ± SD: 253.4 ± 35.2W) which gave each player a heart rate of about 20 beats min^{-1} below the maximal HR at the end of each 2 min bout in normoxia. Between the 2 min exercise periods the players rested sitting on the cycle ergometer until HR was 50 beats min^{-1} lower than maximum HR. The time, from the end of one exercise period to the start of the next, is called rest-time. The HR, work- and rest-times were registered continuously. The $\dot{V}E$ and $\dot{V}O_2$ were measured continuously in the 1st, 4th and 7th exercise and rest periods. Blood samples were taken at the end of the 1st, 4th and 7th exercise periods (Fig. 1b). In order to obtain arterialized venous blood the hand was placed in a small electric blanket for 5 min before and during blood sampling. The blood samples were analysed for whole blood lactate by an enzymatic spectrophotometric method (Lowry and Passoneau, 1972). Haematocrit was measured by a microhaematocrit method. The PO_2 and PCO_2 in blood samples were measured by an automated blood gas and acid-base balance microanalyser (ABL 4, Acid-base laboratory, Radiometer, Denmark) immediately after the blood samples were drawn.

Statistics
Differences between experiments in normoxia and in hypoxia were determined by Wilcoxon ranking test for paired data (Pratt's modification) (Siegel, 1965). A significance level of $P < 0.05$ was chosen a priori.

Results

At the low and high sub-maximal work loads in the pre-test the mean ($\pm$ SD) $\dot{V}O_2$ of 2.30 ± 0.44 and 3.54 ± 0.54 l min^{-1} respectively, were identical in normoxia and hypoxia. The mean heart rates in normoxia were 125 and 155 beats min^{-1}, respectively, while the corresponding values in hypoxia were 133 and 164 beats min^{-1}, respectively. The mean HR during maximal exercise in normoxia was 180 (range: 174-200) beats min^{-1}.

In the 1st, 4th and 7th exercise period of the interval test mean heart rates were higher in hypoxia (Fig. 2); this was also the case in the corresponding rest periods. The mean heart rates at the end of the seven work bouts in normoxia were, on average, 158 beats min^{-1}, which was 8 beats min^{-1} lower than the corresponding value in hypoxia. The $\dot{V}O_2$ during exercise was the same in normoxia and hypoxia. On the other hand, $\dot{V}E$ was increased in hypoxia. Thus, mean $\dot{V}E$ at the end of the exercise bouts was on average about 15 l min^{-1} higher than the ventilation of around 80 l min^{-1} in normoxia (Fig. 2). The $\dot{V}E$ was also increased during rest periods in hypoxia.

Fig. 3 shows the mean values of rest-times. For all seven rest periods the mean time was prolonged in hypoxia. Thus, the average rest-time in normoxia of 0.85 min was increased in hypoxia by 28%.

The individual relationships between the average change in HR [ΔHR = (HR hypoxia) - (HR normoxia)] at the end of an exercise bout and the average change in rest-time [Δ rest-time = (rest-time hypoxia) - (rest-time normoxia)] for each of the rest periods are shown in Fig. 4. The b-value of the regression line and the r-value (=0.70) indicate that factors other than the increased HR in hypoxia are responsible for the prolonged rest-times.

Fig. 5 shows the hand venous blood values for PO_2, PCO_2 and lactate concentration at rest before the interval test and at the end of exercise bouts number 1, 4 and 7. Hypoxia reduced mean PO_2 ($\pm$ SE) to 49 ± 2, 42 ± 2, 45 ± 2 and 45 ± 2 mmHg at rest, and at the end of 1st, 4th and 7th exercise bouts, respectively and blood PCO_2 values

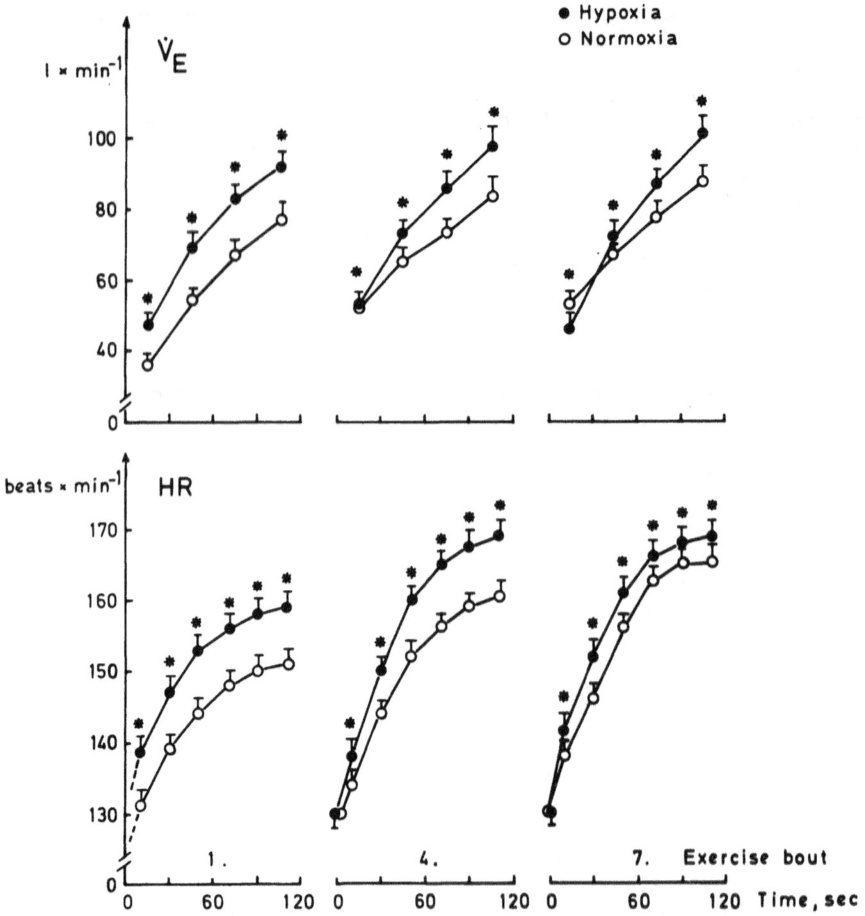

Figure 2. Mean values for ventilation ($\dot{V}E$, l min^{-1}) and heart rate (HR, beats min^{-1}) during 1st, 4th and 7th exercise periods of the interval test in normoxia (mean: 757 mmHg) and in hypoxia (565 mmHg). *denotes significant $P < 0.05$) difference between values in normoxia and in hypoxia

were reduced from 38 ± 1, 42 ± 1, 39 ± 1 and 39 ± 1 to 37 ± 1, 37 ± 1, 33 ± 1 and 33 ± 1 mmHg, respectively (Fig. 5). Since the maximal test at the end of the pretest was carried out only in normoxia, the mean (± SE) lactate concentration before the interval test of 4.6 ± 0.5 mM was higher than in hypoxia (2.8 ± 0.3 mM). As can be seen in Fig. 5 the blood lactate concentrations at the end of 1st, 4th and 7th exercise bouts in normoxia were at the same level as at rest. In hypoxia, however, a continuous increase was seen from one exercise bout to another, and in spite of longer rest periods the values at the end of the 4th and 7th bouts were higher than the corresponding values in normoxia.

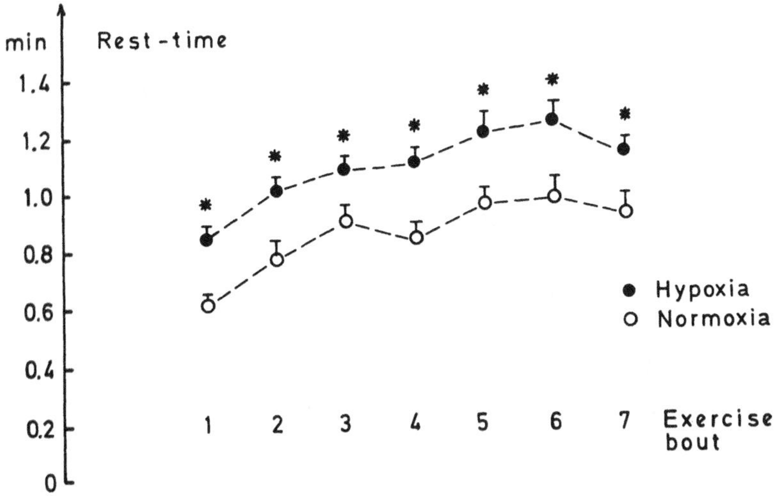

Figure 3. Mean values for the time between each of the seven exercise bouts (rest-time) during the interval test in normoxia and in hypoxia. *denotes significant ($P < 0.05$) difference between values in normoxia and in hypoxia

Discussion

Soccer is characterized by relatively short bursts of exercise at very high intensity alternating with intervals of exercise at high and at relatively low intensity. The relative work load during a soccer game will vary from one player to another, depending on the position in the team, but recordings during soccer games have shown that all players most of the time have hearts rates, which vary between 65-90% of maximum heart rate (see Smodlaka, 1978). The present interval test was constructed to resemble the findings from these field studies. Exercise on a cycle ergometer was chosen because no treadmill was available in the low pressure chamber. However, the physiological response to hypoxia is probably the same during cycling and during running. In order to obtain semi-steady state values of HR and ventilatory variables, the duration of the exercise periods could not be less than 2 min, which is somewhat longer than most of high intensity bursts during a soccer match. The present test did not comprise bursts with maximal intensity, although such bursts are registered during a game (Smodlaka, 1978; Ekblom, 1986). However, the response to hypoxia during maximal periods will probably be at least of the same magnitude as seen within the exercise intensity limits set in the present test.

The increase in HR and ventilation seen in the exercise periods in hypoxia clearly show that the relative strain on the oxygen transportation system was increased. The higher blood lactate concentrations at exercise bouts number 4 and 7 in hypoxia further emphasise that the players were exercising at a higher relative work

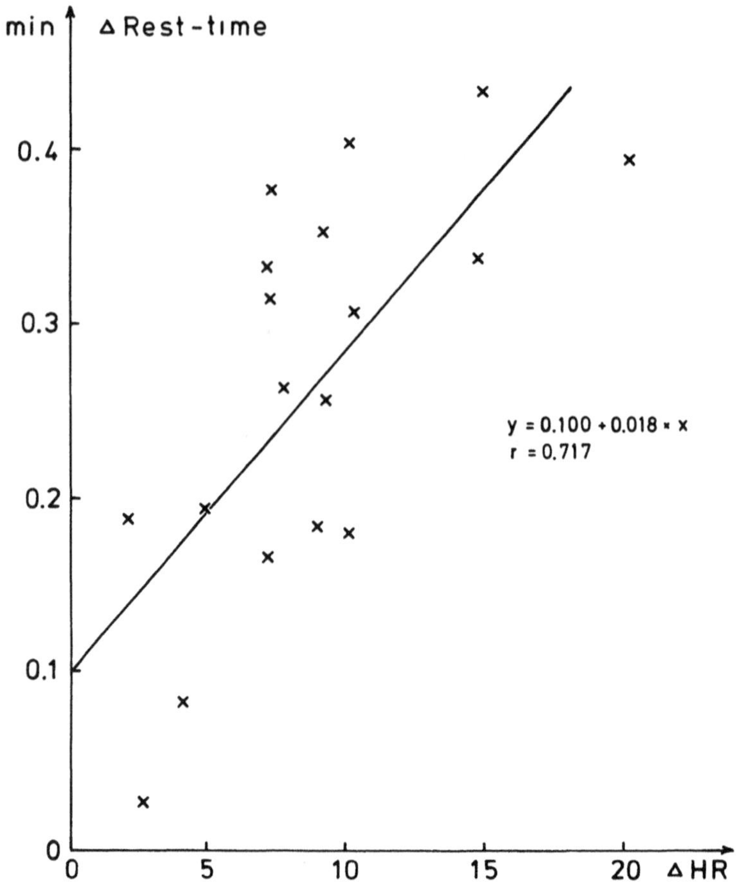

Figure 4. Relation between the average change in HR (ΔHR = (HR hypoxia) - (HR normoxia)) at the end of all exercise bout and the average change in rest-time (Δ rest time = (rest-time hypoxia) - (rest-time normoxia)) for all rest periods. Individual values

load in hypoxia than in normoxia. The increase in relative work load was associated with a substantial increase in rest-time (28%), where the rest-time was defined as the time from end of exercise until HR reached a level 50 beats min^{-1} below maximal HR. As can be deduced from Fig. 4, the changes in rest-time can only partly be explained by the increase in HR during exercise in hypoxia. The slower decrease of HR during the rest periods in hypoxia could be due to a higher concentration of catecholamines in the blood (Bangsbo et al., 1987). The higher ventilation in the rest periods may also contribute to the delayed decrease in HR. The blood lactate values, that were increasing from rest through the 1st, 4th and 7th exercise periods in hypoxia, but were constant in normoxia (Fig. 5), further suggest that the restitution of the players at the end of the rest

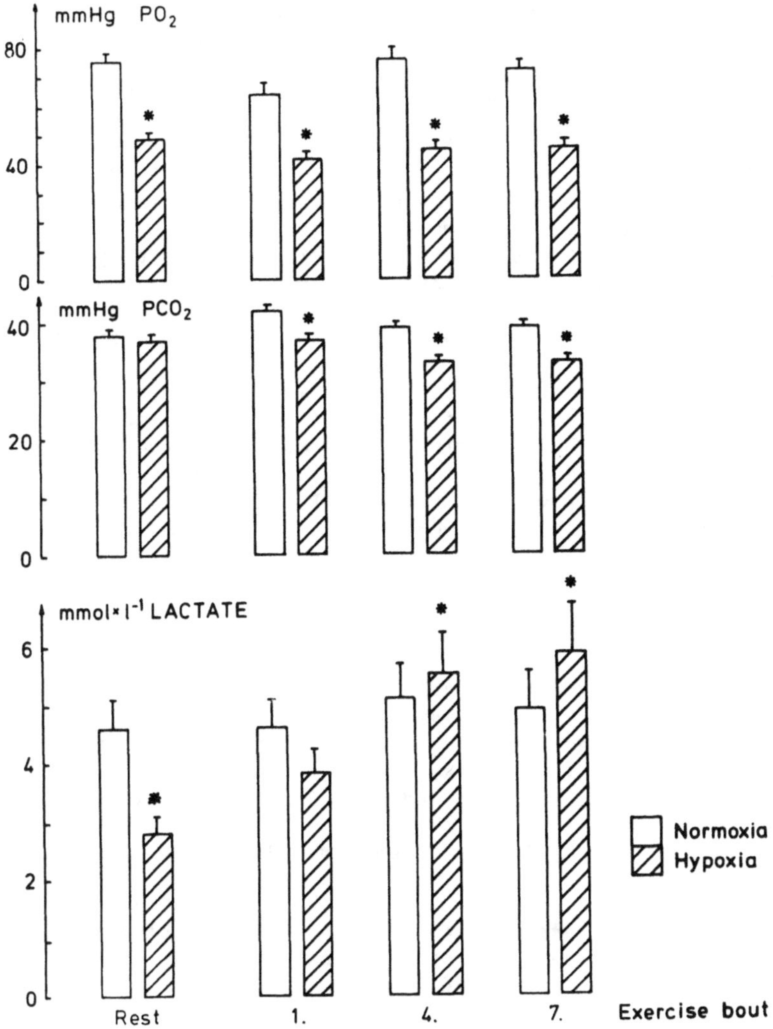

Figure 5. Mean values of PO_2 (mmHg), PCO_2 (mmHg) and lactate concentration ($mmol.l^{-1}$) in hand venous blood at rest before the interval test and at the end of exercise bouts number 1, 4 and 7. *denotes significant ($P < 0.05$) difference between values in normoxia and in hypoxia

periods was less complete in hypoxia than in normoxia. Thus, the lactate values indicate that using HR for the determination of the restitution time in between exercise bouts may underestimate the time it takes to counteract the detrimental effect of hypoxia.

The average response to hypoxia was clear, but there was a large difference in the response of the individual players. Thus, when exposed to hypoxia one subject had an average increase in HR at the end of work periods of 8% and a corresponding elongation of rest-time from 0.85 to 1.24 min (60%), whereas in another subject the same values were only increased 0.3% and 0.4% respectively.

Earlier studies have shown that well-trained persons have a more powerful response to hypoxia (measured as change in $\dot{V}O_2max$) than untrained people (Bangsbo et al., 1987). To evaluate the influence of physical fitness on the response to hypoxia, $\dot{V}O_2max$ was estimated from the two sub-maximal exercise bouts during the pre-test in normoxia (Åstrand, 1960). Individual values of the relation between the estimated $\dot{V}O_2max$ in normoxia and the average increase in HR during the interval test in hypoxia revealed that there was no correlation (r = 0.20) between the two variables.

During the test period it was a common belief among the players that the smaller players would have less trouble in hypoxia than the heavier players. However, no correlation (r = 0.19) was found between body weight and increase in HR during the interval test in hypoxia.

It is concluded that the ability to perform intense, intermittent exercise is reduced, when the players are exercising at a moderately lowered oxygen pressure. Thus, playing soccer at an altitude of 2500m will force the players either to work in shorter periods or with less intensity, or to prolong the rest periods. An acclimatization period at high altitude may, to some extent, counteract this acute effect of hypoxia (Saltin, 1967; Maher et al., 1974).

References

Åstrand, I. (1960) Aerobic work capacity in men and women with special reference to age. Acta. Physiol. Scand., 48 (Suppl.).

Bangsbo, J., Galbo, H., Kjaer, M. and Lortie, G. (1987) Role of hypoxia per se on hormonal responses to dynamic exercise at simulated high altitude in trained and untrained man. J. Physiol., 280, 141P.

Ekblom, B. (1986) Applied physiology of soccer. Sports Med., 3, 50-60.

Hermansen, L. and Saltin, B. (1966) Blood lactate concentration during exercise at acute exposure to altitude. In: Exercise at Altitude (edited by R. Margaria) International Symposium, Milan, September 29th - October, 2nd, 1966.

Lowry, T. and Passonneau, J.V. (1972) A Flexible System of Enzymatic Analysis. New York: Academic Press, 93-108.

Maher, J.T., Jones, L.G. and Hartley, L.H. (1974) Effect of high-altitude exposure on submaximal endurance capacity of men. J. Appl. Physiol., 37, 895.

Saltin, B. (1967) Aerobic and anaerobic work capacity at 2300 meters. Med. Thorac, 24, 205-210.

Siegel, S. (1965) Non-parametric Statistics for the Behavioural Sciences. Tokyo, McGraw-Hill, Kogakusha Ltd.

Smodlaka, V.N. (1978) Cardiovascular aspects of soccer. Physician Sportsmed., 6, 66-70.

Part VII

Match analysis: strategic aspects

THE CABER COMPUTER SYSTEM: A REVIEW OF ITS APPLICATION TO THE ANALYSIS OF AUSTRALIAN RULES FOOTBALL

J.D. Patrick   Div. Computing and Mathematics, Deakin University, Victoria, 3217, Australia.

M.J. McKenna   Department of Physiology, University of Melbourne, Victoria, Australia.

Introduction

Computers are being increasingly used in sports analysis. Specific computer-assisted analyses have been described for a variety of sports, including soccer (Franks et al., 1983), Canadian football (Bedingfield et al., 1982), water polo, fencing, field hockey and wrestling (Franks and Goodman, 1986). Computers have been used in these analyses as their use allows more sophisticated recording and analysis of data. This is achieved in a relatively short period of time. The data collected, however, must be objective and specific to the requirements of the sport (Franks et al., 1986). Further the use of computers reduces the errors involved in a subjective analysis of the game. These include factors such as poor memory of the game events, with the exception of highlights which tend to dominate the memory (Franks et al., 1983).

The way in which information is categorized during the analysis of a game is a major problem for two reasons (Franks et al., 1986). The first is due to difficulties in deciding which information in a game is important. The second problem lies in the efficient recording, storage and printing of large amounts of match related information. As indicated by Franks et al. (1986), the second is not a major problem with the recent introduction of computing skills to game analysis. However, the first problem remains the major barrier to successful and meaningful analysis of sports. This applies especially to complex team sports, such as the different codes of football. These codes of football can be described as 'non-deterministic' sports (Patrick and McKenna, 1986a). That is, they comprise a large number of events with a high degree of player choice of action, combined with a relatively high uncertainty of other players' actions. Australian football, with its additional variability of ball flight, is a good example of a non-deterministic sport. At the other end of the spectrum are the 'deterministic' sports. These require the performance of a highly specific, pre-determined event or sequence of events. Due to the greater complexity of interactions in a non-deterministic sport, analysis of these is more difficult. In addition, the problem of identifying important events during the game is more complicated.

A computer system has been developed which directly addresses both of the major problems in sports analysis identified by Franks et al.

(1986). This paper presents a review of previous work using this sytem in the analysis of Australian Rules football (Patrick and McKenna, 1986a,b) a report on recent research, as well as directions for future research.

The CABER System

Specific computing details of this system, called the CABER system, have previously been reported (Patrick, 1985a,b,c). CABER is a mnemonic for Capture and Analysis of Behavioural Events in Real-time. The CABER system consists of a number of software components which when combined together in an appropriate manner create an application system for the recording and analysis of a particular sport. By the term 'real-time' we mean that the system accepts and analyses the data while the game is actually in progress.

Data recording consists of the entry of quantitative and qualitative data into a CABER system. The quantitative data include all of the actions during the game such as ball possessions and disposals, team events, defensive and offensive actions. These data can also be descriptive, by the inclusion of adjectival qualifiers such as the quality (good, poor), pressure (uncontested, contested), and the location (wings, back pocket). Operation of the system is quite straightforward. One person usually watches and verbalises the game according to the specific football syntax (described below). Data entry is performed on a special football touch-keyboard by the second operator. Storage of the data is performed at the conclusion of the segment of play being analysed, usually every 5-10 s. A print out of all game events, as well as a statistical summary of the match can then be obtained. CABER can be used either at the game, or later from a videotape. The advantage of real-time data entry is that the coach can obtain valuable information whilst the game is in progress. The use of the CABER system dispenses with the need to have a considerable number of observers at the game to record the game information. Thus, the CABER system overcomes the functional problem of game analysis.

The major problem of game analysis, the interpretation of game events, is also addressed by the CABER system. A query language has been inbuilt into the system to enable specific questions to be addressed to the computer. These may include the simple sum of certain relevant statistics. But more importantly, they might include the number of sequences of particular types of plays by one team and the success of these. The query is comprised firstly of a directive to either DISPLAY (on a Video Display Unit), PRINT or REPLAY (on a video-cassette recorder, VCR). A word specifying the number of occurrences of an action is also included (ALL, NEXT, LAST, etc.). Successive actions can also be queried (FOLLOWED BY, PRECEDED BY). Examples of queries that might be addressed to the computer are:-

> DISPLAY ALL Goals kicked by Opposition player # 31
> REPLAY FIRST Kick by Home player # 16 FOLLOWED BY Mark by Opposition.

One of the most striking advantages of the CABER system over other computerised analysis systems, is its linkage with and control over a VCR. This allows the computer to REPLAY any event, or sequences of events during the game on the VCR monitor. Thus, during a quarter break of a game, the coach may look at any actions recorded during the preceding segment of the game. This facility then allows a high degree of dynamic strategy variation by the coach. Post-game analysis will also assist in the critical analysis of the game and in the developent of future strategies.

In order for the computer to understand these actions and sequences of actions, a specific grammar, or set of rules, must be constructed for the sport being analysed. For example, gaining possession of the ball must always precede its disposal. Exceptions to this are 'simultaneous' actions during the game, where a player gains and disposes of the ball in the same action, e.g. a 'Hit-out'. A simplified grammar for use in Australian Rules football is shown in Figure 1. Examples of typical actions during Australian Rules football, using this grammar are:

1. CENTRE BOUNCE UMPIRE 1
2. HIT OUT LEFT EFFECTIVE CONTESTED HOME 26
3. RECEIVE UNCONTESTED HOME 12 (TACKLE INEFFECTIVE OPPOSITION 33) HANDBALL RIGHT
4. PICK UP OPPOSITION 7 KICK RIGHT (SMOTHER POOR HOME 47)
5. MARK CONTESTED OPPOSITION 15 PLAY ON (SHEPHERD OPPOSITION 12 BUMP INEFFECTIVE HOME 19) KICK LEFT GOAL

The CABER System in Australian Football

Several applications of the CABER system in Australian football are presented. These include the description of one player's game performance, of one specific activity, of one team's use of CABER system's findings, and the identification of important factors in team success.

Single Player Performance

The summary of one particular player's game (Patrick and McKenna, 1986a), highlighted the possible importance of this player to the team. Inspection of each action of this player during a game (Table 1) revealed a marked reduction in possessions and in the ability to move the ball quickly, late in the game. This was later found to be associated with the onset of a specific medical problem, with this general pattern of play being repeated in several subsequent games. The most striking fact about this change in performance is that it corresponded to a point in the game where his team was overwhelmed by the opposition. Either the onset of his injury reduced the team's performance substantially, or the player reduced his own performance immediately when his team began losing. Whichever is the true reason, the player was concluded to be a hitherto unrecognised important factor in his team's performance.

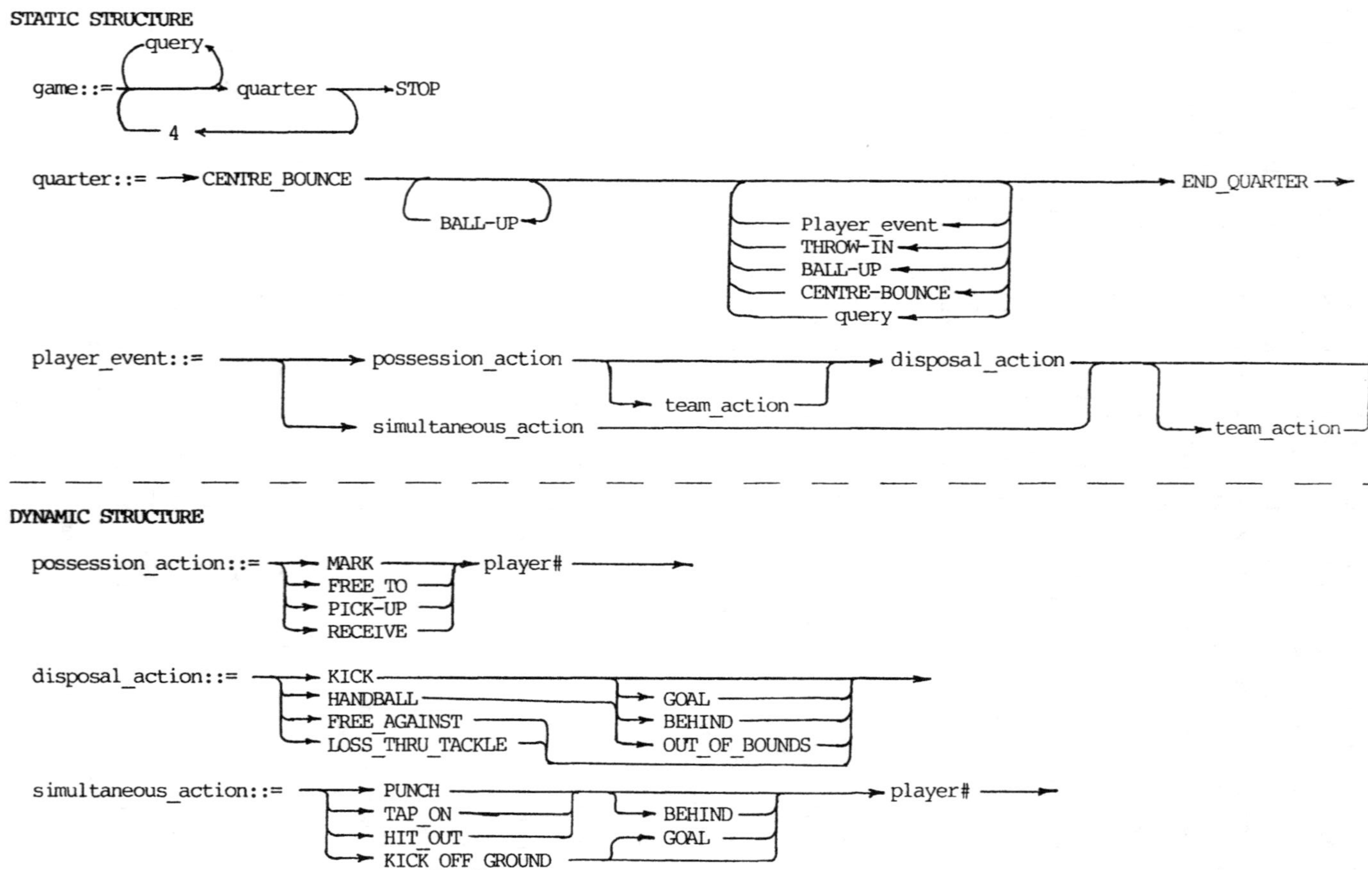

Fig. 1 A simplified syntax for Australian Rules Football showing static & dynamic structures

Table 1. List and summary of each action by one player in an ARF game

No.	Action	Free	Play on	Disposal	Foot	Result	
1.	CENTRE BOUNCE						
2.	MARK			KICK	RIGHT	GOAL	
3	FREE NP	9 OPPOSITION 11		KICK	RIGHT		
4	RECEIVE			KICK	RIGHT		
5	RECEIVE			KICK	RIGHT		
6	MARK		PLAY ON	KICK	RIGHT		
7	MARK		PLAY ON	KICK	RIGHT		
8	MARK			KICK	RIGHT	GOAL	
9	PICK UP			KICK	RIGHT		
10	MARK		PLAY ON	KICK	RIGHT		
END QUARTER							
11	MARK		PLAY ON	KICK	RIGHT		
12	PUNCH						
13	MARK		PLAY ON	KICK	RIGHT	OOB	
14	MARK			KICK	RIGHT		
15	MARK		PLAY ON	KICK	RIGHT		
16	PICK UP			KICK	RIGHT		
17	PICK UP			LOSS THRU TACKLE			
18	PICK UP			KICK	RIGHT		
19	PICK UP			KICK	LEFT		
20	PICK UP			LOSS THRU TACKLE			
END QUARTER							
21	PICK UP			KICK	RIGHT	POINT	HOME
22	PICK UP			LOSS THRU TACKLE			
23	PICK UP			HANDBALL	RIGHT		
24	RECEIVE			KICK	RIGHT	GOAL	
25	PICK UP			LOSS THRU TACKLE			
26	FREE	7 OPPOSITION 4		KICK	RIGHT		
27	FREE	7 OPPOSITION 4		KICK	RIGHT		
28	RECEIVE			KICK	LEFT		
29	FUMBLE						
30	TAP ON						
31	RECEIVE			KICK	LEFT		
END QUARTER							
32	PICK UP			KICK	RIGHT	POINT	HOME
33	PUNCH						
34	RECEIVE			KICK	RIGHT		
35	PICK UP			KICK	LEFT		
END QUARTER							

SUMMARY

POSSESSIONS		%	DISPOSALS		%	SIMULTANEOUS		OTHERS	
Mark	9	30	Kick	25	85	Punch	2	Played on	6
Free-for	3	10	Loss-thru-tackle	4	12	Fumble	1	Goals	3
Receive	6	20	Handball	1	3	Tap-on	1	Points	1
Pick-up	12								
	30			30			4		

Importance of a Specific Activity during the Game.

Specific events during the game can also be analysed using a CABER system. Analysis of every handball was conducted during two important matches from the 1985 season, including the 1985 Grand Final (Patrick and McKenna, 1986b). This analysis revealed a major advantage to one team through a systematic breach of the rules, which was undetected by the umpires. The number of handballs during each match was recorded during a routine CABER analysis. This was subdivided into the number of legal, illegal and suspected illegal handballs, for each team. The numbers for each handball classification are given in Table 2. The proportion of the combined illegal and suspected illegal handballs was significantly greater for Team 1 than for Teams 2 and 3, being 5.19% and 4.76% respectively ($P < 0.05$). When both games were combined, the difference beween the teams was even more apparent ($P < 0.005$). This small difference between the teams gave Team 1 a considerable advantage. Of the 12 non-legal handballs, 6 resulted in a score or a potential goal scoring chance, yielding an average score advantage of 10 points per game.

Table 2. Handball (HB) classification for two matches during the 1985 Victorian Football League season.

Match	Team	Legal HB	Illegal HB	Suspect HB	Total HB
# 1	#1	146	6	2	154
	#2	99	0	0	99
# 2	#1	80	4	0	84
	#3	85	0	0	85

Use of the CABER system in Team Strategy

Analysis of one match revealed a large proportion of the opposition possessions to be gained without being under pressure from the home team. The home team was soundly beaten on this occasion. In the return match, this aspect of the previous game, putting pressure on the opposition, was developed by the coach in order to improve the home teams performance. A much smaller proportion of the opposition possessions were obtained uncontested in this match, with the losing margin being substantially reduced.

The Identification of Important Factors in Team Success

To investigate whether factors might be important to team success over a large number of games, every home game for one team is currently being analysed. Preliminary results reveal that the simple summation of statistics (including possessions, disposals, pressure actions and forced errors) per player and per team, were not reliable predictors of team success. Therefore, traditional analyses of team performance in Australian football do not appear to successfully differentiate between winning and losing matches. Clearly further investigation is required to enable us to identify the most important factors in team success.

Conclusion

Previous applications of CABER systems have shown that the three factors analysed, namely single player performance, systematic breach of the rules, and the pressure placed on the opposition possessions, were all important during those particular games analysed.

However, we have been unable to differentiate between successful and unsuccessful teams on the basis of a simple summation of match statistics. Obviously a complex interaction of many variables affects the outcome of the game.

We are currently investigating this interaction in order to determine the most important factors for team success in Australian Rules football.

References

Bedingfield, E.W., Marchiori, G. and Gervais, P. (1982) Game strategy: film and computer analysis. Coaching Science Update, 23-24.

Franks, I.M., Goodman, D. and Miller G. (1983) Analysis of performance: qualitative or quantitative. Science Periodical on Research and Technology in Sport, GY-1. Ottawa: Coaching Association of Canada.

Franks, I.M. and Goodman, D. (1986) Computer-assisted technical analysis of sport. Coaching Review, May/June, 58-64.

Franks, I.M., Paterson, G. and Goodman, D. (1986) The real time analysis of sport: an overview. Can. J. Appl. Sport Sci., 11, 55-57.

Patrick, J.D. (1985a) The CABER system. Aust. Comp. Sci. Comm., 10-1, 10-2.

Patrick, J.D. (1985b) The capture and analysis of football in real time. Aust. Computer Science Bulletin, May, 9-10.

Patrick, J.D. (1985c) The CABER project: the capture and analysis of behavioural events in real time. Proceedings 1985 ACM Annual Conference, 92-98.

Patrick, J.D., and McKenna, M.J. (1986a) A generalised computer system for sports analysis. Aust. J. Sci. Med. Sport, 18, 19-23.

Patrick, J.D. and McKenna, M.J. (1986b) Computerised analysis of handball in Australian football. Aust. J. Sci. Med. Sport, 18, 24-26.

COMPUTER-VIDEO ANALYSIS OF ACTIVITY PATTERNS IN AUSTRALIAN RULES FOOTBALL

M.J. McKenna, J.D. Patrick*, E.R. Sandstrom, M.H.D. Chennells
Department of Physiology, University of Melbourne, Parkville, 3052, Victoria, Australia;
*Div. Computing and Mathematics, Deakin University, Victoria, 3217, Australia

Introduction

Numerous methods have been employed to assess the game demands on players in different codes of football. Direct observation and charting of the movements was the earlier preferred method of activity analysis of Australian footballers (Nettleton and Sandstrom, 1963). Whilst giving valuable information, the accuracy of this method is limited by the speed of the analysts in keeping up with the game, with no option to either correct errors, or to re-analyse a particular segment of play. Videotapes of a player's movements during a game were subsequently used to enable greater accuracy in the determination of activity patterns (Jaques and Pavia, 1974). However, activity analyses were recorded for only one quarter of a match (approximately 30 min). Consequently, extrapolation of these results to represent full game analysis may introduce a substantial error, since the time period measured may not be representative of the entire match.

Most investigations of both Australian Rules football and soccer have analysed the distance covered during the game, through either short time interval measurements (Jaques and Pavia, 1974; Saltin, 1973), or full game analyses (Reilly and Thomas, 1976; Withers et al., 1982). For the determination of distance covered, ground markings and cues (Reilly and Thomas, 1976), or the stride length and frequency (Withers et al., 1982), have been measured. Possible errors involved in the former approach include the difficulty in quantifying diagonal movement (relative to ground markings), the distance of the recorder from the game and parallax error. In the latter paper, possible errors may occur from changes in gait characteristics during the game. A high reliability (Reilly and Thomas, 1976) and objectivity (Reilly and Thomas, 1976; Withers et al., 1982) have been reported for these methods.

However, the assessment of time spent in each activity mode may be an easier, equally reliable (Mayhew and Wenger, 1985) and more objective measure of activity patterns during a game. The measurement of time involves no estimations or assumptions that are associated with distance determinations. Consequently, the proportion of time spent in, not distance covered, in different activity modes should be the major variable investigated.

Many authors have analysed the percentage time spent in a variety of activity modes for both Australian Rules football (Jaques and

Pavia, 1974; Pyke and Smith, 1975), and soccer (Withers et al., 1982; Mayhew and Wenger, 1985). Few, however, have reported the mean duration spent in each activity type and the work to rest ratios during the game (Withers et al., 1982; Mayhew and Wenger, 1985).

A problem with many previous methodologies is the excessive time requirement for detailed, objective analysis (Withers et al., 1982). Consequently, computerised capture of activity patterns and data reduction is a considerable advantage (Mayhew and Wenger, 1985).

Therefore, assessment of a player's activity patterns during a game should involve video-recording of the player's entire game, with subsequent computerized analysis of the time spent in different activity types. Such an activity analysis for Australian football forms the basis of this paper. The physiological implications of this analysis are discussed and compared with similar analyses of soccer players.

Methods

Subjects

Four Victorian Football League players were videotaped over a complete game. All players were 'rovers' competing in their first grade team. An Australian football rover is a nomadic player, covering a large distance during the game and having a high number of ball contacts (Pyke and Smith, 1975).

Filming

Video filming was conducted from a grandstand located midway alongside the oval playing field. Each player was filmed for a total duration of approximately two hours, comprising four quarters. A three hour videocassette tape was used, allowing uninterrupted filming of the player.

Activity Classification

The activity of each player was classified according to: 1) Movement type and 2) Game related activities (GRA). Movement types used were the same as previously reported (Mayhew and Wenger, 1985), comprising stationary, walk, jog and high intensity run (HIR, stride plus sprint). The GRA class comprised all ball contacts, body contacts including tackles and bumps, and physical efforts such as jumps, dives and fall over/get up. These activities were then combined into 'low intensity' (LI), for stationary, walk and jog; and into High Intensity (HI) for HIR and GRA.

Activity Analysis and Data Reduction

A computer-video system was used in the analysis. A BBC microcomputer was connected to a videocassette recorder (VCR) via a specially designed VCR interface. Analysis was conducted from a videotape replay, although real-time analysis is also possible. Each activity was assigned a specific key on the computer keyboard. To record an event, the appropriate key was depressed, with the event and its duration being terminated by depressing an event marker key. A pause facility enabled the operator to halt the tape, whether to note an error, or to review a particular segment for verification of classification. The event number and type were displayed on the computer monitor during the analysis to enable checks of data entry and to facilitate any error correction.

Data Reduction

Subsequent to the activity classification, a print out of all individual events, their durations and the cumulative total time was obtained. A print-out of statistics was then obtained for each activity classification, for each quarter and for the complete game. These included the number of occurrences, total accumulated time; as well as the mean, variance, minimum, maximum and percentage time. The total time spent in each of the LI and HI categories was summated and used to calculate a mean game work:rest ratio. The ratio was inverted and expressed as LI/HI. The number of occurrences, duration and the work:rest ratio was calculated for each successive HI and LI interval during the game.

Reliability

The complete match of one player was analysed twice by the same operator. The first and last 10 min segment of each quarter was extracted for reliability measurement. A high reliability was found for both the total time (all $r \geq 0.92$) and the number of occurrences (all $r \geq 0.83$) of each activity.

Results

Results of the activity analyses are shown in Table 1.

Table 1. Activity analyses of four Australian football rovers (mean ± standard deviation)

Activity	Percent time	Number	Duration (seconds) Mean	Maximum
Stationary	8.8 ± 3.5	89 ± 42	5.9 ± 2.0	40.7
Walk	44.5 ± 6.2	300 ± 44	9.3 ± 1.7	153.8
Jog	40.9 ± 9.1	308 ± 24	8.4 ± 3.0	52.0
HIR	4.1 ± 0.4	98 ± 13	2.7 ± 0.7	10.4
GRA	2.5 ± 0.8	85 ± 20	1.8 ± 0.2	15.9

The total number of HI efforts during the four games, and the percentage distribution of these into successive 2 s interval durations is shown in Table 2.

Table 2. The duration of all HI efforts during the game (n = 4), distributed into successive 2 s interval durations.

		Duration (seconds)						
		0-2	2-4	4-6	6-8	8-10	10+	TOTAL
Number	$\bar{X}$	33.5	38.0	18.3	9.3	4.4	5.3	108.5
	SD	8.7	8.3	4.6	3.6	3.3	2.2	17.4
Percent	$\bar{X}$	30.5	34.8	17.4	8.8	3.8	4.6	99.9
	SD	3.9	3.7	5.9	4.0	2.8	1.5	0.1

The mean game LI/HI ratio was 14.23 ± 0.86. When the actual LI/HI ratio was calculated for each successive HI and LI interval, a mean number of 108.0 ± 18.4 ratios were found over the complete game. The mean, standard deviation, minimum and maximum of all LI/HI ratios for each quarter and for the complete game, are given in Table 3.

Table 3. Mean (± SD) of all work:rest ratios (LI/HI) calculated per quarter and for the complete game

Quarter	Mean	SD	Min	Max
1	21.9	4.7	0.2	142.2
2	30.5	12.2	0.4	198.5
3	21.1	3.6	0.4	134.8
4	24.6	6.4	0.2	165.9
Game	24.5	-	0.2	198.5

The percentage distribution of these ratios into different levels of intensity is given in Table 4.

Table 4. Percentage distribution of all work:rest ratios during the game

		Ratio LI/HI						
		0-1	1-2	2-3	3-6	6-9	9-12	12+ (s)
Number	$\bar{X}$	8.3	7.3	6.5	12.8	12.8	7.3	53.3
	SD	4.0	2.6	3.4	5.3	5.9	1.7	8.3
Percent	$\bar{X}$	7.6	6.8	5.9	11.8	11.5	7.1	49.4
	SD	3.3	2.1	2.8	4.1	4.2	2.9	0.8

Discussion

Activity patterns have been analysed to give information on energy costs during the game and therefore to enable the development of appropriate training regimes. The computer-video technique presented in this paper is reliable, user-friendly and incorporates advantages of previously published methods.

The rovers analysed in this study were found to spend the vast majority of their playing time (94%) engaged in LI activities. This is consistent with previous findings for Australian football rovers (Jaques and Pavia, 1974). A similar proportion of time is spent in LI activity by Australian soccer players (Withers et al., 1982). In both football codes, playing position was thought to be an important determinant of the work rate, with 'on-ball' or midfield players spending a large proportion of time on the move and consequently covering greater distances during the game, relative to other positional players (Jaques and Pavia, 1974; Reilly and Thomas, 1976). More recently, however, no differences have been shown between midfield and other players in the total distance covered (Withers et al., 1982). This probably represents the current trend towards increased player versatility during the game.

The LI time was comprised of a large number of discrete activities, with a total of 697 LI events. The small proportion of time spent in HI activities was due to a much smaller number of discrete events. The total number of occurrences of each of HIR and GRA was similar to that seen for 'stationary', being approximately 90. The total number of HIR reported in the current study was less than that of 115 to 110, previously reported for two Australian football rovers (Hahn et al., 1979). The mean frequency of HIR occurrence was once every 73 s, somewhat less frequent than the one HIR every 40 s reported for Canadian soccer players (Mayhew and Wenger, 1985). One sprint every 90 s has been reported for English soccer players, although the frequency of HIR occurrence was not reported (Reilly and Thomas, 1976).

A very short mean HIR duration of 2.7 s, with a maximum of 10.4 s, was found for the Australian rovers. The mean HIR distance for two rovers has been reported to be 19 and 12 m, respectively (Hahn et al. 1979). A similar mean HIR duration of 3.7 s and mean HIR distance of

22.2 m was found for Australian soccer players (Withers et al., 1982). However, the maximum duration was 24.3 s and the maximum distance was 105 m for the soccer players: much longer than the corresponding values for Australian Rules football rovers. The maximum HI interval found for Australian Rules football rovers was 21.7 s, similar to the maximum HIR reported by Withers et al. (1982). Thus both of the frequency and mean durations for HIR were greater for the soccer players, with the maximum HI intervals being similar.

An important finding is that approximately 65% of all HI efforts lasted for less than 4.0 s, with 80% being less than 6.0 s. This is in agreement with the findings of Withers et al. (1982) who reported that 75% of all HI efforts lasted for less than 4.8 s.

A low mean duration of less than 10 s was recorded for each of the LI and GRA categories. This reflects the intermittent nature of the game, with a change of event occurring on average every 7.3 s. A similar rate of change was found for soccer players, occurring once every 6.1 s (Mayhew and Wenger, 1985) and 6.4 s (Reilly and Thomas, 1976).

The high event turnover rate, coupled with the regular short bursts of HI activity implies a reliance on both the stored phosphagens and aerobic substrates as sources of metabolic energy. The very short duration of most of the HI efforts implies that energy will be supplied by the degradation of intramuscular ATP and creatine phosphate stores (Hultman and Sjoholm, 1983; Jones et al., 1985). However, since glycolysis is activated within 1.26 s of activity of this intensity (Hultman and Sjoholm, 1983), glycolysis may also be an important metabolic energy source. This is consistent with blood lactate levels of up to 14 mM (Ekblom, 1986) and 16 mM (Agnevik, 1970) reported during soccer matches. With the maximum HIR durations of soccer players being up to 24.3 s and the maximum HI duration for Australian football rovers being up to 21.7 s, respectively, a considerable contribution to energy costs would be drawn from glycolysis.

Despite the relatively long recovery time seen for Australian football rovers, the peak work rates during the game must also be responsible for a metabolic acidosis. The total of 20.2% of all work:rest ratios being less than 3.0 in the current study, suggests that segments of the game must be quite stressful, probably also contributing to any metabolic acidosis. Little work on acid-base balance has been performed on Australian Rules footballers. Some evidence of a metabolic acidosis does exist, however, with findings of an increased anion gap and reduction of bicarbonate levels in the blood (Pohl et al., 1981).

The importance of muscle glycogen stores during soccer is well documented (Saltin, 1973; Currie et al., 1981: Jacobs et al., 1982). The relative contribution of glycogen stores to aerobic and anaerobic metabolism during soccer is only indirectly reflected by blood lactate levels, since the LI exercise may well metabolise the lactate produced during the preceding HI effort (Bonen and Belcastro, 1975). However, both sprinting and jogging distances were reduced with lowered glycogen stores (Saltin, 1973). An increased match distance during indoor soccer (Foster et al., 1986) and reduced distance during indoor soccer (Foster et al., 1986) and reduced muscle glycogen utilisation during a soccer match (Leatt and Jacobs, 1986) have been found following carbohydrate supplementation. The importance of lipid sources to fuel supply during these intermittent sports has not been documented. An important contribution would, however, be expected due to findings in other studies of intermittent exercise (e.g. Essen et al., 1977).

Training for Australian football rovers should closely replicate the intermittent nature of the game. Consequently, training should incorporate a rapid turn-over of activity types, with a high number of both HIR and GRA, mostly of a very short duration. Players should be trained to cope physically with the peak stresses during the game and be able to reproduce a high skill level under these conditions. Thus training should include highly stressful periods, as encountered during the game. An additional feature of the training should be to train players to perform under these peak stresses for longer periods, or more often, during the game. Thus the player's mean work rate during the game would be higher. The principles of training for the two codes of football described in this paper are similar, although the specific activity patterns and skills are somewhat different.

References

Agnevik, G. (1970) Football. Sport Physiology Report Number 7 (Swedish) Stockholm: Trygg-Hansa.

Bonen, A. and Belcastro, A.N. (1975) Lactic acid removal rates during controlled and uncontrolled recovery exercise. J. Appl. Physiol., 39, 932-937.

Currie, D., Bonen, A., Belcastro, A.N., Kirby, R.L., Sopper, M. and Richards, A.R. (1981) Glycogen utilisation and circulatory substrate responses during match play soccer and soccer training sessions (Abstract). Int. J. Sports Med., 2, 271.

Ekblom, B., (1986) Applied physiology of soccer. Sports Med., 3, 50-60.

Essen, B., Hagenfeldt, L. and Kaisjer, L., (1977) Utilisation of blood-borne and intramuscular substrates during continuous and intermittent exercise in man. J. Physiol., 265, 489-506.

Foster, C., Thompson, N.N., Dean, J. and Kirkendall, D.T. (1986) Carbohydrate supplementation and performance in soccer players. Med. Sci. Sports Exerc., 18 (2) suppl., 12.

Hahn, A., Taylor, N., Woodhouse, T., Schulz, G., and Hunt, B. (1979) Physiological relationships between training activities and match play in Australian Rules football rovers. Sports Coach, 3, 3-8.

Hultman, E. and Sjoholm, H. (1983) Substrate availability. In: Biochemistry of exercise. Vol. 13. Int. Series on Sport Sciences. Edited by H.G. Knuttgen, J.A. Vogel and J. Poortmans Champaign, IL: Human Kinetics Publishers, Inc., Champaign, IL.

Jacobs, I., Westlin, N., Karlsson, J., Rasmusson, M. and Houghton, B. (1982) Muscle glycogen and diet in elite soccer players. Eur. J. Appl. Physiol., 48, 297-302.

Jaques, T.D. and Pavia, G.R. (1974) An analysis of movement patterns of players in an Australian rules league football match. Aust. J. Sports Med., 5, 10-21.
Jones, N.L., McCartney, N., Graham, T., Spriet, L.L., Kowalchuck, J., Heigenhauser, G.J.F. and Sutton, J.R. (1985) Muscle performance and metabolism in maximal isokinetic cycling at slow and fast speeds. J. Appl. Physiol., 59, 132-136.
Leatt, P.B. and Jacobs, I. (1986) Effects of glucose polymer ingestion on muscle glycogen utilization during a soccer match (Abstract). Med. Sci. Sports Exerc., 18, Suppl., 6.
Mayhew, J.L. and Wenger, H.A. (1985). Time-motion analysis of professional soccer. J. Human Mov't. Stud., 11, 49-52.
Nettleton, B., and Sandstrom, E.R., (1963) Skill and conditioning in Australian rules football. Aust. J. Phys. Ed., 29, 17-30.
Pohl, A.P., O'Halloran, M.W. and Pannall, P.R. (1981) Biochemical and physiological changes in football players. Med. J. Austr., 1, 467-470.
Pyke, F. and Smith, R. (1975) Football the Scientific Way. University of Western Australia Press, Nedlands: W.A. Harper and Row Publishers.
Reilly, T. and Thomas, V. (1976) A motion analysis of work-rate in different positional roles in professional football match play. J. Human Mov't. Stud., 2, 87-97.
Saltin, B. (1973) Metabolic fundamentals in exercise. Med. Sci. Sports, 5, 137-146.
Withers, R.T., Maricic, Z., Wasilewski, S., and Kelly, L. (1982) Match analyses of Australian professional soccer players. J. Humam Mov't. Stud., 8, 159-176.

COMPUTER-AIDED MATCH ANALYSIS OF SELECTED BALL GAMES (SOCCER AND RUGBY UNION)

Peter John Treadwell
Department of Physical Education and Human Movement Studies, South Glamorgan Institute of Higher Education, Cyncoed Centre, Cardiff, S. Wales CF2 6XD.

Introduction

Coaches and performers are under constant pressure to optimise sporting performance (Franks and Goodman, 1986a). Honest endeavour and enthusiasm are no longer enough to make a coach successful, for effective coaching also depends upon deliberate, structured acts of intervention (Brackenridge and Alderson, 1985). This research examines the structure and function of match analysis systems in selected ball games, using computer and concept keyboards to process match information. The implication is that the statistics gleemed from such a service could make coach interventions more decisive, objective and complement any subjective feelings about player and team performance.

The simplest form of data collection is the pen and paper method, where frequency tallies and outcome information are recorded (Brackenridge and Alderson, 1985). Audio-tape recording using a discrete vocabulary has also been utilized (Baker and Milner, 1985).

However, recording may be immediate but subsequent analysis has proven time-consuming and limited effectiveness and sponsored coach neglect (Hall, 1981). Notational and charting systems have also been developed in selected sports (Sanderson, 1983) which no doubt owe something to the original ideas of Laban and Lawrence (1947), in effort analysis. Video-tape recording has presented the opportunity to extract detailed objective information but this medium still promotes a 'lapsed time' analysis. When used alongside a microcomputer a basic movement analysis laboratory situation is created (Franks and Goodman, 1986a; Hughes, 1985).

Some researchers (Franks and Goodman, 1986b; MacKinnon, 1985) have adapted 'QWERTY' keyboard of the micro-computer or even built keyboards with special ergonomic advantages. Recent studies (Sharp, 1986; Treadwell and Van der Vliet, 1987) have used 'concept keyboards', touch sensitive pads which allow for a greater range of analysis potential and ease of operation. Also, some computer based analytical systems (Treadwell and Van der Vliet, 1987) have moved to 'real time' analysis of sport after a pre-game prioritization of key parameters.

Time and motion analysis centres on the physiological demands of a game and identifies the work rates of players within the team. Mayhew and Wenger (1985) suggested that objective data on movement patterns might be applied to fitness training. Quantitative research regarding player work-rate began with Winterbottom (1959) and Wade (1967) charting a distance covered and categorizing the movement into walking, jogging, running and sprinting.

In soccer Brooke and Knowles (1974), found a range of 3772-6428 m covered (average 4834 m) by English First Division players, and showed a ratio of 3:5:1 when aligned to components of walking, jogging, and sprinting. Players sprinted on average 52 times per game (mean distance 11.4 yd, range 5-65 y). Reilly and Thomas (1976) analysed groups of midfield players in terms of their frequency of movement patterns and ground/aerial activities. Results indicated little time in possession (0.26% to 4.0%, mean 1.73%) and highlighted the predominant aerobic demands within soccer. Withers et al. (1982) determined the intensity of work by studying stride length whilst also collating ball contacts and tackle involvement. Mayhew and Wenger (1985) concentrated on presentability of information and methodology using video and micro-computer to minimise 'data-delay' and highlighted a 1:7 high to low intensity activity ratio with 52.5 s spent in aerobic work to 7.5 s running hard per minute.

In rugby union, an average match has 40 scrums (20 s duration) 50-60 line-outs and 60-80 rucks or mauls (Rugby Football Union, 1978). Using cine-film, Lynch (1974) estimated a total individual player movement of 6329 yards (5787 m) and analysed his sprinting patterns.

The object of this study was to outline methods and procedures used in data collection whilst analysing selected team games and to suggest a format for computer aided study in sport which provides rapid feedback and therefore assists sports strategy and fitness programming.

Method

The hardware used was a BBC 'B' micro computer with information input via an A3 size concept keyboard locked into the game port of the computer. The touch sensitive 'solution' was employed because of initial difficulties encountered when working with the relative inflexibility of the OWERTY keyboard itself, particularly those of confusing layout and key location. The concept keyboard offered a touch sensitive 'pad' divided into 128 cells, each of these cells or group of cells assigned to a word/function, which could be changed by the use of different overlays, according to the programme being used for the match analysis.

The methodology was similar to that of Mayhew and Wenger (1985) where time-motion analysis was structured on time rather than distance covered, lending itself to greater accuracy and the ultimate presentation of time-based data convenient for coach utilization in training regimens. Four movement patterns were identified and specially designed computer programs enabled the following information to be received and sifted:-

MOVEMENT PATTERN	RUGBY FORWARD	RUGBY THREEOUARTER AND/OR SOCCER PLAYER
1	Scrummaging (Time and No.)	Non-Purposive Rest
2	Ruck and Maul (Time and No.)	Purposive Running
3	Non-Purposive Rest	Sprinting
4	Purposive Running	Running with Ball

These movement patterns were grouped into accumulating 0-5 s periods and were displayed in bar graph form on the computer print-out. The computer program encompassed a number of 'clocks' each linked to the movement patterns and were activated and stopped via touching the appropriate cell on the concept keyboard. Each change in movement pattern also employed a simple count mechanism within the program, and these independent 'count' systems existed for collating other physically demanding variables like tackles, jumps, controls and shots. The pilot work involved analysis of individual player performance in five first class rugby union matches in South Wales and five soccer matches, four at collegiate level and one at professional (3rd Division) level. Two games, one from each sport, were recorded live, at the Arms Park, Cardiff, and Ninian Park, Cardiff. This work was carried out after extensive laboratory trials (20 hours) using video tape action, for both the computer program effectiveness and training of two observers. Other matches were videoed from a scaffolding platform 6 m above ground, tracking players using a lightweight National panasonic WVP AIE camera and portable VHS NV 180B video recording system with battery pack. Players being analysed were all unaware that they were the subject of study.

In rugby union the players were also studied as 'groups', in that they often performed in the match situation as part of a unit, i.e. back row/half backs, whilst in soccer, a similar grouping was imposed with each position being analysed for four games and the players randomly selected.

Results

The combined time-motion analysis data for the 24 subjects over 17 soccer games and seven rugby games are shown in Tables 1, 2 and 3. In the case of the soccer analysis a one-way analysis of variance (ANOVA) was computed to consider the difference between positions for each of the four categories of movement taken individually. The results showed significant differences ($P < 0.01$), for 'non purposive running' ($F = 8.43$), purposive running ($F = 12.00$ and 'time with the ball' ($F = 6.69$) but not for sprinting.

A Tukey test was then performed on the three significant movement categories. It was found that in 'non-purposive rest' there was a significant difference between centreback and midfield ($P < 0.01$) and strikers and midfield positions ($P < 0.01$) and between fullback and midfield players.

The 'purposive running' movement category showed a significant difference between midfield and centreback ($P < 0.01$), midfield and forward ($P < 0.01$), and between midfield and fullback ($P < 0.05$).

The 'time with the ball' movement category saw significant

Table 1. Combined time motion analysis for all soccer players

Movement Category	INDIVIDUAL PLAYER POSITIONS Total time (min:s) Full backs	Centre backs	Midfield	Strikers	Mean time (min:s)	% Total time
Non-Purposive Running	62.44	67.01	53.59	65.39	62.11	69.45
Purposive Running	26.28	21.31	33.54	19.25	27.42	28.17
Sprinting	0.45	0.25	0.23	0.39	0.33	0.62
Time with Ball	0.37	3.05	1.00	0.41	1.38	1.49
Changes in Movement Pattern	404	371	377	419		392 (mean total)

'Non-purposive' running included all those types of movement and stationary periods when a player was positively engaged in game play. 'Purposive' running includes jogging and running up to three quarter maximal pace.

Table 2. Combined time motion analysis for all Rugby Union threequarters

Movement Category	INDIVIDUAL PLAYER POSITIONS Total time (min:s) Half backs	Centres	Wings/Full back	Mean time (min:sec)	% Total time
Non-Purposive Running	51.04	55.16	69.24	58.35	73.20
Purposive Running	21.28	14.42	9.54	15.21	19.18
Sprinting	2.16	2.14	0.56	1.49	2.25
Time with ball	1.52	0.20	2.16	1.29	1.85
Changes in Movement Pattern	432	270	296		333(mean total)

Table 3. Combined time motion analysis for all Rugby Union forwards

Movement Category	INDIVIDUAL PLAYER POSITIONS Total time (mins:s) Front five	Back row	Mean time (min:s)	% Total time
Non Purposive Running	47.18	55.10	51.14	63.80
Purposive Running	17.12	18.00	17.36	21.50
Scrummaging (time and number)	9.14(52)	6.28(48)	7.51(50)	9.19
Rucks/Mauls (time and number)	6.32(53)	4.02(56)	5.17(54.5)	6.26
Changes in Movement Pattern	332	320		326(mean total)

differences between centreback and the other three outfield positions.

Discussion

The main purpose of this research was to seek information concerning the amount of time spent by players in both sports, in each of the four movement categories previously specified. It is hoped that the information gleened may be of some practical value in assisting coaches with their planning of training programmes for individuals in set positions in both rugby and soccer. Positions not only require specialist skills they seem to require different types and levels of fitness.

It is clear from the statistics that soccer and rugby players should engage in work that will enhance the aerobic energy system, and that an interval training prescription would prove beneficial as it mimics game demands. Clearly, this is only an initial study as it looked at collegiate and elite performers in both sports, comparing athletes at differing levels of physical and skill performance. However, results do reinforce earlier findings in the studies of Withers et al. (1982) and Mayhew and Wenger (1985). The evidence shows a need to maximise a player's short sprint speed. The number of ball contacts and time with the ball in both games is minimal and, therefore, choice of play makers and tactical style is of paramount importance. In time, this medium for analysis could build a library of standardised data on sport action. They key to analysis is programming flexibility which enables coach and sport scientist to choose and concentrate on the main variables which impinge upon optimal individual and team performance.

Acknowledgement

The author would like to acknowledge the work of Sebastian Van der Vliet in helping to prepare the manuscript.

References

Baker, J. and Milner, K. (1985) Co-operative analysis of strokes used in men's and women's tennis matches. Brit. J. P.E., 16.

Brackenridge, C.H. and Alderson, G. (1985) Interaction Analysis in a team game with particular reference to the use of micro-computers. In: Proceedings of the Sport and Science Conference, Liverpool University.

Brooke, J. and Knowles, J. (1974) A movement analysis of player behaviour in soccer match performance. Proceedings of the British Society of Sports Psychology, Salford University.

Franks, I. and Goodman, D. (1986a) Computer assisted technical analysis of sport, Coaching Review, May/June, pp. 1-9.

Franks, I. and Goodman, D. (1986b) A systematic approach to analysing sports performance. J. Sports Sci., 4, 49-59.

Hall, L.T. (1981) Microcomputer analysis of tennis performance, ISSP 5th World Congress 1980, Ontario, Canada, pp.52-54.

Hughes, M. (1985) Patterns of squash at higher competitive levels. J. Sports Sci., 3, 225-226.

Laban, R. and Lawrence, F.C. (1947) Effort. London: MacDonald & Evans, London.

MacKinnon, G. (1985) Racket sport analysis: computer applications paper to BANC/NCF/BASS workshop Sheffield City Polytechnic, 1985.

Mayhew, S. and Wenger, H. (1985) Time-motion analysis of professional soccer, J. Human Mov't. Stud., 11, 49-52.

Reilly, T. and Thomas, V. (1976) A motion analysis of work rate in differential roles in professional football match-play, J. Human Mov't. Stud., 2, 87-97.

Rugby Football Union (1978) Fitness Training for Rugby. England: Walker Press.

Sanderson, F. (1983) Notation system for analysing squash matches, Physical Education Review, 6, 19-23.

Sharp, R. (1986) National Coaching Foundation Research Project to develop computer software to assist player analysis (badminton). Jordanhill College.

Treadwell, P. and Van der Vliet, S. (1987) Individual and team analysis in selected ball games, unpublished paper, South Glamorgan Institute, Cardiff.

Wade, A. (1967) The F.A. Guide to Training & Coaching. London: Heinemann.

Withers, R.T., Marick, Z., Wasilewski, S. and Kelly, L. (1982) Match analyses of Australian professional soccer players, J. Human Mov't. Stud., 8, 159-176.

Winterbottom, W. (1959) Soccer Coaching. Kingswood: Naldreth.

ASSESSMENT OF THE PLAYING EFFECTIVENESS OF SOCCER PLAYERS

Mitko Chervenjakov, Gueorguy Dimitrov Higher Institute of Physical Culture, 1 Tina Kirkova Str. Sofia, Bulgaria.

Introduction

Current development of soccer is closely related to the successful solution of the problem of assessing activity during play. For the purpose of solving this complex problem a systematic research programme was started in 1971. The established methods for assessing the effectiveness of soccer players were computerized during the years 1974-75, when the author was employed as a soccer coach at the University of Tokai, Japan.

Since 1976, the program 'SOCCER 75' written in 'FORTRAN' and adapted for the 'FACOM' has been applied frequently to the performances of the best Bulgarian teams on behalf of the Bulgarian Football Union. By using the programs developed, specific express processing of the data generated from a given competition was carried out. With the help of mathematical and graphic modelling, the playing activities of the separate players and of the team as a whole were assessed. In 1983, the program was adapted for a personal computer and is now applied to the work of the Central Soccer Club of the Army 'Sredets'.

Methods

An original code is created for recording the playing activities by means of which only one research worker can record all the necessary data on 34 parameters for each player of a given team. With the help of specific modifications, the recording becomes omni-purpose. In particular it was possible, while formalizing the software, to direct attention chiefly to tackling and kicking the ball. The rest of the playing activities, covering about 97% of the competition time of each player, are of a preparatory nature. For the defence the main focus is tackling, and for the attack on kicking the ball with the intention to score, or to pass it to a fellow player who is in a position to shoot at goal, or to pass it to a third player with the same intention. This approach was adopted as the factors of secondary importance to the development of the process which should not be take into consideration when building up the mathematical model. Bearing this in mind it is much easier to quantitatively cover the playing activities during competition, both in the personal and team aspect. The recording of the playing activity looks like the following:

QQ03FQ0311MM010407TQ05060810MQ05KQ0211MQ11MM010208IP08SS010910GM0.

Thus pairs of figures and pairs of letters are recorded in chronological order until the end of the competition. The figures stand for the numbers of the players, and the letters stand for the concrete playing activities of the players, or the recording is done in a format 40A2 on a special form. One can use a dictaphone or record directly on the keyboard of a personal computer placed within a stadium or in the room where a TV - or video - transmission of a soccer match is being received. Two things are required for any one to do the recordings correctly. First it is necessary to distinguish the players, even when not seeing their numbers, second it is essential that the meanings of the pairs of letters, which in soccer amount to 56 have been memorised. Practice shows that learning them is not difficult as they suggest the concrete playing activities. So if one learns to do this, it is possible to use the methods since the rest of the operations are done by the computer, operating according to the instructions of the 'SOCCER 75'. The computer 'reads' the recording and stores the data for each players in two matrices. The data of the first matrix on the basis of which the mathematical modelling is carried out, have 14 parameters.

Table 1. Parameters for mathematical modelling and code of activity according to 'SOCCER 75' program:

1 Total number of ball contacts (L)
2. Number of correctly played balls (P)
3. Number of tackles and correctly played balls (O)
4. Number of cleared balls or tackles but incorrectly played balls (I)
5. Number of shots OFF TARGET (A)
6. Number of shots ON goal (S)
7. Number of violations of the rules/faults (F)
8. Yellow card (Y)
9. Red card (R)
10. Grant for attacking play (BN)
11. Grant for defensive play (BZ)
12. Fair play (C)
13. Goals scored (G)
14. Conceded goals (-G)

Development

In 1972, these parameters received factor weights on the basis of the opinions of a council of experts whose members were coaches of the first and second soccer divisions in Bulgaria at the time. On these grounds, and bearing in mind the specificity of the playing activity in its basic aspects, six mathematical models were worked out. They helped differentiate the playing effectiveness of each player and of the team as a whole in the basic aspects of the game. The models are as follows for an individual player i, with summations made over each member of the team with n = 11:-

(i) Coefficient for activity (KA):

$$KA_i = \frac{L_i}{L}, \quad \text{where } L = \frac{\Sigma L_i}{n}, \qquad i = 1 \text{ to } n$$

This coefficient is based on the reasoning that a higher degree of physical fitness means a greater chance of being the player most often in possession of the ball.

(ii) Coefficient for correctness (KT):

$$KT_i = \frac{P_i}{L_i} = T, \text{ where } T = \frac{\Sigma P_i/L_i}{n}, \qquad i = 1 \text{ to } n$$

The logic here is that the better one's technical preparation, the higher his ability to play with the ball correctly.

(iii) Coefficient for attacking play/tactics,(KN):

$$KN_i = \frac{P_i + A_i + 3S_i \quad BN_i}{N} \quad \text{where} \quad N = \frac{\Sigma\left(P_i + A_i + 3S \quad BN_i\right)}{n}$$

(iv) Coefficient for defensive play/tactics (KZ):

$$KZ_i = \frac{P_i + 2O_i + I_i \quad BZ_i}{Z}, \text{ where } Z = \frac{\Sigma\left(P_i + 2O_i + I_i \quad B_i\right)}{n}$$

(v) Coefficient for fair play/behaviour (KP):

$$KP_i = \frac{1 + 0.1C_i - 0.02F_i - 0.1Y_i - R_i}{P},$$

$$\text{where } P = \frac{\Sigma\left(1 + 0.1C_i - 0.02F_i - 0.1Y_i - R_i\right)}{n}$$

(vi) Total coefficient for classifying every player according to his effectiveness during competition (KE):

$$KE_i = \frac{KA_i + KT_i + KN_i + KZ_i + KP_i}{5}$$

With the help of these mathematical models of playing activity, the assessment is expressed by marks ranging within the values near '1'. The mark '1' reflects a mean level of effectiveness. Marks above '1' show the corresponding degree of increased effectiveness in the given aspect of the play, and the marks below '1' show the corresponding decrease of effectiveness. It is possible to get marks for the team as a whole which reflect not only the different aspects but also the overall game. This allows comparison of the marks of different matches.

The computer arranges and writes out the names of the players according to their marks for playing effectiveness (KE). The player ranking first has the higher degree of playing effectiveness for the given match. The different marks permit the coach to make a thorough quantitative analysis of the activity of every player, accounting for his strong and weak points in the particular match.

Graphic Modelling

Parallel with the selection of the data for storage from the coded record in the first matrix (during which the quantitative modelling of activity is carried out), data for graphic modelling are also selected. These data are stored by the computer in a second matrix. Information related to all playing inter-relations that have been realised during the match (passes of the ball among the players) can be extracted. This tells which player has passed the ball, to which of his team-mates and how many times, as well as which player has received the ball, from whom of his own players, and how often. All the possible playing inter-relations are classified by the computer according to the frequencies noted. This permits a graphic modelling of the playing activity by using strictly defined playing inter-relations e.g. building up a positive model of the playing activity by using only the most frequently fulfilled playing inter-relations (the first 10-15 inter-relations; or building up a negative model of the playing activity by using only the most rarely fulfilled playing inter-relations. It is also possible to build up group models of the playing activity by using only the playing inter-relations between separate groups. A personal model for each player can be drawn by using the playing inter-relations realised between him and his team-mates.

With the help of graphic modelling, coaches can find out and analyse in detail their own as well as the opposing team's organisation of play, the nature of the playing activities within the team, its strong and weak points, the predominant trend and the approach to developing attacks, the zones of most concentration and so on. On this basis it is possible to develop the optimum playing activities of the team, and to draw a precise plan to counter the adversary whose tactics have been previously ascertained using this proposed methodology.

Overview

The application of this methodology to the work of the best Bulgarian soccer players and teams over the years, has facilitated intensive data collection in practical contexts. These have been subjected to different forms of statistical treatment, such as correlation analysis and factor analysis. As a result, a number of norms, normative tables, nomograms and so on were established which considerably ease the work of the coaches in the quantitative assessment of soccer players and teams. The computed programs are multi-purpose. After certain modifications they could be applied to other games, and in this respect some success has been achieved in their modification for rugby. The work in this direction is on-going.

Acknowledgements

The help of M. Maksuo, then Associate Professor in the Institute of Telecommunications at Tokai University, in developing the software in the years 1974-75 is acknowledged. Thanks also are due to D. Svilenov for adapting the program for a personal computer.

FOOTBALL CHANCE: TACTICS AND STRATEGY

Richard Bate,
Notts County Football Club, Meadow Lane, Nottingham, NG2 3HJ, England.

Introduction

Professional football at all levels is concerned with the achievement of victory over opponents, hopefully in a manner that is pleasing to the spectator. It is often stated about soccer that it is 'a game of opinions' and no doubt many coaches and managers have based and will continue to base, strategy and tactics on their own opinions.

Whilst opinions may be both respected and valid, much more than opinion is necessary in the mapping out of a strategy for success. Indeed in fields such as medicine, the military, business and many others, a factual appraisal of the situation is a necessity before any policy is embarked upon. Why should this not be the case in soccer? Should team strategy and consequent results be based on opinion or something more substantial?

A widely held opinion is that 'possession football' (the retention of the ball often accompanied by many consecutive passes being made) is the key to winning soccer matches, especially in many European and South American countries. Whilst keeping possession of the ball may be skilful and even artistic, it is not necessarily effective in producing scoring chances and goals. By playing 'possession football', many team attacks fail to reach the final third ($A\frac{1}{3}$) of the pitch and it is entry into this area of the pitch which is the key to winning soccer matches. If spectators are to be attracted to the game it should be recognised that they are usually entertained by goalmouth incidents and the scoring of goals. As coaches and managers responsible for teams and results, it behoves us to examine those factors that lead to the creation of chances and goals and to consider the possibilities for basing defensive and attacking strategies of the team on the results of this analysis. The classical methodology for data collection and statistical analysis of goal scoring has been provided by Reep and Benjamin, (1968).

This review examines a series of tenets to assess the degree to which generalisation is possible. These are presented as lead statements which are appraised in turn.

<u>The critical scoring area:</u> goals are not scored unless the attacking team gets the ball and one or more attacking players into the $A\frac{1}{3}$ of the field.

Only in unusual circumstances will this statement be proved incorrect. It is not unknown for a goalkeeper to score direct from a kick from his hands past the opposing goalkeeper. Also, in unusual circumstances, free kicks may result in goals scored from outside the $A\frac{1}{3}$, as may goals in free play, but to a high degree of certainty goals are unlikely to be scored from an area further than 40 yards (36m) away from goal.

The number of possessions: the higher the number of possessions that a team has, the greater will be the chance of increasing the number of entries into the $A\frac{1}{3}$.

A possession is defined as originating from the moment that a player gains possession for his team until the time that the team loses possession of the ball to the opponents (Reep and Benjamin, 1968). A possession may therefore involve no passes, one pass or for example 14 or 15 passes before the ball is lost to the opposition. The interception of an opponent's pass followed immediately by a shot, or run and shot resulting in a goal or miss, would be interpreted as a 0 pass move. It is also possible for a team to have two or three consecutive possessions before the opponents gain possession; this would be the case if a passing movement was curtailed by the award of a free kick against a defender. One team would then have had two possessions of the ball consecutively. Generally speaking the number of possessions by each team does not differ greatly since possession usually alternates from one team to another.

Entry into the critical scoring area: entry into the $A\frac{1}{3}$ of the field is the key factor in the scoring of goals and consequently the winning of matches.

The more possessions that a team gains, so the potential chances for moving the ball into the $A\frac{1}{3}$. Also the nearer to the $A\frac{1}{3}$ that possession is gained or regained, then the greater the accuracy and effectiveness in playing the ball into the $A\frac{1}{3}$. If a high number of passes is made within each possession gained outside the $A\frac{1}{3}$, then the total number of possessions gained in the 90 min period of the game is likely to decrease. If the total number of possessions by a team is reduced, then the potential entries into the $A\frac{1}{3}$ will also be reduced. Consequently a team can also reduce the effectiveness of the opposition in attacking its $A\frac{1}{3}$ and therefore winning the game.

The number of passes in a possession: the higher the number of passes in any one possession, the lower will be:- (i) the total number of possessions; (ii) the total potential entries into the $A\frac{1}{3}$; (iii) the chances of gaining a shooting opportunity and scoring a goal.

The theory that 'possession football' and the retention of possession at all costs is the key to winning games should be examined thoroughly, following the analysis revealed here. Whilst football involving a high number of consecutive passes may be very skilful and pleasing to the connoisseurs of the game, its value in the actual scoring of goals should not be over-estimated. Following the World Cup 1982, 106 goals from the total scored were analysed (Table 1).

Table 1. Analysis of 106 goals from the 1982 World Cup

No. of passes -	0	1	2	3	4	5	6	7	8	9	10
No. of goals -	30	19	8	15	12	8	2	7	1	2	2
			84					22			

Goals from 0 passes were scored by: (i) an interception followed by a shot, or a run and shot that scored, where no pass to a team mate was made; (ii) directly shooting the ball into goal from a free kick or penalty; (iii) a shot directly into goal following a clearance etc., where no passes were made to any team-mate.

It should be noted that almost half the goals (48%) came from 0 to 1 pass movements - 49 goals. Altogether 84 goals (79%) were scored from movements of 4 or less passes. No goals were scored from passing movements involving 11 or more passes but there were passing movements of that number in the tournament, The highest number of passes in any one movement was 26.

Further research from two additional sources reveals figures not dissimilar from those above.

The observations of Hughes (personal communication, 1986) looking at 16 international games at all levels of national representation by England (10 matches at Senior level, 2 at U.21 level, 1 at U.18 level and 3 at U.16 level) are summarised in Table 2. Of the 52 goals scored, 49 were scored from movements of 4 or less passes (= 94%) while 3 were scored from movements of 5 or more passes (= 6%).

Table 2. The number of passes, shots and goals in 16 international matches

No. of Passes	No. of Shots	No. of Goals Scored	
0	92	19)	
1	83	8)	
2	70	14)	49 goals
3	32	4)	
4	32	4)	
5	15	2)	
6	11	1)	
7	6	0)	
8	9	0)	
9	1	0)	3 goals
10	1	0)	
11	2	0)	

In the season 1985-1986, Notts County FC in Division 3 of the Football League scored 71 League goals. Of these 71 goals, 37 were video recorded and analysed. The number of passes involved in the scoring of these goals are indicated in Table 3. Altogether 94% of the goals video-recorded came from movements involving 4 or less passes.

Table 3. The number of passes leading to 37 goals scored by Notts County FC

	4 passes or less					4 passes			
Passes	0	1	2	3	4	5	6	7	8
Goals	1	11	11	9	3	1	0	1	0
		35 goals				2 goals			

Observers may come to the conclusion that 0 and 1 pass goals are due to a high-pass build up by a team which results in a strike at goal that may rebound from the goalkeeper or a defender and is then shot into the net by an attacking player. However, Hughes once again, examining the 0-pass goals of which there were 19, in those same 16 international matches, presents the evidence in Table 4.

Table 4. Analysis of 19 0-pass goals (16 England international games)

No. of passes	No. of goals	
0	4)	
1	2)	
2	6)	17 goals
3	0)	
4 (1 penalty)	4)	
5	1)	
6	0)	
7	0)	
8	0)	
9	1)	2 goals
10	0)	
11	0)	
12 (1 penalty)	1)	

The table (Table 4) represents the number of passes made, prior to the 0-pass goal being scored from interceptions, rebounds, set-plays, challenges etc. The 0-pass goals resulted from low passing movements and not from a high number of consecutive passes.

The evidence presented on goals and their relationship to passing movements reveals that at least 80% of all goals and shots at goal come from movements involving 4 consecutive passes or less. The data have been drawn from different segments of high-class soccer (from Senior international level, World Cup Football, international Youth football and from 3rd Division professional soccer in the English Football League).

The theory that 'possession football' produces the results that win games would appear to be based on a highly doubtful premise.

Frequency of attacks: the greater the number of entries into the attacking third ($A\frac{1}{3}$), the greater will be the chances of:- (i) winning set plays in that area; (ii) regaining possession of the ball in that area; (iii) creating the opportunities for a shot at goal; (iv) decreasing the number of entries into a team's defensive third ($D\frac{1}{3}$) by the opponents.

Goals from set-plays (i.e. corner kicks, free kicks, throw-ins, penalties) are a vital source of goals at all levels of the game. As many as 33% of goals scored by Notts County FC in season 1985-86 and video-recorded, came as a result of a set-play in the $A\frac{1}{3}$ of the field. Of 71 goals scored by Notts County in Division 3 in the same season, 33 were the result of set-plays, which represents a figure of 46% of goals scored.

Analysis of 7 England Senior international matches is summarised in Table 5. The figures refer to the gaining of set plays in the $A\frac{1}{3}$ of the field (Hughes, 1987 personal communications).

Table 5. Analysis of set-plays in seven England Senior international matches

	Set-plays from 3 or less consecutive passes	Set-plays from 4 or more consecutive passes
V Denmark	10	6
V West Germany	12	8
V Greece	11	3
V Luxembourg	20	8
V Wales	17 (4 passes or less)	0 (5 passes or more)
V Greece	39	2
V Hungary	21	3
Total	130	30

Further examination by Hughes, of 16 England international matches (Senior, U.21, U.18, U.16 levels) revealed that 87% of all set-plays gained in the attacking third ($A\frac{1}{3}$) of the pitch resulted from movements of 4 or less passes and only 13% of set-plays resulted from 5 passes or more. Similar values were obtained at Notts County FC in that 91% of all set plays gained in the $A\frac{1}{3}$ of the pitch followed movements of 4 passes or less, in a series of 10 League and F.A. Cup matches.

The proposition that 'possession football' precedes the gaining of set-plays in the attacking third of the field is not borne out by the research just described. Once again that evidence is the result of analysing soccer matches from U.16 internationals to Senior League and international level.

It would appear that direct, forward passing, forward running soccer involving a low number of consecutive passes is an effective method of creating shooting opportunities, of scoring goals and of gaining set-play situations in the attacking third of the pitch. So-called 'possession football' (the retention of ball possession at all costs) involving a high number of consecutive passes is not as effective a playing method in terms of creating shooting chances and goals and is not supported by research conducted across a broad cross-section of soccer played at Senior and Youth levels.

Moving the ball with a high degree of accuracy to players in, or moving into the attacking third of the pitch, as quickly as possible on gaining possession of the ball, and then developing the play economically towards a shot on goal is a more effective method of producing shots and goals than basing attacking play on a 'keep-ball' mentality, if winning games is the objective. Whilst there may be times in games that a team deliberately attempts to keep possession at all costs, if the aim is to score goals then the ball must be played forward into the attacking third regularly, accurately and as economically as possible with regard to the number of passes made in each passing movement.

<u>Initiation of scoring moves:</u> 50-60% of all movements leading to shots and goals originate in the $A\frac{1}{3}$ of the field.

These goals and shots will come as a result of:- (i) set plays in the $A\frac{1}{3}$ of the field, (ii) regained possessions in the $A\frac{1}{3}$ of the field.

In Championship and competitive matches at the highest level this figure may rise to 70%. Even in less closely contested games the goal that breaks the deadlock is likely to come from either a set play in the $A\frac{1}{3}$ or a regained possession in that area. It is of more than passing interest to note that in the World Cup Final match in 1974, 1982 and 1986 the opening goal that broke the deadlock resulted from a set-play situation in the $A\frac{1}{3}$ of the field.

Attacking movements that originate in the defending third of the field are unlikely to produce fruitful scoring chances, and goals in the $A\frac{1}{3}$ of the field. To attempt to score goals by constructing passing movements from the defending third of the field involving the goalkeeper and/or outfield players is unlikely to succeed, although there are obvious occasions when there is no other alternative i.e. set-plays.

In seven recent Senior international games involving England, no goals were scored from passing movements originating in the defending third (Table 6).

Table 6. Possessions in the defending third in seven England international matches

	Possession in $D\frac{1}{3}$	Reaching $A\frac{1}{3}$	Shots	Goals
V Denmark	87	22	3	0
V West Germany	64	17	3	0
V Greece	73	17	0	0
V Luxembourg	22	14	1	0
V Wales	69	14	3	0
V Greece	34	15	2	0
V Hungary	62	23	2	0
	411	122	14	0

In these international matches only 1 in every 3.5 possessions actually reached the attacking third of the field. Only 14 shots at goal were produced and no goals were scored. However, when those seven games are analysed on the basis of regaining possession of the ball in the attacking third of the field, then a much different picture appears (Table 7).

Table 7. Regained possessions in the attacking third

	Regained Possessions in $A\frac{1}{3}$	Shots	Goals
V Denmark	30	8	2
V West Germany	37	6	1
V Greece	21	5	1
V Luxembourg	55	17	6
V Wales	34	10	2
V Greece	68	7	0
V Hungary	46	9	2
Total	291	62	14

Whilst delivering the ball into the $A\frac{1}{3}$ is the key to producing shots and goals, it is essential that a team then pushes players forward to regain the ball if it is lost to opponents in that area. To concede possession in the $A\frac{1}{3}$ and to make no attempt to regain the ball in that area reduces considerably the number of shots and goals that a team will have in any game. Being prepared to commit players into a forward position to gain possession of the ball is a most important factor in the winning of soccer matches.

A high number of entries into the attacking third is vital in the strategy of winning games. However, teams must work on delivering the ball forward accurately into that area and also commit players into forward positions to support the pass and to regain possession of the ball if possession is conceded. Failure to do this reduces a team's overall effectiveness.

The relationship between shots, goals and origin of attack is markedly different when one examines the thirds of the pitch in which attacks commence.

Table 8. Possessions - Shot - Goal ratio in relation to areas of the pitch

Area of field	Shots to Possessions	Ratio Goals-shots	Goals to Possessions
Defence (D)	1 : 65.1	1 : 11	1 : 716
Midfield(M)	1 : 24	1 : 9.5	1 : 228
Attack (A)	1 : 5.2	1 : 5.1	1 : 26

It can be seen clearly from the figures of Hughes in research with the England Senior team that to gain or regain possession of the ball in the A$\frac{1}{3}$ of the pitch is 13 times more productive in terms of shots at goal, than to commence attacks from the D$\frac{1}{3}$ (Table 8). It will pay teams great dividends to attempt to regain possession of the ball in the A$\frac{1}{3}$ rather than to concede possession and to fall back in order to win the ball in the defending half of the pitch. The more a team retreats, the less become the chances of scoring, on gaining possession nearer to one's own goal.

In 16 England international matches involving teams at Senior, U.21, U.18 and U.16 levels almost 9 times more goals were scored from attacks originating in the A$\frac{1}{3}$ than in the D$\frac{1}{3}$. It can be seen in Table 9 that twice as many goals are scored from moves originating in the attacking third (A$\frac{1}{3}$) than in both the two other areas of the field.

Table 9. Outcome of possessions originating from the three areas of the pitch in 16 international matches

Area of Field	Possessions	Shots	Goals	%
D	2,865	44	4	7.5
Midfield	3,203	133	14	26.5
A	939	179	35	66.0

<u>Set plays and regained possessions as sources of goals</u>: as many as 60-70% of all goals are scored from a combination of (i) set-plays; (ii) regained possessions in the A of the field.

In the season 1985-86 at Notts County FC, 50% of shots and goals were the result of set-play situations and regained posessions in the A$\frac{1}{3}$ of the field. It is crucial in the preparation of teams that coaches should be mindful of this from both an attacking and a defending viewpoint.

The importance of moving the ball into the attacking third of the pitch economically and regularly is crucial to the winning of soccer matches. Developing strategies to take advantage of any resultant set play situations in that area of the field is also of vital importance. Additionally, an overall team strategy to regain possession of the ball in the A_3^1 or as early as possible, is productive in generating shooting opportunities and in scoring goals.

One cannot under-estimate the importance of entering the attacking third of the pitch as regularly, as economically and as accurately as possible. The evolution of team play to then take advantage of all shooting situations, set-play situations and losses of possession becomes crucial to the winning of matches.

Conclusion

In order to increase the number of entries into the attacking third of the pitch, a team should:-

- (i) play the ball forward as often as possible;
- (ii) reduce to a minimum, square and back passes;
- (iii) increase the number of long forward passes and forward runs with the ball of 40 yards (36 m) or more;
- (iv) play the ball into space behind defenders as early and as often as possible.

Acknowledgement

This paper owes much to the work conducted by Charles F.C. Hughes, the Assistant National Coach of the Football Association. The lead statements reflect his work; the data are from his unpublished research, except where Notts County Football Club is referred to. Without the co-operation of C.F.C. Hughes this paper could not have been presented in its present form.

Reference

Reep, C. and Benjamin, B. (1968) Skill and chance in association football. Journal of the Royal Statistical Society, Series A, 131, 581-585.

A STATISTICAL ANALYSIS OF TACTICAL MOVEMENT PATTERNS IN SOCCER

A.H. Ali
Department of Physical Education, University of St. Andrews, Scotland.

Introduction

Soccer is not only a game, but a professional sport, the object of scientific research, an exciting spectacle and a commercial activity. As in most professional sports today, the political, sociological and economic aspects of the game have assumed an importance which reaches far beyond the mere practice of the sport and performance of the players.

Relatively little research has been carried out on soccer (e.g. Winterbottom, 1959; Wade, 1967; Saltin, 1973; Agnevik, 1970; Vinnai, 1973; Brooke and Knowles, 1974; Reilly and Thomas, 1976). Much of this research has been concerned with the distance covered by players in a game with the aim of quantifying their work rate. The main purpose of this study is to identify attacking patterns of play and assess their success. The main questions which the study raises are:-

(i) Are there specific patterns of attack which can be identified in the game?
(ii) How successful is each individual pattern in influencing the result of the match?

Methods

The attacking moves of a Scottish Premier Division soccer team were observed and analysed. Thirteen basic factors of the game were assigned a shorthand symbol (Figure 1).

The researcher was in a stand close to the centre line. As soon as the match started, the movement of the ball in the visitors' half of the pitch was noted on diagram sheets, using the designated notation. This occurred when the home team had possession of the ball and started to build up an attack in this half. These movements were all noted down, each attack being drawn on a separate diagram sheet.

----->	Dribbling	----lGK	Ball intercepted by goalkeeper
...s..>	Short pass	::::::::)	Header on target
...L..>	Long pass	==)==)	Kick off target
.....O	Goal	...s..IDF	Short pass intercepted by defender
(OFF)	Off-side	..L...IDF	long pass intercepted by defender
====)	Kick on target	::::)::::)	Header off target

\+ Indicates position of free-kicks, throw-ins or corner-kicks

Figure 1. Shorthand symbols used in the analysis

Data collection

For the purpose of analysis, a grid of 26 squares long by 32 squares wide, was drawn and superimposed on the diagram of half the pitch. Each square was 2 x 2 m, thus representing an area four square metres. The length of half the pitch was represented by 26 squares. The width of the pitch was represented by 32 squares. Each attack was analysed with respect to the separate, constituent moves and by using the grid, the starting and finishing points of each move were noted down in terms of their X axis and Y axis co-ordinates. The data obtained were fed into a computer.

A separate file was created to hold the data for each match using the format described. Set-plays which occurred in each match were examined separately from ordinary attacks. The attacks were converted through the same procedure into separate sets of data and fed into the computer as above.

Data analysis

Given a large number of attacking movements, the aim was to obtain a scatter diagram of points, each point representing one attack, attacks which are similar to one another being represented by points that are close together. The aim was achieved in two stages:-
(i) a measure of dissimilarity between each pair of attacks;
(ii) a configuration of points is obtained, with the property that the distance between any pair of points approximates their pairwise dissimilarities.

Once all 18 League matches had been observed, drawn on the diagram sheets and converted into data, 18 graphs were produced. Each graph was subjected to a visual cluster analysis, thereby grouping similar patterns of attack with each other. The method was supplemented by comparison of the original diagram sheets of the attacks within each cluster. From each cluster for each individual match, an attack was selected which represented the mean of that particular cluster. This attack, termed the optimum attack pattern for that cluster, was selected by visual analysis.

The optimum attacks chosen from all 18 League matches were grouped into a new data set. The same program as used previously was run for these data. Using a similar cluster analysis technique to that already described, these optimum attacks were classified into 7 major clusters. Each attack, from each match, could then be classified into one of the 7 major clusters.

A similar procedure was adopted for set-plays. The pattern-types for corner-kicks and throw-ins from left and right sides of the pitch, were clustered separately. For free-kicks these points were so spread out on the graph there was no obvious clustering. These have consequently been regarded as belonging to a single pattern type. Each attack was also analysed in terms of its final action (Table 1).

Table 1. Symbols of final actions

1............	Goal
2............	Shot on target saved
3............	Shot off target
4............	Lost possession
5............	Corner-kick
6............	Throw-in
7............	Off-side
8............	Penalty
9............	Free-kick

Having obtained a grouping of the set of movements into classes of similar attacks, each attack was then categorized by one of the nine final actions. The method of correspondence analysis (Greenacre, 1984) provided a means of extracting information from such data. This method represents a set of points in a scatter diagram, one point for each type of pattern and one point for each final action. Such scatter diagrams provide the following types of information:-

(i) types of pattern which have a similar profile of final actions are represented by points that are close together:

(ii) final actions that have a similar profile of types of pattern are represented by points that are close together:

(iii) a type of pattern point will tend to be attracted to an area of the plane containing the points for those final actions that occur relatively more often in that type of pattern.

Results

Seven major types of pattern were identified. Each of these types of pattern occurred in a number of attacks (Figure 2).

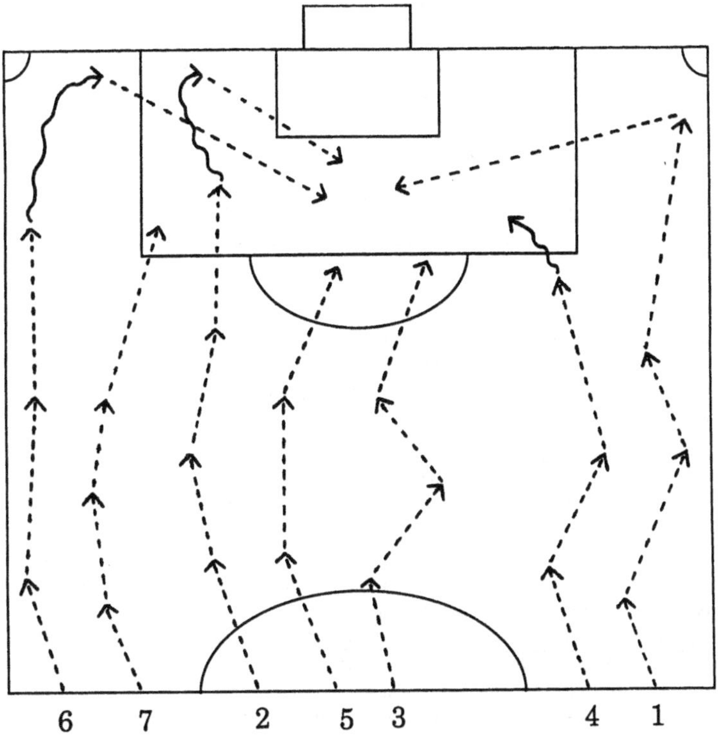

Figure 2. Seven types of attacking patterns

An analysis of the association between the types of pattern and final actions, after frequency analysis and tabulation was carried out using the chi square test. This indicated a significant relationship ($\chi^2 = 66.37$; $P < 0.0001$). From the relationship between the types of the pattern and the final actions it was possible to determine which patterns were most and least successful. The relationship of final actions and types of pattern with the number of long passes, number of short passes and dribbling sections in each of these moves was investigated using similar techniques. Only three were found to be statistically significant as shown in Table 2.

The results indicated that for set-plays only corner-kicks which include short passes were significantly associated with final actions (chi-square = 25.83; $P < 0.01$).

Table 2. Indicates the relationship of types of pattern and final actions with the number of long passes, the number of short passes and dribbling sections

Variable	Final actions χ^2	P value	Types of pattern χ^2	P value
Number of long passes	15.09	0.05	4.13	N.S.
Number of short passes	11.33	NS	60.62	0.001
Dribbling sections	3.24	NS	28.94	0.001

Discussion

Of the 7 major types of attacking pattern found, those patterns which proceed along the length of either wing are more successful than the others. They provide more scoring and shooting opportunities. There are a number of possible reasons for this:-

(i) The strategy of the team. It is possible that the team has repeated these particular types of pattern in practice more often than it has the others, believing that these patterns fit better into the particular style of play that the team employs.

(ii) Individual players. The team has possibly utilised its best players in creating these patterns, since such players would have enough skill to perform them successfully.

(iii) The weather and condition of the ground. It may be that these patterns are more successful on wet and muddy pitches, especially those patterns which included long crosses.

These could cause difficulties for the defending team due to a relative inability to balance and turn quickly on this type of pitch and in this sort of weather. This would present the attacking team with more favourable scoring opportunities.

(iv) Style of long pass and short pass. The suitability of the particular combination of long and short passes within these patterns may have been such that it helped towards keeping possession of the ball and thus gave advantages in scoring and shooting opportunities.

Analysis of the association between final actions and the number of long passes showed that the greater the number of long passes within a single move, the more likely it was to end in final action 7 (which represents off-side). Possible reasons for this are:-

(i) Penetration into the opposition territory. This can be achieved more easily and an attack can be launched at speed. This appears to be one of the most important factors in modern-day soccer. For this the team often used a number of long passes for its attacks. This style of play, however, requires greater passing skills since it is obviously more difficult to make a long and accurate pass than it is to make a short accurate one. Besides, with the frequent occurrence of long passes there is a greater risk of losing possession of the ball and the attack will stop very quickly. However, the players in the team did not all have the requisite skill; thus the forwards are often played off-side as a result of a long pass.

(ii) Players' judgement of off-side. For an attacking player to be judged on-side, he must be in front of his own goal-side at least two defending players in the opponent's half of the pitch when the pass is made. The nearer the possessor of the ball is to another attacking player, the easier it will be to judge whether or not this second player is still on-side should a pass be made. Consequently, an attacking situation in which the attacking players are close to one another (therefore primarily involving short passes) is less likely to result in a player's being caught off-side. Similarly, an attacking situation that requires one or more long passes implies some distance between the passer and receiver of the ball. The greater the distance, the more likely it is for the passer either to mis-judge whether another attacking player would be off-side, or to notice the forward movement of another player too late and so delay the pass.

The number of long passes and instances off-side may be due to errors in the timing of the pass to coincide with the forward movement of another attacking player. The errors would increase as the distance between passer and receiver increases.

For set-plays it was found the corner-kicks which included a greater number of short passes would provide more goals. There are a number of possible reasons for this:-

(i) Frequency of short corner-kicks used. It is possible that because a lower frequency of the short corner-kicks was used, this caused confusion among the opposing defenders as to how to cope with this situation.

(ii) The opponents, goalkeepers and defenders. Since most of the opposing goalkeepers were tall and had the advantage over an attacking forward in gaining possession of a high long cross, it may be that corner-kicks that utilised short passes tended to be more successful, because the danger of losing possession was not so great.

However, there must be some reasons for the lack of statistical significance out of all the possible relationships for the throw-ins. This leads to a number of speculations:-

(i) The strategy of throw-ins. Coaches differ in their instructions for bringing the ball back into play in the throw-ins. For example, 'Take the throw quickly', 'Throw to an unmarked man', 'Throw it so it is easy to control.'

(ii) The rules. In the throw-in the ball has to be brought into the game by a throw according to the rules. Obviously the throw-in does not have the same effects as the kick. Teams pay most attention to bringing the ball into play and not losing possession, which always starts as an ordinary attacking move.

In the light of the experiences gained in this study further studies should be conducted dealing with defensive situations. Analysis of more teams of different standards in the game is also recommended.

References

Agnevik, G. (1970) Fotboll. Idrottsfysiologi, Rapport No. 7 Stockholm, Trygg-Hansa.

Brooke, J.D. and Knowles, J.E. (1974) A movement analysis of players' behaviour in soccer match performance. Paper presented at the British Society of Sports Psychology Conference, Salford.

Greenacre, M.J. (1984) Theory and Applications of Correspondence Analysis. New York: Academic Press.

Reilly, T. and Thomas, V. (1976) A motion analysis of work-rate in different positional roles in professional football match play. J. Human Mov't. Stud., 2, 87-97.

Saltin, B. (1973) Metabolic fundamentals in exercise. Med. Sci. Sports, 5, 136-146.

Vinnai, G. (1973) Football Mania. London: Ocean Books.

Wade, A. (1967) The F.A. Guide to Training and Coaching. London: Heinemann.

Winterbottom, W. (1959) Soccer Coaching. Kingswood, Surrey: The Naldrett Press.

THE QUANTITATIVE COMPARISON OF PLAYING STYLES IN SOCCER

Richard Pollard — Department of Mathematics, The University of the South Pacific, Fiji.
Charles Reep — 16 Sconner Road, Torpoint, Cornwall, England.
Simon Hartley — Hillside, Milford Lane, Tamerton Foliot, Plymouth, England.

Introduction

The objective analysis of team performance in soccer has long been hindered by the continuous and fast-moving nature of the game. No such difficulties exist for sports such as tennis, baseball and American football, where the action is broken down into a series of discrete events, relatively easy to record, and from which performance can be assessed and strategies and tactics developed. A comprehensive shorthand system for recording the action of a soccer game has, however, been in existence since 1950. The use of this 'Reep system' of performance analysis by Wolverhampton Wanderers during the mid-1950s has been well documented (Reep, 1982) and many other professional teams in England have since made successful use of the performance analysis of data provided by this system, an outline of which is given in Pollard (1986).

Basically, the 'Reep system' breaks down the continuous movement of a soccer game into a series of discrete on-the-ball events (such as a pass or a shot) for which a detailed categorization has been developed, together with a shorthand recording code. With the accumulation of such data from many matches, it becomes possible to isolate those particular sequences of events most likely to be associated with successful attack and defence. Tactics and strategies making use of this knowledge can hence be developed. The computer analysis of the 'Reep system' began in 1968, since when several other computer-aided methods of soccer performance analysis have been attempted (Figueiredo and Rodrigues, 1983; Franks, Goodman and Miller, 1983; Gould and Gatrell, 1979; Ali, 1986). Thomson (1985) has suggested ways in which performance analysis can be put to good use by soccer coaches.

The intention of this paper is to use the 'Reep system' of performance analysis in order to develop a computer-aided method enabling a quantitative comparison of different playing styles to be made.

Methods

Using the 'Reep system' of recording team performance, data were obtained from two sets of matches:- 32 games from the 1982 World Cup in Spain and 42 from the First Division of the Football League in

England during 1984-85. Teams seen on only one occasion were excluded, restricting the analysis to 32 teams (10 in the World Cup all seen at least three times) and all 22 teams from the First Division (all seen at least twice).From the performance data recorded, a comparison of the 32 teams was made based on the following measures, calculated for each team, and each representing a different strategy or style of play:-

(i) Long forward passes: the number of passes (excluding goal clearances) taking the ball at least 30m closer to the opponents' goal line, expressed as a percentage of the number of possessions further than 50m from the opponents' goal line.

(ii) Long goal clearances: the number of long forward goal clearances made by a goalkeeper after picking up the ball, expressed as a percentage of all goal clearances.

(iii) Centres: the number of centres expressed as a percentage of the number of attacks reaching the opponents' half of the field. This indirectly indicates how much use a team makes of the width of the field. A centre if defined as a cross, made at an angle of less than 45°, taking the ball into the central 20m of the penalty area. Very occasionally centres may also be counted as long forward passes.

(iv) Regaining possession in attack: the number of occasions that a team regains possession of the ball within 35m of the opponents' goal-line, expressed as a percentage of the number of times possession is lost in that area. This is an indirect measure of the determination with which a team mounts its attacks.

(v) Possession in defence: the number of movements of three or more completed passes that a team makes in its own half of the field, expressed as a percentage of all movements originating in its own half. This and the following measure are both indicators of the importance that a team attaches to possession of the ball.

(vi) Multi-pass movements: the average number of passes per game in all movements containing over three completed passes.

These procedures have certain limitations. The data for many of the teams were based on only two or three recorded matches. Since teams can modify their usual style in response to the opposition, players available for a particular match and the state of the game, a larger sample of games would have produced more reliable results. Furthermore, only six general style variables were used and there is obvious scope for extension and refinement of these variables.

A data matrix consisting of 32 rows (teams) and 6 columns (style variables) was therefore used for the analysis, the purpose being to compare the teams according to similarities of playing styles as measured by the variables. Factor analysis was used to do this: it was anticipated that this technique would allow a meaningful interpretation and display of the results by reducing the 6 variables to 2 or more factors and by displaying the resulting team factor scores graphically.

The analysis was carried out using the SPSS computer package. All six principal components were initially extracted; those retained were then rotated using the varimax criterion and the resulting two main factors, each representing a particular aspect of playing style, used for the interpretation. Factor scores were obtained for the 32 teams on each of these factors. The teams were then plotted on a graph with the two factors as axes, comparison of the teams being made from this graph.

The teams used in the analysis together with their code in Fig. 1 were as follows:- Brazil (BR), England (ENG), France (FR), Italy (IT), Northern Ireland (NI), Poland (POL), Scotland (SC), Spain (SP), Soviet Union (USSR), West Germany (WG), Arsenal (AR), Aston Villa (AV), Chelsea (CH), Coventry City (CV), Everton (EV), Ipswich Town (IP), Leicester City (LE), Liverpool (LV), Luton Town (LU), Manchester United (MU), Newcastle United (NEW), Norwich City (NR), Nottingham Forest (NF), Queen's Park Rangers (QPR), Sheffield Wednesday (SW), Southampton (SO), Stoke City (ST), Sunderland (SU), Tottenham Hotspur (TH), Watford (WAT), West Bromwich Albion (WBA) and West Ham United (WH).

Results

Table 1 lists the six style variables and those teams with either very high or very low performance on each variable. Long forward passes were most used by Ipswich, Sheffield Wednesday and Watford and least by France and Brazil. Of the World Cup teams, England, Scotland and Northern Ireland made most use of long passes while Norwich and West Ham were the least frequent users in the First Division. The use of long goal clearances was the variable for which the difference between the two sets of matches was most marked. Southampton (78%) had the lowest Division 1 figure, well above the highest World Cup figure (USSR, 44%). England and Spain made most use of the centres, Newcastle the least, Southampton and West Ham being the most frequent users in the First Division. West Bromwich Albion was the least effective in regaining possession in attack, while West Germany and Luton had the highest figures. There were large differences in the two closely related variables measuring short possession play. All World Cup teams were high, Brazil and France especially so, England and Poland the least. West Bromwich was the highest in Division 1 with Sheffield Wednesday and Watford the lowest.

Table 1. Teams with very high or low figures on each variable used to describe style

	Variable					
	Long forward passes	Long goal clearances	Centres	Regaining possession in attack	Possesion in defence	Multi-pass movements
High	Ipswich Sh.Wed Watford	Leicester Newcastle Sh.Wed Chelsea Luton Watford	England Spain S'hampton West Ham Brazil Scotland	Luton W.Germany France Poland Watford Chelsea	France Brazil Scotland N.Ireland W.Germany	France Brazil Scotland
Low	France Brazil Spain USSR	W.Germany Brazil France England	Newcastle Luton Coventry France USSR	WBA QPR Sunderland	Sh.Wed Arsenal Watford	Watford Sh.Wed Chelsea Newcastle

The first three principal components extracted by the analysis accounted for 92.5% of the variation in the data matrix (60.0%, 18.8% and 13.8% respectively). Table 2 gives the loadings on these three factors after varimax rotation and they can be interpreted as follows.

Table 2. Variable loadings on rotated factors

Variable	Factors 1	2	3
1 Long forward passes	0.811	0.336	0.157
2 Long goal clearances	0.904	0.335	0.117
3 Centres	0.166	0.934	0.143
4 Regaining possession in attack	0.123	0.128	0.981
5 Possesion in defence	0.952	0.216	0.078
6 Multi-pass movements	0.946	0.194	0.065

Factor 1 clearly distinguishes between those teams relying on short passing and possession (variables 5 and 6) and those that prefer long passes (variables 1 and 2). A team concentrating on multi-pass attacks with few long passes will score high on this factor, while a team using many long passes and short sequences of passing movements will score low. This factor can be said to distinguish between an elaborate style (high scores) and a direct style (low scores).

Factor 2 primarily measures the use of centres (variable 3).

Factor 3 represents regaining possession in attack (variable 4).

Plotting the team factor scores for Factor 1 and Factor 2 enables a comparison of the 32 teams to be made on the basis of the two playing style factors that distinguish team differences to the greatest extent.

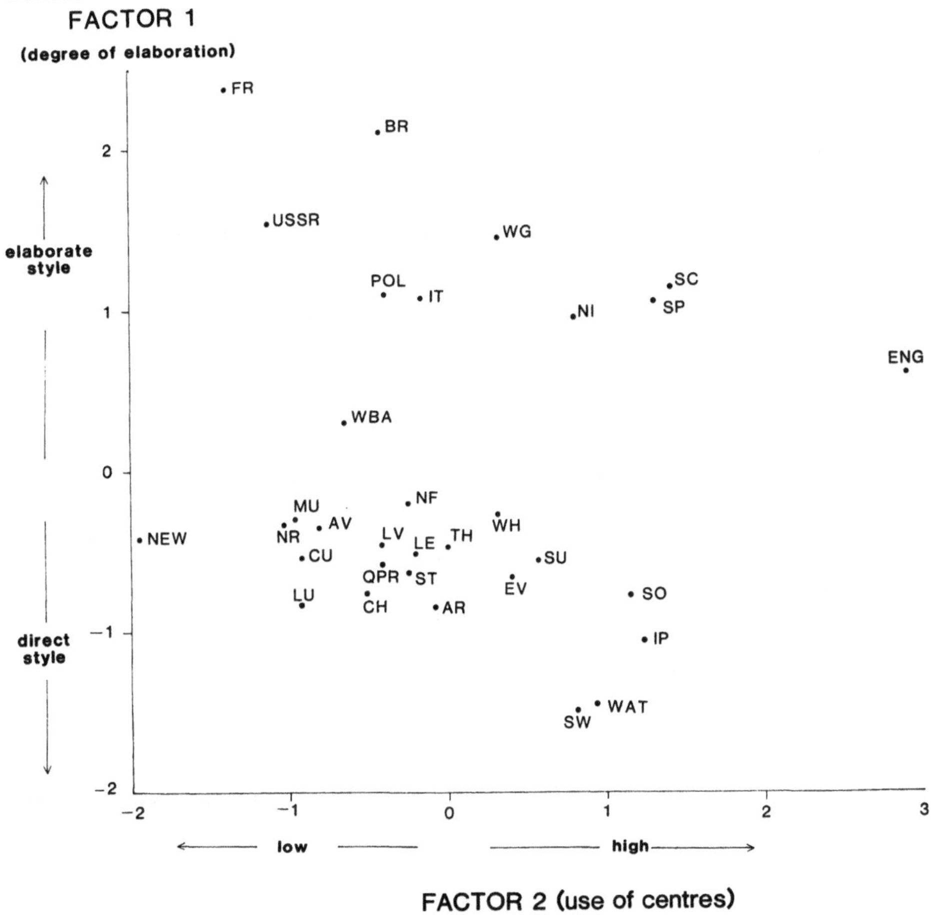

Figure 1. Representation of World Cup and English League teams according to two factors of playing styles

As can be seen from Fig.1, Factor 1 allows a complete distinction between the two sets of matches, all World Cup teams having higher scores (and hence more elaborate styles) than the 22 First Division teams. France and Brazil had the most elaborate styles, Watford and Sheffield Wednesday were the most direct. England had the least elaborate style of the World Cup sample, slightly above West Bromwich, easily the least direct of the England club sides. Factor 2 allows greater separation of the teams to be made. England's style is further distinguished from other World Cup teams by its relatively high use of centres, while the combination of a multi-passing style with few long passes and few centres sets France apart in the opposite direction. The bulk of Division 1 teams are clumped closely together, indicating broadly similar playing styles. The exceptions are Watford and Sheffield Wednesday (much more direct, slightly more centres), Ipswich and Southampton (greater use of centres with Ipswich also more direct than most other teams), Newcastle (much lower use of centres) and West Bromwich (much more elaborate than other teams).

Conclusion

The analysis described can be considered a first step towards a comparison of playing styles based on objective quantitative measures instead of the more usual subjective assessments. Despite being based on a small number of matches for most teams and on only 6 measures of style, the analysis has produced some clear differences, both between the two sets of matches and between individual teams within each set. The method has clearly isolated Sheffield Wednesday and Watford whose styles were causing much attention and controversy during 1984-85. Refinement and extension of the playing style variables will allow the method to pick out less obvious differences in style, as will the inclusion of more than two factors in the interpretation. For example, plots using Factor 3 separate out Queen's Park Rangers and Sunderland as a result of their attackers failing to regain possession of the ball in the matches seen.

With the widespread availability of match video recordings, it would now be possible for a coach rapidly to build up style profiles of other teams in his League using performance analysis and subsequent style analysis. This should enable him to back up or modify his own subjective views on opponents' playing styles, from which tactics for his own team can be planned for a particular match.

Acknowledgment

I am grateful to David Johnson for helpful advice. Support was provided by the Research Fund of the University of the South Pacific.

References

Ali, A. (1986) Statistical analysis of tactical movement patterns in association football. Unpublished master's thesis; University of St. Andrews, Scotland.

Figueiredo, M.A.C. and Rodrigues, L.E.S. (1983) Isolamento e definacao de algumas situacoes caracteristicas para compor um instrumento de avaliacao do rendimento de equipes de futebol Arquivos Brasileiros de Psicologia, 39, 185-206.

Franks, I.M., Goodman, D., and Miller, G. (1983) Analysis of performance: qualitative or quantitative. Science Periodical on Research and Technology in Sport GY-1 (March). Ottawa: Coaching Asociation of Canada.

Gould, P. and Gatrell, A. (1979) A structural analysis of a game: the Liverpool v Manchester United cup final of 1977. Social Networks, 2, 253-273.

Pollard, R. (1986) Soccer performance analysis and its application to shots at goal. Research Bi-annual for Movement, 4, 19-27.

Reep, C. (1982) The great Magyar myth exploded. Times, May 29 p.18.
Thomson, B. (1985) Anatomy of a season. Science Periodical on Research and Technology in Sport GY-1 (November). Ottawa: Coaching Association of Canada.

GAME SYSTEMS IN SOCCER FROM THE POINT OF VIEW OF COVERAGE OF SPACE

J.F. Grehaigne
Laboratoire d'Etude et de Recherche Sur la Performance Sportive, UER-EPS de Dijon BP 138, 21004 Dijon Cedex, France.

Introduction

The game system is defined as the general form in which players' attacking and defensive actions are organised, by establishing a precise arrangement of certain tasks (positions and field coverage) and certain principles of co-operation between them. The game system is the basic structure of collective team tactics (Teodoresca, 1965) In soccer, these arrangements refer most often to a formal distribution of positions and field coverage among various players, as expressed in team structure. These are described in systems such as WM, 4-2-4, and 4-4-2 (Frantz, 1975; Talaga, 1977; Morris, 1981), which illustrate with more or less precision the strategy the trainer has chosen. Quite obviously, a system which objectively quantifies the movements of performers within the game situation would be a valuable tool to aid the coach in evaluating team performance.

Tools of Observation

To study this problem, a system was developed which recorded the effective space covered by a specific player (Buono and Jade, 1976; Merand, 1976; Grehaigne, 1986). In these studies:- (i) the reference system for the space effectively covered by a given player was composed of boundary lines surrounding the regulation playing area; (ii) the observed variable was player position (recorded every 30s - although intervals of 10s and 15s have also been tested [Grehaigne, 1986; Winkler, 1984]). This provided a 'cloud' of 180 positional points per player. By linking the positional points it was possible to delimit the effective space coverage of the performer; (iii) the player's action zone was defined as being composed of those squares where the athlete's frequency of appearance is equal to 80% ± 5% of the positional points. This is an arbitrary choice, but it does seem to reflect the space coverage trends rather well. The remaining 20% of the positional points are deemed outside the players' action zone and reflect areas where the player executes tasks which are either ancillary to structured position or are infrequently performed. Undoubtedly, games may be often won or lost by the events in the 20% of positional points outside the action zone. However, this area does not reflect the predominant coverage of space by each individual which is the subject of the present study.

Although the configuration defined by the 'cloud' of positional points provided indications of the positions of players within the team structure, this type of analysis was considered too general since it cannot distinguish between spaces which have been subjected to heavy or light occupation. Thus, for a more detailed spatial analysis the field was divided into 40 equal squares (see Figure 1). This follows procedures established elsewhere (e.g. Roberts 1979; Zerhouni, 1980). The specific question examined in the present study concerned the frequency of player dispersion within the established structure of the team strategy. For example, is it possible to objectively characterise the distribution of player positions in open match play according to team strategy? It is feasible that this system of movement notation may provide valuable feedback to the soccer coach relating to the positional efficacy of individuals within the team composition.

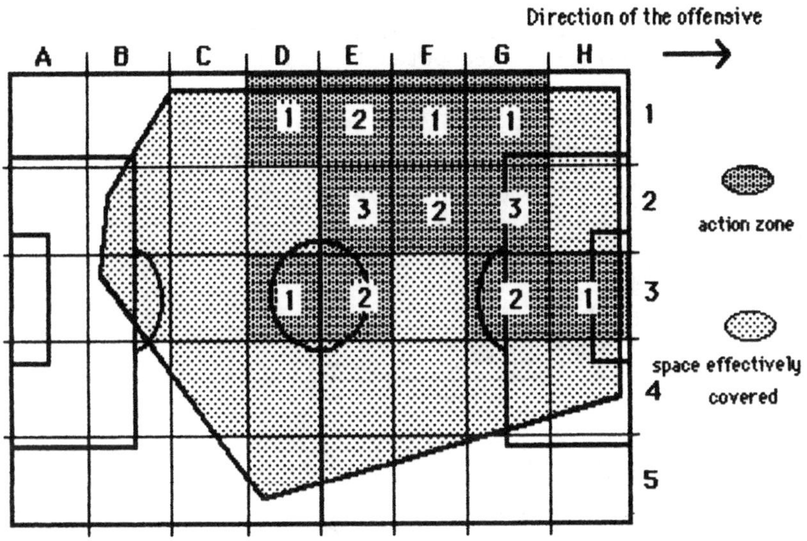

Figure 1. The space effectively covered by Garande (Auxerre). (Garande's action zone is compared with the space effectively covered by him)

Method

To study the way players disperse around the playing area, a theoretical distribution where the variable X (the player) obeys a theoretical law of uniform probability was hypothesised. It is often affirmed in modern soccer that 'everyone attacks, everyone defends' (Kowacs, 1975). Taking this strictly, it is assumed that it is equiprobable for a player to appear in one square as it is in another. This hypothesis was tested against a sample of positions taken up by players in observed matches. The problem is, thus, to consider the gap between observed and uniform theoretical distributions. Five professional teams were analysed in different seasons:- Auxerre (1982), Italy vs Brazil (1982) and Auxerre vs Marseilles (1984). Chi-square analysis was used to confirm or invalidate the hypothesis of uniform distribution of player movement. If the chi-square observed is greater than 55.8 ($P < 0.05$; 39 degrees of freedom), it can be concluded that the observed and theoretical distributions differ significantly.

Results

In all of the teams, the chi-squares of all the players exceeded 55.8, ranging from 136 to 852. All of the distributions were non-uniform. Studying the player data more closely, major deviations in the dispersion of the chi-square values were found. To find if the differences were as great between teams, the mean values found in the chi-square test for each team were compared and the extreme values plotted (Figure 2).

For the professional teams, a mean chi-square value of around 400 was consistently found, which seems to be a key threshold value (Figure 2). For the deviations (computed by taking the difference

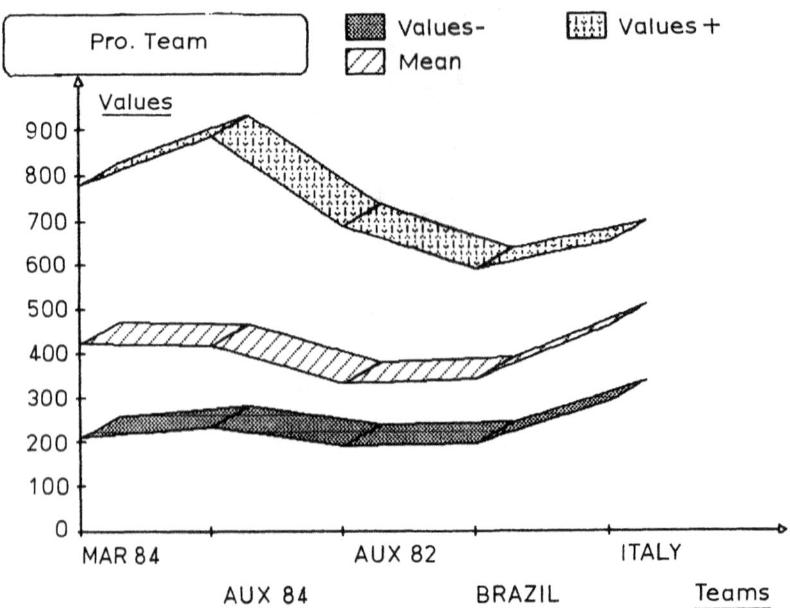

Figure 2. Mean chi-squares and the extremes

between the highest and lowest value for a team), a very large range was noted, but still hovered around this figure. It seems that four patterns emerge from these data:

i) Mean χ^2 > 400 with large difference between extremes: this is a model where <u>many</u> players occupy fixed positions, doubtless following precise instructions to this effect, but a few move widely around the playing field. The first set of players remains relatively central around a small space while the latter group interlinks the various areas of play and thus covers much more space.

ii) Mean $\chi^2 > 400$ with little difference between the extremes: this indicates a pattern where all the players are distributed around relatively fixed areas of the field. The team moves as a whole with respect to position of the ball.

iii) Mean $\chi^2 < 400$ with a large difference between extremes: this indicates a model where few players occupy fixed positions, according to precise instructions (in particular the key positions of defensive and attacking central players) while all the others move over the entire field of play. The former remain centred on a bounded space while the latter play in different areas of the field.

iv) Mean $\chi^2 < 400$ with little difference between extremes: in this model all of the players move about; but the team is kept stable by an organised interchange of positions, giving rise to a relative homogenicity in the x^2 values. It is still true that certain positions, which determine the stability of a team, are regularly occupied by the same player.

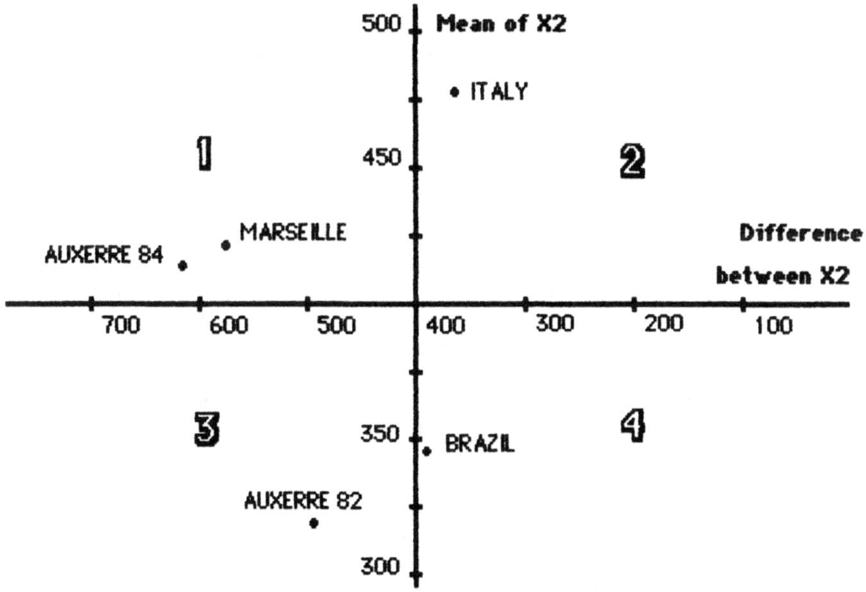

Figure 3. Groups of models and distribution of teams in relation to models

To facilitate the analysis below, these models can be characterised by a pair of mean coordinates defined as follows, using M to denote the mean value of the χ^2 variable and E to denote the mean excursion of the variable:-

[M450; E550] for model 1
[M450; E250] for model 2
[M350; E550] for model 3
[M350; E250] for model 4

Players' action zone

Using this method the movements of the Auxerre team were analysed in a match versus Marseilles. The points for each player were grouped by tens, up to a total of 145 ± 5, to obtain 80% of the points. The number 1 in a given square represents a frequency of appearance between zero and ten points of [0; 10], the number 2 indicates a frequency between 21 and 30 [21; 30] and so on. An example of the action zone for a player is incorporated in Figure 1. This action zone provides information on the exact boundaries of the preferential space occupied by a soccer player. It gives greater precision than does the concept of a space effectively covered by examining areas of concentration in the cloud of points. It can be seen that the space effectively covered gives an idea of the area within which a footballer plays, whereas the action zone tells more about the density of play inside this area.

It is possible to model this by using the action zone. By analyzing the chi square data for the professional team players, space occupation models for each position can be proposed. In such a representation, the densities of a performer's zone depend on the match configuration, the individual's style, changes in the score, tactical instructions and the importance of the game.

Discussion

The purpose of this investigation was to study game systems in soccer on the basis of the space covered in a match. To do this, a player's effective space coverage was measured. The game models identified were further developed by studying the action zone of each player to arrive at space coverage models for each position. This helps sum up the analysis of the confrontation of two teams, characterises the actual distribution of the players and thereby determines the game system used.

The actual game system of a team can be defined as the resultant of several interacting factors, such as:- (i) the general order derived from the general strategic choices of the team (team composition); (ii) the positions assigned to be covered according to the particular instructions each player receives in training; (iii) the effective positions taken in reaction to an adversary in a game situation.

In a given soccer match, then, the two teams are most often two interacting non-uniform systems. With a longitudinal analysis of a given team, constants in behaviour could be found, apart from the conditions of competition. Analysing a greater number of matches would provide further and more precise information on the game systems actually used and on the reliability of the models generated.

Finally, using these tools and currently available models, the study should be extended to further investigation of the principles at work in the game of soccer. At the moment, this technique of analysis seems rather crude, but it is a preliminary step. In future, such a method could be used to study positional changes in relation to team strategy, to scores, and also to injury of a particular player. Moreover, it can help coaches to categorise playing patterns and adopt new ones in order to gain tactical advantages via flexibility.

References

Buono, A. and Jade, R. (1976) Le Football a Montreal. Paris: Sport et Plein Air.

Frantz, P. (1975) Le Football. Mulhouse: L'Alsace.

Grehaigne, J.F. (1986) Des outils d'observation pour le jeu de football. DIRE en APS, 19, 23-29.

Kowacs, S. (1975) Football Total. Paris: Calman levy.

Merand, R. (1976) L'educateur face a la haute performance. Paris: Sport et Plein Air.

Morris, D. (1981) The Soccer Tribe. London: Jonathan Cape.

Roberts, G. (1979) Trois lecons sur les fondements du jeu. Ligue du Sud-ouest.

Talaga, J. (1977) Fussball-taktik. Berlin: Sport Verlag.

Teodorscu, L. (1965) Principes pour l'etude de la tactique commune aux jeux sportifs collectifs. Actes Colloque Vichy sur les Sports Collectifs.

Winkler, W. (1984) Sport strategie als lehrfach. Leistungssport, 2, 5-13.

Zerhouni, M. (1980) Principes de Base du Football Contemporain. Orges: Fleury.

SPACE, TEAMWORK AND ATTACKING SUCCESS IN SOCCER

S. Harris : Faculty of Physical Education and Research, University of New Brunswick, Fredericton, N.B. Canada.

T. Reilly : Department of Sport and Recreation Studies, Liverpool Polytechnic, Byrom Street, Liverpool L3 3AF, England.

Introduction

Multiple player interactions, fast often weaving movements and unpredictable game patterns are typical features of field invasive sports such as soccer. Indeed part of these games' fascination is the conjecture generated among spectators about what might have been the outcome had a particular alternative strategy been adopted. In soccer, observers tend to form independent subjective opinions about the determinants of a game's progress and generally they vary greatly in their conclusions.

Suggestions have been made to employ computerised methods of monitoring match tactics (e.g. Franks et al., 1986), though such techniques are mainly restricted to the production of descriptive data. The work of Reep and Benjamin (1968) concentrated on the scoring of goals and attempted to isolate the important antecedents of goal-scoring. Goals provide few data points in complete games so it may be more fruitful to study broader aspects of success within the game. In this respect success can be viewed as producing attacking moves (or sequences of passes) that culminate in a shot at goal. It may also include negating the opposition's attacks or denying the opponents space to set up scoring opportunities.

Players depend on their colleagues for support in attacking manoeuvres by creating gaps in the opposition's defence or by running into space to create an opportunity to shoot. Conversely, defenders are vulnerable without covering team-mates to help to neutralise attacks. The astute use of space and regular maintenance of a favourable configuration of players is characteristic of good team work. The aim of this study was to investigate the contributions to attacking success of selected variables associated with this aspect of teamwork and the use of space on the pitch.

Methods

Derivation of measures of attacking potential

A summary of terms and definitions is given in Table 1. A prime concern was to derive a measure of attacking potential using the concept of configuration. It was measured at the start and end of each 'unit of play' which reflected an individual's contribution to the attack while possessing the ball. The change in configuration during a 'unit of play' in turn reflected the additional contribution from team-mates by strategic movements and positioning. A configuration index (CI) was first proposed which reflected the principles:- i) the greater the ratio of attacking (A) to defending (D) players, the more positive is the attack's potential for success; ii) the fewer the number of defending players, the more space is available to the attackers, thereby enhancing the opportunity for success. The formula adopted for calculating the index was:-

$$CI = A(12-D)/11(D) + [(D-6)/11]^3$$

The ratio A/D needed refining as it did not take into account that a situation with two attackers versus two defenders has relatively greater potential for success than say a configuration of 9 versus 9. The factor (12-D)/11 considers this, its value increasing as the number of players decreased and consequently the amount of attacking space increased. The final term in the equation was found empirically to correct for potential error, for example in extreme conditions when defending players number 1, 2, 10 or 11.

Table 1. Definition of major concepts and terms

Attack:	occurs during a team's possession in which the ball and player(s) move towards the opponent's goal.
Success:	the level of effectiveness of an attack is graded:- successful (A): an attack concludes with a shot on target; intermediate (B): the attack ends with a shot but it is off-target; unsuccessful (C): the attack ends without a shot being taken.
Unit of play:	begins when the attacker tries to make contact with the ball and ends when his contribution to the attack is known. Each attack consists of one (or more) units of play, during each of which one player has possession.
Data point:	a single action within a unit of play by an individual attacker i.e. a component of a 'unit of play'.
Configuration:	describes the potential of an attack for success. It considers the ratio of attacking to defending players in the immediate area of the play and the relative advantage or disadvantage this gives to the attacking team.

The second parameter was the space available. The distance (m) between the nearest pressurising defender and the attacker in possession of the ball was calculated at the moment the ball was received. For short distances the playing figures were used as reference cues: for longer distances markings on the pitches were employed e.g. penalty spot, 16.5 m line and so on.

Sample

Video taped recordings of 24 first class soccer matches were analysed. Attacks where the camera angle did not adequately catch the configuration were not used in the analysis. The teams selected were top European club teams and national sides. Altogether 180 attacks, spread equally between the three hierarchical success categories (Table 1) were monitored.

Procedure

Each attack was chosen randomly from the match video recording. The Cl value was calculated at two points in each unit of play - as soon as the attacking player attempted to win possession, and again when he lost possession or transferred it to a team-mate. It was thus possible to calculate the change in configuration between these two points. The functional variables selected for analysis were: i) the initial configuration, the final configuration and the change in configuration for the final unit of play of the attack; ii) the average value of the initial configuration and final configuration, and the overall change in configuration during the course of an attack.

The variables associated with space availability were treated as follows. First the mean distance between attacker and nearest defender during an attack was calculated. Second, the distance from the nearest defender at the final data point of an attack was employed.

Statistical analysis

A one-way analysis of variance was performed to investigate differences between the levels of attacking success for all four variables selected for examination. Specific differences for post-hoc purposes were studied using t-tests. One-way analysis of co-variance was also used to examine the configuration indices with the effect of the initial attacking potential used as the covariate.

Results

Configuration

On average each attack contained 5.3 units of play. For the attack as a whole the configuration indices (Cl) were significantly higher in successful attacks (category A) than for the failures (category C) at the initial Cl ($P < 0.05$); the difference between A and B attacks were only apparent in the final Cl values ($P < 0.05$). Values for B were significantly better than for C at the initial configuration and at the final configuration but the change in configuration was similar for both these types of attack (Table 2). When the initial Cl was used as covariate, no significant differences were found at the final configuration using ANCOVA. The results for the change in configuration were found to be significant in both sets of analyses, ANOVA and ANCOVA ($P < 0.05$). Localisation of differences using t-tests established that the most successful attacks were different from the other two categories ($P < 0.05$), which were similar to each other.

Table 2. Mean configuration indices for the attack as a whole and for the final unit of play at the three levels of attacking success

	Whole attack		Final unit of play	
	Initial Cl	Change in Cl	Initial Cl	Change in Cl
On target (A)	0.341	0.164	0.434	0.063
Off target (B)	0.347	0.086	0.394	-0.004
No shot (C)	0.295	0.079	0.349	-0.033

When the final unit of play in all attacks was analysed, differences between the failed attacks (C) and the others were apparent as at the outset ($P < 0.05$). The most successful (A) differed significantly from B only in the final Cl. When the change in configuration was examined significant results were apparent in all the comparisons of the three levels of success.

Space

Table 3. Mean (±SD) distance (m) from the nearest defender during an attack and at the final unit of play (FUP) for the three success categories

Category	Attack	FUP
On target (A)	3.27±1.61	2.62±2.52
Off-target (B)	3.21±1.50	2.77±2.59
No shot (C)	2.44±1.58	0.93±2.42

Results for space available to attackers during a whole attack (Table 3) indicated that more shooting opportunities arose when the distance between the attacker in possession and the nearest defender increased. Analysis of variance showed that category A and B attacks did not differ significantly in this respect but both had significantly higher values for space available than those attacks (C) that ended in failure. When the final unit of play was analysed results were found to be similar for the attacks that produced a shot, both A and B attacks having significantly higher values than category C ($P < 0.05$).

Discussion

The descriptive data of this study show how teamwork, expressed as the relative dispersal of players close to the area of ball-play, and the use of space on the field contribute to the success of attacking moves in soccer. The configuration index employed to describe how players congregate around the immediate play provided a useful, albeit crude measure which could be refined in further research.

The initial configuration values successfully discriminated between attacks which resulted in a shot at goal and those which ended with a shot off target or no shot at all. This demonstrated that attacks which started with a good potential or were soon able to attain such a position, and maintained it, tended to be the more successful. Teams should, then, try to initiate attacks in positions of good potential, or upon gaining possession quickly try and attain a position of high potential and then try to maintain or improve upon it. One method of achieving this is to pressurize opposing players near to their own goal to try and dispossess them while they are unprepared and out of position to defend a counter-attack. Franks et al. (1983) stressed the importance of this strategy in their report. A second strategy, as proposed by Bauer (1975), is to quickly transfer defence into attack. The team gaining possession attempts to create a position of high attacking potential by moving the ball quickly forward and bypassing defenders. A third strategy is to play long passes directly into scoring areas and hope to maintain or regain possession through skill, chance or defensive error.

Attacks which concluded with a shot on goal were discriminated from unsuccessful attacks by a change in attacking potential. As the configuration value was designed to take account of the effects of relative changes in attacker to defender ratios, this factor was an indication of the effects of teamwork on success. The improved ratio of attacking to defending players was probably achieved by team mates advancing forward to support the player in possession and secondly the ball being passed through or behind the defensive players to another team member. The effect of the first tactic is to disperse and weaken the defence's resources and the effect of the second is to make a number of the defensive players temporarily redundant. Teamwork, then, successfully discriminated between successful attacks and intermediate or unsuccessful attacks.

The ANOVA showed that significant differences existed between the configuration values attained at the end of the final unit of play. This indicated first that successful attacks tended to experience a positive shift in potential (i.e. an attacking player passes an opponent before shooting), and second, unsuccessful attacks experienced a negative shift in attacking potential (i.e. an attacking player passes away from the danger area or slows the attack down, allows the defence to recover and is dispossessed). The data seemed to suggest that it was in the final unit of play that teamwork was critical. Although teamwork has been shown to be crucial, it is unlikely that teams at the top level of play would be able to significantly outwork each other during the approach play and, hence, it was probably the maintenance of attacking potential and the utilization of the players and the space available (attacking potential) which was more critical to success.

The final configuration value discriminated between the hierarchical success categories. This lent support to the original theory upon which the configuration value was developed. During the unit of play the successful attacks experienced significantly greater positive changes in configuration. This vindicated the importance of forwards getting past defenders. It should be noted, however, that in only one-third of the successful attacks did a player pass a defender. Attacks experiencing intermediate levels of success achieved positive potential changes in one-fifth of the cases and unsuccessful attacks in approximately one-eighth of the cases.

The second major factor to be examined was the space available to attackers. Attacks which culminated with a shot at goal were characterised by a greater average distance being maintained between the player in possession and the closest marking defender throughout the attack. Soccer theorists have long recognised the importance of creating space as an aim in attacking play (Conrad, 1966) and the present data vindicate this. A coaching implication is that players should be instructed in the best methods of running to support the attack and drawing defending players away from the man in possession. Further, players should be coached in how to create space for themselves when receiving the ball and how to make space for themselves when closely marked.

Attacks which culminated without a shot being produced were characterised by having a significantly smaller distance from the nearest pressurizing defender during the last movement of the attack. This emphasised the need to create space for the attacking players to enhance the probability of a shot at goal. Attacking players with little space in which to manoeuvre tended to be prevented from shooting.

Logically the space available should be related to the success of an attack. The greater the distance between the man in possession and the nearest pressurizing defender, the more time a player has to decide what to do with his possession, and the greater his error tolerance in ball control without losing possession. Surprisingly the distance from the nearest pressurizing defender failed to discriminate between those attacks which finished with a shot off target and those which finished with a shot on target. It is likely that the critical factor in the ultimate success of a shot, judged either by its accuracy on target or the scoring of a goal, is the skill (accuracy and timing) of the shooter.

A schema for attacking success has been outlined where the attack is initiated in a position of good potential. The team must maintain this potential during its approach play. The attack concludes with possession being transferred to a forward in space who shoots at goal, to a forward who passes his marker, or passes the ball through or behind the defence for another forward player to move on to.

In summary this study looked at the contribution of collective and individual use of space to attacking success, evaluated as producing opportunities for a shot at goal rather than in terms of goals scored. Data showed that both strategic aspects were important discriminators of the level of attacking success. Results emphasised that team members should concentrate on creating space when attacking and denying it when defending, supporting each other in attack and in defence, and trying to dispossess opponents while they are vulnerable in defence. Attacking players gain advantage in penetrating the defence by passing the ball through it to an on-rushing team-mate or penetrating the defence by dribbling past a marker and so gaining space. The overall attacking aim should be to outnumber the opposition in crucial areas of the field, particularly in the attacking third, or by dislocating defenders provide one or more key attackers with a good opportunity to score.

References

Bauer, G. (1974) Football. Wakefield: EP Sport.

Conrad, L. (1966) Understanding Soccer Tactics. London: Faber and Faber.

Franks, I.M. and Goodman, D. (1986) A systematic approach to analysing sports performance. Sports Sci., 4, 49-59.

Franks, I.M., Goodman, D., and Miller, G. (1983) Human factors in sport systems. An empirical investigation of events in a team game. Proceedings from the Human Factors Society 27th Annual Meeting. Norfolk, Virginia. 10-14th October, pp.383-385.

Reep, C. and Benjamin, B. (1968) Skill and chance in Association Football. Royal Stat. Soc. Series A. General, 131, 581-585.

MEASURING MOVEMENT SPEEDS AND DISTANCES COVERED DURING SOCCER MATCH-PLAY

J. Ohashi*, H. Togari*, M. Isokawa** and S. Suzuki***
* Department of Sports Sciences, University of Tokyo, Japan.
** Department of Physical Education, Tokyo Metropolitan University, Japan
*** Department of Sports Sciences, Seikei University, Tokyo, Japan.

Introduction

During a match, soccer players must move in many directions and at various speeds for their team's success. Their movements in the field are based on various physical abilities such as aerobic or anaerobic capacity and others. In order to study physiological characteristics of soccer, the analysis of the mode of movements of players during a match is needed. Using the published data of Whitehead (1975), Reilly and Thomas (1976), and Withers et al. (1982), Ekblom (1986) summarized that players cover approximately 10km in a match, of which 8 - 18% is at the individual's top speed. However, the values obtained by these investigators were not consistent. Ekblom (1986) suggested that one of the reasons for this was the different methods used for estimating the distances covered. Most investigators were estimating distances by observing modes of players' movements at pre-determined levels of speed. It seems that such estimations reduce the precision or objectivity of the observations.

The present authors have recently devised a new method of recording and analysing movement speeds and distances covered by a player during match-play, in which triangular surveying methods linked to a computer provided the system of analysis. It was found that they possess a high practical value compared with previous methods. In this presentation, the authors would like to describe the method and report some of the results obtained.

Methods

Two VTR cameras each attached to a tripod which was equipped with potentiometers, were set up on two spots at 10-20 m away from the corner flag on the extended goal line outside the field. A subject was followed at the same time by the two cameras during a match. Signals of angles obtained by potentiometers were sequentially converted into digital data and recorded on a data tape recorder at 0.5 s intervals (Fig. 1).

Four elite soccer players were used as subjects. Two of them were Japanese national team players and their movements were recorded during two regular matches of the Japan Soccer League (JSL). The other two were JSL players and their movements were interchangeably measured -5 minutes each 8 times for 40 minutes- during the whole period of a practice match before the JSL season.

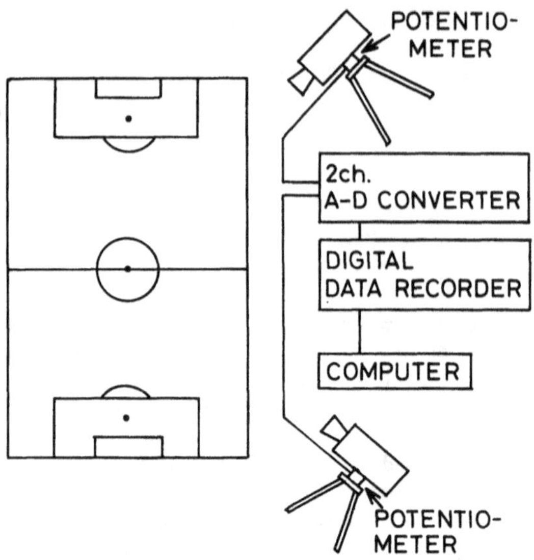

Figure 1. Diagramatic view for measurements

The data were input into the computer memory and each value of angle at every 0.5 s was smoothed by the method of a three-points moving average to correct the lateral error due to centering the subject with a camera. Every X, Y co-ordinate of a player was calculated from two angle data and the distance between two cameras: then the distance between consecutive two X,Y co-ordinates was continuously calculated.

Results

Figure 2 shows the changes of movement speeds with the passage of time during a match. The total distances covered by two national calibre players, which were measured during a match, were 9303m and 10387m respectively. From the distances covered in 40 min during a practice match by the other two players, the total distances in 90 min would be 11601 m and 10046 m, respectively.

The distribution histogram of distance covered at each movement speed during 1st and 2nd halves is shown in Figure 3. The mean distances covered during 1st and 2nd halves for 4 players were 5373 m and 4968 m respectively.

The percent total distance covered and percent total time spent at each movement speed are shown in Table 1.

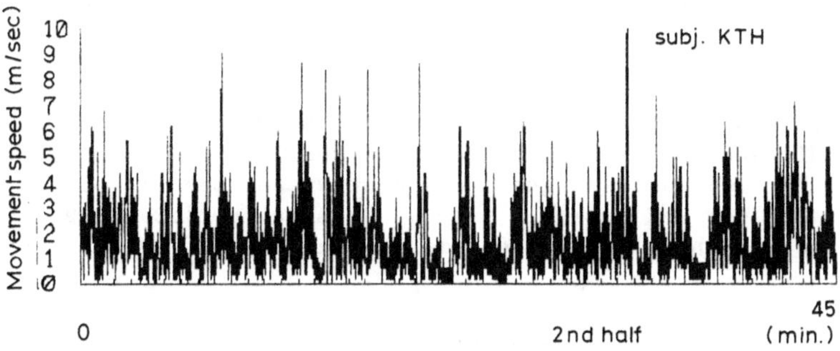

Figure 2. Changes of movement speed during a match

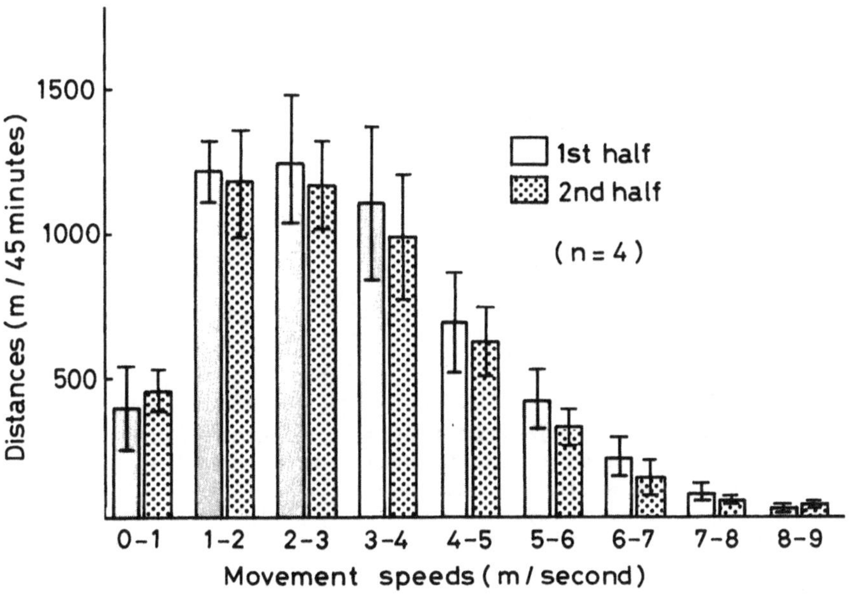

Figure 3. The distribution of distance covered at each movement speed

Discussion

From this study it can be said that, if this method is applied, it is possible to measure very precisely the movement speeds and distance covered with the passage of time during soccer match-play (Fig. 2). In this study, the total distances covered by players during a match ranged from 9303 m to 11601 m. These values closely corresponded with those reported previously by Reilly and Thomas (1976) and Withers et al. (1982).

As shown in Table 1, distance covered at the speeds of over 7 m s^{-1} was 2.5%, over 6 m s^{-1} was 5.8% and over 5 m s^{-1} was 12.8% of the total distance covered. According to Reilly and Thomas (1976), sprinting, defined as the highest movement speed, was 11% of the total distance covered during a match. This ratio closely agrees with the one for the distance covered at the speed of over 5 m s^{-1} in this study.

Table 1. Ratios of distance covered and time spent at each speed (n = 4)

speed range (m s^{-1})	% total distance	% total time
0 - 1	8.0	30.5
1 - 2	23.1	30.5
2 - 3	23.3	18.3
3 - 4	20.2	11.3
4 - 5	12.6	5.5
5 - 6	7.1	2.5
6 - 7	3.4	1.0
7 - 8	1.4	0.4
8 - 9	0.8	0.0
9 - 10	0.1	0.0
total	100.0	100.0

Withers et al. (1982) reported that sprinting was 5.8% of thetotal distance covered and high intensity work (striding and sprinting) was 18.8%. The ratio of sprinting agreed with that for the speed of over 6 m s^{-1} (5.8%) in this study, and that of high intensity work seemed to fall between those ratios at the speeds of 4 m s^{-1} (24.4%) and 5 m s^{-1} (12.8%).

Mayhew and Wenger (1985) measured the time spent in each mode of movement and reported that the running at the highest speed of movement was 11.3% of the total time. This ratio almost agreed with the one attained at the speed of over 4 m s^{-1} in this study.

As already described, it might be possible to compare the results obtained in this study with those reported by other investigators. However, the data previously reported seem to have been derived from gross observations whose techniques were not precisely devised. Those data are gross estimations of the distances covered on a field through arbitrarily defined categorizations of the mode of movements and the speeds.

On the contrary, the method and technique used in this study were much more sophisticated than those previously applied. Although the system of observation and analysis of data seems to be complicated, it is possible to obtain data on the distance covered at each level of speed in a very precise way. Therefore, it is suggested that it should be applied when trying to observe and analyze the movements of players on a field during match-play for further physiological and technical purposes.

References

Ekblom, B. (1986) Applied physiology of soccer. Sports Med., 3, 50-60.

Mayhew, S.R. and Wenger, H.A. (1985) Time-motion analysis of professional soccer. J. Human Mov't. Stud., 11, 49-52.

Reilly, T. and Thomas, V. (1976) A motion analysis of work-rate in different positional roles in professional football match-play. J. Human Mov't. Stud., 2, 87-97.

Whitehead, N. (1975) Conditioning for Sport. pp.40-42, Yorkshire: E.P. Publishing Co. Ltd.

Withers, R.T., Maricic, Z., Wasilewski, S. and Kelly, L. (1982) Match analyses of Australian professional soccer players. J. Human Mov't. Stud., 8, 159-176.

TIME AND MOTION ANALYSIS IN TOP CLASS SOCCER GAMES

K. Yamanaka, S. Haga, M. Shindo, J. Narita, S. Koseki, Y. Matsuura and M. Eda
Institute of Health and Sport Science, University of Tsukuba, Sakura, Niihari, Ibaraki, 305, Japan.

Introduction

In soccer, each game lasts a total of 90 min, 45 min for each half. During a game in which defence and offence alternate repeatedly, players, using various ball techniques, perform a variety of actions ranging from some at a low speed to others at full speed. Furthermore, the players are free to move widely throughout the field. In planning training programmes for soccer players, therefore, it is important to study movements in the game in order to establish the type of physical fitness required.

Research on soccer has included analysis of the game from the viewpoint of technique and tactics. Such studies have focussed on the frequency with which each tactic or technique is used in an actual game, its continuity (Yamanaka, 1968), and the number of times offensive and shooting skills are used in games (Akai, 1977, 1978). Many studies report the maximum oxygen intake of players, the relative metabolic rate or heart rate response to soccer play (e.g. Reilly, 1979; Togari, 1979; Yamaoka, 1956). Many analyse the motions of players in actual games. Ohashi (1983), for example, reported on the distance covered by players competing in the World Club Championship. Reilly and Thomas (1976) and Mayhew and Wenger (1985), examining the players of professional teams, reported the distances covered by the players during games and their patterns of motion. This study attempted to classify field players' movements into fundamental modes of motion that reflected the exercise intensity and study the time spent on each mode and the frequency of each mode in order to provide a data base on which training programmes could be founded.

Methods

This survey was conducted on a total of 49 players including:- 10 field players who participated in the European-South American Cup in December, 1984 (Group A), 19 players who participated in the Japan Emperor Cup (Group B) and 20 players who participated in the Japan Inter-college Soccer Championship in November, 1984 (Group C). Each player was individually audio-taped by one observer, who recorded every motion of the player during a game. Soccer players from universities were assigned to the testers, who were previously trained to observe each player's motions in a simulated game.

The modes of motion of players during games were classified as follows:- i) Standing; ii) Walking: iii) Jogging: a state of running at a low speed; iv) Running: a state of running with a clear goal or aim, intermediate between sprinting (dashing) and jogging: v) Sprinting (Dashing): a state of running at full speed. In this study, the sprint (dash) included dribbling at top speed and keen (one on one) man-to-man offensive and defensive plays.

The objectivity of the data generated was assured in the following manner. A university midfielder who played in one of the games of the Japan Kanto University Soccer League held in November, 1984 was selected for study. Five experimenters collected data on the movements of this player by means of the afore-mentioned method for 45 min to confirm the objectivity of the data, multiple t-tests were applied to the values obtained by the experimenters. During the analysis of the data, while replaying the tape in which the entire game of 90 min was recorded, the time spent on each mode of motion and the frequency of each mode were obtained by using a specially programmed personal computer.

Results

The time spent in each of the five modes of activity are reported in Table 1 for each group. The percentage of the total time spent on each mode of motion according to the three groups is shown in Figure 1. The mean value of the time ratio of each mode on the whole showed a common tendency among the three groups. The values for the different modes in the three groups were in the order of:- walking > jogging > running > standing > dashing (sprinting). The time ratio occupied by running and sprinting in group A was low compared to that of group B or group C.

Table 1. Time(s) spent in the various modes of motion for the three groups of players - A: European-S. American Cup; B: Japan Emperor Cup; C: Japan Inter-College

	A	B	C
Walking	2990±480	2588±353	2575±350
Jogging	1767±569	2034±443	1889±498
Running	308±124	371±122	425±150
Standing	232±160	262±183	379±123
Sprinting	104± 53	262±183	143±120

The total numbers of movements according to the five modes used during a single game were 736 in group A, 882 in group B and 956 in group C. The professional team tended to have lower changes in activity. The percentage of each mode is expressed in Figure 2 as a percentage of the total observed during a single game.

The frequency values for jogging, walking, running, standing and sprinting in Group A were 298, 226, 98, 78 and 35 respectively. In

Group B, the figures were 334, 281, 144, 71 and 52 respectively. The corresponding frequencies in group C were 328, 310, 150, 116 and 35, respectively.

A common tendency was found among the three groups: that is, the frequencies were in the order:- jogging > walking > running > standing > sprinting. The number of runs and sprints (dashes) in a game tended to be less in Group A than in Groups B or C.

When the time spent on each mode was rearranged by positions (Defence, DF; Midfield, MF; and Forward (FW) (Figure 3), the results for Group A were:- MF < DF(P < 0.05) and MF < FW (P < 0.01) in standing, MF < DF(P < 0.01) in walking and MF < DF(P < 0.01) in jogging. In group C findings were:- MF < FW (P < 0.01) in walking, conversely MF < FW(P < 0.05) in jogging. Thus MF spent less time in standing and walking and more in jogging than did DF and FW players.

When the frequency of each mode was rearranged by positions (Figure 4), the results of statistical significance were:- in group A, MF < DF(P<0.01) in standing, MF < DF(P<0.01) and MF < FW(P<0.01) in walking. On the other hand in Group B findings were:- FW < DF(P< 0.01) both in standing and walking: In Group C results were:- MF < DF(P<0.01) and MF < FW(P<0.05) in jogging. In this case also frequencies for MF were lower in standing and walking and higher in jogging than noted in the other groups.

Discussion

From the point of view of time spent in the various activities the rank order was:- walking > jogging > running > standing > sprinting. This result was common among the three groups. The time ratio in a game is mostly occupied by walking and jogging (83% - 88%), less by running and sprinting (7% - 10%) and least by standing (4% - 10%). Mayhew and Wenger (1985) surveyed three professional players to study their motions in a game. Walking, jogging, running and standing occupied 46.4%, 38.0%, 11.3% and 2.3%, respectively of the total time. Present results replicate their findings.

In a soccer game, various types of motions, actions or exercises are attempted intermittently and at different speeds. Balls travel a great distance because of the space available and the duration which balls stay in one area is short. Generally players must play the ball and manoeuvre their own position within a limited time. They are mostly jogging or walking. They are, in other words, in a perpetual state of preparedness to fully execute their ball playing abilities. From the viewpoint of physical fitness, it is suggested that it is essential to possess a satisfactory level of aerobic work capacity to move continuously for a full 90 min. On the other hand, the time spent on running at speed occupies only a small proportion of time compared to that spent jogging or walking. Running and sprinting are attempted during the phases which are decisive and directly related to play, as in receiving the ball, shooting and guarding an opponent.

Furthermore, manoeuvres attempted during such occasions are at a high intensity, albeit sometimes momentarily. The ability a player displays during these phases is directly connected to the scoring potential of his team and may be the deciding factor in the game.

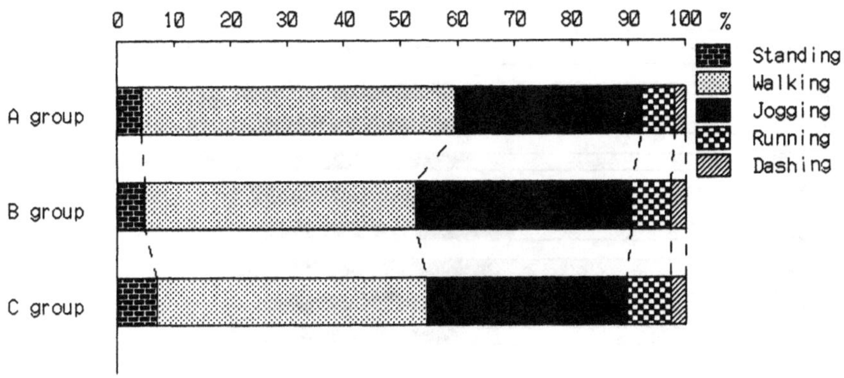

Figure 1. Time and motion analysis by groups

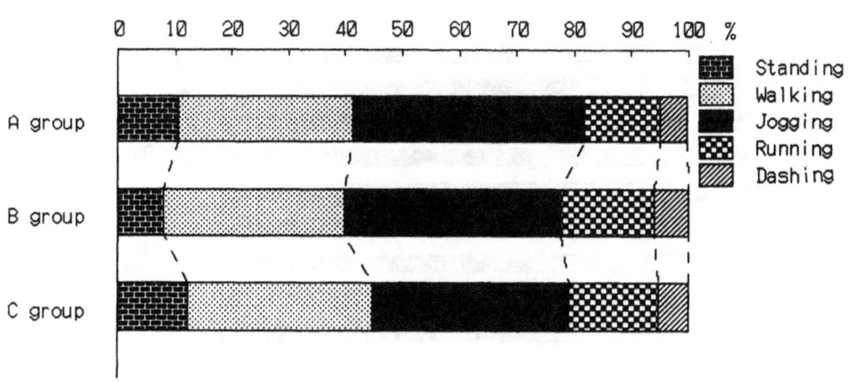

Figure 2. Frequency motion analysis by groups

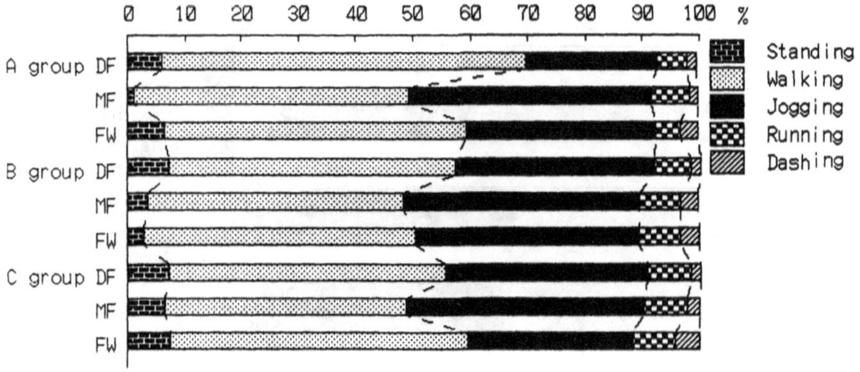

Figure 3. Time and motion analysis by playing positions

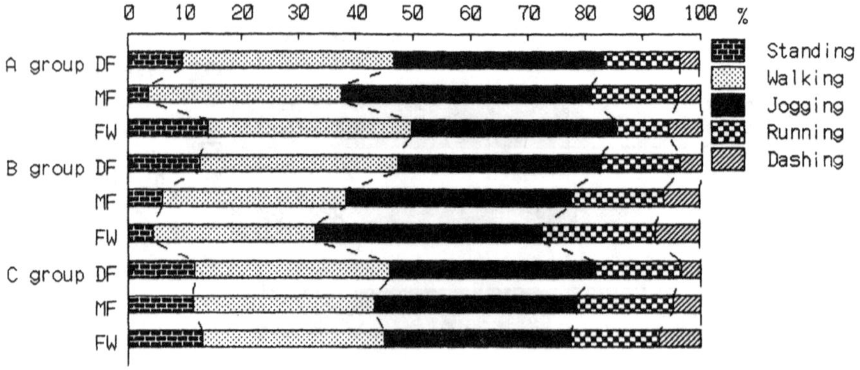

Figure 4. Frequency-motion analysis by playing positions

This ability can therefore be crucial, even though it may be expressed in a brief moment. This suggests that whole-body and ball manoeuvring ability and a high degree of anaerobic capacity are needed to supplement a player's endurance capacity.

Our results regarding the frequency of observation of each mode of motion in a game are similar to those obtained by calculations from Mayhew and Wenger's (1985) report. Their results agreed with those of Reilly and Thomas (1976). The J.S.L. players of Group B and college teams of Group C attempted running or sprinting very competitively about once every five modes of activity. This indicates how intense the game of soccer is. The professionals (Group A) showed a conspicuously lower frequency of running than did the other groups. Taking into consideration that the professional team is presumably high in tactical, technical and scoring ability, its low frequency of all-out runs suggests how efficiently the professional players move and manoeuvre the ball.

With regard to positional differences, MF players spent less time in standing and walking than DF and FW players and spent more time jogging than DF and FW players. Midfield players are required to cover a wide area constantly, because they are supposed to support the offence and play an important role in defence: this explains their lower frequency of standing and their higher frequency of jogging bouts compared with defenders and forwards. More motion is expected of MF players than in the other two positions.

Though various kinds of motion are attempted intermittently by players, walking and jogging predominate. This study suggests that it is crucial to train the endurance capacity so that players can move continuously for a full 90 min. On the other hand, momentary motions during periods of high intensity, such as running and sprinting, are also involved in a game of soccer. That is, anaerobic power and anaerobic capacity are also important.

References

Akai, I. (1977) A study of shooting in football games (in Japanese). The Journal of Human and Cultural Sciences, Musasi University, 9, 1-14.

Akai, I. (1978) A study of shooting in football games: 2 (in Japanese). The Journal of Human and Cultural Sciences, Musasi University, 10, 57-72.

Mayhew, S.R. and Wenger, H.A. (1985) Time-motion analysis of professional soccer. J. Human Mov't. Stud., 11,49-52.

Ohashi, J. (1983) The distance moved by players during soccer games at the European/South American Cup and at Japan Vs Korea (in Japanese). Proceedings of Scientific Research Division of Japan Football Association, 53-59.

Reilly, T. and Thomas, V. (1976) A motion analysis of work-rate in different positional roles in professional football match-play, J. Human Mov't. Stud., 2, 87-97.

Togari, H. (1979) The study on work intensity during the playing of soccer (in Japanese). Proceedings of Division of Sport and Medical Research. Japan Sports and Athletic Ass., 285-295.

Yamanaka, K. (1968) A study on game analysis in soccer (in Japanese). Jap. J. Phys. Ed., 13, 271.
Yamaoka, S. (1956) The study on energy metabolism of sports (II) (in Japanese). Jap. J. Phys. Ed., 1, 123-126.

ANALYSIS OF MOVEMENT PATTERNS OF REFEREES DURING SOCCER MATCHES

T. Asami, H. Togari and J. Ohashi
Department of Sports Sciences, College of Arts and Sciences,
University of Tokyo, 3-8-1, Komaba, Meguro-ku, Tokyo, 153, Japan.

Introduction

Presently, soccer matches proceed at a quick tempo, and soccer players are required to move quickly and to cover a wide range on a playing field in the course of a game. Referees, who control such games, are also required to cover a wide range on a playing field while making good judgements. Various time-motion analyses of soccer games have been done (Ohashi and Togari, 1981; Ohta et al., 1969; Reilly and Thomas, 1976; Togari, 1967; Saltin, 1973; Mayhew and Wenger, 1985; Withers et al., 1982) and reports conclude that soccer players travel 8-12km (about 10km on average) during a 90 min competition. However, no data have been collected concerning referees. The purpose of this study was to investigate the movement pattern of referees in soccer games by tracing their movements on a playing field and to obtain data for the consideration of fitness characteristics which are essential to refereeing.

Methods

Six Japanese top class referees (including 4 FIFA registered referees) and 7 foreign FIFA referees were used as subjects. Ten games in the 1st Division of the Japan National Soccer League refereed by Japanese referees and 7 international matches of world class level (including the Toyota Cup) refereed by foreign referees were analyzed.

Tracing methods (Ohta et al., 1969; Togari, 1967) were used for the movement analysis. Movements of the referees were traced on a scaled (1:350) map of a soccer playing field by four well-trained observers. Observations were made from a seat located at the top of the main stand. Every 5 min each sheet was changed for a new one. Thus 9 records of movement were obtained during each of the 1st and the 2nd halves of the game (45 min), resulting in 18 records in total being obtained for a game of 90 min. Fig. 1 shows an example of the movement tracings.

In 11 of the 17 games, movements of the referees were classified into 3 categories - walking, jogging and running.

After the games, the lengths of the traced lines were determined by a curvimeter. Distances covered were totalled for each 15 min period, for each half of the game (45 min), and for every whole

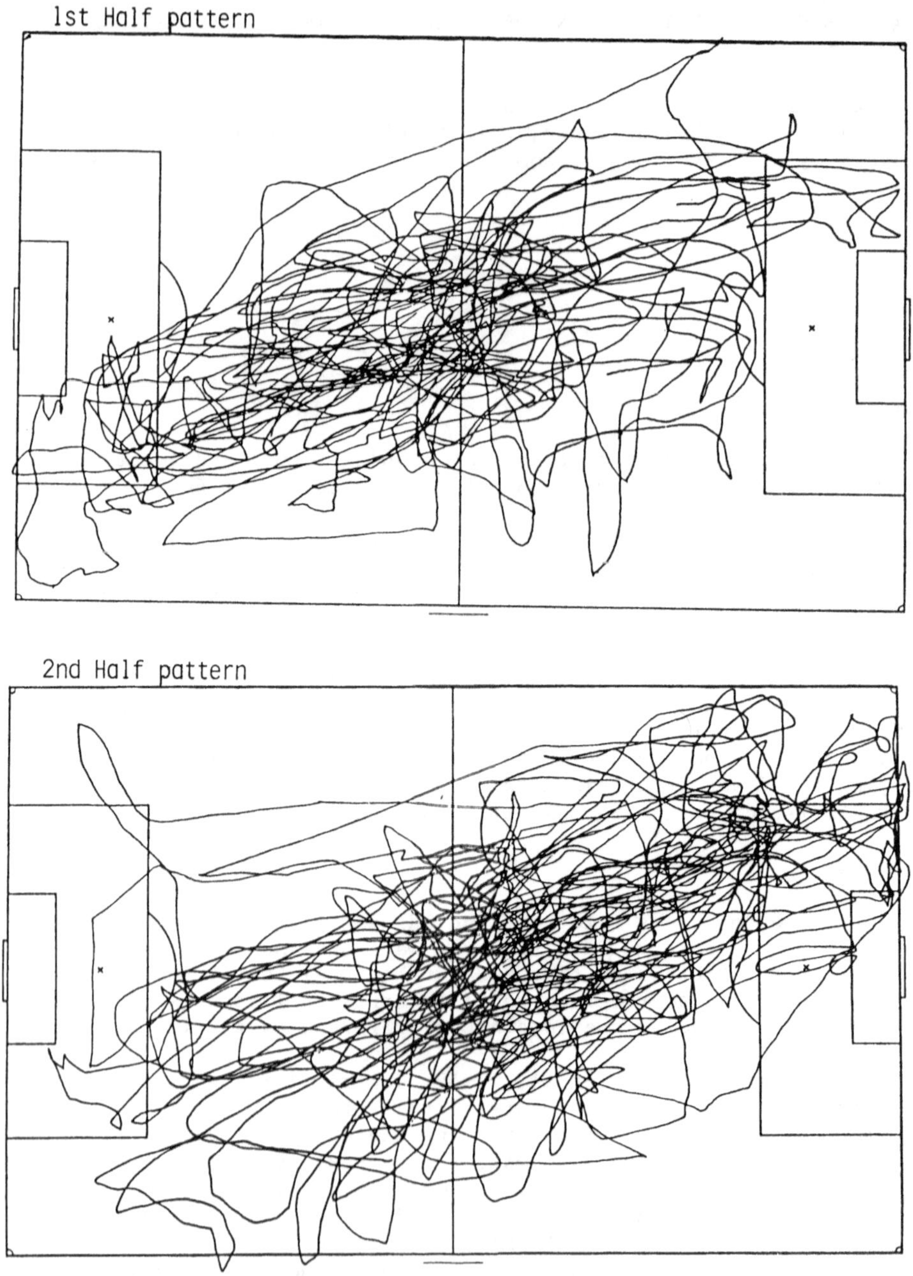

Figure 1. Movement chart of a soccer referee
Referee: Luis P. Siles Calderon; Game: 3rd Toyota European/South American Cup Aston Villa F.C. (England) vs. C.A. Penarol (Uruguay) 0:2 (0:1);
Date: 1982, 12.12.

period (90 min). The mean and standard deviation of each time period were then calculated.

Results and Discussion

Means of distances covered by Japanese referees, foreign referees and the combined subjects during the 1st half, the 2nd half and the whole game are shown in Table 1.

Table 1. Maximum, minimum, mean and SD of distances (m) covered by referees during soccer matches of 17 high level games

	n		1st half	2nd half	Total	Minimum	Maximum
Foreign		mean	4826	4910	9736	8054	10498
referees	7	SD	523	589	1077		
Japanese		mean	4920	5248	10168	8768	11180
referees	10	SD	425	408	756		
Total	17	mean	4881	5109	9990	8054	11180
		SD	470	518	927		

Distances covered in the whole game (90 min) for Japanese and foreign referees ranged from 8-11km with the mean value about 10 km. This value is similar to those of players reported by Ohta et al. (1969), Togari (1967), Reilly and Thomas (1976), Ohashi and Togari (1981) and Withers et al. (1982). The mean distance covered by Japanese referees was a little longer than that of foreign referees in each half (45 min) and whole game period (90 min), but the difference was not statistically significant ($P > 0.10$).

Distances covered in the 2nd half of the games were longer than those of the 1st half both for the Japanese and foreign referees, but the difference was also not statistically significant ($P > 0.10$). Analysis of data for individuals showed that 9 out of 17 referees covered longer distances in the 2nd half than in the 1st half by over 100 m; in another 6, differences in distances between the 1st and the 2nd half were within 100m and only 2 referees covered shorter distances in the 2nd half by over 100m. This result was contrary to the results of studies on soccer players (Ohashi and Togari, 1981; Reilly and Thomas, 1976 and Withers et al., 1982) which showed that distances covered by the players in the 2nd half of the games were shorter than those of the 1st half.

Mean distances of walking, jogging and running in 11 games are shown in Table 2. Jogging shared the highest percentage of 48.5% of the total distance covered, followed by walking (33.8%) and running with a fairly high speed acconted for 17.7%. This result is not much different from that of players reported by Withers et al. (1982). However, Reilly and Thomas (1976) reported that the distance covered cruising and sprinting by players shared 32% of the total distance, a percentage which is larger than that of the present study.

Table 2. Mean and SD of distances covered by referees for each movement criterion in 11 high level soccer games

		1st half	2nd half	Total	%
Walk	mean	1671	1714	3385	33.8
	S.D.	345	281	614	
Jog	mean	2319	2532	4851	48.5
	S.D.	555	441	946	
Run	mean	856	916	1772	17.7
	S.D.	459	374	792	
Total	mean	4846	5162	10008	100.0
	S.D.	471	498	899	
Backward step	mean	544	537	1081	10.8
	S.D.	196	270	434	

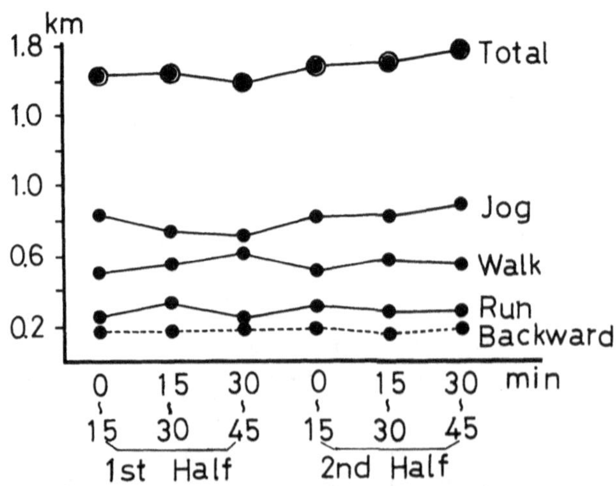

Figure 2. Variation of movement distances for each criterion in process of time

The total distance covered using backward steps in walking, jogging and running was 1081 m per game on average, which accounted for 10.8% of the total distance. This ratio for referees is higher than that for players, (6.4%) as reported by Reilly and Thomas (1976)

and (7.6%) Withers et al. (1982). These results suggest that backward stepping is more important for referees than for players as a component of movement in soccer games.

Variations of distances for each criterion (walking, jogging, running and so on) as the game progresses are shown in Fig. 2. The whole time period of a game (90 min) was divided into consecutive 15 min periods. Distances of jogging and running were apt to decrease and distances for walking were apt to increase in the last 15 min period of the 1st half; however, these decreases and increases were not statistically significant. Variations in distances covered jogging, walking, running, backward steps and total distances among 15 min time periods were rather small. It seems that referees continued to move constantly throughout the whole game.

These results mentioned above suggest that in soccer games, like players, referees are also required to move about throughout the whole game (90 min). Although the distance for sprinting is not as long as that in players, anaerobic physical fitness, as well as aerobic physical fitness is nevertheless essential for referees.

References

Mayhew, S.R. and Wenger, H.A. (1985) Time motion analysis of professional soccer. J. Human Mov't. Stud., 11, 49-52.

Ohashi, J. and Togari, H. (1981) Change of moving distance in football match-play (in Japanese). Proceedings of the Departmentof Physical Education, College of General Education, University ofTokyo, 15, 27-34.

Ohta, T., H. Togari and Y. Komiya (1969) Game analysis of soccer. (in Japanese). Soccer (by Japan Football Association), 92, 31-43.

Reilly, T. and Thomas, V. (1976). A motion analysis of work-rate in different positional roles in professional football match-play.J. Human Mov't. Stud., 2, 87-97.

Saltin, B. (1973) Metabolic fundamentals in exercise. Med. Sci.Sports, 5, 137-146.

Togari, H. (1967) Asian elimination round for Mexico Olympics froma scientific viewpoint (in Japanese). Soccer Magazine, 12, 86-89.

Withers, R.T., Maricic, Z., Wasilewski, S. and Keily, L. (1982)Match analysis of Australian professional soccer players. J. Human Mov't. Stud., 8, 159-176.

SYMMETRY AND ASYMMETRY IN SHOOTING DEMONSTRATED BY ELITE SOCCER PLAYERS

Wlodzimierz Starosta
Institute of Sport, Department of Sports Kinesiology, 01-809 Warsaw, Ceglowska 68/70, Poland.

Introduction

Soccer is a specific sport in which utilization of the upper limbs is minimised by the rules and extremely high demands are made on the lower limbs under variable external conditions. The performer is required to demonstrate good technique and endurance throughout play. In view of the wide range of techniques and tactics in this sport, it is generally believed that top performance may be achieved only by players with great versatility and co-ordination.

The notion of versatility may be interpreted in many ways. Some authors (e.g. Grabda, 1980; Karwowski, 1978; Starosta, 1975, 1986) argued that it involves the ability to use both feet during play. Perhaps that is why in the U.S.S.R. footballers are required to practice precision in shooting at goal with both the right and left foot, in order to achieve sports class awards. It is also worth mentioning that using only the dominant foot during play is a cause of injury to the other foot (Cirok, 1980).

Extensive literature on soccer (e.g. Gagajeva, 1973; Gorski et al., 1978; Reilly, 1979; Reilly and Thomas, 1977; Talaga, 1960, 1978: Thomas and Reilly, 1979) fails to provide a model of versatile technical preparation in which symmetry (or asymmetry) of movement stimulates appropriate concern and debate. It is not known which model of preparation is preferable - uniform development of fitness of both feet or on dominance of one. This study sought an answer to this question, by looking at what happens in practice. It was decided to concentrate on perhaps the most important technique, shooting at goal.

Materials and Methods

Material was based on 298 soccer players, a majority of which (53.4%) were World Championships participants; of these 134 were soccer of the top ten teams of 1978, and 26 were the best scorers of 1986. The other subjects were football league players of the Polish first (n = 121) and third divisions (n = 17). Tests for establishing the dynamic strength of the legs and accuracy of shooting at goal were employed. The main methodology was observation of shots at goal with left and right legs during 29 matches. Precise registration was effected by using a coding system, dividing the soccer field into four areas and having the observations made independently by two investigators. Differentiation of disagreement was resolved by replaying the match on video. The footballers shooting at goal and the place from which this was done were noted.

Results

Polish League

The studies began with observations of 121 players of the Polish 1st Division during 11 matches (Karwowski, 1978; Starosta, 1986). Analysis of the performances in shooting at goal revealed that out of 416 shots, 64.2% were performed with the right foot (39.7% scored), 20.5% with the left foot (13.7% scored) and 15.3% strikes were performed with the head (11.7% scored). In the individual matches (Fig. 1) of the Polish 1st Division (n = 121) the shots with the right and left foot ranged from 27.2% to 87.5% and 4.3% to 50% of all the shots (including heading), respectively. The ability to shoot well with both feet was demonstrated only by a small number of players, including Deyna, Boniek and Szoltysik. Deyna and Boniek were among the best scorers in the 1st Division during the period of observation.

Table 1. Variation on length of kick by advanced soccer players ($\bar{x}$ of three trials) n = 17

Players	Dominant leg	Ball flight length right leg (m)	Ball flight length left leg (m)	Difference in flight length with right and left leg (m)	Difference in flight length with right and left leg %
M.A.	R	43.65	39.85	3.80	8.7
K.R.	R	44.30	38.35	5.95	13.4
B.E.	R	41.35	34.35	7.00	16.9
K.O.	R	48.90	40.50	8.40	17.0
M.I.	R	43.45	33.50	9.95	23.1
S.U.	R	43.35	39.15	6.20	13.7
K.A.	L	39 10	41.40	-2.30	-5.6
K.Ar.	R	39.85	34.70	5.15	12.9
L.A.	R	44.50	37.15	7.35	16.5
G.R.	R	47.15	35.35	11.80	25.0
G.E.	R	39.15	36.20	2.95	7.5
K.R.	R	41.50	33.65	7.85	18.9
A.N.	R	49.85	39.85	10.00	20.1
G.R.	R	39.35	33.25	6.10	15.5
B.A.	R	38.35	35.80	2.55	6.6
J.A.	R	40.50	38.50	2.00	4.9
B.U.	R	37.85	35.30	2.55	6.7
Mean		42.60	36.87	5.73	13.5

The goals scored in proportion to the number of shots performed was adopted as the index of practical effectiveness. This index was

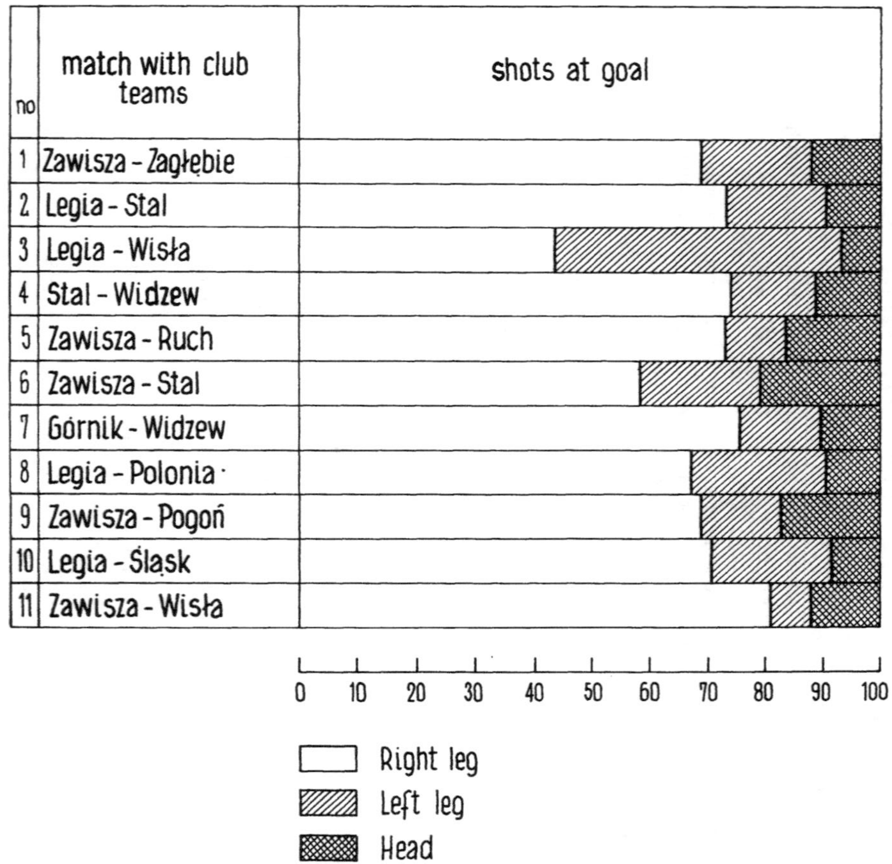

Fig. 1 Shots at goal performed with right leg, left leg and head (%) by players of various Polish First Division teams (n = 121)

Table 2. Analysis of performance of shots at goal and practical effectiveness (ratio of the number of shots to that of goals) of teams marked in order of performance during 1978 World Championships (n = 134)

Team	Number of shots					Number of goals					Practical effectiveness %			
	L	R	H		Total		L	R	H	Total	L	R	H	Total
Argentina	36	28	13	88	5	3	3	11	18.88	10.71	23.07	14.28		
Holland	11	26	11	48		4	1	5	15.38	9.09	10.41			
Brazil	21	47	3	71		7		7		14.89		9.86		
Italy	9	21	8	38			1	1		12.50	2.63			
FRG	3	19	8	30			2	2		25.00	6.66			
Poland	18	69	15		102	1	4	1	6	5.55	5.79	6.66	5.88	
Peru	8	11		19										
Mexico	10	12	4	26		2		2	16.66	7.69				
Tunisia	9	12	5	26		3		3	25.00	11.54				
Sweden	6	7	2	15		1		1	14.28	6.66				
TOTAL	131	252	69		452	6	24	8	38	4.58	9.52	9.52	8.40	

L - left leg; R - right leg; H - head.

lower for the right (61.8%) than for the left foot (66.8%) for all shots from different areas of the field. On the other hand, the values for shots made from the penalty area were similar for both feet (65.7% for the left and 69.9% for the right foot), suggesting great effectiveness for the left foot even in situations demanding immediate action. It may be assumed, therefore, that planned improvement of shooting ability with the left foot may lead to further benefits in performance.

In a specific test measuring the distance covered by the ball after shooting with both feet performed by 17 players, an average difference of almost 6 m was observed: 16 players attained a better result with the right leg and one with the left leg. The range of variation of the dynamic leg strength as indicated by the length of kick (Table 1) suggests a possibility of attaining a similar proficiency in both legs. The test of accuracy in shooting at goal, performed twice, revealed that the right leg was more accurate in 12 players, while 5 players demonstrated identical values for both feet. Variation between limbs reached 28.1% in favour of the right leg. In summary, the results obtained during observations of Polish players suggest functional differences of lower extremities probably resulting from the orientation of training. During competition, utilization of the right leg in movements associated with strength was predominant. High values for the left leg were obtained only in situations under constraint - while carrying out an immediate strike from close to goal, even in cases of the top players.

1978 World Cup

Further interesting information on functional symmetry and asymmetry of soccer players (Grabda, 1980; Starosta, 1986) was obtained from analysis of shots at goal made at the 1978 World Championships: 134 finalists of the best teams were observed during 44.5 hours in 18 matches. Out of a total of 452 shots (Table 2), 252 were performed with the right leg (55.8%), 131 with the left leg (29.0%) and 69 with the head (15.2%). As many as 94.5% shots with the left leg were missed. Among the top teams, the highest index of effectiveness (the ratio of goals to shots) was demonstrated by players of Argentina, Holland, Federal Republic of Germany, Brazil and Poland. The most successful right-footed players were the members of the Dutch (15.3%), Brazilian (14.8%) and Argentinian (10.7%) teams. At the same time, the Argentinian team demonstrated the highest index of practical effectiveness of left-footed players (13.8%) and therefore total effectiveness of the right and left leg.

Analysis of the effectiveness of shots made from different areas of the field (Table 3) showed that the highest effectiveness of shots with the right leg from the penalty area was demonstrated by the players of Brazil (68.4%) and Poland (38.2%) and in the case of shots with the left foot - by the teams of Argentina (29.7%) and Holland (22.2%) who met in the final. A high index of effectiveness of left-footed players may have been instrumental in the ultimate success of the teams.

The corresponding values for shots made from the middle area of the field showed that the team of the Federal Republic of Germany was foremost (100%) in terms of shots made with the right foot, the

Table 3. Analysis of performance of shots at goal during 1978 World Championships according to the field area n = 134

	Team	Total	penalty area L	R	H	Total	middle area L	R	Total	peripheral areas L	R	Total
1	ARG	77	11	13	13	37	24	14	38	1	1	2
2	HOL	48	4	3	11	18	7	23	30			
3	BRA	71	3	13	3	19	11	36	47	2	3	5
4	ITA	38	3	5	8	16	6	14	20		2	2
5	FRG	30	3	3	8	14		12	12		4	4
6	POL	102	6	13	15	34	11	53	64		4	4
7	PER	19	2	3		5	6	4	10		4	4
8	MEX	26	2	3	4	9	5	8	13	1	3	4
9	TUN	26	1	5	5	11	7	6	13	1	1	2
10	SWE	15	2	1	2	5	5	3	8	1	1	1
	Total	452	37	62	69	168	82	173	255	6	23	29
	%	100	8.2	13.7	15.2	37.1	18.1	38.3	56.4	1.3	5.1	6.4

Shots performed with left leg (L) and right leg (R); H - Heading the ball.

Argentinian team with the left foot. The latter team obtained a very high effectiveness index (63.2%), almost three times as high as that of the next team (23%). The shots made from the peripheral areas of the field were considerably less effective.

The members of the teams of Poland, Peru, Italy, Federal Republic of Germany used only the right leg, while those of Argentina (50%) and Brazil (40%) frequently also used the left foot. The victorious team, Argentina, had the highest number of missed shots (85.7%) and, at the same time, scored the highest number of goals, i.e. eleven (left foot, 45.5%; right foot, 27.3%). The Argentinian and Dutch teams included outstanding players who used their left foot (Table 4). In the winning team Passarella had 8 shots with the left foot, Kempes had 20 shots with his left foot and 1 shot with the right foot. Kempes was the top scorer of the Championships and made a significant contribution to the success of his team. It is possible that his individual play as the left-sided striker was crucial for his high effectiveness. The left-footed specialist of the Dutch team was Rensenbrink: he had 6 shots with the right and 2 shots with the left foot and was ranked second best on the list of scorers.

The Argentinian (Olguin, Bertoni, Ortis, Larros, Houseman, Luque) and Dutch (Rep, R. and W. van de Kerkhof, Hann, Poortvliet) players demonstrated a high level of symmetry by being two-footed. Their versatility, permitting varied technical and tactical actions, might have been of importance for the success of their teams in the World Championships.

Table 4. Shots with the right and left leg performed by the top football players - scorers of the 1978 World Championships (n = 30)

Player	Country	Number of shots performed with rt.leg	Number of shots performed with left leg	% ratio of shots performed with rt.leg	% ratio of shots performed with left leg	number of games	dominant leg R	dominant leg L
Kempes	ARG	1	20	4.8	95.2	6		+
Rensenbrink	HOL	2	6	25.0	75.0	5		+
Luque	ARG	7	1	87.5	12.5	4	+	
Rep	HOL	2	1	66.7	33.3	3	+	
Rummenige	FRG	3		100.0		3	+	
Roberto	BRA	8	3	72.7	27.3	3	+	
Dirceu	BRA	2	4	33.3	66.7	3		+
Boniek	POL	9		100.0		2	+	
Lato	POL	7	3	70.0	30.0	2	+	
Flohe	FRG	1	1	50.0	50.0	2	+	+
Rossi	ITA	2		100.0		2	+	
Bettega	ITA	5		100.0		2	+	
Nelinho	BRA	4	1	80.0	20.0	2	+	
Brandts	HOL	2		100.0		2	+	
Haan	HOL	10	1	90.9	9.1	2	+	
Passarella	ARG		8			1		+
Tarantini	ARG	1		100.0		1	+	
Houseman	ARG	5	1	83.3	16.6	1	+	
Reinaldo	BRA	4	3	57.1	42.9	1	+	
Zico	BRA	6		100.0		1	+	
Tardelli	ITA	3	1	75.0	25.0	1	+	
Zaccarelli	ITA	2		100.0		1	+	
Causio	ITA	2	2	50.0	50.0	1	+	+
Szarmach	POL	5	5	50.0	50.0	1	+	+
Deyna	POL	26	4	86.7	13.3	1	+	
Abramczik	FRG	1		100.0		1	+	
Holzenbein	FRG	1		100.0		1	+	
Van de Kerkhof W.	HOL	4	1	80.0	20.0	1	+	
Van de Kerkhof R.	HOL	1	1	50.0	50.0	1	+	+
Poortvliet	HOL	1	1	50.0	50.0	1	+	+
Mean		4.4	3.4	74.6	41.8	1.9	70.0	13.3

Note: Only those football players whose motor abilities were recorded during observations are included in the table RL - 16.7%

Table 5. Proportion of left-legged players among the top scorers of the 1986 World Championships, n = 26

Player	Country	number of games	dominant leg R	L	R	L
Lineker	ENG	6	–		5	
Butragueno	ESP	5	–			
Careca	BRA	5		–		
Maradona	ARG	5		–		4
Altobelli	ITA	4		–		
Bielanow	URS	4	–			
Elkjer-Larsen	DEN	4		–		
Valdano	ARG	4		–		
Ceulemans	BEL	3	–			
Claesen	BEL	3	–			
Olsen	DEN	3		–		
Voeller	FRG	3	–			
Allofs	FRG	2		–		
Burruchaga	ARG	2	–			
Cabanas	PAR	2	–			
Caldero	ESP	2		–		
Jaremczuk	URS	2	–			
Josimar	BRA	2	–			
Khari	MAR	2		–		2
Papin	FRA	2	–			
Platini	FRA	2		–		2
Quirarte	MEX	2	–			
Romero	PAR	2	–			
Scifo	BEL	2		–		
Socrates	BRA	2	–		1	
Stopyra	FRA	2	–			
n			15	11		
%			57.7	42.3		

The greatest number of players who shot with both feet was in the Argentinian team - 7 out of 11 shots at goal. Other teams also had a number of such players (Holland, 6; Poland, 7; Italy, 5; Brazil, 6). The proportion of shots with both feet was varied. Some players (16.7%) demonstrated ability in using both feet with equal efficiency (Flohe of the Federal Republic of Germany, Causio of Italy, Szarmach of Poland, R. van de Kerkhof and Poortvliet of Holland). Altogether, as many as 66.7% top scorers of the 1978 World Championships performed shots with the left foot (66.7%). As regards left-footed players, as many as 75% performed shots with the right foot (Table 4). This suggests that technical versatility of top players may be developed on the basis of using both feet; at the same time the existence of the dominant foot should not be excluded.

1986 World Cup

Similar, though less detailed observations, made during the 1986 World Championships (Table 5) suggest an increasing number of left-footed players, among 26 top scorers they accounted for 11 (42.3%). The ability to use both feet, with the right dominant (e.g. Butragueno, Ceulemans) and left leg dominant (e.g. Allofs, Platini) was also observed. However, the material available does not confirm the changes in the symmetry of football shots, i.e. its increase or decrease.

Conclusions and Recommendations

These observations suggest that development of symmetry in a shooting should be included in the preparation of top world soccer teams. In this respect practice is ahead of theory, since the literature on the subject has neglected the analysis of symmetry in technique and lacks the essential evidence for developing appropriate models. This descriptive study is an attempt to start filling the gap.

These observations also show the higher efficiency of shots at goal performed by the left-footed players, resulting from different motor abilities to which their right-footed counterparts are unable to adapt themselves rapidly enough. Ambidexterous players demonstrated even higher efficiency, using this feature of versatility not only as a technical but also as a tactical factor.

The main recommendation is that basic technical elements should be developed symmetrically at all stages of sports instruction. Part of the training time, especially during the preparatory period, should be devoted to technical improvement of the 'poorer' foot with due attention being paid to regularity, proper assignment of tasks, their regular control and evaluation of performance.

In the course of improving performance of the dominant foot, the efficiency of the support leg should be also maintained. One of the methods of improving the 'weaker foot' may be to play in a position which forces the player to use the other foot e.g. a right-footed player has to play on the left wing of the attack.

Selection of candidates for various stages of sports instruction should give preference to left-footed players. Each team should benefit from including two or three such players, especially at the highest levels of performance.

References

Cirok, L. (1980) Lateralita ako jeden z limitujúcich faktorov úrazovosti vo futbale. Teor. Praxe tel. Vych., 28, 239-243.
Fidelus, K. (1982) Zastosowanie biomechaniki do analizy skutecznosci treningu w pilce noznej. Sport Wyczynowy, 11, 3-10.
Gagajeva, G.M. (1973) Psychologia gry w pilke nozna. Warszawa: Sport i Turystyka.
Gorski, K., Jakusyn, M., Kaćalin, G., Simonian, N. (1978) Porady trenerów. Kraków: Sport i Turystyka.
Grabda, M. (1980) Analiza techniki gry czolowych druzyn świata w pilce noznej z punktu widzenia symetrii i asymetrii czynnościowej. Praca magisterska. Biala Podlaska: Filia AWF.
Karwowski, A. (1978) Analiza akcji ofensywnych w pilce noznej z punku widzenia symetrii i asymetrii ruch. Praca magisterska. Biala Podlaska: Filia AWF.
Kowal, H. and Zuchora, K. (1962) Asymetria morfologiczna, dynamiczna i czynnosciowa u pilkarzy w wieku 14-18 lat. Kultura Fizyczna, 11, 835-839.
Klyszejko, W. (1961) Proba analizy skutecznosci akcji ofensywnych w pilce noznej. Kultura Fizyczna, 9, 631-638.
Reilly, T. (1979) What Research tells the Coach about Soccer. Washington: AAHPERD.
Reilly, T. and Thomas, V. (1977) Effects of a program of pre-season training on the fitness of soccer players. Journal of Sports Med. Phys. Fit., 17, 401-412.
Starosta, W. (1975). Symetria i asymetria ruchu w sporcie. Warszawa: Sport i Turystyka.
Starosta, W. (1982) Symetryzacja ruchów mlodych zawodników jako element mistrzostwa sportowego. Miedzynarodowa Konferencja Naukowa "Wychowanie fizyczne i sport dzieci i mlodziezy". Wybrane materialy. Warszawa: AWF, 147-159.
Starosta, W. (1983) Movement coordination as a sport selection element. In: Genetics of Psychomotor Traits in Man. Int. Soc. Sport Gen. Somat. Warszawa: PWN, 247-271.
Starosta, W. (1984) Movement symmetrization as a method of coordination improvement in children. International Congress 'Child and Sport', Urbino.
Starosta, W. (1986) Symmetria und asymmetrie der Sporttechnik in Manschaftsspielen. In: Beitrage zur Sportspielforschung (edited by R. Andresen) pp.100-113. Ahrensburg bei Hamburg: Verlag Ingrid Czwalina.
Starosta, W. (1986) Simmetria ed asimmetria della tecnica dei giochi sportivi. Rivista di Cultura Sportiva, 6, 11-17.
Talaga, J. (1960) Próba analizy strzalu na bramke w pilkarskich rozgrywkach I ligi. Kultura Fizycyzna, 7/8, 556-565.
Talaga, J. (1974) Pilka nozna. Warszawa: Sport i Turystyka.
Talaga, J. (1978) Rozwazania nad wspolczesna pilka nozna. Kultura Fizyczna, 5, 196-202.
Thomas, V. and Reilly, T. (1979) Fitness assessment of English League soccer players throughout the competitive season. Brit. J. Sport Med., 13, 103-109.

RELIABILITY OF VIDEO OBSERVATION OF INDIVIDUAL TECHNIOUES USED IN SOCCER

Pekka Luhtanen
Department of Biology of Physical Activity, University of Jyvaskyla, SF 40100, Jyvaskyla, Finland.

Introduction

In ball games, players can move with or without the ball with varying patterns of motion. These actions vary in duration, space, speed, direction, technique used, and the tactical goal: thus each ball contact by a player can be considered as a random skill test. The skill output of such tests can be evaluated using video recording and written instructions for coding the actions with respect to technique used, duration, speed and direction.

Analyses of video recordings have been used to study game actions in soccer both qualitatively and quantitatively (Dufour, 1982; Withers et al., 1982). The distance covered by the player without the ball has been evaluated in terms of his mode of motion, speed, direction and the purpose of movement (Mayhew and Wenger, 1985; Reilly and Thomas, 1976; Withers et al., 1982).

Multiple correlation coefficients between two observations have been used to estimate reliability and objectivity. The reliability coefficient in one study was 0.966 for evaluating walking, 0.962 for jogging, 0.915 for sub-maximal running, and 0.971 for sprinting (Reilly and Thomas, 1976). Objectivity in establishing the distance covered was examined by regression analysis where the distances were calculated using two different methods. The coefficient of objectivity was found to be 0.970.

Establishing reliability in running at sub-maximal and maximal velocities seems to be most difficult. The product moment correlation coefficients between two observers were 0.745 for sub-maximal and 0.813 for maximal running in the study of Withers et al (1982). The other reliability correlations were greater than 0.904.

In an analysis of the mode of motion by Mayhew and Wenger (1985) the coefficients of reliability and objectivity were 0.97 and 0.95, respectively. The different individual techniques used in soccer matches and the reliability of establishing these measurements have not been reported in the literature. Therefore, the purpose of this study was to determine the level of agreement between two observers about the techniques used and the player's movements when controlling the ball during play.

Methods

Two Finnish national level junior teams (under eleven years) participated in this study. They played one official match, nine players per team with two halves of 20 min, and rules relevant to their age. The players were identified according to their colours, numbers and special tape markers on their socks. The size of the field was 70 m x 50 m: it was divided into coordinates (x, y) with 10 m x 10 m squares for localization of the players and the ball (± 2.5 m).

All actions with the ball in the match were recorded with a Hitachi VHS colour video camera recorder, which included a timer (± 0.04 s), from a height of 12 m and a distance of 25 m from the halfway line. Using video playback, slow motions and still frames of the skill manoeuvres, two trained assistants coded the second half of the match on a data sheet according to written instructions (Luhtanen et al., 1986). The technical aspects examined were receiving, passing, dribbling, shooting, scoring, tackling, and dead ball situations for all players. These were analyzed with respect to the team, player, position, location on the field, time spent in a single manoeuvre, technique used, speed, and direction of the manoeuvre. These aspects of the different skills were divided into categories which have been reported in detail before (Luhtanen et al., 1986). The numbers of these categories for each of the skills are shown in Table 1.

Table 1. Numbers of the categories of the selected variables in different manoeuvres

	Skill manoeuvres				
Variable	Receiving	Passing	Dribbling	Shooting	Goalkeeping
Technique used	9	9	4	6	7
Speed of player	4	4	4	5	5
Direction	4	4	4	10	6
Result of manoeuvre	6	9	8	5	6

The variable termed 'Result of manoeuvre' is defined as the classified alternatives available when receiving, passing, dribbling, shooting or goalkeeping has been performed successfully or unsuccessfully. When measuring passing distances, intervals of 5 m were used.

The coded data were processed with a UNIVAC 1100 computer. The reliability coefficients were calculated as Pearson Product Moment correlations between two independent observers using the numbers of the classified data (n_{ij}) as observation values (Table 2). The significance of the correlations was examined using a t-test of the independent correlation coefficients. For the statistical analysis, SPSS software was used.

Table 2. Number of observations in the different categories of the variables

Observer	Category of variable 1	2	3	j
i=1	n_{11}	n_{12}	n_{13}	n_{1j}
i=2	n_{21}	n_{22}	n_{23}	n_{2j}

Results

The total match included more than 600 separate manoeuvres. The second half involved 302 and 305 manoeuvres coded per observer. The total amount of trials in different manoeuvres were:- receiving 264, passing 208, dribbling 40, shooting 8, goalkeeping 15, and dead ball situations 33.

Identification of the players and all the dead ball situations was complete. The coefficient of reliability for the distance of the passes was 0.674 ($P < 0.001$). Selected coefficients of reliability and their statistical significance are shown in Table 3.

The observations were in complete agreement when evaluating directions of the ball for receiving, passing, and goalkeeping, and result of the manoeuvres in shooting. The lowest coefficients of reliability were for evaluating the speed of the players in receiving, passing, and shooting. For localization of the players and ball the coefficients of reliability were 0.968 ($P < 0.001$) for field players and 0.807 ($P < 0.01$) for goalkeepers.

Table 3. The reliability coefficients between two observers when evaluating selected variables in different manoeuvres

Variable	Receiving	Passing	Dribbling	Shooting	Goalkeeping
Technique used	.997[c]	.998[c]	.997[c]	.982[b]	.884[b]
Speed of player	.640	.784	.987[b]	.783 (d)	.825[b]
Direction of ball	1.000[c]	1.000[c]	.986[b]	.663 (d)	1.000[c]
Result of Manoeuvre	.990[c]	.998[c]	.999[c]	1.000 (a)	.962[b]

Significance levels: (a) $P < 0.05$, (b) $P < 0.01$, (c) $P < 0.001$.

Discussion

The validation of the methods used for estimating output of skill manoeuvres required the establishment of its reliability or objectivity. The research design entailed the comparison, manoeuvre by manoeuvre and variable by variable, between two estimates of performance according to pre-established criteria. These variables were defined before the measurements were made in this study (Luhtanen et al., 1986). According to the written guidelines, two observers coded all the manoeuvres when players were working with the ball. The difference between the totals of the detected manoeuvres was only 1%. In dribbling, shooting and goalkeeping there were no differences between observers. Thus, the problem of the reliability was not in the quantity of the detected manoeuvres but more in the evaluation of quality in the classified variables.

The reliability coefficients were greatest when evaluating the direction of the ball in receiving, passing and goalkeeping. The reliability coefficient for shooting was not high because of the precise division in scaling and the low number of shots. Collecting data from several matches may increase its reliability.

In evaluating the technique used and the result of the manoeuvres in receiving, passing, dribbling, shooting and goalkeeping, the reliability coefficients were highly significant. This meant the structure in the classification of these variables was acceptable.

The lowest reliability coefficients were found in evaluating the speed of the players especially in receiving, passing, and shooting. This was due to the difficulties in evaluating the running speed during striding or sprinting. Additionally, the speed, either accelerating or decelerating, might have been correct at the critical ball contact phase, which meant the transition phase from striding to sprinting was incorrectly evaluated. During the phases of constant speed these problems did not often exist. In previous reports (Reilly and Thomas, 1976; Withers et al., 1982); Mayhew and Wenger 1985) the reliability coefficients have been higher than in the present study. The reason might lie in the longer sampling times for evaluating individual motions divided into walking, jogging, striding, and sprinting. The method used for assessing the speed of players during manoeuvres could be improved if the observers could know the relation between running speed, step frequency and step length characteristics of each player.

In conclusion, the results indicated that observing skills in soccer with video is reliable as far as the techniques used, direction of the ball, and result of the skill manoeuvres are concerned, but is less reliable in assessing the speed of the players during different manoeuvres. The research methodology introduced could be useful in evaluating the developemnt of individual and team skills in match conditions.

Acknowledgement

This research has been carried out by the grant from the Finnish Ministry of Education.

References

Dufour, W. (1982) Les proceeds, d' objectivation du compartment, moteur le scouting en football. Paper presented at the 1st World Congress of Biological Sciences Applied to Football, Barcelona.

Luhtanen, P., Nieminen, K., Helimaki, E., Westerlund, E. and Makinen, P. (1986) Qualitative and quantitative analysis of team games by computer. Series A 19, 1-54. University of Jyvaskyla, Department of Physical Education, Jyvaskyla, Finland.

Mayhew, S.R. and Wenger, M.A. (1985) Time motion analysis of professional soccer. J. Human Mov't. Stud., 11, 49-52.
Reilly, T. and Thomas, V. (1976) A motion analysis of work-rate in different positional roles in professional football match play. J. Human Mov't. Stud., 2, 87-97.
Withers, R.T., Maricic, Z., Wasilewski, S. and Kelly, L. (1982) Match analysis of Australian professional soccer players. J. Human Mov't. Stud., 8, 159-178.

Part VIII

Match analysis: World Cup soccer 1986

COMPARISON OF PATTERNS OF PLAY OF SUCCESSFUL AND UNSUCCESSFUL TEAMS IN THE 1986 WORLD CUP FOR SOCCER.

M. Hughes, K. Robertson and A. Nicholson
Department of Sport and Recreation Studies, Liverpool Polytechnic, Byrom Street, Liverpool L3 3AF, England.

Introduction

The need for accurate and objective feedback has been well researched and documented (e.g. Franks et al., 1983). Notation systems have been utilised in a number of sports (Downey, 1973; Reilly and Thomas, 1976; Sanderson, 1983). The development of the microcomputer has led to rapid, objective 'easy-to-use' systems that can produce large amounts of data post-event (Franks et al., 1983; Franks and Goodman, 1986; Hughes, 1985a; 1985b). Recent work on soccer by Church and Hughes(1987) reported elsewhere at this Congress, demonstrated that Liverpool F.C. in the 1986 season played in the same pattern whether winning or losing. Different teams may therefore have their own unique pattern of play. There is some debate within the game about the significance of the observation that the majority of goals are scored from three-pass attacking moves. Although this statistic is a result of an analysis of attacking moves only, its interpretation has promoted a particular style of play (Reep and Benjamin, 1968). This study set out to differentiate between successful and unsuccessful teams by examining the main characteristics of their play when in possession of the ball.

Methods

Successful teams were defined as those that reached the semi-finals of the 1986 World Cup. Unsuccessful teams were those eliminated after the first round pool of matches at the Mexico World Cup finals. The eight matches of the successful teams were balanced as much as possible with those of the unsuccessful teams, in terms of wins and losses and also with respect to playing in 'pool' matches compared to playing in the knockout matches of the later rounds.

A BBC microcomputer was used in conjunction with a concept keyboard as an easier way to input information into the computer. An overlay was used delineating the pitch into 18 positional cells; each penalty area was further divided into four sub-cells. For ease of interpretation, the length of the pitch was also divided into six strips, each containing three positional cells. The players were identified by shirt numbers and the play described by the variables shown in Table 1.

Table 1. The 24 action variables and their relevant code for the concept keyboard

Action Variable	Code on Concept Keyboard
Goalkeeper - kick	GK
Goalkeeper - throw	GT
Goalkeeper - save	GS
Goalkeeper - catch	GC
Foul	FOUL
Dribble	DRIB
Run	RUN
Clear	CLEAR
Pass	PASS
Lost possession	LOST POSS
Throw in	THROW IN
Free kick	FREE KICK
Corner	CORNER
Penalty	PEN
Shot	SHOT
Shot : high	HIGH
Shot : wide	WIDE
Shot : blocked	BLOCK'D
Shot : rebound	REB
Saved	SAV'D
Goal	GOAL
End of possession	END POSS
Crosses	CROSSES
Headed	HEADED BALLS

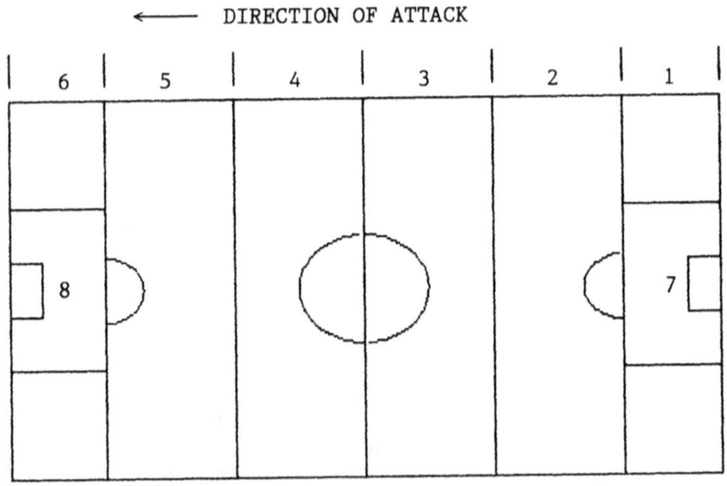

Figure 1. Diagram showing the sub-divisons of the pitch

These areas started with '1' in defence and progressing to '6' in attack, as shown in Fig. 1. In addition, the two penalty areas were examined separately as areas of special interest; these were denoted areas of '7' (central defence) and '8' (central attack). The software developed aggregated the eight matches and printed out the frequencies of each of the variables on representations of the pitch. Chi-square analysis was used to test for levels of significance in the differences of the frequency distributions.

Results and Discussion

Pictorial representations of all 24 variables on the computer facilitated interpretation of the data. For the sake of brevity a summary of the significant results is presented in Table 2.

It is not surprising that unsuccessful teams took more goal kicks than successful teams; this was supported by the observation that the successful teams had significantly more shots at goal. The differences in the distribution of fouls for the two sets of teams showed more fouls occurring out on the wings for the unsuccessful teams. This was probably due to the fact that the unsuccessful teams dribbled and ran with the ball out of defence towards the wings. The successful teams drove up the middle of the pitch, while the unsuccessful teams were forced to play up the flanks.

Table 2. Comparison of action variables that had significant differences in frequency distributions for successful and unsuccessful teams

	Area of pitch with significant differences	Successful Teams			Unsuccessful Teams		
		Left Wing	Centre	Right Wing	Left Wing	Centre	Right Wing
Goal kick	1^b	1	94	1	3	164	1
Foul	2^a	3	9	2	6	1	7
Dribble	3^b	8	13	7	11	10	14
Run	2^b	27	38	20	38	29	44
Run	3^a	47	53	28	32	39	47
Pass	2^a	110	239	117	169	239	157
Pass	3^b	126	280	105	104	274	198
Pass	4^b	124	265	122	195	200	161
Pass	5^b	76	166	63	80	101	101
Lost Possession	1^b	3	4	1	7	1	6
Lost Possession	6^a	14	41	15	22	60	30
Shots	Attack Pen.Area	-	50	-	-	21	-

KEY a: $P < 0.05$
b: $P < 0.01$

This playing 'up the middle' was further reinforced by the observation on passes originating from areas '2' - '5' of the pitch. The pass distribution patterns showed clearly that the successful teams dominated the centre of the field. Unsuccessful teams showed patterns of passes out to the wings more as they approached goal.

Results indicated a significant pattern in lost possessions, these being the defending and attacking 'sixths' of the pitch. It was in these critical areas that unsuccessful teams lost significantly more possession.

The touches of the ball per possession were aggregated over 15 min periods of the match. Both sets of teams showed a drop in touches per possession in the mid-third of each half. The average number of touches per possession (5.59) was significantly higher for the successful teams ($P < 0.01$) than that of the unsuccessful teams (5.22). Successful teams, seemingly played more possession football than unsuccessful teams. Top teams that have sufficient players to sustain controlled possession can afford to play with the ball and wait for a dislocation in the defensive formation before using a longer or quicker 'through ball' as a tactical variation. For coaches or sports scientists, to suggest that teams should in the main aim to restrict their possessions to three successive passes, or less, would therefore seem a simplistic approach to winning.

A summary of the main observations is as follows:-

i) Successful teams played significantly more touches of the ball per possession than unsuccessful teams.

ii) The unsuccessful teams ran with the ball and dribbled the ball in their own defensive area in different patterns to the successful teams. The latter played up the middle in their own half, the former used the wings more.

iii) This pattern was also reflected in the passing of the ball. The successful teams approached the final sixth of the pitch by playing predominantly in the central areas while the unsuccessful teams played significantly more to the wings.

iv) Unsuccessful teams lost possession of the ball significantly more in the final sixth of the playing area both in attack and defence.

v) Successful teams had significantly more shots from within the penalty area than had the unsuccessful; this difference was not observed when shots from outside the penalty area were examined.

References

Church, S. and Hughes, M. (1987) A computerised approach to soccer notation analysis. First World Congress of Science and Football Abstracts (Liverpool), April 1987, pp. 20.

Downey, J.C. (1973) Winning Badminton Singles. Wakefield: E.P. Publishing

Franks, I.M. and Goodman, D. (1986) A systematic approach to analysing sports performance. J. Sports Sci., 4, 49-59.

Franks, I.M., Goodman, D. and Miller, G. (1983) Analysis of performance: qualitative or quantitative? Science Periodical on Research and Technology in Sport, GY-1. Ottawa: Coaching Association of Canada.
Hughes, M.D. (1985a) Patterns of squash at higher competitive levels. J. Sports Sci., 4, 225-226.
Hughes, M.D. (1985b) A comparison of the patterns of play of squash. In: Ergonomics International 85 (edited by I.D. Brown, R. Goldsmith, K. Coombes and M.A. Sinclair), pp.139-141. London: Taylor and Francis.
Reep, C. and Benjamin, B. (1968) Skill and chance in association football. J. Roy. Stat. Soc. Series A, 131, 581-585.
Reilly, T. and Thomas, V. (1976) A motion analysis of work-rate in different positional roles in professional football match play. J. Human Mov't. Stud., 2, 87-97.
Sanderson, F.H. (1983) A notation system for analysing squash matches. Phys. Ed. Rev., 6, 19-23.

A NEW APPROACH TO THE VIDEO ANALYSIS OF TACTICAL ASPECTS OF SOCCER

W. Winkler
Institut für Sportwissenschaften, Georg-August-Universität Göttingen, Sprangerweg 2, 3400 Göttingen, West Germany.

Introduction

Football training is a process which must be based on methodical, pedagogical and psychological considerations. These are applied according to the aims of the trainer and players. The main goal is to develop and improve each player's abilities within a team framework, as well as his psychological stability.

The aim of coaching is based on and encompasses the realisation of external factors, complementary information (e.g. information about sources of error in the last game and, if possible, through replay of video sequences, information about the next opponent),the avoidance of destructive elements (e.g. too much alcohol, poor diet or the avoidance of destructive criticism) and systematic observation and evaluation. Needless to say, the main emphasis is placed on "feed back" from all possible sources, through systematic game analysis (Fig. 1).

Systematic game analysis may only be possible if: i) the aims of the observation are clearly defined; ii) appropriate methods of observation are applied, including the use of technical aids (such as video equipment and computer facilities; iii) a viable means of evaluating the observation is developed and then applied, e.g. computerised fixation of the mean of all relevant points with regard to each player's range of action (Winkler, 1985); iv) the results are presented in the form of video sequences, computer plotted materials, e.g. figures, graphs and tables; v) the results are interpreted, then stored for later reference. In the following sections two aspects of a systematic approach to game analysis will be described. Observations are based on the 1986 World Cup Final in Mexico.

Methods

Analysis of the team's system of play

To gain insight into tactical aspects of soccer matches various methods of observation have been developed. These have previously been described in the literature (Winkler, 1984 and 1985). If something is to be said about the system of play of a team, each individual player's range of action must be studied. A player's range of action during any given time span can be determined by noting down the number corresponding to the minute of play

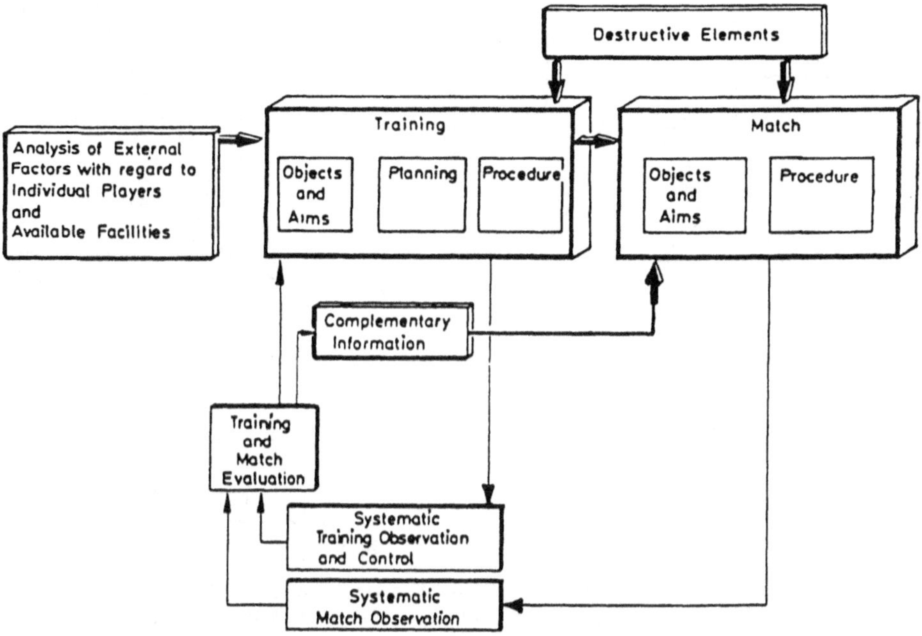

Figure 1. Model of control and regulation for the independent relationship between football training and match play

(superimposed on the video-tape) at the point on the diagram of the field which corresponds to the player's exact location. If at that point in time the player has the ball, the number is circled. If he dribbles less than 10 m, the number is noted at the half-way point. For longer runs, the start and end points are noted. The same holds true for movements without the ball. Figure 2 (a and b) show Burruchaga's range of action from the 1st - 30th minute in comparison to his range of action from the 1st - 45th minute in the 1986 World Cup final. The similarity is obvious. Therefore, it is only necessary to show the ranges of action of the players from the 1st - 30th minute. A range of action is the result of several factors:

i) a basic system (e.g. 4 - 4 - 2);
ii) tactical measures (e.g. standard situations, variation of a player's function) agreed upon before and during a game;
iii) chance, which of course is dependent upon the opponent, at least in part.

Taken as a whole the ranges of action form an objective basis for the concept of a system of play. A system of play can be defined as the way in which a team actually distributed the ranges of action among its individual players on the field. A mean value of all points noted for a particular player can either be estimated or better still calculated by finding the mean value of all co-ordinates.

The distribution of these focal points can be used to graphically

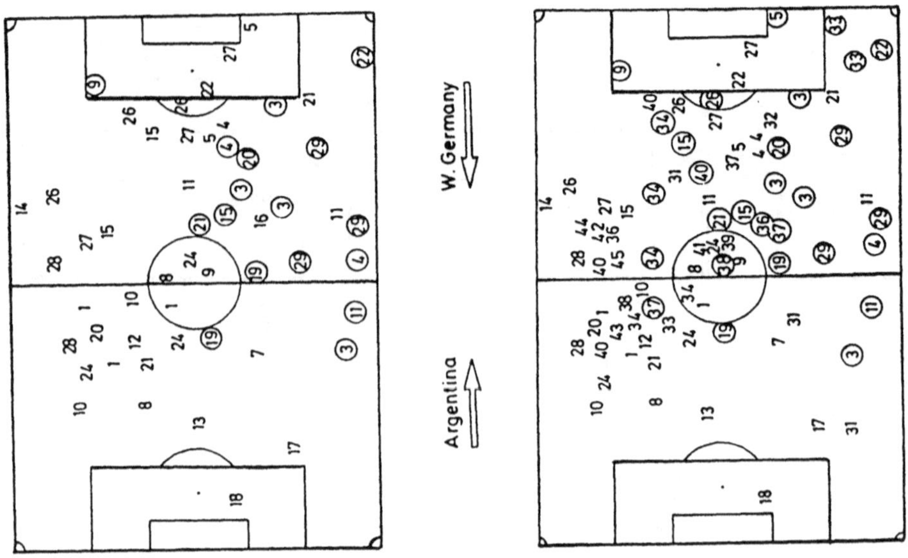

(a) (b)

Figure 2. Burruchaga's range of action in the 1986 World Cup final 1986 for a) 1st-30th minute; b) 1st 45th minute

depict a team's system by placing each player, i.e. his name and number, at his respective point on the field diagram. This in turn presents us with the possibility of describing the system with a combination of numbers. It is not always possible, however, to label the resulting groups (i.e. groups of players whose focal points are either in different areas in their own half of the field or in the opponent's half of the field) with a definite set of numbers, e.g. '1-2-4-3' because the ordering of the groups is often a question of personal interpretation.

Analysis of the defensive behaviour of both teams

In order to be able to describe the defensive behaviour of the players on both teams during each offensive attack, observations were made as to which offensive players came into contact (in the broadest sense of the word) with which defensive player(s), either consecutively or concurrently. The percentages representing the frequency of contact between two players were recorded. Unfortunately, the data do not provide enough information about the actual and intentional 'marking - behaviour' of a defensive player because the percentages can also be the result of unintentional contacts with defensive players who are momentarily covering for team-mates.

Therefore, the percentage of times a defensive player directly defends against or attacks all offensive players was noted. These figures help identify the offensive player(s) that is(are) of interest for a particular defensive player and which are not.

Results and Discussion

Characteristics of specific Argentinian and German players

The Argentinian forwards (Valdano, Maradona and Burruchaga) had, in comparison to the 2 German forwards - during the last 30 min Germany played with 3 forwards - an extremely large range of action longitudinally. The former also better fulfilled their defensive assignments in their own half of the field.

Burruchaga was active in what can roughly be described as an elliptical area. He defended on the left side and had a lot of ball contacts on the right side of the field between the goal area and midfield. He often received the ball as he ran diagonally into areas poorly covered by the German defence. In addition, it was possible to observe the formation of the following blocks within their defensive behaviour. There was a rear centrally-located block consisting of a sweeper (Brown) and two man-to-man defensive players (Cociuffo and Ruggeri).

Observation of the ranges of action of Brown, Ruggeri and Cociuffo as well as their defence behaviour supports this statement. Ruggeri marked Rummenigge 87.1% and Cociuffo was found to mark Allofs 84.6% of the time whilst Brown abstained from man-to-man coverage.

At this point the connection between the system of play of a team and the 'covering behaviour' of each player is obvious. On the right and left sides there were double blocks (Valdano and Guisti and Burruchaga and Olarticoechea, respectively). Finally, there was also a middle block formed by Maradona, Enrique and Batista.

The German team was not as successful in distributing defensive assignments for its zones nor in forming blocks until the 64th minute of play. Not until then did Brehme switch to the left side where he could give Briegel support both on offence and defence. On the whole, the distribution of assignments and ranges of action for Förster, Matthäus, and above all Eder and Brehme did not prove effective.

The system of play and the defensive behaviour of both teams

Using the numbering system already described to label the Argentinian system of play, it was found that the Argentinian players began with a '1-2-4-3-' (Brown - Cociuffo, Ruggeri - Guisti, Enrique, Batista, Olarticoechea - Valdano, Maradona, Burruchaga; and then they changed to a '1-4-4-1' system (Brown - Cociuffo, Ruggeri, Batista, Olarticoechea - Valdano, Guisti, Enrique, Burruchaga - Maradona) during the last 30 min of the game. Germany had replaced Völler with Allofs at the beginning of the second half and then substituted Hoeness for Magath in the 60th minute, giving them three forwards. This was done for obvious reasons, namely to overcome an Argentinian lead by increasing offensive pressure. Argentina's answer was the aforementioned '1-4-4-1' defensively oriented playing system. The new focal points of the ranges of action monitored these changes. During the same periods of time the German players used a '1-3-4-2' (Jacobs; Brehme, Matthäus, Förster; Berthold, Eder, Magath, Briegel: Rummenigge, Allofs) and then a '1-2-4-3' playing system (Jacobs; Förster, Briegel; Berthold, Eder, Matthäus, Brehme-Rummenigge, Hoeness, Völler).

In order to be able to make a statement about a "man-to-man" defence, it is necessary to observe a particular defensive player closely. The number of encounters with an opponent can then be determined. One could see that if, for example, all of the contacts between Matthäus and Argentinian players during Argentinian offensive attacks were counted, it is clear that he 'covered' Maradona in 76.9%, Burruchaga in 13.5% and Valdano in 5.8% of the cases.

Furthermore, one can recognise that both team played a 'mixed' defence (zone and man-to-man). The opposing forwards (Maradona, Valdano, Rummenigge, Allofs and in the 2nd half Völler and Hoeness), as well as the German midfield player Magath (in the first 45 min of the game), were 'covered' man-to-man in at least 60% of the cases. When these 'covering-percentages' fall below 60%, it is difficult to speak of 'man-to-man' coverage.

Who 'covered' whom varied in some cases during the course of the game: for example, Ruggeri "covered" Rummenigge in 87.1% of the cases during the first 45 min and then Hoeness in 66.6% of the cases during the last 30 min of the game. These interactions could be shown in a comprehensive matrix. In some instances more extensive observations of other games are necessary because a high percentage of encounters is not necessarily proof of a man-to-man defence, since it could, for example, be the result of two ranges of action being almost identical.

If, in the future, one wants to give exact and differentiated information about defensive behaviour, it will be necessary to make a quantitative statement; therefore, a particular man-to-man defence could be described, e.g., as a 60% or 80% man-to-man defence. This type of systematic approach is also useful for analysing many other tactical aspects, including i) tactical mistakes (Winkler, 1985) and ii) further examinations of systems of play.

References

Winkler, W. (1984) Zur Taktik im Fußballspiel. Leistungssport, 2, 5-13.

Winkler, W. (1985) Fußball analysiert: Hamburger SV gegen Inter Mailand I, II und III. Spielanalyse im Leistungsfußball mit Hilfe von Video-Aufzeichnungen. In: Fußballtraining 9/10, 22-25, Fußballtraining 11, 25-30, Fußballtraining 12, 19-22.

AN ANALYSIS OF GOAL SCORING STRATEGIES IN THE WORLD CHAMPIONSHIP IN MEXICO, 1986.

E. Olsen
The Norwegian College for Sport and Physical Education,
Sognsveien 220, 0807 Oslo, Norway.

Introduction

There are several indicative trends in modern soccer. Play has become faster and the player in possession of the ball has less time and space at his disposal. Even sides with a defensive structure based on marking (priority to the work of third defenders) have during the last few years given higher priority to pressurising the player with the ball. In sides with a defensive structure based on zonal methods the pressurising is harder than ever before.

The World Championship in Mexico in 1986 represented an interesting case since there was an obvious influence of climatic conditions. Few teams initiated pressure in the attacking third of the field, unless there was an instant and specific demand. Usually teams retreated to their own half before pressurising the player on the ball. Since all the defenders were behind the ball, thus providing balance and depth, there should have been few opportunities for attacking players to create space in the final third of the field. However, since there was a significantly large number of goals scored during the final stages of this tournament, the indications are that there was a high degree of attacking skill and team work in evidence. In order to analyse this aspect of play at this elite level it was decided to study the use of space and time in attacking movements leading to goals. In particular the following key features of play were notated:-

(i) the number of touches on the ball required by the goal scorer;
(ii) the amount of space the goal scorer had;
(iii) the number of touches used by the assisting player before the final pass;
(iv) the amount of space he had at the moment of passing;
(v) the number of passes involved in the scoring move;
(vi) the number of goals scored from set plays;
(vii) the specific type of set play leading to a goal e.g. corner, free-kicks, throw-ins, penalties;
(viii) the number of goals resulting from the breakdown of a move;
(ix) the location on the field in which moves break down.

Method

Recordings of the final 52 matches in the 1986 World Championship in

Mexico were observed. Goals (n = 132) were scored in 48 of these games. Where possible the complete move resulting in a goal was video recorded for detailed observation in slow motion. This resulted in insufficient data for 21 of the goals and these were discarded from the analysis. The data were coded and stored on file in a computer system by two experienced observers.

Complete agreement was required before the data were stored. In some cases detailed discussions preceded the recording of data. Numerical and positional data of defensive players were also recorded around the location of the ball. The only limitation here was the angle of view permitted by the television camera.

Results

In Tables 1, 2, 3 and 4 the information derived from the video observations by two experienced observers is displayed.

Table 1. The number of touches on the ball and the amount of space for scorers at the moment of scoring

No. of touches	No. of goals (%)	Space (m)	No. of goals (%)
⩾ 4	8 (6)	⩾ 4	35 (29.2)
3	9 (6.8)	3	15 (12.5)
2	22 (16.7)	2	16 (13.3)
1	93 (70.5)	1	30 (25)
		< 1	24 (20)
Total	132		120*

* Penalties filtered out

Table 2. The number of touches on the ball and the amount of space at the moment of passing for players assisting

No. of touches	No. of goals (%)	Space (m)	No. of goals (%)
⩾ 4	19 (18.5)	⩾ 4	31 (29.8)
3	13 (12.5)	3	16 (15.4)
2	21 (20)	2	19 (18.3)
1	51 (49)	1	26 (25)
		< 1	12 (11.5)
Total	104*		104*

*Penalties filtered out

Table 3. Number of passes in scoring movements

No. of passes	No. of goals	%
⩾ 7	27	22.5
6	11	9.2
5	4	3.3
4	10	8.3
3	19	15.8
2	33	27.5
1	12	10
0	4	3.3
Total	120*	99.9

*Penalties filtered out

Table 4. Number of passes in scoring moves after the last restart or a breakdown

No. of passes	No. of goals	%
⩾ 5	25	20.8
4	11	9.2
3	18	15
2	27	22.5
1	27	22.5
0	12	10
Total	120*	100

*Penalties filtered out

Information is provided on the following problems:-

(i) The number of touches on the ball by the goal scorer and the amount of space (in metres) at the time of scoring;
(ii) The number of touches on the ball by the assisting passer and the amount of space at the time of passing;
(iii) The number of passes in a scoring move;
(iv) The number of passes in a scoring move after a breakdown of the opponent's move.

Discussion

As can be seen from the descriptive data provided in Tables 1 - 4 there are a number of interesting features of play at such an elite level of competition. Most goals are scored with one touch on the ball. This is the case even if set pieces are discarded from the analysis. Very few goals are scored after more than three touches on the ball by the goal scorer. This suggests that dribbling into a scoring position is no longer a critical feature of the modern game at international level. More than 90% of goals were scored from within a distance of 16m of the goal. Every fifth goal was scored under what can be termed as severe defensive pressure. In situations where the scorer uses more than one touch, the first touch is critical for setting himself up.

The passing player used more touches on the ball than goal scorers. In 66 of the 104 goals recorded, the passer had at least 2m of space at the moment of passing. In approximately 50% of the goals, only one touch was used to provide the 'assist'. Obviously the opportunity for effective penetration exists for only a fraction of a second and a first time pass is the most successful means of providing an 'assist'. Passing players had more space than the goal scorer because most teams did not use a zonal defensive strategy but instead used a man-to-man marking system which restricted the space available to the attacker. In approximately 30% of the goals the passer had at least 4m or more space at his disposal.

Table 3 reveals that few goals are scored in a multi-pass movement. When penalties are filtered out, only about 20% of the goals are preceded by five or more passes. In fact most of the goals are scored after two passes or less.

Scoring from a set-play was defined as a score occurring less than 5 s after a re-start. With this definition 34 goals occurred from set pieces. Hughes (1980) estimated that 40% of goals at international level are scored from set pieces; this is significantly higher than the 25% figure provided by the 1986 World Championships.

If penalties are disregarded about 50% of the remaining goals were scored after a passing movement had broken down. In this study a breakdown was defined as an interception and scoring counter-attack by the opposition. Despite the low pressure style dominating in Mexico, it is surprising that more than 50% of the breakdowns occurred in the attacking third of the field.

In conclusion, it is clear that such exercises in notation are needed if the soccer coach is to gain valuable insight into correct strategies at work at elite levels of play. In this way experience may be made to work for the athlete in an unpainful and vicarious manner.

References

Hughes, C. (1980) The Football Association Coaching Book of Soccer, Tactics and Skills. London: The Football Association.

Svenska Fotbollförbundet (1976) Bättre Fotbol, Taktic. Uppsala: Almquist and Wiksell.

ANALYSIS OF THE REFEREEING DECISIONS DURING THE WORLD SOCCER CHAMPIONSHIP IN 1986 IN MEXICO

R. Van Meerbeek, D. Van Gool and J. Bollens
Department of Physical Education, Katholieke Universiteit, Leuven, Belgium.

Introduction

Since soccer competitions have been broadcast on television, often faulty rulings made by the referee can be irrefutably shown by means of slow motion replay. Spectacular miscalculations by the referee are willingly analysed at full length by the media. However, the many right decisions are all but ignored. In Germany, Heisterkamp (1979) investigated the objectivity of sportswriters about referees' arbitrations and came to the conclusion that 77% of the commentary was spent on negative criticism, 16% was neutral and in only 7% of the cases was the referee praised for his action. It is the aim of this paper to attempt a preliminary analysis of the percentage of correct and incorrect decisions made by top class referees during competition. By analysing video recordings of soccer games, the number of right and wrong decisions made by the referee may be registered. Nevertheless, not all errors are shown on television. That limited number of offences has not been considered in this investigation and it is assumed that the referee made the correct decision.

Sixteen competitions were analysed. These included all the games which were played during the soccer World Championship (1986) in the second round, i.e. from the 'last sixteen' to the final. This gave the opportunity to see 14 referees at work, of which two referees acted twice. The extra-time periods were not taken into account in order to enable a comparison between games.

Method

While observing games, all situations which required the referee to make a decision were registered. Clearly, the observer engaged in a numerical analysis of action in soccer is open to subjective bias. However, this was assumed to be minimal due to the use of three experienced observers.

Decisions were divided into four categories:

i) Fouls;
ii) Misconduct;
iii) Duration of the game;
iv) Ball out of play.

Fouls

An attempt was made to distinguish between:-

i) fouls, registered and whistled by the referee;

ii) fouls, registered by the referee, yet advantage was played:

iii) fouls not noticed or misjudged by the referee and consequently not whistled;

iv) actions perceived as fouls and whistled wrongly by the referee.

The fouls observed in this investigation are those mentioned in the 'Laws of the Game' (FIFA 1979). Nine fouls are penalized by means of a direct free-kick - kicking or attempting to kick an opponent, tripping an opponent, jumping at an opponent, charging an opponent in a violent or dangerous manner, charging an opponent from behind, striking or attempting to strike an opponent, holding an opponent, pushing an opponent and handling the ball.

Six fouls are penalized with an indirect free-kick - playing in a manner considered by the referee to be dangerous, charging fairly, with the shoulder, when the ball is not within playing distance, intentionally obstructing an opponent when not playing the ball, charging the goalkeeper, fouls of the goalkeeper (e.g. taking more than 4 steps) and off-side.

Misconduct

Misconduct punished with a booking or an exclusion is whistled as a foul, unless there is 'ball advantage'. However, misconduct can also be punished at times when the ball is out of play.

Timekeeping

This is the application of rules Vc and VIIa which state that the referee 'acts as timekeeper' and allows the full or agreed time, adding thereto all time lost through accident or other cause. At the end of each period the referee decides how much lost time he must add to prescribed time. Referees are also required to make decisions concerning whether the ball is or is not out of play.

From the four categories of decisions that a referee has to make during a soccer game, judging 'fouls' is the most difficult aspects, especially when decisions are required immediately. The great advantage of analysing a video recording is, of course, the possibility of repetitions, slow-motion and if necessary static pictures. This method of investigation permits a reasonable level of objectivity since all three experienced soccer observers, in this study, were required to agree before a decision was made upon the referee's decision.

Results

Number of decisions in a game

Overall in 16 games, 2167 decisions were registered. Those decisions also included the perceived fouls which were deemed by the observers to be wrongly whistled by the referee.

Fouls

Between different games there was a large amount of variation in the categories 'fouls' and 'ball out of play' (Table 1).

In the category, 'playing advantage', mainly push and shove duels (i.e. charging 40.3%; holding 39.0%; charging in the back 36.6%;

Table 1. Average number of decisions made by a referee in a game (N=16)

	N	%	S.D.	Min.	Max.
Fouls	77.4	57.1	16.15	49	118
Ball out of play	56.9	42.0	12.06	33	78
Misconduct	1.1	0.8	1.40	0	5

Table 2. Different kinds of decisions made by the referees for the various fouls (N = 16)

	Whistled correctly		Advantage ball		Not Whistled		Whistled wrongly		Total
	N	%	N	%	N	%	N	%	
Direct free-kick									
Kick	44	64.7	17	25.0	7	10.3	0	0.0	68
Trip	73	77.6	9	9.6	11	11.7	1	1.1	94
Jump	5	-	1	-	9	-	0		8
Charge	80	38.8	83	40.3	42	20.4	1	0.5	206
Charge in back	97	56.7	63	36.6	11	6.0	1	0.6	172
Strike	2	-	1	-	2	-	0	-	5
Hold	35	45.5	30	39.0	11	14.3	1	1.3	77
Push	196	61.1	73	22.7	45	14.0	7	2.2	321
Hand	25	65.8	5	13.2	7	18.4	1	2.6	38
Total	557	56.3	282	28.5	138	14.0	12	1.2	989
Indirect free-kick									
Play dangerously	11	-	4	-	4	-	0	-	19
Charge, ball not playing distance	1	-	4	-	2	-	0	-	7
Obstruction	11	18.6	20	33.9	26	44.1	2	3.4	59
Charge goal-keeper	14	-	2	-	4	-	1	-	21
Fouls goal-keeper	2	-	0	-	5	-	0	-	7
Off-side	115	16.2	0	0.0	3	2.2	18	13.2	136
Total	154	61.8	30	12.0	44	17.7	21	8.4	249
Total	711	57.4	312	25.2	182	14.7	33	2.7	1238

pushing 22.7%) were permitted by the referees.

The number of decisions judged as wrong (n = 215) consisted mainly of fouls that were not whistled (n = 182, 84.6%). For obstructing an opponent the percentage of unwhistled fouls amounted to 44.1%. Direct free-kicks were on average incorrectly whistled in 15.2% of cases. For the indirect free kick category this amounted to 26.1% although obstruction was seldom whistled. In this group of elite referees the best performance was 11% wrong decisions; the worst performance amounted to 34.6% wrong decisions.

Table 3. Number of correct and incorrect decisions by the referees for the various fouls (N = 16) as judged by the observers

	Correct		Incorrect		
	N	%	N	%	Total
Direct free-kick	839	84.8	150	15.2	989
Indirect free-kick	184	73.9	65	26.1	249
Total	1023	82.6	215	17.4	1238

Ball out of play

Table 4. Ball out of play (N = 16)

	N	$\bar{X}$	%	S.D.	Min.	Max.
Throw-in	467	29.2	51.3	11.04	14	55
Goal-kick	291	18.2	31.9	4.44	10	25
Corner-kick	153	9.6	16.8	3.03	5	16
Total	911	56.9	100	12.06	33	78

On average a ball is put out of play 57 times per match. The number of times a ball is played over the touch-line or the goal-line has an approximate probability of 0.5, although there is a large amount of inter-game variation.

Misconduct
In 16 games there were 50 bookings (± 3 per game) and 2 dismissals (sending-off). The fairly small number of bookings were mainly for tackling from behind, arguing with the referees and tripping opponents.

Timekeeping
The extremely low actual playing time (55'08") is quite striking. In a similar investigation on this problem, Kuhn et al. (1977) found an average actual playing time of 59'20" in the World Championship (1974) and Willekens (1979) came to an average actual playing time of

60'01" for the World Championship in 1978.

Table 5. Average full duration of the game (N = 16) in min(') and s('')

	$\bar{X}$	Min.	Max.
1st period	45'38"	44'51"	46'50"
2nd period	46'02"	44'59"	47'27"
Total	91'41"	90'00"	93'23"

Table 6. Average actual playing time (N = 16)

	$\bar{X}$	Min.	Max.
1st period	28'23"	24'30"	32'26"
2nd period	26'43"	19'48"	31'09"
Total	55'08"	44'18"	63'10"

The range between the minimum and the maximum actual playing time was also greater in 1986 (18'52") than in 1978 (16'56") and 1974 (14'48").

Discussion

During the 16 games that were analysed, the referees made on average three decisions every 2 min. This entailed a decision every 40s, illustrating that a referee must focus full attention for every moment of the game.

Observers (n = 3) deemed that 17.4% of the decisions made were wrong. However, it should not be forgotten that essentially the best referees in the world were at work here. More than half of the faults were noted in close physical skirmishes which tend to be actions in which a referee is likely to award a playing advantage.

The finding that actual playing time is reduced to 66% of the prescribed duration of the game is not new. Apparently it is more important that there is a range of variation of 19 min. This means that the opportunity to create equal chances is not the same for each team in large scale competitions. In sports competitions each team should perhaps get the same amount of time to score or ... to have a score against it. Therefore, it is feasible that a 'running clock' of 30 min duration for each half would result in equal opportunities to score or let in goals. This is obviously a speculative idea which may enhance the value of soccer as a spectator sport.

References

FIFA Handbook (1979) The Laws of the Game. Zurich: FIFA.

Heisterkamp, G. (1979) Untersuchungen zur Objektivität von Schiedsrichter-beurteilungen durch Sportredakteure. Leistungssport, 9, 384-393.

Kuhn, W., Maier, W. and Wiepking, W. (1977) Untersuchung zur Problematik der Spielzeit im Fussbal. Leistungssport, 7, 22-30.

Willekens, B. (1979) Wereldkampioenschap voetal 1978, onderzoek naar de effectieve spelduur. Leuven: K.U.Leuven.

Part IX

Biomechanics and football equipment

IMPACT CHARACTERISTICS OF TWO TYPES OF SOCCER BALLS

T.A. Levendusky, C.W. Armstrong, J.S. Eck, J. Jeziorowski* L. Kugler**
Physical Education Department, Southern Methodist University, Dallas, Texas 75275, U.S.A.
*Applied Biomechanics Laboratory, University of Toledo, Toledo, Ohio 43606, U.S.A.
**Physical Education Department, Point Loma Nazarene College, San Diego, California 92106, U.S.A.

Introduction

Considerable attention has been focused on the treatment and prevention of the injuries that occur in the game of soccer. Most of this attention has been directed at injuries involving the lower extremities. Recently, several authors have discussed the incidence of injury to the head, due to both intentional and incidental contact between the ball and the head (Schneider, 1984; Smodlaka, 1984). While injury rates for the head are considerably less than those for the lower extremities, the potential harmful consequences of head injuries are often much greater. Although the occurrence of catastrophic head injury in soccer is relatively rare, it does happen. Beyond this, there is evidence that repeated exposure to head impact, as typically occurs in soccer may produce degenerative changes in the cervical spine that may ultimately lead to impaired function (Tysvaer and Storli, 1981).

Although head and neck injuries are not as prevalent in soccer as in American football or boxing, for example, there have been reported cases of injury. The injury to the head and neck may be either acute or chronic to the musculoskeletal system and soft tissues of the body. Verdaguer (1982) reported retinal detachments caused by the impact of soccer balls in twenty patients. Burke et al., (1983) reported further on 24 eye injuries resulting from impact with soccer balls. Sandyk (1983) reported on two boys who were struck on the head accidentally during a game. The impact blow was of sufficient magnitude to cause immediate migraine attacks in the boys.

Kross et al., (1983) studied electroencephalographs (EEG) of players heading a soccer ball. They indicated that cerebral damage cannot be assumed in general, although predisposed persons may have microtraumas and sub-clinical cerebral dysfunction caused by heading. They also indicated that long term studies should be performed to determine the risk of permanent cerebral damage in soccer players. Tsyvaer (1985) described a case of a cervical disc herniation occurring in a soccer player who headed the ball in the wrong manner. The injury caused various symptoms afterwards and the medical advice for this 29 year old First and Second Division player was to terminate his soccer career. In another related study, Sortland et al. (1982) examined 43 former players for the National Football Team of Norway both clinically and radiologically for degenerative changes in the cervical spine. The comparisons with non-players showed onset of degenerative changes 10 to 20 years earlier for players. The type of player who headed the ball often also had a higher frequency of subjective complaints and clinical findings, such as reduced cervical range of motion. Tysvaer and Storli (1981) also surveyed Norwegian First Division clubs and found a low percentage of traumatic head injury due to heading. However, fifty percent of the players surveyed indicated that they had had acute symptoms due to heading, sixteen percent complained of protracted symptoms and five percent had permanent symptoms due to heading.

The characteristics of impact, associated with head injury, have been well documented for several sports. The studies of impact with sports equipment have included cycling helmets (Bishop and Briard, 1984), American football helmets (Bishop, Norman and Kozey, 1984) and boxing and karate gloves (Smith and Hamill, 1985). In soccer, the ball in motion is responsible for producing impact that is sometimes directed to the head. In spite of the worldwide popularity of soccer, little is known about the characteristics of this impact. Such information may be of value in decreasing the incidence of impact-related injury, through alterations in game rules and ball design. Thus, the objectives of this study were twofold: (1) to document selected impact characteristics of soccer balls travelling at game-like velocities, and (2) to determine how two standard methods of soccer ball construction differentially influence ball impact.

Methods

Twenty different soccer balls, representing two methods of construction (moulded and stitched) were selected for the study. Moulded soccer balls have cover panels which are either bonded to a moulded rubber lining or the entire cover is moulded and the panel designs are painted on the surface. Stitched soccer balls typically have covers which are hand-sewn panels of leather, or synthetic material which simulates leather (Tucker, 1979). The laws of the game, established by the Federation Internationale de Football Association (FIFA) state that the outer casing or cover of the ball should be leather or another approved material which does not prove dangerous to players. The ball circumference of 27 to 28 inches (68.5 - 71.1 cm) and ball weight of 14 to 16 ounces (396.89 - 453.59 g) are also stated within the rules established by FIFA (1986, p.7).

The 20 soccer balls (moulded = 10; stitched = 10) were inflated to an inflation pressure of 9 pounds per square inch (62052 N m^{-2}). The inflation pressure was regulated by a pressurized nitrogen tank fitted with a Matheson single stage regulator (Model 8-580) and two gauges. All balls were kept in the testing site overnight to stabilize the tempeature (29 degrees Celsius), and were inflated immediately prior to the testing session. The balls were then weighed on an Ohaus balance scale to the nearest 0.5g. Ball motion and impact were produced by dropping the balls from a height of 18.09 m on to a rigid flat surface. The surface contained a force recording system AMTI Biomechanics force platform (Model OR6-5-1) which recorded the vertical force applied by the ball to the platform. The output voltage from the platform was amplified and sampled at a rate of 1000 Hz by a Cyborg Issac data acquisition system interfaced to an Apple IIe microcomputer. Software was written to evaluate specific characteristics of the impact generated waveform.

The four impact characteristics identified for this study were peak force, impulse, duration and rise time to peak force. The peak force, recorded in Newtons (N), represented the maximum force which the ball imparted upon impact. The impulse, recorded in newton-seconds (N:s) was the product of the average net force and the time interval, and represents the change in momentum produced during the brief time of contact. The duration was the time period from fifty percent of the maximum peak force on the rise until fifty percent of the maximum on the downside of the pulse. The duration was referred to as the full width, half maximum time period and was recorded in milliseconds (ms). The rise time to peak force, also recorded in milliseconds (ms), was the time period from ten percent of the peak force until ninety percent of the peak force and was an indication of how quickly the ball reached the maximum force upon impact with the platform. A diagram indicating an actual waveform and the four impact characteristics studied in this project is shown in Figure 1.

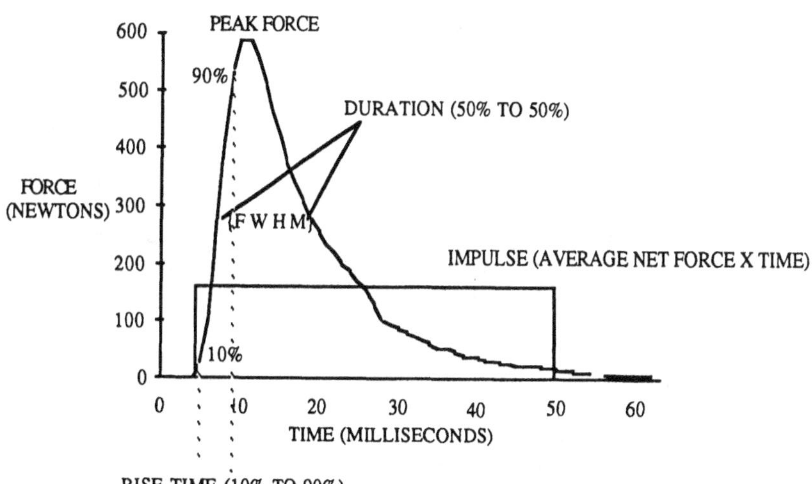

Fig. 1 Data graph illustrating impact characteristics

The force platform was secured to a steel mounting plate directly beneath the drop site. On a catwalk near the building's ceiling a ball holder was mounted consisting of a funnel 17.78 cm in diameter and positioned such that the large opening faced downward. The funnel was embedded into a wooden frame to prevent any movement when the soccer ball was moved upwards into the funnel opening. The ball valve was centred and positioned facing upwards to provide a standard drop placement procedure. The ball was held in place by a single fingertip of a researcher prior to release.

The height of 18.09 m was selected to ensure ball velocities typical of those achieved in game conditions. Pilot testing established that this height would result in velocities in the range of 17 to 18 m/s. Each ball was dropped repeatedly until five successful direct hits (full ball on the centre of the platform) were recorded. The platform was 18 x 20 inches (40.7 x 50.8 cm). Due to variability in the flight paths of the balls, produced by aerodynamic factors, on average 75 drops per ball were necessary to achieve the goal of 5 direct hits. The aerodynamic drag forces and Magnus effect cause such erratic flight patterns that a large number of drops was necessary to collect enough direct hits for each ball for data analysis. The data were then analyzed with one-way analysis of covariance (ANCOVA) for peak force and impulse, using ball mass as the covariate. A one-way analysis of variance (ANOVA) was used to evaluate duration and rise time, as pilot studies had established that the temporal measures were not influenced by ball mass.

Results

The two groups of balls (moulded and stitched) were compared to evaluate differences between group means for the four dependent variables of peak force, impulse, duration and rise time. The mean mass of the moulded soccer balls was 426.7 g and the mean mass of the stitched soccer balls was 437.7 g. This difference was statistically significant at the 0.05 level of significance.

The ANCOVA for peak force indicated a significant ball type effect, $F_{1,18} = 12.67$, $P < 0.01$. The overall correlation between dependent variate and covariate was $r = .81$. The mean peak force for the moulded balls was 851 N, and the mean peak force for the stitched balls was 912 N. The ANCOVA for impulse indicated a significant ball type effect, $F(1,18) = 31.17$, $P < 0.01$. The overall correlation between dependent variate and covariate was $r = .72$. Mean impulse was 12.43 N:s. for the moulded type of ball and mean impulse for the stitched type of ball was 13.72 N:s Table 1 provides the results of the ANCOVA for peak force and impulse.

Table 1. Analysis of covariance for peak force and impulse

Source	SS	df	ms	F
Peak Force				
Between Groups	5304.26	1	5304.26	12.67[a]
Within Groups	7113.43	17	418.43	
Total	12417.69	18		
Impulse				
Between Groups	3.71	1	3.71	31.17[a]
Within Groups	2.02	17	.11	
Total	5.73	18		

[a] indicates $P < 0.01$

The dependent variable which involved the impact characteristic of time of contact was duration. The mean duration for the moulded ball group was 10.24 ms and the mean duration for the stitched ball group was 10.76 ms. These data were analyzed with a one-way ANOVA. The analysis indicated a significant ball type effect, $F_{1,19} = 10.99$, $P < 0.01$. The mean rise time for moulded type balls was 3.265 ms and the mean rise time for stitched balls was 4.168 ms. The ANOVA yielded a significant ball type effect, $F_{1,18} = 62.31$, $P < 0.01$. The summary of the analysis for duration and rise time is presented in Table 2.

Table 2. Analysis of variance for duration and rise time

Source	SS	df	ms	F
Duration				
Between Groups	1.374	1	1.374	10.99[a]
Within Groups	2.252	18	1.252	
Total	3.627	19		
Rise Time				
Between Groups	4.073	1	4.073	62.31[a]
Within Groups	1.176	18	.065	
Total	5.25	19		

[a] indicates $P < 0.01$

Discussion

The results of this study establish that the peak force and impulse produced during impact of soccer balls moving at velocities common to game conditions are of sufficient magnitude to warrant serious attention. Hodgson and Thomas (1981) reported that a peak force of 784 N occurring for 6 ms was sufficient to produce concussion. Hodgson and Nakamura (1981) found fractures of cadaver zygoma (cheek bone) at peak forces of 670 to 1100 N. Additionally, they reported that the location of force application was a critical factor influencing the likelihood of injury. The forehead, in some cases, was able to withstand peak forces of 1700 to 4000 N and the side of the head could withstand up to 890 to 3340 N before fracture occurred. In the present investigation, the mean values of peak force for the moulded balls and stitched balls were 851 and 912 N, respectively. This is clearly in a range that represents the potential to produce injury. As peak force is a function of both ball mass and velocity, it would be expected that the risk of injury would increase when velocities greater than those tested in this study occur. In comparison to the approximate velocity of 18 $m\ s^{-1}$ in the present study, other soccer ball velocities have been recorded from both kicked and thrown balls. Velocities from kicked soccer balls included 21.52 $m\ s^{-1}$ for ten male collegiate players in America

(Abo-Abdo, 1980), 25.60 m s^{-1} for professional players, 25.25 m s^{-1} for collegiate players and 19.92 m s^{-1} for unskilled players (Stoner, 1980). Velocities for the soccer throw-in have also recorded the following: 18.31 m s^{-1} for collegiate players in America (Levendusky et al., 1985) and 21.10 m s^{-1} for a highly skilled professional (Kline, 1980). Variability in ball velocity is likely to be a function of age, skill level and intent of the player. These current data suggest that the peak impact forces present in soccer may range from below a level that could cause injury, to well within the range known to cause injury.

Brancazio (1984, p205) described impulse as "a sudden force of relatively brief duration which describes the effect of a force that acts for a finite (and usually short) period of time." The impulse is a measure of the change in momentum which occurs during impact and a larger change may be more desirable in terms of performance. In relation to injury levels, Hirsch (1966) studied concussive level impulse values and noted that approximately 22N:s of impulse would be nearing the injury intensity of the human head. The values for moulded and stitched soccer balls for impulse in this study were 12.43 and 13.72 N.s, well below the concussive levels. However, in typical heading skills, the impulse would increase greatly due to the momentum of the player's head being imparted to the incoming ball. Thus, although the impulse of a soccer ball contacting a non-moving platform is relatively small, the change in momentum will be much greater when the ball contacts a moving body part like the head.

The two temporal characteristics of duration and rise time to peak force have not been studied often, so comparative values of other impacts are lacking. It would appear to be favourable for a soccer ball to have larger temporal values in terms of reducing the likelihood of injury. The stitched soccer balls had significantly larger duration and rise time values (10.76, 4.168 ms) than the moulded soccer balls (10.23, 3.265 ms). Of these two temporal characteristics, perhaps the rise time is most important to consider. As the rise time decreases, the time available to dissipate the force as it approaches its peak value decreases. Thus, shorter rise time periods would be associated with an increased likelihood of injury. While no data have been published previously indicating typical rise times to peak force for soccer balls, the values found in this study appear to be relatively short (moulded = 3.265 ms; stitched = 4.168 ms). These values would be likely to change in an actual collision between a soccer ball and the player's head, such that compliance of the human tissues would increase the values.

In addition to documenting the characteristics of impact produced by soccer balls, the objective of this study was to compare the responses of moulded and stitched soccer balls. For each of the four impact characteristics studied, the differences between moulded and stitched balls were statistically significant at the 0.01 level of significance. The mean peak force for stitched soccer balls was 7.2% greater than that for moulded balls. Similarly, the mean impulse for stitched balls exceeded that of the moulded balls by 9.5%. While the practical significance of these differences has not been determined, the data suggest that there are differences between these two types for peak force and impulse. The durations of contact for the stitched soccer balls were 5% greater than the moulded ball duration periods.

In terms of practical significance, the rise time of the stitched soccer ball was 27.6% greater than the moulded soccer balls. As a representation of soccer ball compliance and force dissipation, both desirable in terms of injury prevention, the stitched ball is favourable with respect to rise time to peak force. Beyond the relationship of this measure of rise time to injury considerations, this may be important in the response of the ball to a player's feet and other body parts. The stitched balls tend to be subjectively favoured over moulded balls because they possess a better feel or "touch" to play with. Such differences in rise time between types of soccer balls may enable a player to exert greater control in passing and dribbling.

While it is difficult to draw firm conclusions from laboratory testing that can be applied to actual game conditions, the results of this study are certainly thought-provoking. It may be that soccer players utilized techniques of heading that diminish the intensity of the impact levels well within tolerable levels. If this is the case, inexperienced players who have not developed these strategies and abilities may be at increased risk of injury. This would be particularly true when inexperienced players are matched with veteran players who possess the capacity to produce faster ball velocities. In contrast, certain aspects of heading may actually increase the magnitude of the impact. When heading is used to purposely redirect the ball, as in attempting to clear a ball or shoot on goal, the head is generally accelerated towards the ball prior to contact. Since the ball and the player's head both possess momentum, but in opposite directions, the resulting impact would reflect the combined effect of these forces. Likewise, a player running in one direction who is struck on the head by a ball moving towards him would experience the same phenomena. The result in both cases would be an impact of a magnitude significantly greater than those recorded in this study. These situations may be the more frequent circumstances under which injuries occur. Schneider (1984) alluded to the uniqueness of actual game conditions in stating that extrapolation of the results from experimental conditions to the real game-like situations may indeed show that heading could cause cerebral concussion and possibly irreversible brain injury.

While it is premature to conclude that one type of ball is safer than another, the results of this study indicate that ball construction influences characteristics of impact that have been associated with injuries. This information may be particularly important in establishing procedures for evaluating the safety of various types of soccer balls. Additionally, it may be useful in assisting soccer ball manufacturers in developing construction techniques to maximise safety. Beyond this, the results of the study indicate that serious attention needs to be given to the potential that exists in soccer for head and cervical spine injury due to ball impact. This may have implications for teaching and training techniques as well as for rules limiting heading for selected at-risk populations.

References

Abo-Abdo, H (1980) Mechanical analysis of the soccer instep kick, NCAA performer. In: Biomechanics Symposium Proceedings (edited by J.M. Cooper and B. Haven). Bloomington, Indiana, Indiana University.

Bishop, P.J. and Briard, B.D. (1984) Impact performance of bicycle helmets. Canad. J. Appl. Sport Sci., 9 94-101.

Bishop, P.J., Norman, R.W., and Kozey, J.W. (1984) Evaluation of football helmets under impact conditions. Amer. J. Sports Med., 12, 233-236.

Brancazio, P.J. (1984) Sport Science: Physical Laws and Optimum Performance. New York: Simon and Schuster.

Burke, M.J., Sanitato, J.J., Vinger, P.F., Raymond, L.A. and Kulwin, D.R. (1983) Soccerball-induced eye injuries. J. Amer. Med. Ass., 249, 2682-2685.

Federation Internationale de Football Association. (1986) Laws of the Game and Guide for Referees USSF. English edition. Zurich; Switzerland: FIFA. p.7.

Hirsch, A.H. (1966) Current problems in head protection. In: Head Injury Conference Proceedings (edited by W.F. Caveness and A.E. Walker). pp.37-40. Philadelphia: J. B. Lippincott Company.

Hodgson, V.R. and Nakamura, G.S. (1968) Mechanical impedance and impact response of the human cadaver zygoma. J. Biomech., 1, 73-78.

Hodgson, V.R. and Thomas, L.M. (1981) Boxing gloves compared using dummy head acceleration response. (Report to the New York State Athletic Commissioner, November 13, 1981).

Kline, L. (1980) Analysis of the soccer throw-in. Paper presented at the National Soccer Coaches Association of America conference. Philadelphia, Pennsylvania. January 18, 1980.

Kröss, R. Ohler, K. and Barolin, G.S. (1983) Cerebral trauma due to heading-computerized EEG-analysis of football players. EEG-EMG, 14, 209-212.

Levendusky, T.A., Clinger, C.D., Miller, R.E. and Armstrong, C.W. (1985) Soccer throw-in kinematics. In: Proceedings of ISBS 1985: Biomechanics in Sports II. (edited by J. Terauds and J.N. Barham). Del Mar, California: Academic Publishers.

Sandyk, R. (1983) Footballer's migraine - a report of two cases. S. Afr. Med. J., 63, 434.

Schneider, K. (1984) The risk of brain-injuries in soccer-header. Unfallheilkunde, 87, 40-42.

Smith, P.K. and Hamill, J. (1985). Karate and boxing glove impact characteristics as functions of velocity and repeated impact. In: Proceedings of ISBS 1985: Biomechanics in Sports II (edited by J. Terauds and J.N. Barham). Del Mar, California: Academic Publishers.

Smodlaka, V.N. (1984) Medical aspects of heading the ball in soccer. Physician Sportsmed., 12, 127-131.

Sortland, O., Tysvaer, A.T. and Storli, O.V. (1982) Changes in the cervical spine in association football players. Brit. J. Sports Med., 16, 80-84.

Stoner, L.J. (1980) Instep soccer kick of skilled and novice performers. In: Biomechanics Symposium Proceedings (edited by J.M. Cooper and B. Haven). Bloomington, Indiana. Indiana University.

Tucker, V. (1979) What it takes to make a soccer ball and Understanding the manufacturers' terms. Soccer World, 6, 26-30.

Tysvaer, A. and Storli, O. (1981) Association football injuries to the brain: A preliminary report. Brit. J. Sports Med., 15, 163-166.

Tysvaer, A. (1985) Case report: Cervical disc herniation in a football player. Brit. J. Sports Med., 19, 43-44.

Verdaguer, J. (1982) Juvenile retinal detachment: Pan American American Association of Opthalmology and American Journal of Opthalmol. Lecture. Amer. J. Opthalmol., 93, 145-156.

INFLUENCE OF INFLATION PRESSURE AND BALL WETNESS ON THE IMPACT CHARACTERISTICS OF TWO TYPES OF SOCCER BALLS

C.W. Armstrong*, T.A. Levendusky**, J.S. Eck, P. Spyropoulos, L. Kugler*
* Applied Biomechanics Laboratory, University of Toledo, Toledo, Ohio 43606, U.S.A.
** Physical Education Department, Southern Methodist University, Dallas, Texas 75225, U.S.A.

Introduction

Various authors have expressed concern over the potential for head and cervical spine injury that exists in soccer (Hess and Huberty, 1985; Kross et al., 1983; Sortland et al., 1982; Scoppetta and Vaccario, 1978). Ball-to-head contact, through heading, is an intended part of the game. Beyond this, incidental ball to head contact is a relatively frequent occurrence, especially among children and other inexperienced players. The intensity of the impact resulting from ball-to-head contact is influenced by many factors. Included are ball velocity, ball mass, angle of impact, and the elasticity of the ball. Not only are these variables affected by the dynamics of the game, but also by the conditions under which the game is played.

Two factors, considered to be potential determinants of the intensity of impact, are ball wetness and inflation pressure. Soccer is routinely played under conditions that result in the ball accumulating moisture. Tysvaer (1985), Mathews (1972) and others have commented on the increased risk of injury associated with heading a wet ball. The second factor, inflation pressure, is regulated to some degree by FIFA. It is specified that balls should be inflated to between 8.5 and 15.6 pounds per square inch (psi): 1 psi = 6975 Pa. While this range is quite broad, it is likely that in actual practice inflation pressure may vary even beyond this range. Vinger (1985) has suggested that inflation pressure may be a factor in head injury, particularly that involving the eye.

Both inflation pressure and ball wetness are factors that can be controlled. Additionally, the effect that they produce may be partially a function of the type of ball used. For this reason it is important to identify the degree to which they influence the characteristics of ball impact. Thus, the purpose of this study was to investigate the influence of variability in both ball wetness and inflation pressure on selected impact characteristics in two types of soccer balls.

Methods

Twenty different soccer balls (size 5) were selected for the study. They represented two styles of construction, moulded synthetic and stitched leather. Based on a review of the ranges for inflation pressure suggested by the manufacturers of the balls, a value of 9 psi was chosen as the standard value. Two additional inflation pressures were chosen for use in the study; 12 psi and 6 psi. During testing all balls were inflated from a tank of pressurized nitrogen, using a precision regulator that permitted inflation to the exact specified pressure. Ball wetness was induced by immersing the balls in water for a prescribed period of time. This time period was determined by evaluating the typical increase in ball mass, due to water retention, resulting from an extended period of play on a wet field. A soaking period was then determined that would produce an increase in ball mass similar to that produced through actual play.

Ball impact was measured by dropping the balls from a height of 6 m onto an AMTI force platform. This was interfaced to an Apple IIe microcomputer that sampled data at 1000 Hz through a twelve bit A-D converter. The raw digital values were processed to provide the following measures:- peak force - a measure of the maximum force applied by the ball to the force platform, rise time - a measure of the time from ten per cent of the peak force to the actual peak force, impulse - a measure of the area under the force curve. Peak ball velocities immediately prior to impact were determined by a photoelectric timing system, and ranged from 9.60 to 9.84 m s^{-1}.

The experimental format involved a 2 x 2 x 3 design with repeated measures; i.e. two ball types (moulded and stitched), two moisture conditions (wet and dry), three inflation pressures (6, 9, 12 p.s.i.), and three trials for each ball at each condition. The conditions were administered in the following order: (1) 6 psi dry, (2) 9 psi dry, (3) 12 psi dry, (4) 12 psi wet, (5) 9 psi wet, (6) 6 psi wet. Within each of the six conditions the twenty balls were tested in a random order. The mass of each ball was measured before the first trial in the dry condition, and before and after every trial in the wet conditions. It was determined that there was no significant loss of moisture due to the testing during the wet conditions. Data were analyzed with a three-way analysis of variance. Post-hoc comparisons were made using the Fisher's Protected Least Square Difference method.

Results and Discussion

Listed in Table 1 is a summary of the means for the analysis of main effects for the four variables. In addition to the significant main effects indicated there were numerous significant interactions.

Table 1. Datas summary

Variable	Peak force (N)	Impulse(Ns)	Rise time(ms)	Duration(ms)
Ball Type				
Moulded	516.04	8.016	3.745	11.938
Stitched	557.79[a]	8.882[a]	4.565	12.126[b]
Wetness				
Dry	523.11	8.243	4.163	12.060
Wet	550.72[a]	8.655[a]	4.146	12.000
Inflation				
6 psi	511.80	8.297	4.321	12.402
9 psi	540.91[a]	8.481[a]	4.121[a]	12.020[a]
12 psi	558.05	8.568	4.023	11.673

[a] denotes significant difference at the 0.01 level
[b] at the 0.05 level

It has been suggested that the moisture which a ball accumulates during play may influence its impact characteristics and, as such, increases the likelihood of injury. The results of the analysis support this conclusion. The mean peak force for all balls in the wet condition exceeded that of the dry condition by 5.01%. Further, when the interaction of ball type and wetness was considered, the difference was even more pronounced. While the peak force for moulded balls increased only 2.76%, that of the stitched balls increased 8.46%. These increases, due to ball wetness, can perhaps best be explained on the basis of the influence of ball mass on peak force. Moisture retention adds mass to the ball. In the case of the moulded balls, the mean increase in mass due to soaking was 1.31%. In contrast, the mean mass of the stitched balls in this condition was 7.46%. This difference may be a function of the material (synthetic versus leather) and/or the construction process (moulded versus stitched). In addition to the increase in peak force, there was also an increase in total impulse. The mean impulse for the wet condition was 4.76% greater than for the dry condition. Since the difference between the wet and dry conditions for the variable of duration was non-significant, the difference in impulse is most likely a function of an overall change in the total force. This, again, appears to be due to the increase in ball mass. When ball type was considered, as with peak force, the stitched balls in the wet condition produced the greatest impulse. Since there was no significant interaction between ball type and wetness, for the variable of duration, these results can best be explained on the basis of change in ball mass. The stitched ball retained the most moisture, producing the greatest gain in mass, and as a result had the greatest impulse. Ball wetness did not appear to influence the variable of rise time.

As with ball wetness, ball inflation pressure appears to be subject to considerable variability. It is reasonable to assume that quite frequently balls are used that fall outside of the range recommended by the international organisation (FIFA) and/or the ball manufacturer. It has been speculated that inflation pressure may influence characteristics of ball impact. The results of this study support this contention. The increasing levels of inflation used in the study (6, 9, 12 psi) produced increasing levels of peak force, with each level significantly different from the other. Since the mass of the balls did not change appreciably across the levels of inflation, the change in peak force is perhaps best explained by examining the changes in rise time. As inflation pressure increased, rise time decreased significantly (6.9% decrease from the 6 psi condition to the 12 psi condition). Rise time reflects the rate of deceleration that the ball experiences upon impact. Decreased rise time values indicate increased rates of ball deceleration. As force is a product of mass times acceleration, increases in acceleration would be reflected by increases in peak force. The rise time of a ball would appear to be primarily a function of its elasticity. Gases, such as nitrogen, are highly elastic. The overall elasticity of the ball is a function of the amount of gas contained within it (represented by inflation pressure), and the elasticity of the material from which it is constructed. Thus, increases in inflation pressure enhance ball elasticity causing a decrease in rise time upon impact, resulting in an increase in peak force. Additionally, examination of the main effect for ball type, on the variable rise time, suggests that ball construction may be of importance. Moulded balls had significantly lower rise time values (17.96% lower) than stitched balls. This would suggest that, disregarding the effects of mass, moulded balls would produce greater peak force values. The fact that this did not occur in this study is best explained by examining the mean mass of the stitched balls (437.5 g) and that of the moulded balls (426.5 g). Apparently, the mass of the ball influenced the peak force sufficiently to negate the effect of differences in acceleration as expressed by rise time.

In addition to the changes in peak force produced by variations in inflation pressure, total impulse was also affected. As inflation pressure increased, there was a significant corresponding increase in total impulse. This is somewhat surprising, in view of the theoretical relationship between inflation pressure, impact duration, and total impulse. It would be expected that increases in inflation pressure, by increasing elasticity, would produce decreases in impact duration. The analysis of the variable duration indicated that this did occur. Additionally, it would be expected that decreases in duration would produce decreases in total impulse. This did not occur. It may be an indication that force, which increased as inflation pressure increased, influences total impulse to a greater extent than does duration.

Conclusions

The results of this study indicate that selected characteristics of ball impact are influenced by variability in both ball wetness and inflation pressure. As balls accumulate moisture, the intensity of the impact that is produced when they contact an object is increased. This is more pronounced in the stitched balls than in the moulded balls. Although statistically significant, the practical significance of a four to five percent increase (in peak force or impulse) may be questionable. However, the level of moisture retention and ball velocities under actual conditions of play, may well exceed those employed in this investigation. Thus the effect of moisture retention under actual playing conditions may be much more pronounced than has been demonstrated. This points to several areas of consideration. First, ball manufacturers should endeavour to improve the moisture repellant characteristics of their balls, through modification in materials and construction techniques. Secondly, it may be inappropriate for at-risk populations, children and un-conditioned adults to play soccer under conditions that promote water retention in the ball.

With regard to inflation pressure, the intensity of impact appears to increase with increases in the inflation pressure of the ball. Rise time is the primary variable influencing this. Additionally, rise time reflects the amount of time available to the individual being struck by the ball to attenuate the impact force as it approaches its peak. Factors that decrease rise time diminish force attenuation. The result is that the potential negative consequences of a given force are increased. Perhaps the most obvious practical implication of this is that care should be exercised by players, coaches, and referees to ensure that balls are not over-inflated. Beyond this, it may be prudent to use under-inflated balls in practice and with populations that may be particularly susceptible to impact related injury.

References

Hess, H. and Huberty, R. (1985) Soccer injuries. In: Sports Injuries: Mechanisms, Preventions, and Treatment (edited by R.C. Schneider, J.C.Kennedy, and M.L. Plant), pp.163-177. Baltimore: Williams and Wilkins.

Kross, R., Ohler, K., and Barolin, G.S. (1983) Cerebral trauma due to heading: computerized EEG-analysis of football players. EEG-EMG, 14, 209-212.

Matthews, W.B. (1972) Footballer's migraine. Brit. Med. J., 2, 326-327.

Scoppetta, C., and Vaccario, M.L. (1978) Central cervical cord syndrome after heading a football. The Lancet, pp. 1269.

Sortland, O., Tysvaer, A.T., and Storli, O.V. (1982) Changes in the cervical spine in association football players. Brit. J. Sports Med., 16, 80-84.

Tysvaer, A. (1985) Case report: cervical disc herniation in a football player. Brit. J. Sports Med., 19, 43-44.

CONSTRUCTION TECHNIQUES FOR WINTER GAMES PITCHES

S.W. Baker
The Sports Turf Research Institute, Bingley, West Yorkshire,
BD16 1AU, England.

Introduction

The soils and drainage system of a football pitch control the number of games the pitch can sustain during a season, the playing quality of the surface and the risk of cancellations because of adverse weather conditions. Traditional construction techniques have usually been restricted to adding a pipe drainage system to the native soil. On most soils heavy usage will cause compaction in the surface layer and, in particular, the volume of large soil pores will be reduced. This will limit rates of water infiltration (Canaway, 1978), lead to an unfavourable environment for the grass roots (van Wijk et al., 1977) and cause poor playing conditions (Baker and Isaac, 1987b). Indeed, for Local Authority sports grounds, where most of the pitches are restricted to pipe drainage systems, Ward (1983) found that 44% of the pitches had a drainage problem and on 20% of pitches there were regular cancellations of matches between November and March.

In the last twenty years techniques of sports field construction have improved considerably. This has been brought about by either the use of slit drainage to allow surface water to by-pass compacted soil or the creation of highly permeable rooting media, either as sand-soil mixes or in a pure sand construction. In this paper the technical background of these developments is reviewed.

Slit Drainage

In a slit drainage scheme vertical bands of highly permeable granular material are used to conduct water away from the soil surface, by-passing the main body of the soil. One of the first examples, for which published information is available, was at the Rugby Union ground at Twickenham in 1966-67 (Clark, 1970). Since then, there have been many technical developments in equipment and now three main categories of slit drainage can be recognised:-

(i) Excavated slits where soil material is excavated with a trenching machine and the spoil is removed, leaving channels typically 50-75 mm in width. These channels are filled with either sand or a layer of sand over gravel.

(ii) Sand injection, where deep bands of sand typically 15-20 mm in width run from the surface either into the under-drainage or into more permeable soil horizons. No soil excavation takes place, but instead a cutting blade forces the soil apart and sand is added to the resulting fissure. The early work at Twickenham would fall into this category.

(iii) Surface grooving where shallow slits are inserted to a depth of 75-100 mm. The principal use is to restore continuity between the soil surface and existing slit drains which have been capped by soil.

The spacing of the slit trenches must be chosen to prevent water accumulating between the slits and Adams (1981) suggested that 1 m is about the maximum to prevent ponding. For excavated slits, the Sports Turf Research Institute (1978) suggested a spacing of 0.45-0.9 m and Baker (1982) stated that 0.6 m would be a typical value. For surface grooving the slit spacing is closer, generally 0.2 m.

The design of a slit drainage system must allow for the layout of the underlying pipe drainage system, surface gradients, the dimensions of the slits, the permeability of the soil and slit materials, likely rainfall intensities and the consequences of the design rainfall being exceeded. It is particularly important that there is adequate lateral transfer of water along the slits and a modification of the Hooghoudt steady-state drainage formula can be used for this aspect of drainage design (Baker, 1982).

Sand-soil Mixes for Rootzone Layers

If sand is added to a soil in large quantities, a rootzone material can be created which is free-draining even after the effecs of compaction. However, the success will depend on the use of a uniform sand, for which the particles will not interpack, and achieving the correct mixing ratio of soil to sand.

The amount of fine material in the soil must be diluted below prescribed limits. A minimum specification is that sufficient sand should be added so that the final mix has less than 20% total fines (particles < 0.125 mm diameter), less than 10% silt + clay (particles < 0.05 mm diameter) and less than 5% clay (particles < 0.002 mm diameter) (Baker, 1985).

Where higher design objectives are to be satisfied, proportionally more sand is required. For re-constructions at Everton F.C. in 1981 and Sheffield Wednesday F.C. in 1984 clay contents were reduced to 2-3% and there were no more than 12% of particles less than 0.125 mm in diameter. Uniform medium-fine sands were used for reconstruction and the distribution of particles has been concentrated into the range 0.125-0.5 mm diameter. At Everton's ground 80% of the material occurs in this size range and at Sheffield Wednesday's the figure is 75%.

In 1970, in contrast, rootzone analyses for 17, mainly First and Second Division Football League Clubs had a much higher percentage of fine material (Thornton, 1978). The average clay content was 10% and the quantity of material less than 0.125 mm diameter was 33%. Only 44% of the material was within the 0.125-0.5 mm diameter size range. To attain comparability with the amount of fine material at Everton's and Sheffield Wednesday's grounds a soil with 10% clay and 33% of the material less than 0.125 mm diameter would have to be mixed with sand in the ratio of one part soil to three parts sand by volume.

Water infiltration rates are critical for the performance of winter games pitches. These rates will decline with time and vary with maintenance treatments. Table 1 shows changes in infiltration rates for rootzone mixes containing varying proportions of sandy loam soil and a medium-fine sand. Details of the rootzone analyses and the construction, maintenance and wear are given by Baker and Isaac (1987a).

Infiltration rates for the mixes with 2 soil : 1 sand and 1 soil : 1 sand declined rapidly and were $\leqslant$ 5 mm h^{-1} in March 1985. Infiltration rates for the mixes of 1 soil : 2 sand fell more slowly but by March 1986 were only 3 mm h^{-1}. For winter pitches of the highest standard and intensity of use infiltration rates should be sufficient to deal with rainfall intensities approaching 20 mm h^{-1} with a duration of 30 minutes (Adams, 1981): this was only achieved on the pure sand rootzone.

Table 1. Changes in infiltration rates with time for four rootzone materials

Mixing Ratio	October 1984 (pre-wear)	March 1985	August 1985	March 1986	August 1986
		Infiltration rate (mm h^{-1})			
2 soil : 1 sand	60	2	1	1	5
1 soil : 1 sand	24	5	1	1	7
1 soil : 2 sand	57	18	5	3	15
All sand	274	487	512	291	260

Compaction and sealing of the surface layer by fine mineral and organic matter (Adams, 1981) combine to lower infiltration rates. Maintenance procedures aim to reverse these deleterious effects. The infiltration rates in Table 1 represent a 'worst case' in that no spiking had taken place since the last wear treatment. Regular spiking can increase water infiltration; for example, Baker (1981) found that hand-forking on a Rugby ground increased infiltration rates from 2 mm h^{-1} to values in range of 30-66 mm h^{-1}, while Canaway et al. (1986), comparing spiked and unspiked treatments on a sand construction, found spiking increased infiltration rates by a factor of 1.5 to 2.6 during the period of wear.

More severe mechanical decompaction treatments are also available. The increase in infiltration rates recorded in August 1986 probably reflects the use of a vibratory decompaction treatment, two weeks earlier, in which narrow fissures were cut into the turf to a depth of 150 mm at a spacing of 230 mm.

Dilution of any fine material or organic matter that accumulates at the soil surface is also required if high infiltration rates are to be sustained. Sand dressings are normally used and Ward (1983) found that First Division Football League Clubs added 80 tonnes of sand per pitch each year, while the clubs in the lower divisions added between 23-39 tonnes.

Sand Constructions

Although sand-soil mixes can produce a free-draining rootzone layer there are disadvantages, particularly in that small deviations from the recommended mixing ratio can have severe consequences and that migration of the finer material can impede infiltration of water. A number of construction techniques therefore use sand without soil as the rooting medium. In some cases this sand may be modified by the inclusion of various organic and inorganic materials (Paul et al., 1970). The selection of sand must consider water retention and the stability and traction properties of the surface; uniform medium-fine sands (0.125-0.5 mm diameter) are therefore preferred (Baker, 1984).

Three basic types of sand constructions can be recognised:

(i) Sand carpet pitches (e.g. Fig. 1). A layer of sand, usually 100-150 mm deep, overlies the native soil which is intensively drained. The sand serves as a free-draining surface layer but the grass roots are able to penetrate into the underlying soil which acts as a source of water and nutrients. This type of construction has been used successfully in Northern Ireland since 1966 (Mulqueen and Prunty, 1972).

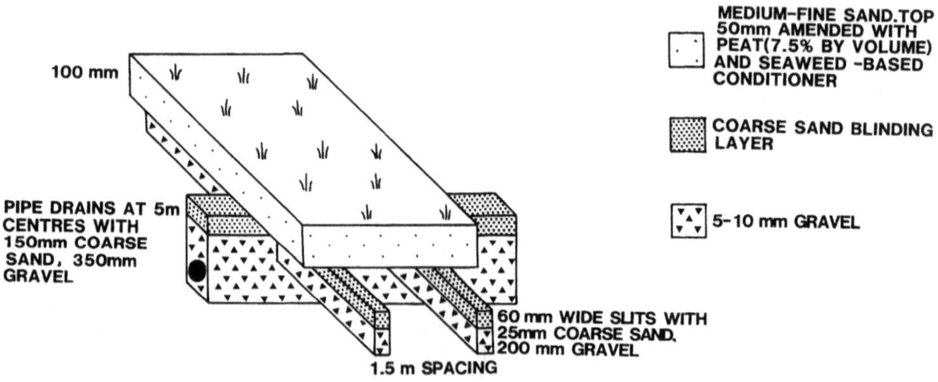

Figure 1. Constructional details of a sand carpet pitch (Birchwood Complex, Warrington 1985)

(ii) Suspended water table constructions (e.g. Fig.2). The rootzone layer of 250-300 mm medium-fine sand is placed over a coarse blinding layer and a gravel drainage carpet. High drainage rates are ensured and the textural break between the sand and gravel improves water retention in the rootzone layer (Radko, 1974).

(iii) Sand surrounded by an impermeable membrane (e.g. Fig.3). This is useful where water conservation is at a premium as the system allows control of the water table in the rootzone layer and re-cycling of water as long as this does not contribute to salinity problems.

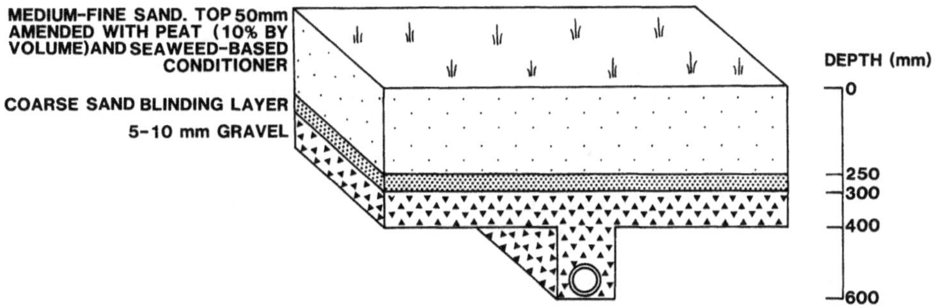

Figure 2. Constructional details of a sand-based suspended water table pitch (Metropolitan Police, Imber Court, London, 1984

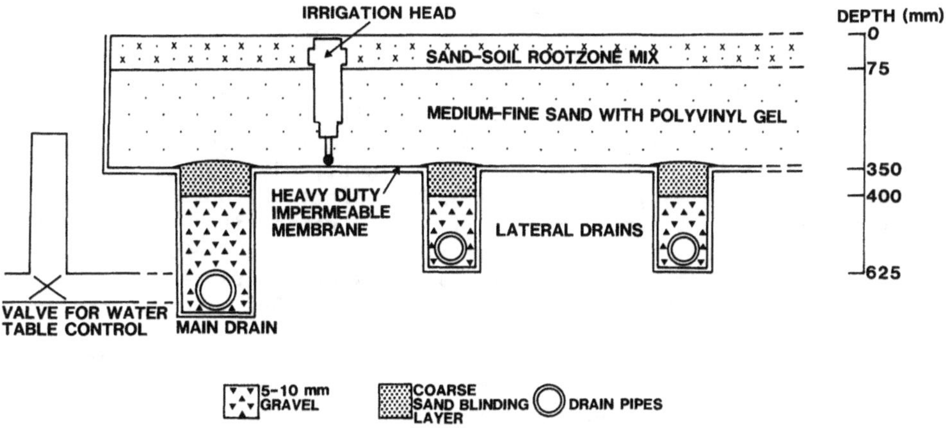

Figure 3. Constructional details of a sand-based pitch with an impermeable membrane and water table control (Gizan, Saudi Arabia, 1987)

Overview

In the last twenty years, construction techniques have developed to the extent that drainage should not be the limiting factor for the performance of winter games pitches, as long as scientific design criteria are used and construction materials are selected to published specifications. However, sports turf is a dynamic system and drainage performance will deteriorate in the absence of appropriate management. In the long run it is therefore aspects of groundsmanship which will determine whether the investment in pitch drainage will result in the hard-wearing surface that is required for a high quality sports pitch.

Acknowledgements

The author wishes to thank Miss S.L. Thornton for her help in the production of the figures.

References

Adams, W.A. (1981) Soils and plant nutrition for sportsturf: perspective and prospects. In Proceedings 4th International Turfgrass Research Conference (edited by R.W. Sheard) pp. 167-79. Guelph, Canada, Ontario Agricultural College/International Turfgrass Society.

Baker, S.W. (1981) The effect of earthworm activity on the drainage characteristics of winter sports pitches. J. Sports Turf Res. Inst., 57, 9-23.

Baker, S.W. (1982) Regional variation of design rainfall rates for slit drainage schemes in Great Britain. J. Sports Turf Res. Inst., 58, 57-63.

Baker, S.W. (1984) The science of sand. In Sand Constructions for Sports Pitches (edited by Pl. Crewdson) pp. 4-9. National Turfgrass Council Workshop Report No.3.

Baker, S.W. (1985) Topsoil quality: relation to the performance of sand-soil mixes. In: Proceedings 5th International Turfgrass Research Conference (edited by F. Lemaire) pp. 401-409. Avignon, France, Institute National de la Recherche Agronomique.

Baker, S.W. and Isaac, S.P. (1987a) The effect of rootzone composition on the performance of winter games pitches. I. Sward characteristics. J. Sports Turf Res. Inst., 63, 57-66.

Baker, S.W. and Isaac, S.P. (1987b) The effect of rootzone composition on the performance of winter games pitches II. Playing quality. J. Sports Turf Res. Inst., 63, 67-81.

Canaway, P.M. (1978) Trials of turfgrass wear tolerance and associated factors: a summary of progress 1975-77. J. Sports Turf Res. Inst., 78, 7-14.

Canaway, P.M., Isaac, S.P. and Bennett, R.A. (1986) The effects of mechanical treatments on the water infiltration rate of a sand playing surface for Association Football. J. Sports Turf Res. Inst., 62, 67-73.

Clark, H.E. (1970) Drainage at Twickenham. J. Sports Turf Res. Inst., 46, 14-16.

Mulqueen, J. and Prunty, J.P. (1972) Constructing all-weather sports grounds. Parks, Golf Courses and Sports Grounds, 37, 428-30.

Paul, J.L., Madison, J.H. and Waldron, L. (1970) Effects of organic and inorganic amendments on the hydraulic conductivity of three sands used for turfgrass soils. J. Sports Turf Res. Inst., 46, 22-32.

Radko, A.M. (1974) Refining green section specifications for putting green construction. In: Proceedings 2nd International Turfgrass Research Conference (edited by E.C. Roberts) pp. 287-97. Blacksburg, U.S.A., American Society of Agronomy.

Sports Turf Research Institute (1978) Slit drainage of winter pitches. Sports Turf Bull. 121, 5-6.

Thornton, D.J. (1978) The construction and drainage of some specified sports field playing surfaces. Unpublished Ph.D. Thesis. University College of Wales, Aberystwyth. 594 pp.

van Wijk, A.L.M., Verhaegh, W.B. and Beuving, J. (1977) Grass Sportsfields top layer compaction and soil aeration. Rasen-turf-gazon, 6, 77-83.

Ward, C.J. (1983) Drainage of sports turf areas: results of a questionnaire survey. J. Sports Turf Res. Inst., 59, 29-45.

GROUND REACTION FORCES DEVELOPED ON ARTIFICIAL TURF

Gordon A. Valiant
Nike Sport Research Laboratory, 9000 S.W. Nimbus Drive, Beaverton, OR, 97005, U.S.A.

Introduction

Injuries to the lower extremity frequently occur in sports which involve a large amount of lateral movement. For example, soccer players experience a relatively high number of injuries to the knee and ankle (Muckle, 1981). American football, with its high frequency of hitting and collisions, is probably the sport that accounts for the greatest percentage of lower extremity injuries (DeHaven and Lintner, 1986). Many of the knee injuries are caused by large torques that are developed at the interface between the foot and playing surface. Excessive traction due to the type of shoe (Torg and Quedenfeld, 1974) or due to the type of playing surface (Morehouse and Morrison, 1975) has often been implicated in many of these injuries.

The need to develop forces against the ground to run fast, start and stop quickly and make rapid cuts necessitates sufficiently high traction characteristics of athletic footwear. There is thus an apparent compromise between skilled performance and protection from potentially harmful situations in the design of shoe outsoles. Therefore, it was the objective of this study to describe the pattern of ground reaction force development during lateral movements and to use these force measurements to determine the minimum traction needs of a shoe outsole on a dry artificial playing surface.

Methods

Six components of ground reaction forces and moments were measured at 500 Hz per channel on eight recreational and former college soccer players during straight-line running and during two different lateral movements. All testing was conducted in an area covered with an artificial playing surface (Astroturf) with a separate section of Astroturf securely fastened to the force measuring platform. The two lateral movements investigated were a rapid stop with the right foot followed by a 90 degree cut to the left, and a rapid stop with the right foot followed by a 180 degree pivot medially and a push-off in the direction opposite to the original run-up. Running speed during the final 4 m approach to the force platform averaged 4.3 m s^{-1}. These lateral movements were simple to perform and to repeat within and between all subjects. They incorporated components that required several different traction needs, including posteriorly directed translational traction forces during rapid stopping, anteriorly directed translational traction forces during straight-line push-offs, laterally directed translation traction forces during 90 degree cuts, and rotational traction forces during 180 degree pivots.

Placement of the foot on the force platform was determined by filming at 148 frames per second the image of the dorsal aspect of the foot in a mirror suspended above the force platform and angled 45 degrees to the horizontal. Digitization of two markers spaced 38 mm apart along the midline of the shoe in the forefoot region and markers fixed on the force platform was initiated at the first frame where both heel and forefoot were down. Digitization was ended when the image of the shoe markers became hidden by the shank as a result of dorsi-flexion. Approximately 5 frames were digitized for the running trials, 30 frames for the pivotting and the entire support period was digitized for the cutting movements. Using the angle of foot placement on the force platform calculated from digitized shoe markers, the shear components of the ground reaction forces were expressed as mediolateral (F m-l) and anteroposterior (F a-p) force components and the centre of pressure of the resultant ground reaction force vector was expressed in terms of the shoe placement. It was assumed that during the running trials the angle made by the foot on the force platform remained unchanged during the support phase and so the shear forces were resolved in terms of shoe axes for the entire support period.

For each trial, F m-l/Fz, F a-p/Fz and 1000 Mz'/Fz were calculated to give dimensionless expressions of maximum translational and rotational friction during the support phase of each of the three movements. Fz and Mz' are the vertical force and the free moment about the vertical axis, respectively. Data from five trials of each of the three movements by each subject were normalized to the mean time of support and averaged. Peak force components and peak force ratios were determined for each of the three movements. Ratio peaks were not calculated for vertical forces which were less than 0.10 body weights (BW).

All subjects wore the same pair of indoor soccer shoes. The right shoe of this pair was tested on an Astroturf surface by a physical traction testing device. The device closely simulated the normal loads acting and velocities of the shoe on the surface during actual sports movements. A more detailed description of the physical traction testing device can be found in Valiant (1987).

Results

The average peak forces and the average times of occurrence are reported in Table 1. Propulsive force components for the pivotting movement were not determined because shoe markers were hidden in the last half of the movement when the foot placement angle was continually changing. The peaks plotted in the averaged force curves are less than the tabulated peaks due to the attenuation that occurs when averaging curves whose peaks do not occur at exactly the same time.

Table 1. Mean ground reaction force peaks [BW] and the relative times of occurrence [% of support period] during braking (brake) and propulsive (prop) phases of the movements

	F m-l				F a-p			
	brake		prop		brake		prop	
run	-0.06	14%	-	-	0.66	14%	-0.34	74%
cut	-1.55	11%	-0.97	42%	1.85	9%	-	-
pivot	-1.46	9%	NA		1.60	8%	NA	

	Fz			
	brake		prop	
run	2.46	12%	2.84	40%
cut	3.45	10%	1.82	32%
pivot	3.02	9%	-	-

Mean ground reaction force components for the cutting and pivotting movements are plotted in Figure 1. When performing the 90 degree cuts, subjects planted their right foot on the force platform in front of and to the right of their body. Thus, the mediolateral impulse is developed entirely in the lateral direction, initially as a braking impulse and then as a propulsive impulse. The mean centre of pressure path for the 90 degree cuts, plotted in Figure 2, shows primarily an anterior progression down the midline of the shoe: however, there was considerable variation between subjects, as demonstrated by the high standard deviations. There was a tendency to make initial contact with the ground nearer the medial edge of the rear of the shoe, largely because the foot plant, as indicated above, was to the right of the body. The resultant ground reaction force vector during the propulsive phase was located near the midline of the forefoot region and then moved in a medial direction.

The ratios of mean mediolateral and anteroposterior forces divided by the mean vertical force for the cutting and pivotting movement are plotted in Figure 3. The peak mediolateral force ratio during the cutting movement averaged 0.62. The mean anteroposterior ratio during the cutting movement was greater, however, averaging 0.80. This peak ratio always occurred during the braking phase, at a mean support period time of 14%. The peak anteroposterior force ratio during pivotting averaged 0.79 and occurred at a mean support period time of 5%. The peak of the mediolateral force ratio during pivotting also occurred during the early braking phase, averaging 0.61 at 9%. Mean peaks are averages of individual trials, not peaks from average curves.

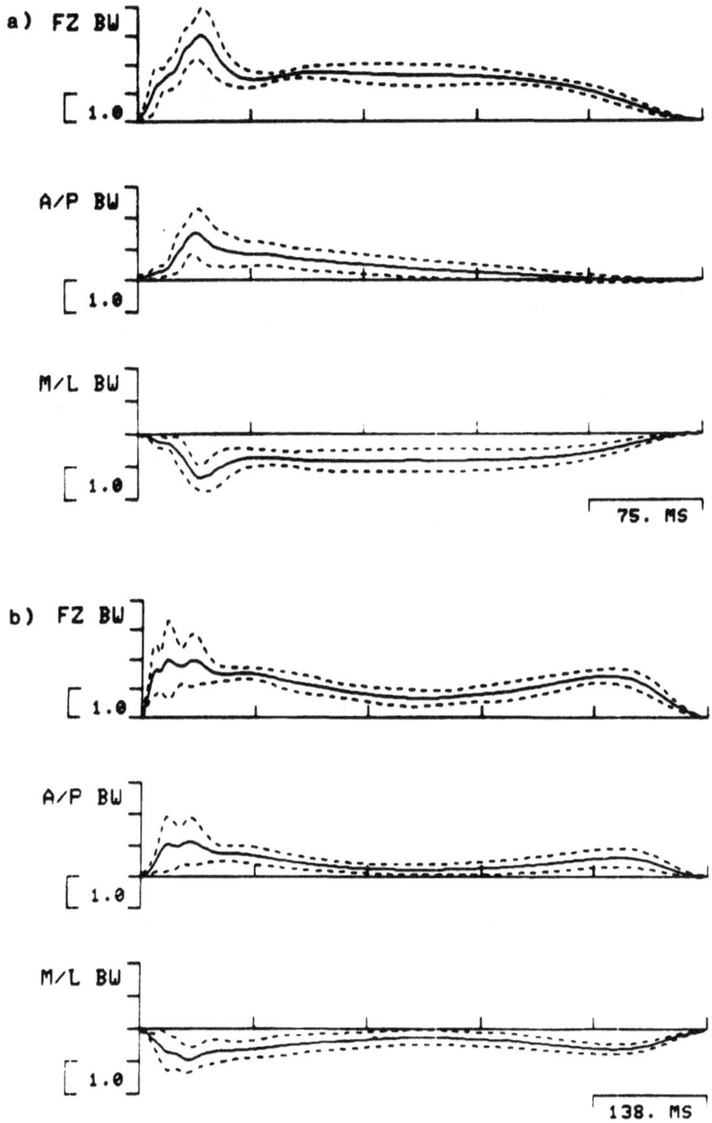

Figure 1. Mean ground reaction force components in mediolateral (m-l), anteroposterior (a-p), and vertical (Fz) directions normalised to subjects' body weight during a) cutting (n=37 trials) and b) pivotting movements (n=33 trials). Dotted lines represent ± 1 standard deviation. Positive a-p forces are directed anteriorly and negative m-l forces are directed laterally. Shear forces were resolved for the pivotting movement for only the first 39% of the support phase.

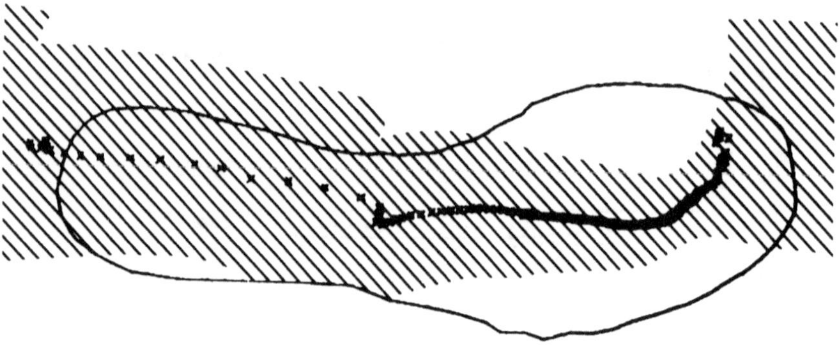

Figure 2. The centre of pressure pattern

The mean free moment during pivotting is shown in Figure 4. The peak moment averaged -17.2 Nm. As the developed moments generally increase with increased normal loading, these moments were normalized with respect to normal load. This peak normalized free moment averaged -25.6 mm. When normalized with respect to normal loading, the expression of resistance developed during pivotting is about four times greater than during running, which averaged 6 mm.

When tested on the physical traction testing device, -48 Nm of torque resisted medial rotation of the soccer shoe on an Astroturf surface. Also measured on the physical traction test was the coefficient of kinetic friction for the shoe on Astroturf and it was found to be 1.6. Results of these two physical traction tests are summarized in Figure 5. Images in the overhead mirror revealed very small amounts of relative movement of the foot with respect to the Astroturf and it was therefore felt that a physical measure of the kinetic coefficient of friction was more applicable in this study than a measure of the static coefficient of friction. The physical traction device gave more reliable measures of the kinetic

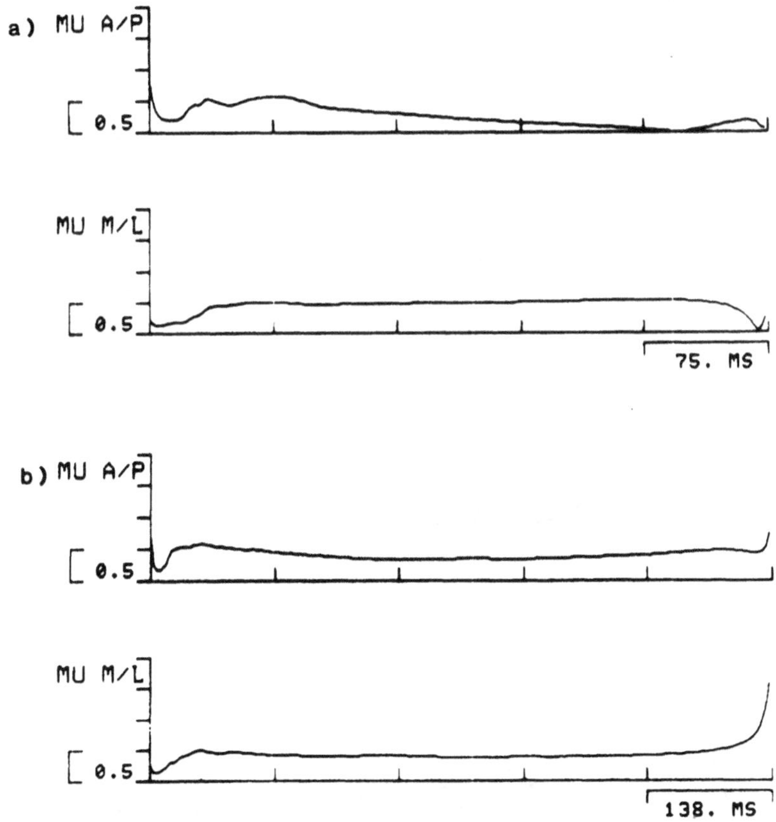

Figure 3. Ratios, labelled mu, of the absolute value of mean shear force components divided by mean vertical force components for the a) cutting and b) pivotting movements

coefficient of friction, but, as can be seen from Figure 5, estimates of the static coefficient of friction, which exceed the kinetic coefficient, can also be made.

Discussion

The greatest shear forces were developed in an anterior direction and occurred during rapid stopping. The peak anterior shear forces were the same regardless of whether the subjects were stopping their forward progression to make a cut or to make a pivot. The high laterally directed shear forces developed during the cutting movement also had the greatest peaks during the braking rather than the propulsive phase. Thus, when making lateral movements, the force peaks developed when the subjects in this study stopped themselves were greater than the force peaks created when initiating a change of direction and propelling themselves in that new direction.

It was found that in most cases, the force ratios (shear/vertical) were greatest during the braking phase. This is in spite of high

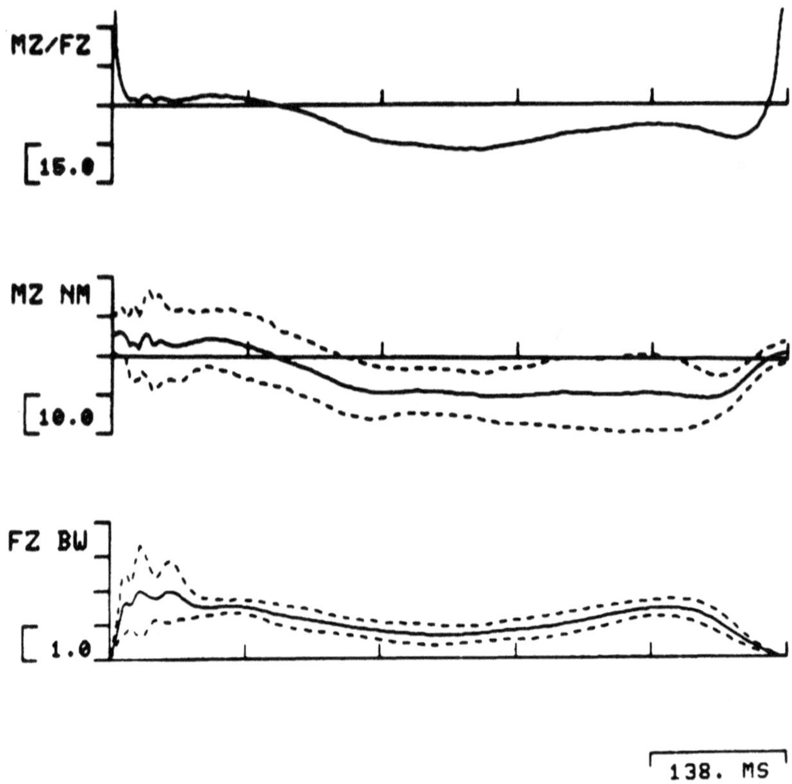

Figure 4. Mean free moment (Mz) and ± 1 standard deviation developed during the pivotting movement (n=33 trials). A negative moment resists medial rotation of the right foot. The normalized moment in units of mm equals the mean free moment divided by the mean normal load

vertical forces, exceeding 3 BW, developed during the braking phase. The ratios calculated with the forces acting along the longitudinal axis of the shoe exceed those ratios calculated with the forces acting along the transverse axis of the shoe. This further suggests that the traction needs of the soccer shoe worn are greater for movements that involve anteriorly directed forces, such as those during stopping, than for movements involving laterally directed forces, such as those developed in making a change in direction.

The outsole on the shoe that was used in this study is made of

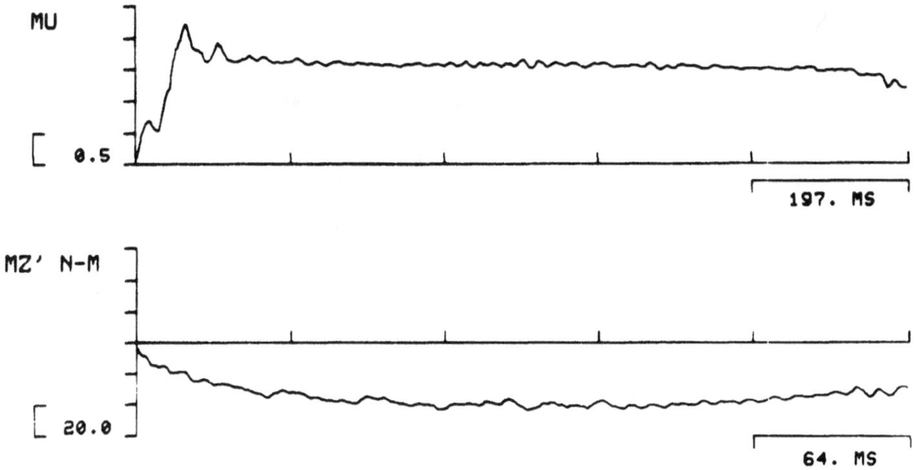

Figure 5. Coefficient of friction (mu) and free moment of rotation (Mz') developed by the soccer shoe used in this study on Astroturf. The physical traction testing device pulled the shoe in an anterior direction at an average velocity of 0.37 m s^{-1} , or rotated the shoe medially at an average velocity of 6.62 rad s^{-1}. Normal loading for both tests averaged 740 N

rubber with 56 individual projections with varying cross-sectional dimensions extending downward 5 mm from the outsole. The -48 Nm of torque developed by this shoe when physically tested in medial rotation agrees closely with torques reported by Bonstingl et al. (1975), by Van Gheluwe et al. (1983) and by Andreasson et al. (1986). The former group reported 23-32 ft lb (31-43 Nm) of torque developed by multicleated soccer shoes when tested in rotation on Astroturf. The second group of investigators reported a range of 35-50 Nm of resistance to rotation of soccer shoes with similar outsole designs on Astroturf. The latter group of investigators reported torques developed while sliding on an artificial turf which were as high as 50 Nm for some shoes. The coefficient of kinetic friction measure of 1.6 was as much as 60% higher than the translational friction measures reported by Van Gheluwe et al. (1983). It should be kept in mind that the shoes in all of the above tests, as well as the tests themselves are different, and direct comparisons of results, both rotational and translational, are difficult to make.

The high kinetic coefficient of friction for the test shoe indicates that its translational traction characteristics may be overspecified. This is because the highest mean translational traction requirement measured during any of the movements studied was a force ratio of 0.80. The highest mean force ratio for any one subject was 0.97 and the highest force ratio measured on any single trial in an anterior direction was 1.14.

The rotational traction characteristics of the shoe, which should be at a minimum, may actually be too high. The free moment of -48 Nm resisting rotation is high, and is capable of resisting the torques that subjects develop voluntarily during pivotting movements. Situations other than voluntary pivots that develop higher rotary forces between the shoe and the playing surface can arise, especially when contact with opposing players is made, and especially when played on artificial surfaces where the traction is very high. High resistance to rotation implies that much of this rotary force can be transmitted to skeletal structures such as the knee joint. If the rotational friction characteristics of this shoe were lower, it would be less likely to place the athlete in a potentially injurious situation.

Thus, because the outsole of the shoe probably exhibited more translational traction than was necessary, its frictional characteristics could be reduced, thereby reducing the resistance to rotation as well. In that case, the shoe would still exhibit adequate translational traction, but it would also exhibit better rotational traction characteristics. The results of this study have shown how the measurement of ground reaction force components can be used to identify the traction needs of shoes used for the movements studied. Implications for outsole design include a means for reducing resistance to rotation without jeopardizing the development of sufficient friction forces in translation, particularly for movements of the shoe in an anterior direction.

References

Andreasson, G., Lindenberger, U., Renstrom, P. and Peterson, L. (1986) Torque developed at simulated sliding between sport shoes and an artificial turf. Amer. J. Sports Med., 14, 225-230.

Bonstingl, R.W., Morehouse, C.A. and Niebel, B.W. (1975) Torques developed by different types of shoes on various playing surfaces. Med. Sci. Sports, 7, 127-131.

DeHaven, K.E. and Lintner, D.M. (1986) Athletic injuries: Comparison by age, sport and gender. Amer. J. Sports Med., 14, 218-224.

Morehouse, C.A. and Morrison, W.E. (1975) The artificial turf story. In: Penn State HPER Series (edited by M.J. Haverbeck): The Pennsylvania State University.

Muckle, D.S. (1981) Injuries in professional footballers. Brit. J. Sports Med., 15, 77-79.

Torg, J.S. and Ouedenfeld, T. (1974) Effect of shoe type and cleat length on incidence and severity of knee injuries among high school football players. Res. Ouart., 42, 203-211.

Valiant, G.A. (1987) Effects of outsole pattern on basketball shoe traction. In: Biomechanics of Sport III and IV (edited by J. Terauds, B.A. Gowitzke and L.E. Holt), pp.29-37. Del Mar, CA: Academic Publishers.

Van Gheluwe, B., Deporte, E. and Hebbelinck, M. (1983) Frictional forces and torques of soccer shoes on artificial turf. In: Biomechanical Aspects of Sports Shoes and Playing Surfaces (edited by B.M. Nigg and B.A. Kerr), pp.161-168. Calgary, Canada: University Printing.

DESIGNING A FOOTBALL BOOT: A THEORETICAL AND EXPERIMENTAL APPROACH

R. Rodano*, P. Cova** and R. Vigano**
*Centro di Bioingineria, Politecnico di Milano - Fondazione Pro Juventute Don Gnocchi, Milano, Italy
**Istituto Ortopedico "G. Pini", Italy

Introduction

A modern approach to sport shoe production cannot do without scientific research. Significant examples are supplied by Cavanagh (1980). The aim of this study is to illustrate the scientific approach adopted in the design and production of a football boot and to describe some original solutions introduced to improve the boot's technical characteristics. In football, more than in other sports, the footwear plays a fundamental role in influencing the athlete's performance. It must be stable, have a good fit and properly contain the rearfoot. It must moreover allow the player to run freely and help him play correctly by not interfering with his movement and running style, since the very nature of this sport involves heavy stress on the player's legs and feet.

Materials and Methods

A correct basis for football boot design is provided by the study of the ground foot interactions mediated by the footwear during football play according to the scheme of Fig. 1. In order to analyse these interactions correctly the researcher should know the major elements in the system, i.e. the locomotor apparatus and the typical sports movements. In this section the methods used to study the locomotor apparatus, football typical movements and their mutual biomechanical interactions, as well as how these affect the footwear are described.

The locomotor apparatus and in particular the player's foot

A clinical analysis protocol was worked out on the basis of the data collected from the literature, from a series of interviews with 50 professional soccer players concerning the dynamic stress imposed on the locomotor apparatus by the various game skills, as well as with experimental measurements of the athlete's lower limb and foot. The aim of this study was to define the most common morphotypes in a sample of top professional footballers and eventually identify any pathological disorders directly associated with football practice.

The protocol included:

i) a visit by a specialist in bone and joint diseases and collection of data on the footballer's history:

ii) the measurement of standard foot parameters - length, instep and metatarsal region and

    IMD intermalleolar distance;
    MH distance between the medial malleolus apex and the bearing surface;
    LH distance between the lateral malleolus apex and the bearing surface;
    MD distance between the medial malleolus apex and the heel rear profile tangent plane;
    LD distance between the lateral malleolus apex and the heel rear profile tangent plane;

iii) lower limb postural photos by a special set-up;

iv) photopodogram according to the usual medical technique.

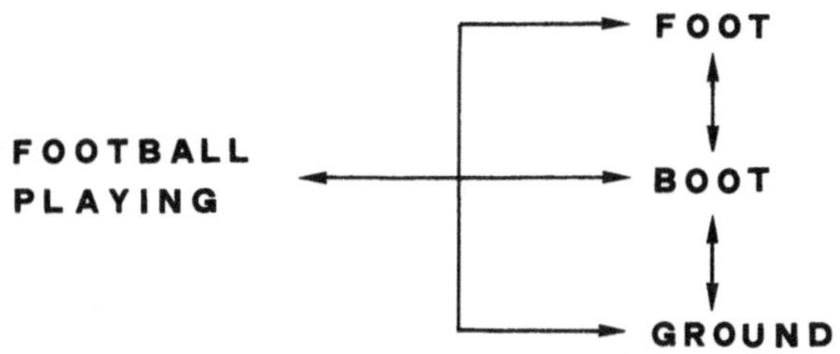

Figure 1. Interaction foot-footwear-ground

Definition of football fundamental movements

A special technique for TV image analysis was developed to identify football fundamental movements and qualitatively define their technical characteristics. This particular system consisted in filming selective shots of the players' lower limbs during championship matches.

The films thus obtained underwent an editing process aiming at highlighting the aspects of movements which might escape ordinary observation. Thus, the major features of running, dribbling, kicking and tackling were defined and some typical movements identified which better lent themselves to biomechanical laboratory studies.

Biomechanical studies and foot-ground interaction analysis

Three fundamental points were considered:-

i) the loading on the locomotor apparatus during various game skills as a function of kinematics and dynamics;

ii) the distribution of local loading on the foot and footwear soles;

iii) the measurement of ground reaction forces during simulated impacts.

Each point was studied in an experimental set-up consisting of:-i)an automatic TV image processing unit (ELITE) for the on-line acquisition of the space coordinates of a number of joint points of reference through markers fitted on the players' joints (Ferrigno and Pedotti, 1985);

ii) a force-platform for the measurement of ground reactions at foot impact and production of the corresponding vector diagrams (Boccardi et al., 1978);

iii) a piezoelectric polymer transducer insole for the measurement of vertical loading on the footsole bearing points (Assente et al., 1985);

iv) an impact simulator and force platform for the measurement of ground reaction forces resulting from the various types of footwear.

Due to the variability of playing surfaces it was not possible to test samples of all existing surfaces. Therefore, to make results homogeneous, laboratory tests were carried out on synthetic grass.

Results

Morphological aspects

The clinical, photographical and podographical survey described above allowed the authors to identify the characteristic typologies of soccer players and collect a series of data which could be of use in re-designing football boots.

With respect to the plantar arch, the analysis of the data on the 50 subjects indicated that 68% were normal, 32% showed signs of pes cavus while no sign of flatfoot was observed. An 8% overloading on the first metatarsal bone head was demonstrated by the development of painful corns at this site.

Circumferential measures of the infoot and metatarsal region showed that in the test sample these tend to be the same for each player, the mean difference between the two measures being 0.3%.

Table 1 shows the data relating to the malleolus space of the players' feet for the sizes of 7½ (44% of sample players), 7(10%) and 8(20%).

Table 1. Mean values and standard deviations (in mm) of the coordinates of the foot anatomical points. The data refer to the most common phases

		IMD	MH	LH	MD	LD
7	$\bar{x}$	72	86	60	104	43
(10%)	SD	2	3	5	6	8
7½	$\bar{x}$	75	88	63	105	43
(44%)	SD	2	4	4	7	8
8	$\bar{x}$	76	89	63	107	45
(20%)	SD	4	6	4	8	10

Characteristics of various game skills

The TV analysis indicated the following movements as major points of interest:-

i) Running which is substantially different from other sports like jogging, because a) weight bearing is mainly on outwardly rotated forefoot, b) at impact on rearfoot, the foot is outwardly rotated, especially in passes, c) the player's feet are wider apart.

ii) Kicking: while the player prepares to kick and especially in crosses, his weight bearing foot is subject to extensive stress due to outward rotation and abduction with extreme talipes valgus position of the rearfoot.

iii) Dribbling is characterized by continuous stress on the rearfoot which twists continuously from valgus to varus position and tends to loose footing.

iv) Tackling produces a predominance of horizontal stress on the foot in all directions.

Biomechanical aspects and foot-ground interactions

Kinematics: Fig. 2 shows the stick diagram of a player's lower limb during kicking. Thus an overall view of the movement was obtained and derived amplitudes, angles (Fig. 3), speed and acceleration were calculated using a suitable lower limb mathematical model. Thus use of these measurements for both the weight bearing and kicking foot lead to the quantification of the range of angle variation for each joint and particularly the ankle, and of the effect of these variations on the football boot.

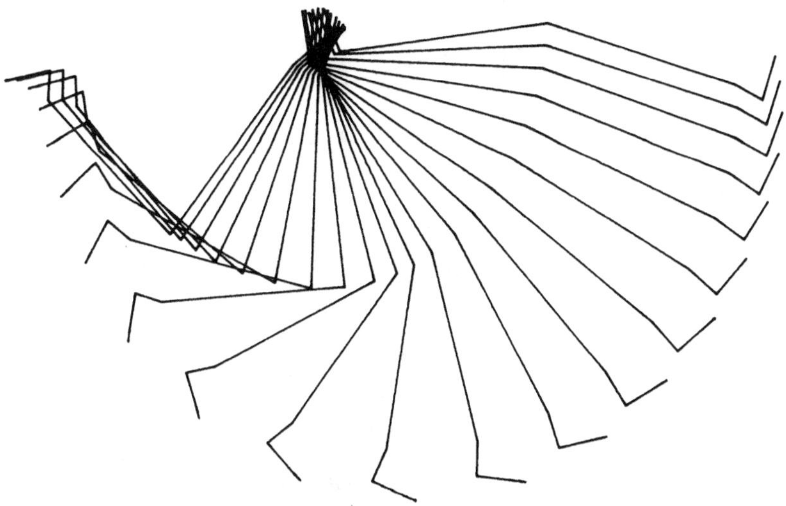

Figure 2. Stick-diagram of the football player's kicking limb

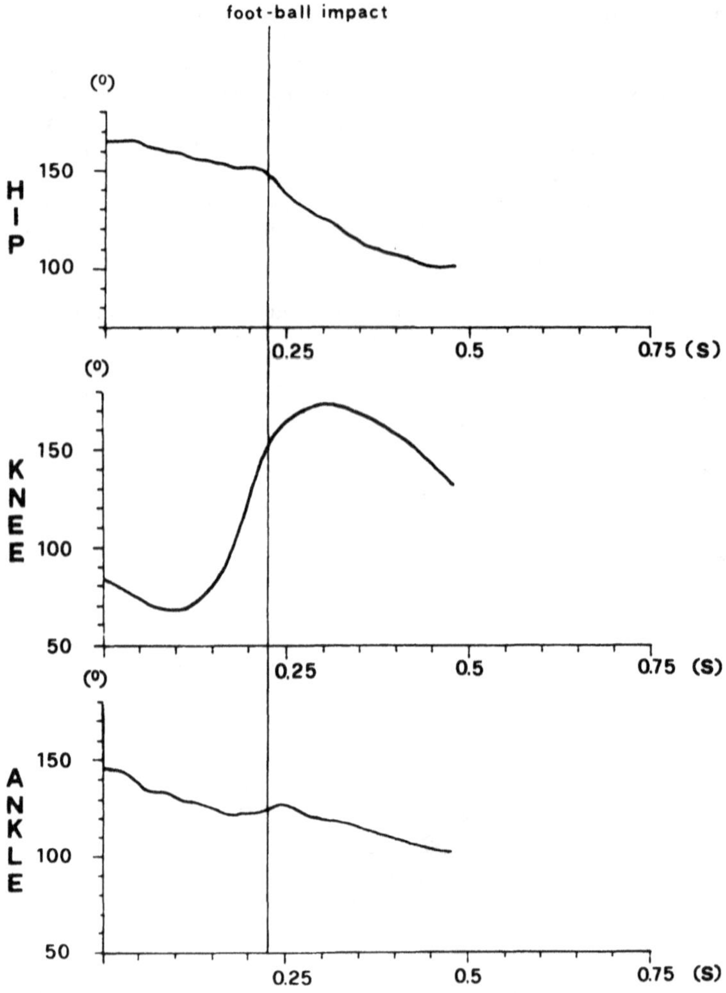

Figure 3. Curves of the kicking limb hip, knee and ankle joint angles

Dynamics: the analysis of ground reactions was used to quantify the load on the bearing foot (Fig. 4). It was thus observed that at kicking the vertical component (Rz) is 1.93 to 2.36 times the body weight and the horizontal components (Ry and Rx) are 0.88 to 0.50 times the body weight. Peak reaction is generally reached before the kicking foot touches the ball (0.12-0.08 s).

Another interesting result is the remarkable breaking effort (sticks inclined against travelling direction) the athlete performs to reduce his speed near to zero before kicking.

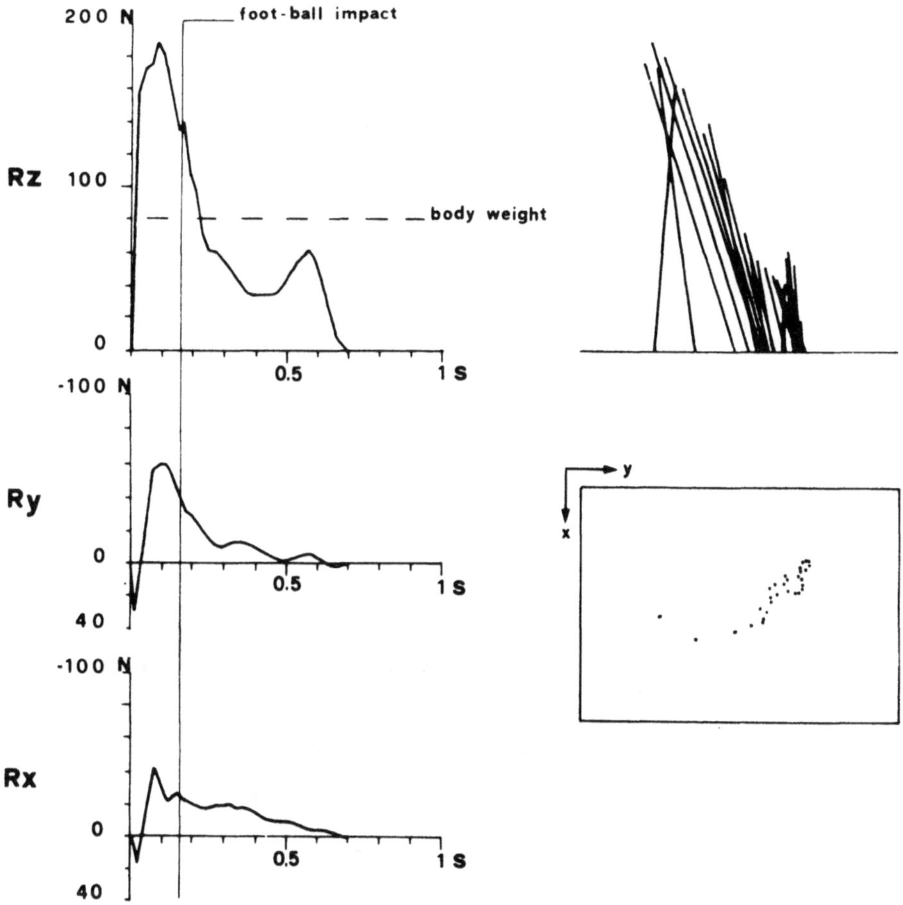

Figure 4. Ground reaction forces, sagittal vector-diagram and time course of the point of application recorded for the bearing limb during kicking

The stick distribution indicated that for the player's weight bearing foot, the highest forces are applied to the rear and midfoot. The shift in the point of application of force confirms the quick movement of load from the heel to the midfoot, with the foot outwardly rotated position with respect to the player's travelling line, in agreement with the data supplied by TV recordings.

Local load distribution: the players were required to perform simple and easily repeatable movements, but involving dynamic elements which would allow researchers to refer results to soccer match-play. Fig. 5 shows the curves obtained by using a piezoelectric polymer insole of 16 round transducers (0.6 mm) located on the anatomical points indicated in the Figure. The movement required of players was take-off with rebound on the same foot.

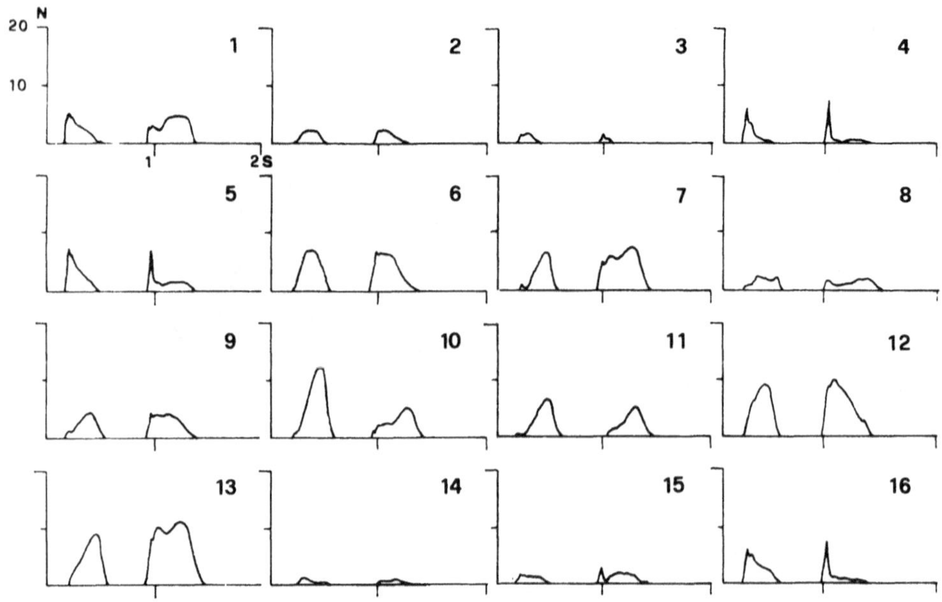

Figure 5. Loads recorded behind selected areas of the foot during take-off and subsequent landing. The numbers on the curves identify the foot as follows:
heel: 1 - medial heel, 2 - anteriomedial heel, 3 - posteriomedial heel, 4 - posteriolateral heel, 5 - anteriolateral heel, 6 - lateral mid foot,
metatarsal heads: 7-fifth, 8-fourth, 9-third, 10-second, 11 and 12-first,
toes: 13 and 14 big toe, 15-third, 16-fifth.

Curve analysis shows differences in shape, duration and time distribution depending on both the movement the player performs and the anatomical point concerned. At take-off the curves referring to the metatarsal region are rounded with load mainly bearing on the 1st, 2nd and 5th metatarsal bone heads; as to the rearfoot, curves show quick initial peaks depending on the kind of impact of this area with the ground. Load is mainly distributed on the mid- and anteriolateral portions of the heel.

During falling with rebound, the impact is less controlled than at take-off, as shown by peaks on all transducers. Most of the load is borne by the 1st and 5th metatarsal bone heads and the load tends to be concentrated medially. These tests were repeated several times changing cleat models and distribution and the results were used to work out criteria for cleat location and shaping.

Cushioning: load distribution on the locomotor apparatus at foot/ground impact depends on a number of factors, for example movement, player's morphotype and ground quality. The materials used in boot manufacturing are of a fundamental importance in order to reduce loading. Attention was focused on the physical characteristics of the material. The need to consider the football boot as a whole (functional unit) and eliminate possible confounding factors in comparisons induced the authors to adopt an impact simulator where the boot was fitted onto an artificial foot and hit the surface of a force platform. Foot inclination and impact energy are thus under strict control. The measurement of ground reactions at impact can be performed on a wide range of boot models and materials under the same experimental conditions and the various constructive options can be objectively compared. Ground reaction curve analysis (amplitude of peaks, durations, integral of force in time and discontinuity) was used to identify the manufacturing options which could ensure the best shock absorption and depression of vibrations without hindering the efficiency and precision of movement.

Conclusions and Proposals

The test procedures described above have helped to better understand many aspects of the function of the footwear as a force mediator. In this connection, the major elements are the footwear shape, the upper, the sole and the insole.

The shape Shape designing involves no major problems since, as indicated above, the morphotype of sample soccer players was not significantly different from the average youth's. But football boots should be close-fitting and slender as indicated not only by the experience and preference of the players but also by the statistical data showing the almost constant equivalence of circumferential instep and metatarsal region measures.

The upper Though fashioned in a rigid mould, the upper must in fact adjust to the live foot variations in position and morphology, which can be obtained by studying an appropriate design of components and choosing suitable materials. From a biomechanical point of view, foot and footwear are to be considered as a functional unit and it is the upper which should bind the unit, and at the same time, avoid friction. In soccer, load-bearing is mainly on the outwardly rotated forefoot involving greater stress on the upper outside section which should also ensure good and graded flexibility in the metatarsal region in agreement with the sole, without producing creases or hollows or foot-footwear incongruity. It must contain the rearfoot without friction on the Achilles tendon or the malleoli, especially the lateral one.

Lacing must favour steadiness without producing painful sensations at instep level and this may be obtained by stiffening and strengthening the tongue which, in association with a rational design of lacing, should ensure maximum tension and distribution of force on the widest possible instep surface.

The sole and cleats The football boot sole should resist torsional stress along its central line lengthwise in order not to lose stability and produce harmful stresses on some sectors of the foot. This is the reason why it should have transverse bending lines, the position of which greatly depends on cleat position.

There are two main types of sole. Firstly, the sole with a small number of cleats is recommended for wet slippery play areas because it ensures better footing. As cleats should be positioned as off-centre as possible for stability reasons, the best solution was thought to be the adoption of the seven cleat formula, with five fore- and two rear-cleats as illustrated in Fig. 6. It is worth noting the position of the rear-cleats was meant to favour running and the inclination of some cleats was meant to ensure better footing and stability.

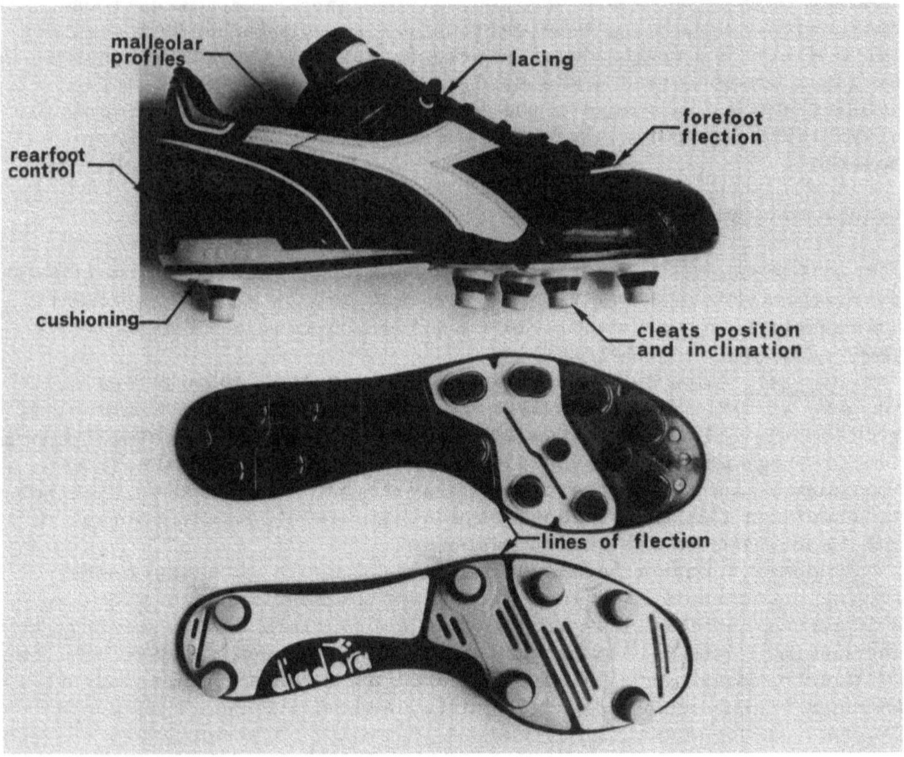

Figure 6. Football boot and soles with the main problems involved

The sole with a larger number of cleats is recommended for hard play areas as it avoids concentration of pressure and unstable footing. Because of the cleats reduced height, it was not possible to modify their inclination to improve stability, the section of the cleats bearing the greatest functional stress was modified (Fig. 6).

Insole The insole should meet two partly contradictory needs, absorbing shocks and limit vibrations. This cannot be achieved with one material only, as shock-absorbing materials produce vibration effects while vibration-depressing materials have practically no elastic qualities. An association of materials (EVA and NOENE) was therefore attempted which proved to ensure the predominance of one or the other of their respective qualities according to the stress applied to the foot with minimum interference of the shock-absorbing over the vibration-depressing function and vice versa.

References

Assente, R., De Rossi, D., Pedotti, A., and Rodano, R. (1985) Application of a piezoelectric polymer in gait analysis to measure the loads in selected foot areas. In: Biomechanics: Current Interdisiplinary Research (edited by S.M. Perren and E. Schneider) pp. 645-650. Dardrecht: Martinus Nijhoff Publs.

Boccardi, S., Pedotti, A., Frigo, C., Rodano, R., and Santambrogio, G.C. (1978) Analysis of some athletic activities by means of vector diagrams. In: Science in Athletics (edited by J. Terauds and G.G. Dales) pp. 183-192. Del Mar: Academic Publs.

Cavanagh, P.R. (1980). The Running Shoe Book. Mountain View: Anderson World Inc.,

Ferrigno, G. and Pedotti, A. (1985) ELITE: a digital dedicated hardware system for movement analysis via real-time TV signal processing. IEEE Trans. on Biomed. Eng., Vol. BME 32, No. 11.

Part X

Biomechanics of football skills

MAXIMAL BALL VELOCITY AND PEAK TORQUES OF HIP FLEXOR AND KNEE EXTENSOR MUSCLES

M.V. Narici, M.D. Sirtori and P. Mognoni,
Centro Studi Fisiologia del Lavoro Muscolare, CNR, via Mangiagalli 32, 20133, Milano, Italy.

Introduction

Isokinetic ergometry is often utilized for testing muscle function in soccer players (Oberg et al., 1984). Some authors maintain that this kind of measurement is useful for the prediction of muscle injuries typical of this game (Grace, 1985). Maximal torque values of isokinetic contractions are usually read at joint angles and angular speeds which are different from those encountered in the actual movement of kicking when ballistic torques (BT) are maximal (Huang et al., 1982; Robertson and Mosher, 1983). Furthermore, while several studies have been carried out for knee extensor muscles (KEM), little attention has been paid to hip flexor muscles (HFM) which have been shown to play a determinant role in ballistic conditions (Huang et al., 1982; Robertson and Mosher, 1983).

The aim of the present study was to measure isokinetic torques of KEM and HFM at the nearest possible angular speed to that reported for the ballistic movement of kicking and to correlate the obtained data to ball velocity attained during a powerful kick.

Material and Methods

Eleven male subjects (age 25.1±5.0 yrs; weight 76.1±10.8 kg; height 1.74±0.07 m) were studied; three of them were Fifth Division soccer players while the others were unaccustomed to this game.

According to standard technique, isokinetic testing of KEM is carried out in a sitting position, starting with a knee angle of 1.57 rad and that of HFM in supine position, starting with a hip angle of 3.14 rad. The above technique was modified in three details. First, the starting angle of movement was changed by increasing the excursion by 0.53 rad for both articulations; second, HFM were tested in an upright position; third, flexion of HFM was immediately preceded by a counter-movement. The rationale for these changes was to achieve a better simulation of the actual kicking and to produce higher torques. The angular speeds chosen were 3.14 rad s^{-1} for HFM and 5.23 rad s^{-1} for KEM. These speeds correponded to those evaluated under ballistic conditions for HFM, but was lower for KEM because a higher speed could not be achieved with the isokinetic dynamometer we used (Cybex II, Lumex Inc.). Both peak torques (PT) and values at angles corresponding to peak BT (IT) were read. These angles were 1.31 rad from full extension for KEM and 0.26 rad from the vertical for HFM. All torque values were corrected for gravitational effect (Winter et al., 1981).

To measure maximal ball velocity, the sounds generated by ball impact with foot and a 1.5 m^2 barrier, 10 m away, were recorded on an audio cassette whose output was fed into a graphic recorder to obtain time intervals between impacts.

Results and Discussion

Data for peak torque, angle at peak torque and angular velocity obtained with isokinetic ergometry and from ballistic measurements (Huang et al., 1982) are summarised in Table 1 for both the dominant(D) and non-dominant(ND) limbs.

Table 1. Means ± SD; for KEM angles (rad) from full knee extension, and for HFM from the vertical

		PT			IT			BT		
		Nm	rad	rad s^{-1}	Nm	rad	rad s^{-1}	Nm	rad	rad s^{-1}
	D	103	0.93	5.23	88	1.31	5.23	90	1.31	7.85
KEM		±21	±0.18		±22					
	ND	99	0.97	5.23	80	1.31	5.23			
		±24	±0.20		±24					
	D	147	0.19	3.14	135	0.26	3.14	260	0.26	3.14
HFM		±33	±0.28		±30					
	ND	140	0.20	3.14	123	0.26	3.14			3.14
		±35	±0.16		±37		3.14			3.14

The IT always occurred before PT and the percentage difference between the two ranged from 8% (HFM of the dominant limb) to 19% (KEM of the non-dominant limb). No statistical difference can be observed between torques developed by dominant and non-dominant limbs. The IT of HFM was higher than that of KEM (36% for dominant and 38% for non-dominant, $P < 0.001$). On the contrary Poulmedis (1985), who studied players from the National Greek team, found that at an angular speed of 3.14 rad s^{-1}, PT of KEM and HFM were 126±26 Nm and 95±17 Nm. The difference between ours and Poulmedis's data on the HFM is due to the different angles where IT was read in the two studies: as a matter of fact, Poulmedis by starting hip flexion without a counter-movement could not detect the real peak torque which we showed to occur with the hip still extended. The disagreement between the data regarding KEM is due to the different testing speeds chosen. Indeed, at a higher speed of contraction a lower torque is produced according to the classical force-velocity concept.

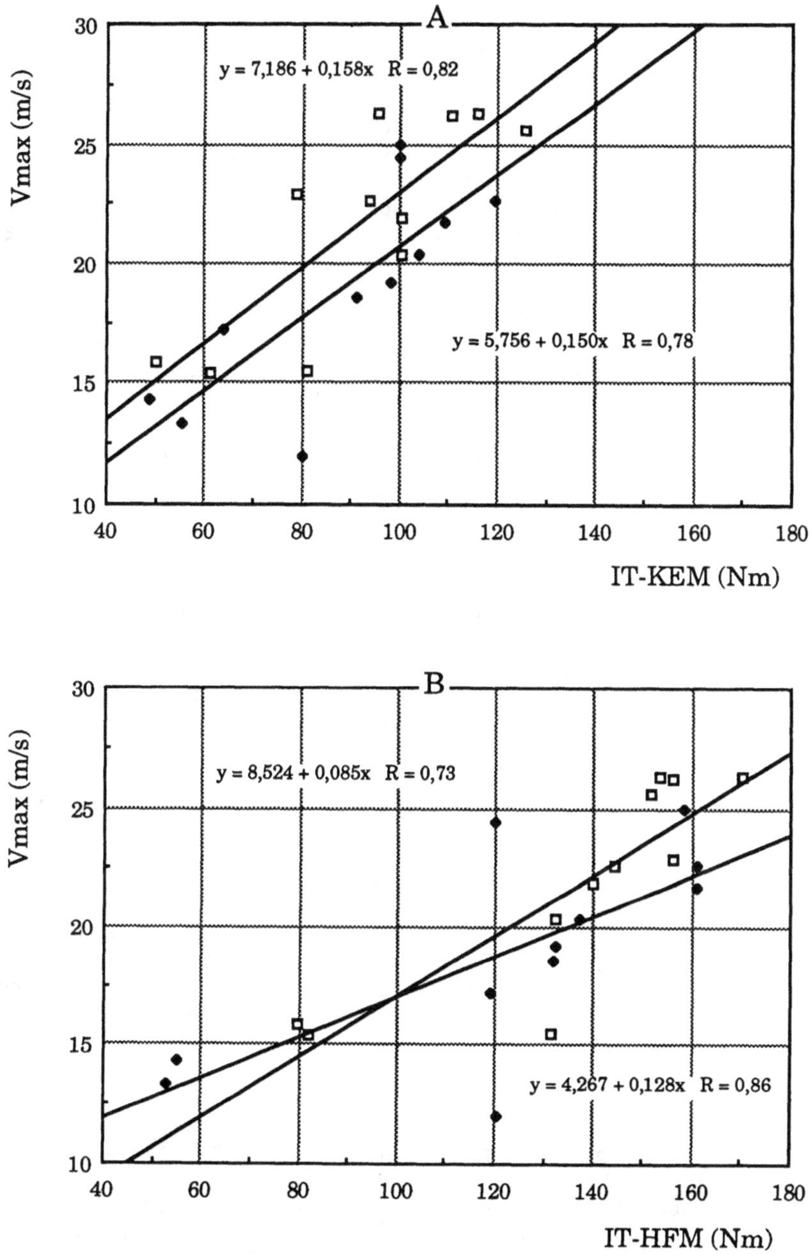

Figure 1. The relationship between IT and maximal ball velocity for the dominant (open squares, lower curves) and non-dominant limb (filled squares, upper curves) for KEM(A) and HFM(B)

In ballistic conditions an elite soccer player develops during a powerful kick a peak torque of 90 Nm for KEM and of 260 Nm for HFM. As far as the data of KEM are concerned, higher values might have been expected for isokinetic contractions since the angular speed at which this group was tested (5.23 rad s^{-1}) was lower than that measured in ballistic contractions (7.85 rad s^{-1}). On the other hand it must be pointed out that our subjects were not quite 'elite' players. The IT of HFM was definitely lower than in ballistic conditions. A possible explanation for this discrepancy might be that maximal torque was underestimated in isokinetic conditions. We are not aware of any neurophysyiological study showing different EMG activities in agonist and antagonist muscles due to different temporal patterns of hip angular speed or to different numbers of recruited muscle groups acting on a single limb. It should be remembered, however, that for a soccer player the kicking of a ball is a much more natural movement than an isokinetic contraction might be for any subject, thus a different degree of recruitment might be present in the two situations.

This speculation could be supported by our values of maximum ball velocity from dominant and non-dominant limbs, i.e. 20.0 ± 3.6 m s^{-1} and 17.7± 2.2 m s^{-1}; the difference is significant ($P < 0.001$) while no difference in torque was observed. This observation might imply that under ballistic conditions the dominant limb is able to produce a higher torque. However, it is worthwhile remembering that the product of average torque and time of torque application is a determining factor for maximal ball velocity while a single torque value is an indirect index. Nevertheless, a high correlation between IT and maximal ball velocity (Figure 1A and B) was found.

In this study the isokinetic torque of ankle dorsi-flexors was not investigated since ballistic measurements have shown that their contribution is negligible (Huang et al., 1982).

Conclusions

This study has shown that high correlation exists between maximal ball velocity and isokinetic torque produced by HFR and KEM. The hip flexor muscles prove to play a more important role in kicking than knee extensors even if their contribution appears lower than that found by Huang et al. (1982) and Robertson and Mosher (1983). From a practical point of view it seems reasonable to suggest that strength training should be particularly focused on hip flexors.

References

Grace, T.G. (1985) Muscle imbalance and extremity injury: a perplexing relationship. Sports Med., 2, 77-82.

Huang, T.C., Roberts, E.M. and Youm, Y. (1982) The biomechanics of kicking. In: Human Body Dynamics. Oxford Medical Engineering Series (edited by D.N. Ghista), pp. 409-443, New York: Oxford University Press.

Öberg, B., Ekstrand, J., Möller, M. and Gillquist, J. (1984) Muscle strength and flexibility in different positions of soccer players. Int. J. Sports Med., 5, 213-216.

Poulmedis, P. (1985) Isokinetic maximal toque power of Greek elite soccer players. J. Orthop. Sports Phys. Therapy, 5, 293-295.

Robertson, D.G.E. and Mosher, R.E. (1983) Work and power of leg muscles in soccer kicking. In: International Series on Biomechanics, Vol. 5B - Biomechanics IXB (edited by D.A. Winter, R.W. Norman, R.P.Wells, K.C. Hayes and A.E. Patla), pp. 533-542. Champaign, Illinois: Human Kinetics Publishers.

Winter, D.A., Wells, R.P. and Orr, G.W. (1981) Errors in the use of Isokinetic Dynamometers. Eur. J. Appl. Physiol., 46, 397-408.

MUSCLE ACTIVITY IN THE SOCCER KICK

E. De Proft, J.P. Clarys, E. Bollens, J. Cabri and W. Dufour
Depts. of Experimental Anatomy & Physical Education, Free University of Brussels, Laarbeeklaan 103, 1090 Brussels, Belgium.

Introduction

In recent years the measuring technique of electromyography (EMG) has been strongly promoted, not only by virtue of its technical improvements, but also because of its applications in kinesiology and sport research. Research in soccer has been developed also, but few investigations have been exclusively concerned with muscle activity in the soccer kick motion. Most electromyographical reports have described muscle activity of agonist muscle groups (McCloy, 1946; Yamashita and Kumamoto, 1976; Osternig, 1975). Some investigations (Clarys et al., 1984) have reported that extensor muscles are likely to be active during the flexion movement and vice versa, the so-called 'soccer paradox.' The purpose of the present investigation was to check muscle activity and synchronisation during a standard soccer kick movement, by means of electromyography (EMG) and video monitoring.

Procedures

Thirteen well trained soccer players (from RSC Anderlecht) and 12 subjects active in other sport disciplines, all Caucasian young men between 18 and 23 years of age, took part in the experiment (Table 1). The electrical activity of the six muscles was registered by

Table 1. Descriptive data of the subjects (N = 25)

	N	Age (years)		Height (cm)		Weight (kg)	
		Mean	SD	Mean	SD	Mean	SD
Soccer players	13	21.2	1.1	179.6	4.8	73.4	8.8
Non-soccer players	12	22.0	1.5	178.1	4.0	71.7	11.1

active surface electrodes in combination with an on-line data acquisition system (Clarys and Publie, 1987). The signals were amplified for tape-recording and attenuated for ink writing of the raw EMG and linear envelope. Data were normalised versus the maximal voluntary contraction using a semi-computerised Kintron - Ibas I system. In order to identify all EMG patterns, video recordings of the kick movement were made simultaneously with the EMG registration using a series of voltmeters for synchronising movement and electrical activity (Fig. 1). The choice of six leg muscles (m. vastus medialis, m. vastus lateralis, m. tibialis anterior, m. gluteus maximum, m. semitendinosus and the m. semimembranosus) was based on previous investigations.

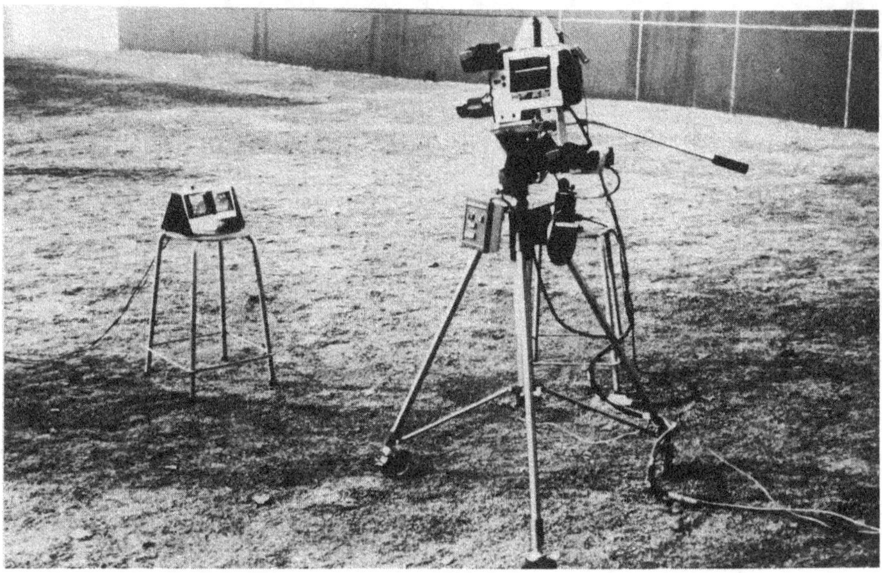

Figure 1. Synchronisation EMG-VIDEO-Voltmeters

All shots were performed in a standardized way. The players were asked to shoot at a fixed goal, which was divided in eight rectangular compartments. They always had to shoot towards the same compartment lower left for those who shoot with the right foot and vice versa (Fig. 2). The distance of the kick was measured on the field by means of a tape-measure.

Results and Discussion

For a simple evaluation of the results, the kick movement was divided into six phases as shown in Fig. 3. Phase 1 was the first stride, phase 2 the second stride, phase 3 the loading phase, phase 4 the swing phase, phase 5 the kick phase and finally the follow through.

The soccer players (Fig. 4)
Phase 1 showed minor activities (30% of MVC) of all muscles: the m. tibialis anterior even showed an activity less than 10% of MVC. This

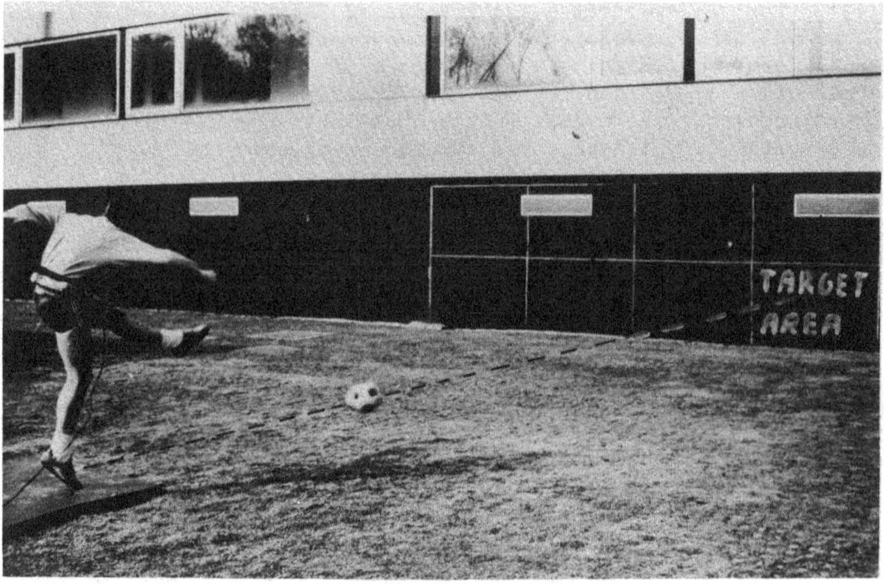

Figure 2. Standard shot procedure

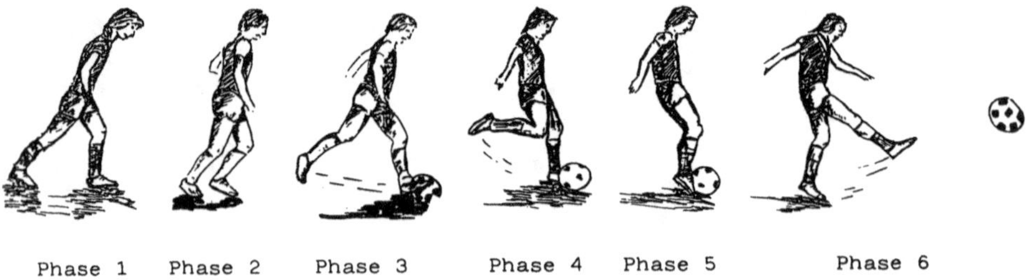

Figure 3. The six phases of a soccer kick

m. tibialis anterior really gets activated during the second stride of the player (up to 50% of MVC). This is a concentric, agonistic action because at that point, the foot of the kicking limb is in dorsi-flexion. The activities of the other muscles at this time were very low (10% of MVC) and not important.

At the time the kicking limb is preparing for the kick, through loading backwards (phase 3), important muscle activities were registered. The agonistic muscles at this time (m. gluteus maximus, m. semitendinosus and m. biceps femoris) were working at 70% of MVC. The antagonists m. vastus lateralis (70% of MVC) and the m. vastus medialis (90% of MVC) showed even greater activity. This is a first indication of the importance of antagonistic muscle activity through eccentric work, but this trend was not continued in the following phase of the movement. At the time the kicking limb swings forward (phase 4), there is an activity level of 80% of MVC for both

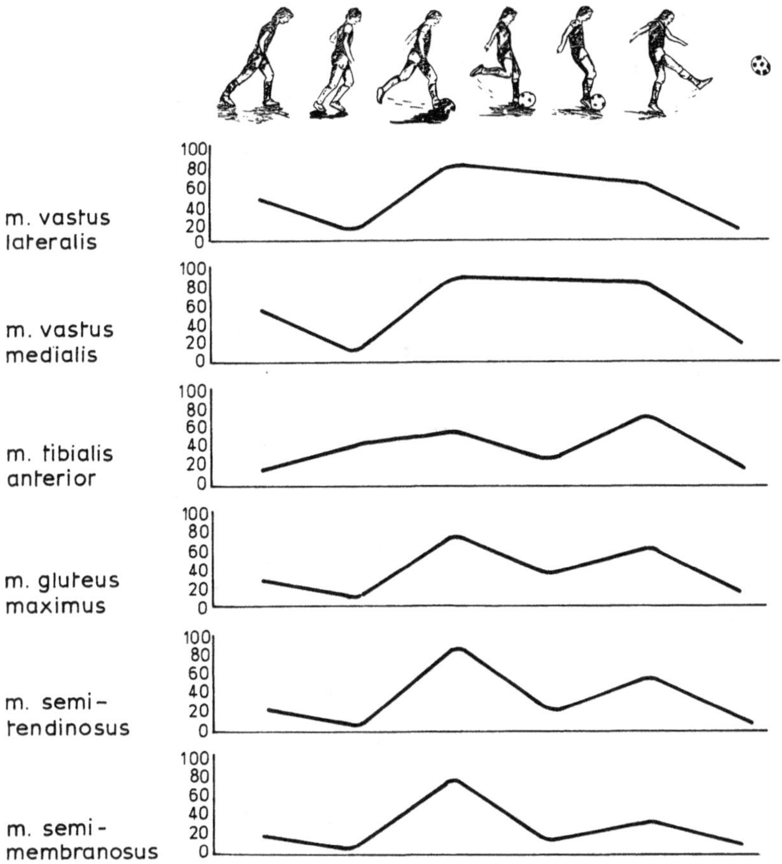

Figure 4. The normalized EMG patterns of six muscles during the soccer kick (soccer players)

the agonistic vasti. The other muscles, which are antagonists during this swinging phase, showed 30% of MVC activity. This can be explained by the fact that at the beginning of this phase (turning from loading backwards to swinging forwards) little or no strength is needed. The movement starts automatically through gravity. Nevertheless, the agonists (both vasti) showed a high amount of activity in preparation for the kick, at speed, towards the end of the movement.

During phase 5, the actual kicking of the ball, identical activities were noted in agonistic and antagonistic muscles. The concentric agonistic activity of both vasti was about 80% of MVC. Also m. gluteus maximus and m. tibialis anterior showed an activity level corresponding to 80% of MVC. This is the antagonistic activity through eccentric work. The other antagonist (m. biceps femoris) was less active, with only 40% of MVC.

Finally, during phase 6, in which the leg is swinging through, the electrical potentials were negligible. The leg swings further forward (continues its trajectory) through the mechanical forces, without much application of muscle strength.

The non-soccer players (Fig. 5)
Non-soccer players showed broadly similar patterns of activity to those of the soccer players. The discriminating feature was that the agonists were always more active than the antagonists.

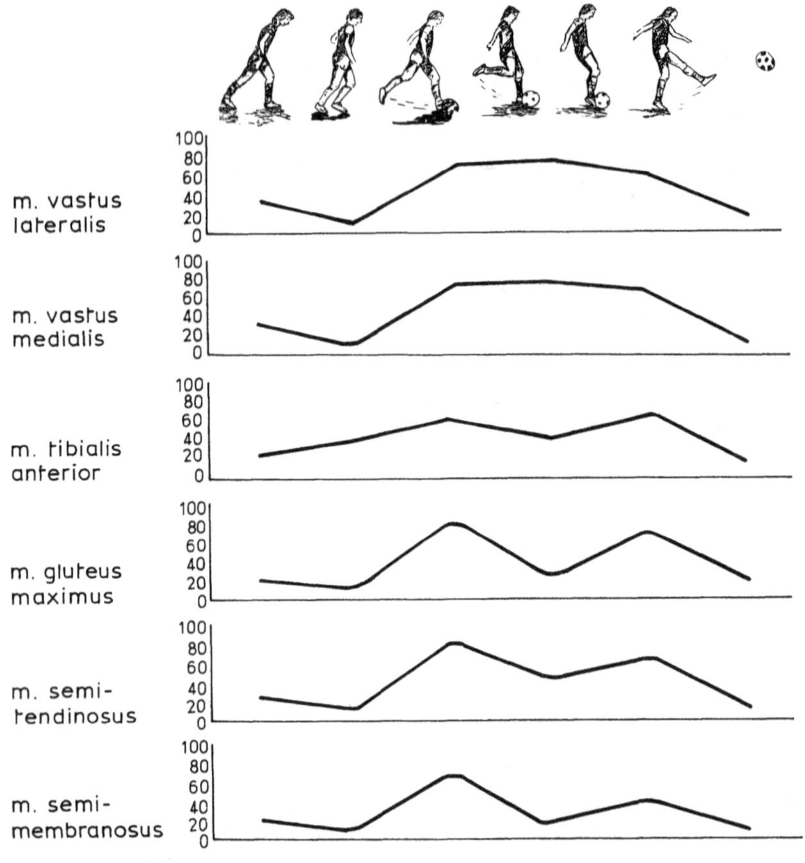

Figure 5. The normalized EMG patterns of six muscles during the soccer kick (non-soccer players)

Phase 1 showed only minor activity in all muscles. During phase 2, only the m. tibialis showed an activity of 60% of MVC. This level was identical to that observed in the soccer players.

When the kicking leg is loaded, in phase 3, agonists as well as antagonists showed a high electrical activity of 60-70% of MVC similar to that noted in soccer players. In contrast to the soccer players, where the antagonistic m. vastus medialis showed the highest activity (90% of MVC), here the highest muscle activity was produced by an agonist, the m. semitendinosus (90% of MVC).

In phase 4, when the kicking leg comes forward, only the agonists showed notable activity. Again this was identical to the finding in soccer players, but the level of activity was lower (60% compared to 80%).

When the ball is hit, in phase 5, agonists and antagonists were active. The agonistic vasti showed electrical activity corresponding to 70% of MVC. The antagonists, m. gluteus maximus and m. biceps femoris, had an activity level of only 50% of MVC, which is less than that for the soccer players. During phase 6, the follow through, no important activities were registered ($< 10\%$ of MVC).

Comparing the muscle activities during the complete movement (all phases together) via integration of the overall linear envelopes, and for all six muscles together, the non-soccer players showed more activities than the soccer players. These differences were significant ($P < 0.05$) (Fig. 6).

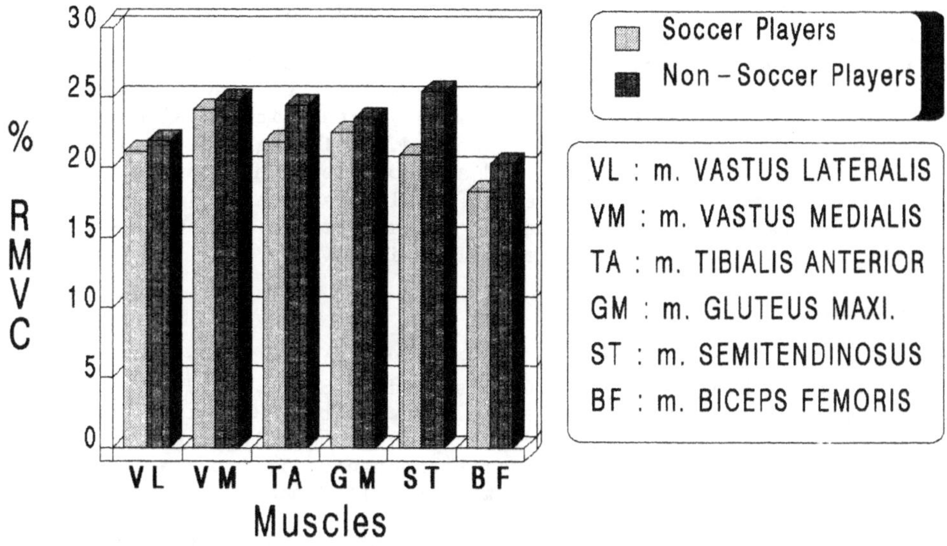

Figure 6. Muscle activity during the kick

Kick performance

Soccer players kick the ball much further than non-players. Mean distances (± SD) were 52.5 (± 2.7)m and 33.1 (± 4.2)m respectively for the two groups. We know from earlier investigations (De Proft, 1984) that the technique of kicking a ball is very important in this matter. Our results showed that muscle activity also plays a part. Agonists as well as antagonists showed high levels of activity during a soccer kick. Soccer players kick the ball much further than non-soccer players, although the soccer players have less general muscle activity but more antagonistic activity. We believe that the antagonists, which are synergists to the movement, through eccentric work, are very important in defining and controlling the kicking motion.

The synergistic work of antagonistic muscles is not just a passive way of permitting the movement, but involves active cooperation. This results in eccentric action, through which the muscles can create a stronger force than concentrically.

It is suggested that the agonist - antagonist co-operation is not just based on the force of the agonistic muscles and the degree of stretch in the antagonists, but on a synchronisation of force and flexibility of both agonists and antagonists. This could explain the frequent appearance of paradoxical muscle activities.

Applications

Our findings have primarily an informative and descriptive value, but it is clear that the data allow for specific training applications. One implication is the importance of specific muscle training, additional to the normal training programme. Agonists must be trained concentrically, antagonists eccentrically.

At the time the foot kicks the ball, the knee extensors and hip flexors are agonists. They must be trained mainly concentrically, although the eccentric force may not be neglected, because in other parts of the movement these muscles are antagonists.

At the same time, the knee flexors and hip extensors are antagonists, and must be trained mainly eccentrically although their concentric strength may not be ignored. Building a strong equilibrium between agonists and antagonists with a combination of concentric and eccentric strength should mean that injuries will be less frequent, the neuro-muscular pattern of the kick will be enhanced and kick performance will be improved.

References

Clarys, J.P., Dufour, W. and Pynaert, M. (1984) Electromyography of 3 soccer kick movements. Geneeskunde en Sport, 17-21.

Clarys, J.P. and Publie, J. (1987) A portable EMG data acquisition system with active surface electrodes for monitoring kinesiological research. In: Biomechanics X, International Series on Biomechanics Vol. 6. Champaign, III,Human Kinetics Publ; (in press)

De Proft, E. (1984) Voetbal, De wreeftrap: Een biomechanisch en electromyografisch onderzoek, Masters thesis, Vrije Universiteit, Brussel.

McCloy, C.H. (1946) Some notes on differential actions of partite muscles. Res. Quart., 17, 254-262.

Osternig, L.R. (1975) Optimal isokinetic loads and velocities producing muscular power in human subjects, Arch. Phys. Med. Rehabil., 56, 152-155.

Yamashita, N. and Kumamoto, M. (1976) Force generation in leg extension. In: Biomechanics V-B, Proceedings of the 5th International Congress of Biomechanics, (edited by P.V.Komi), pp. 41-45. Baltimore: University Park Press.

KINEMATICS AND KINETICS OF MAXIMAL INSTEP KICKING IN JUNIOR SOCCER PLAYERS

Pekka Luhtanen
Department of Biology of Physical Activity, University of Jyvaskyla, SF 40100 Jyvaskyla, Finland.

Introduction

In performing kicking movements the dominant extremity functions as an open kinetic chain system. In this segmental link system the internal muscle torques act between the individual links, which in soccer kicking are thigh, shank and foot. These body segments move by rotating around an imaginary axis of rotation that passes through the articulation of the segments. The motion of rotating body segments in kicking can be described in terms of angular position, displacement, velocity or acceleration. The linear velocity of the rotating foot hitting the ball is directly proportional to the sum of both the angular velocity and the radius of rotation of the consecutive body segments. The timing of these consecutive rotational movements is important in relation to the impact of the foot with the ball when maximizing the release velocity of the ball in kicking. The linear momentum of the kicking leg transfers to the ball according to the relationship between the force impulse and the change of linear momentum.

The angular acceleration of the segmental link system in the kicking leg depends on the external motive moment (torque) of the muscles producing the rotation of the thigh, shank and foot and on the resistance provided by the rotational inertia of these leg segments being moved by the motive moment. The inertial resistance of the thigh, shank and foot is determined by the distribution of the mass relative to the axis of rotation.

The described kicking movements have been studied with film analysis from the point of view of kinematics and kinetics in senior football players (Roberts and Metcalfe, 1968; Zernicke and Roberts, 1976), kinetics (Roberts et al., 1974), and kinematics concerning the development of the kicking skills in soccer (Bloomfield et al.,1979). Variation in movement pattern with professional soccer players has been related to the kinetic energy of the body segments when executing long and medium range in-step kicks (Stoner and Ben-Sira, 1976). Studies using film analysis and force platform technique on loading of the support leg in senior football players were done by Kermond and Konz (1978) and Asami and Nolte (1983).

The purpose of the present research was to study the release velocity of the ball in maximal in-step kicking in junior soccer players at different ages, to explain the produced resultant forces and their movements in the hip, knee and ankle joints of the kicking leg and ground reaction forces in the support leg.

Methods

Twenty-nine volunteered, skilled junior soccer players trained to perform maximal in-step kicks with run-up of two steps on a force platform (Komi et al. 1974). The subjects were divided into three different age groups with age class intervals EF: 9-11, CD: 12-14 and AB: 15-18 years. For film analysis and ground reaction force analysis subjects performed a minimum of three successful kicks. The fastest kick of every subject was selected for detailed analysis. Anthropometric data for the subjects are provided in Table 1. Each kick was filmed with a Canon Scoopic 16 mm camera, which operated 65 fps. The frame frequency was determined by a digital timer. The camera was placed perpendicular to the plane of motion of the kicker and the ball. Small black markers were placed on the following body land marks: greater trochanter, lateral epicondyle of femur and lateral malleolus of the ankle. The same ball was used in all measurements (m = 450 g, pressure = 98 000 Pa).

Table 1. Number of subjects, their age and selected anthropometric characteristics ($\bar{X} \pm$ S.D.) in different groups

Group	Number of Subjects	Age (Years)	Height (cm)	Weight (kg)	Thigh (cm)	Shank (cm)	Foot (cm)
AB	13	17.1 ±2.3	175.1 ±4.5	64.1 ±6.4	39.3 ±1.9	42.5 ±1.5	22.1 ±1.1
CD	8	13.4 ±1.1	160.2 ±5.7	46.6 ±7.1	36.9 ±1.9	40.4 ±1.5	21.1 ±1.0
EF	8	10.3 ±0.9	143.0 ±6.4	32.8 ±3.6	33.1 ±1.5	35.0 ±2.2	20.3 ±1.5
		$P<.001$	$P<.001$	$P<.001$	$P<.001$	$P<.001$	$P<.01$

Digitized coordinates of markers were recorded from the film by a Vanguard Motion Analyzer interfaced with a HP 21 MX computer. These coordinates were used to compute the centre of gravity locations, mass moment of inertia relative to the segments' centre of mass (Dempster, 1955) and the angular inclinations of segments. Linear and angular kinematic data were smoothed by the digital filtering method (Winter et al., 1974).

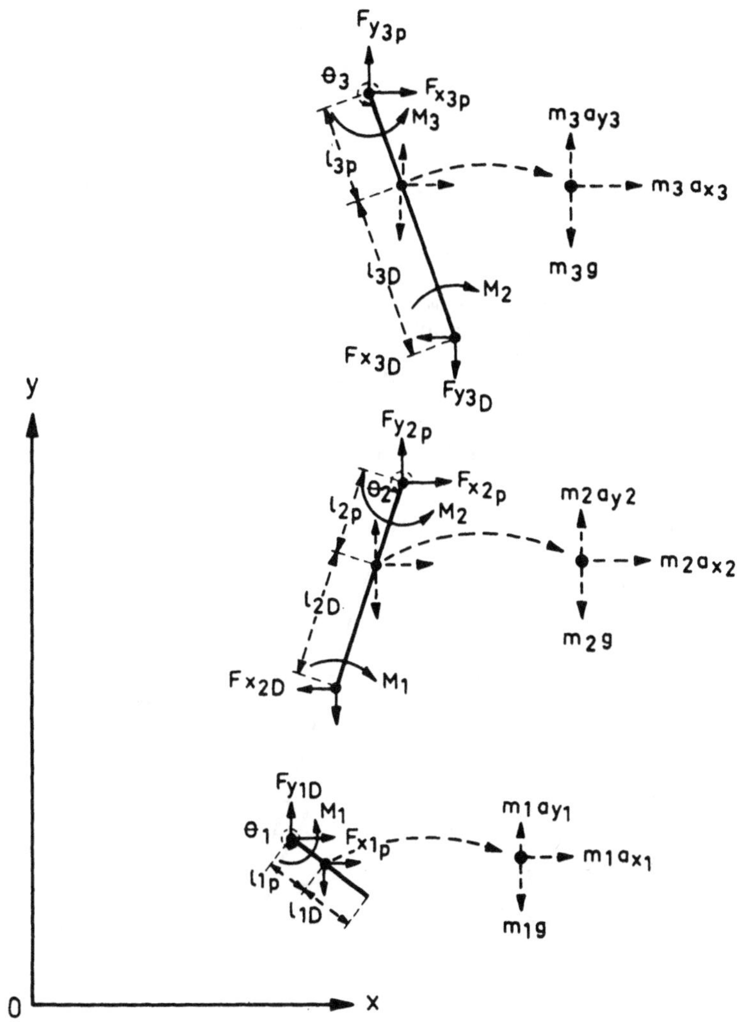

Figure 1. Free body diagram of the thigh, shank and foot in the kicking leg

The non-weight bearing phase of the kicking leg motion was assumed to be 2-D motion. Equations of motion consisted of the following:-

(1) $$\Sigma F_{x_{ij}} = m_i a_{x_{ij}}$$

(2) $$\Sigma F_{y_{ij}} = m_i a_{y_{ij}}$$, and

(3) $$\Sigma M_{ij} = I_i \alpha_{ij}$$

where, $\Sigma F_{x_{ij}}$ = sum of horizontal forces of segment i in frame j

m_i = mass of segment i

$a_{x_{ij}}$ = acceleration of segment i in frame j

$\Sigma F_{y_{ij}}$ = sum of vertical forces of segment i in frame j

$a_{y_{ij}}$ = acceleration of segment i in frame j

ΣM_{ij} = sums of moments relative to the center of mass of segment i in frame j

α_{ij} = angular acceleration of segment i in frame j

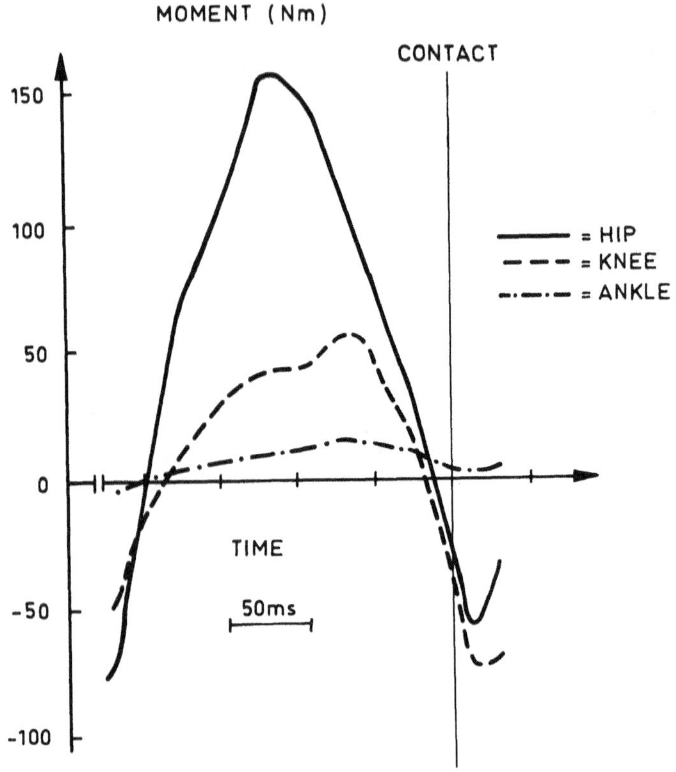

Figure 2. Typical moments of a selected in-step kick in the hip, knee and ankle

In the kicking motion the lower extremity segments formed an open linkage system and the force at the end of the distal segment was zero. The equations of motion were derived and unknowns solved. Free body diagrams for the foot, shank and thigh segments are shown in Figure 1. In Figure 2 are shown the typical moments of the proximal ends of the thigh (hip), shank (knee) and foot (ankle) in the kicking leg.

For statistical analysis a one-way analysis of variance was employed with respect to the three age groups. A multiple correlation matrix between anthropometric, kinematic and kinetic variables was calculated. For statistical analysis a UNIVAC 1100 computer and SPSS software were used.

Results

The release velocities of the ball were 14.9 ± 1.7, 18.4 ± 2.3, 22.2 ± 2.3 m s^{-1} in EF, CD and AB groups, respectively ($P < 0.001$). Vertical and lateral ground reaction forces differed significantly both in the maximal forces and in the forces when foot and ball contact existed. The forces ranged in the maximal vertical forces from 1170 ± 275 N to 1589 ± 87 N ($P < 0.01$), in the maximal lateral forces from 236 ± 55 N to 629 ± 196 N ($P < 0.001$) and in the forces during foot and ball contact in vertical direction from 550 ± 73 N to 1169 ± 218 N ($P < 0$ .001) and in lateral direction from 189 ± 30 N to 561 ± 208 N ($P < 0.01$). Angular velocities and accelerations differed significantly between all groups. In timing when the phases of maximal angular velocity occurred there was no significant different. The average of the phase of maximal angular velocity in the shank was 9 ms before the contact of the foot and ball.

Three different phases were selected for comparing resultant forces and their moments in the proximal end of thigh, shank and foot as follows: i) the phase when the first contact of the support leg occurred = CSL; ii) the phase when the knee angle was in its minimum = MKA, and iii) the phase when the contact of kicking with foot and ball occurred = CKL. The resultant forces of these phases in different groups are shown in Table 2.

Table 2. The resultant forces of the proximal end of thigh (hip) and shank (knee) in CSL, MKA and CKL phases (X ± S.D.)

		Resultant force (N)					
	Number of	Thigh			Shank		
Group	subjects	CSL	MKA	CKL	CSL	MKA	CKL
AB	13	297	283	578	252	139	492
		±54	±78	±108	±39	±44	±95
CD	8	159	220	341	142	90	288
		±49	±51	±97	±33	±41	±69
EF	8	119	128	250	92	63	196
		±25	±39	±74	±17	±33	±76
(x)= P < 0.001		(x)	(x)	(x)	(x)	(x)	(x)

The maximal moments of the forces in different joints can be seen in Table 3.

Table 3. The maximal moments in different proximal joints of the kick leg (X ± S.D.)

Group	Number of subjects	Moment (Nm) Thigh	Shank	Foot
AB	13	61 ± 15	25 ± 11	7 ± 2
CD	8	104 ± 31	44 ± 17	11 ± 4
EF	8	194 ± 33	83 ± 21	20 ± 4
		$P < 0.001$	$P < 0.001$	$P < 0.001$

Figure 3 presents the ranges of directions of the resultant forces and moments in the proximal end of the thigh, shank and foot in the selected CSL, MKA and CKL phases.

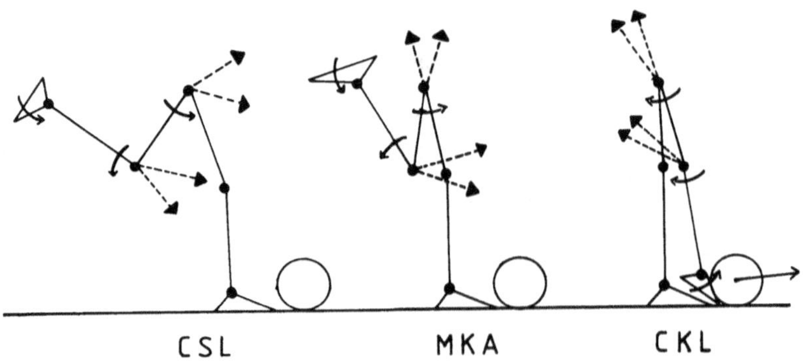

Figure 3. The ranges of directions of the resultant forces and moments of the kicking leg in the selected phases

The direction angles between the arrows of the resultant forces decreased when the foot ball contact approached. Before this contact the directions of the moments turned, except the moment of the foot. The release velocity of the ball correlated significantly to the body weight - $r = 0.928$, height $r = 0.911$, and age $r = 0.902$. The highest correlations were found between the release velocity of the ball and the maximal proximal moments in the thigh - $r = 0.932$, shank $r = 0.937$ and foot $r = 0.935$. The correlation coefficients between the proximal resultant forces of the thigh and shank and the release velocity of the ball were higher than $r = 0.900$ in the phases of CSL and CKL.

Discussion

The results concerning the angular velocities, accelerations and timing of the thigh and shank were in agreement with the fast kicking pattern, where the angular velocity of the thigh reached its maximum before the knee extension and maximum velocity phase of the shank (Roberts and Metcalfe, 1968; Zernicke and Roberts, 1978; Putman, 1983). Also, the resultant force values and moments of force of the eldest juniors were close to the values of the senior players in the kicking leg reported by Roberts and Metcalfe (1968), Roberts et al. (1974), and Zernicke and Roberts (1976 and 1978).

Bloomfield et al. (1979) studied development of the kicking pattern in 2 - 12 year old boys. According to this study the seven year old boys were able to take a run-up for kicking. The back swing of the kicking leg, knee flexion, good thigh and shank timing and follow through were observed at the age of eight years. Almost perfect timing in the total kicking performance was detected in eleven year old boys.

In this study the players performed the maximal in-step kicks with a run-up of two steps. The kicking pattern studied was the phase from the first contact of the support leg beside the ball to the contact phase of the foot and ball. The results indicated that angular moments of the thigh and shank were the largest, fastest and most accelerating in the eldest group ($P < 0.001$). The timing pattern did not differ significantly in the studied age groups. The maximal angular velocity of the shank was reached on the average 9 ms before the contact of the foot and ball.

The average for timing for the three selected phases of the moments applied in joints was similar in all subject groups. The directions of moments were counter-clockwise in CSL and MKA phases and clockwise in the CKL phase. Thus the difference between the age groups was mainly in the magnitude of the force production ($P < .001$). The force production was also due to the direction applied. In CSL and MKA phases the distributions of the directions of the resultant force applied was larger than in the CKL phase. This may mean that in all age groups the pattern in skilled kicking movements is similar in type and timing. The pattern had more variation in the first phases of the leg swing. In the MKA phase the forces applied to the hip might be directed slightly forward or backward (Fig. 3). In the CKL phase the directions of the forces, both in the hip and knee, were slightly backward, which meant proper timing is needed to get high linear velocity for the foot and ball.

According to this study the release velocity of the ball with respect to timing had the strongest relationship to the maximal moments produced during the hip flexion, knee extension and ankle stabilization in the kicking leg. Also the relationship between the maximal resultant forces of the thigh and shank and the release velocity of the ball was strong but less than mentioned above. The relationships between the release velocity of the ball and age was high but less than with weight or height.

Acknowledgement

This study has been supported by the grant from the Finnish Ministry of Education.

References

Asami, T. and Nolte, V. (1983) Analysis of powerful ball kicking. In: Biomechanics VIII - B (edited M. Matsui and K. Kobayashi), pp. 695-699, Champaign, Illinois: Human Kinetics Publishers.

Bloomfield, J., Elliot, B.C. and Davies, C.M. (1979) Development of the soccer kick: a cinematographical analysis. J. Human Mov't. Stud., 5, 152-159.

Dempster, W.T. (1955) Seated requirements of seated operator. WADC Technical Report, Wright - Patterson Air Force Base, Ohio, U.S.A. pp 55-159.

Kermond, J. and Konz, S. (1978) Support leg loading in punt kicking. Res. Ouart., 49, 71-79.

Komi, P.V., Luhtanen, P. and Viljamaa, K. (1974) Measurement of instantaneous contact forces on the force platform. Research Report 5/1974 from the Department of Biology of Physical Activity, University of Jyvaskyla, Jyvaskyla, Finland.

Putman, C. (1983) Interaction between segments during kicking motion. In: Biomechanics VIII - B, (edited by M. Matsui and K. Kobayashi), pp 668-694. Champaign, Illinois: Human Kinetics Publishers.

Roberts, E.M. and Metcalfe, M. (1968) Mechanical analysis of kicking. In: Biomechanics II, (edited by J. Wartenweiler, E. Jokl and M. Hebbelinck) pp. 315-319, Basel, Switzerland: S. Karger.

Roberts, E.M., Zernicke, R.F., Youm, Y. and Huang, T.C. (1974) Kinetic parameters in kicking. In: Biomechanics IV, (edited by R.C. Nelson and C.A. Morehouse) pp. 157-162, Baltimore: University Park Press.

Stoner, L.J. and Ben-Shira, P. (1976) Variation in movement patterns of professional soccer players when executing a long range and a medium range in-step soccer kick. In: Biomechanics VII - B, (edited by A. Morecki, K. Fidelus, K. Kedzior and A. Wit) pp. 337-342, Baltimore. University Park Press.

Winter, D.A., Sidwall, H.G. and Hobson, D.A. (1974) Measurement and reduction of noise in kinematics of locomotion. J. Biomech., 7, 157-159.

Zernicke, R.F. and Roberts, E.M. (1976) Human lower extremity kinetic relationships during systematic variations in resultant limb velocity. In: Biomechanics V - B, (edited by P.V. Komi) pp. 20-25, Baltimore: University Park Press.

Zernicke, R.F. and Roberts, E.M. (1978) Lower extremity forces and torques during systematic variation of nonweight bearing motion. Med. Sci. Sports, 10, 21-26.

A BIOMECHANICAL ANALYSIS OF THE INSTEP KICK MOTION IN SOCCER

Masanori Isokawa : Department of Sports Science, Tokyo Metropolitan University 1-1-1, Yakumo, Meguro-ku, Tokyo 152, Japan.

Adrian Lees : Department of Sport and Recreation Studies, Liverpool Polytechnic, Byrom Street, Liverpool L3 3AF, England.

Introduction

The instep kick is one of the more fundamental and frequently used skills in the game of soccer. As many players perform the instep kick, it is often performed approaching from a diagonal.

In earlier investigations on the kicking motion of the instep kick, Asami et al. (1968) have suggested that the power of knee extension has an effect on the ball velocity. Togari (1972) has reported on the difference between top players and minor players in the swing motion kinematics obtained from film analysis.

Roberts and Metcalf (1968) have taken a cinefilm of the kicking motion in three dimensions (above, side and front) by means of 16mm high speed cameras, and suggested that the factors which govern the swing velocity are mainly hip rotation at the start of kicking, hip flexion and then knee extension just before impact.

Aitchison and Lees (1983) have reported that in successful kicking the position of the leg and the foot at impact is important. Kermond and Kong (1978), Bloomfield et al. (1979) and Elliot et al. (1980) have investigated the development of the punt kick, and the relation between performance parameters obtained from the cine film and the ball distance kicked. Lindbeck (1983) has suggested that muscles are pre-stressed during impact as the result of the impulsive moments occurring in the hip joint, and Hoshizaki (1984) has determined the relative influence of isokinetic quadriceps leg strength on motor coordination in maximal kicking. Plagenhoef (1971) has reported on the relation between the swing velocity, striking mass at impact and the ball velocity obtained from film analysis. Togari (1972) has reported on the importance of the supporting leg position and knee joint angles in successful kicking, and Isokawa (1981) and Kermond and Kong (1978) have reported the relation between the ball velocity and ground reaction force.

However, in the literature, there are few studies which investigate the relative influence of approach angle on ball velocity. The purpose of this study was (1) to determine the relationship between the kinematic data (velocity of toe, ankle, knee and hip) and ball velocity at different approach angles and (2) to determine the relationship between the kinetic data (ground reaction force and moment) and ball velocity at different approach angles.

Methods and Procedures

Six male soccer players ranging in age from 20 to 36 years were selected as subjects. The subjects were asked to perform a maximal instep kick with a one step approach to the kick.

The approach angle was set so that zero degrees represented the direction in which the ball was kicked. The subjects were asked to perform the kick three times each at approach angles of 0, 15, 30, 45, 60 and 90 degrees.

The kicking motions were recorded from the side by a 16mm Locam camera operating at 150 frames per second. This camera was set on a tripod and was positioned at right angles to the plane of the kicking. In the camera view were the subject, trial identification number, and horizontal and vertical reference lines. A conversion factor for changing film distances into real-life measurements was determined by filming a reference marker of known length in the plane of movement.

The force platform was used to consecutively measure the ground reaction force of the supporting leg from the landing to the end of the follow through. The vertical, frontal and lateral forces were measured as well as the torque about the vertical axis. The force signals were recorded and analysed by computer to determine the peak force and torque during the forward swing, the impact force and torque, and the integral of force from the landing to the impact. Measures of the ball velocity and the velocity of the kicking leg markers on the toe, ankle, knee, and hip were obtained from a film motion analyser (NAC Movias 200AEH).

Results

Kinematic analysis

The peak velocities of the toe, ankle, knee and hip during the instep kick with one step approach were measured at each approach angle. The results are presented in Table 1.

Table 1. The peak velocity of striking limb and ball

Approach angle (degrees)	Toe $m\ s^{-1}$ Mean	SD	Ankle $m\ s^{-1}$ Mean	SD	Knee $m\ s^{-1}$ Mean	SD	Hip $m\ s^{-1}$ Mean	SD	Ball $m\ s^{-1}$ Mean	SD
0	18.08	0.74	12.79	0.18	7.36	0.51	2.78	0.20	18.73	0.95
15	18.29	0.94	12.61	0.42	7.14	0.69	3.13	0.45	19.12	1.23
30	18.32	0.96	13.07	0.36	6.70	0.48	2.72	0.12	19.87	1.14
45	18.01	0.45	12.14	0.29	6.25	0.48	2.42	0.23	20.14	1.58
60	18.09	0.90	12.28	0 27	6.09	0.39	2.29	0.20	19.46	1.59
90	15.38	0.76	10.77	0.33	4.11	0.46	1.48	0.21	19.13	1.64

Peak hip velocity occurred as the supporting foot landed on the force platform, and then gradually reduced with flexion of the hip joint. The peak velocity of the hip was maximum at an approach angle of 15 degrees, but reduced as approach angle increased.

Knee velocity reached its peak between 40-70 ms after peak hip velocity was reached. The peak velocity of knee was maximum for the straight approach and gradually reduced as the approach angle increased.

Ankle and toe velocities reached their peak just before impact, and from 40-50 ms after the peak velocity of knee. The peak velocity of ankle and toe was at 30 degrees.

The maximal ball velocity was at an approach angle of 45 degrees. This was 0.37 $m\ s^{-1}$ faster than the ball velocity which was generated at maximum ankle velocity at an approach angle of 30 degrees. It was noted that the approach angle required to gain the maximum ball velocity was 15-30 degrees larger than that of the maximum ankle velocity.

Kinetic analysis

Figure 1 shows a typical example of the ground reaction forces recorded at an approach angle of 15, 45, 60 and 90 degrees and peak values are given in Table 2. The peak vertical force during forward swing did not change noticeably with approach angle. The difference between the maximum and minimum vertical force was less than 92N. However the peak lateral reaction force tended to increase as the approach angle increased while the peak of frontal reaction force tended to decrease.

Table 2. The peak of three dimensional ground reaction force and torque during forward swing

Approach Angle (degrees)	Vertical Force (N)		Frontal Force (N)		Lateral Force (N)		Peak of Torque (Nm)		Torque at Impact (Nm)	
	Mean	SD	Mean	SD	Mean	SD	Mean	SD	Mean	SD
0	1362	124.2	398	77.5	68	29.9	1.2	5.0	7.5	4.1
15	1395	154.6	388	77.3	212	60.5	-1.7	5.7	4.4	5.2
30	1410	202.1	377	82.3	328	76.5	-4.8	5.4	3.4	7.0
45	1432	178.6	306	88.7	433	127.2	-8.1	3.8	2.4	6.8
60	1439	212.6	243	72.0	489	104.4	-8.9	4.6	-1.4	6.9
90	1454	294.8	63	92.2	583	114.8	-11.4	2.6	-1.8	2.2

The mean time from the landing of the supporting leg to ball impact was measured at each approach angle but this showed no change. However, there was a difference between subjects which was caused by their different kicking patterns. There might be two kicking patterns in the performance of the instep kick with one step. One of them used a large back swing and this resulted in a longer kicking time. The other used a small back swing and moved the lower leg forward sharply by knee extension and this resulted in a shorter kicking time (Table 3).

The integral of the force from the landing of the supporting leg to impact was determined at each approach angle. The integral of vertical and lateral force tended to increase slightly as approach angle increased, but the integral of frontal force decreased as approach angle increased.

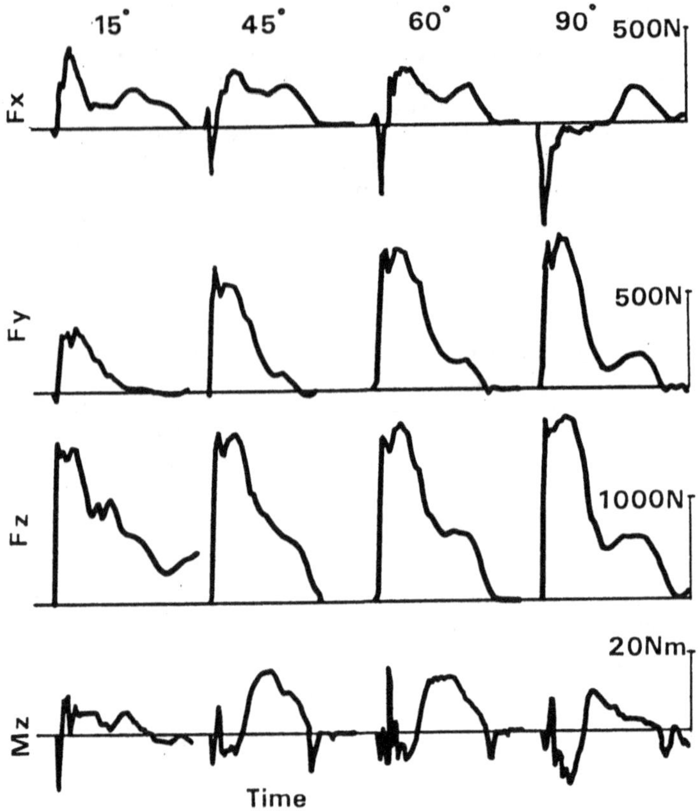

Figure 1. The raw data shown are examples of three dimensional force and moments at 15, 45, 60 and 90 degrees approach angle

Table 3. The integral of three dimensional ground reaction force and swing time from landing of supporting leg to impact

Approach Angle (degrees)	Vertical (Ns) Mean	SD	Frontal (Ns) Mean	SD	Lateral (Ns) Mean	SD	Swing Time (ms) Mean	SD
0	155.4	11.2	35.9	11.9	6.9	1.9	134.6	10.6
15	153.4	17.2	33.8	11.5	22.8	8.1	135.6	17.3
30	157.4	19.2	31.5	13.2	35.7	9.4	136.2	17.8
45	161.0	24.0	22.1	10.8	46.8	14.5	141.2	14.5
60	177.3	32.9	14.4	10.6	60.8	14.5	143.7	10.4
90	195.2	44.9	-17.3	2 6	71.3	15.4	150.0	6.1

Discussion

Kinematic analysis

There have been few studies which have investigated the effect of approach angle on ball velocity in soccer. Plagenhoef (1971) and Asai et al. (1980) have investigated the effect of straight and diagonal approaches on ball velocity and leg swing velocity. These studies emphasized that the diagonal approach caused greater ball velocities and leg swing velocities than the straight approach. It was considered that there might be an optimum approach angle to produce a maximum ball velocity and leg swing velocity. In this study, the peak ankle velocity, taken to be swing velocity, was maximum between an approach angle of 0 and 30 degrees. On average, the maximum swing velocity was at an approach angle of 30 degrees, but the peak of ball velocity was maximum within the range of 30-45 degrees, with a maximum velocity at 45 degrees. Togari (1972) and Isokawa (1980) have reported that the ball velocity was significantly related to the swing velocity (r = 0.80), but in these studies, the approach angle was constant in all trials. Plagenhoef (1971) suggested that both swing velocity and striking mass have an effect on the ball velocity. Fixation of knee and ankle joints at impact changes as the approach angle changes, and the striking mass also changes, therefore the resulting ball velocity changes too.

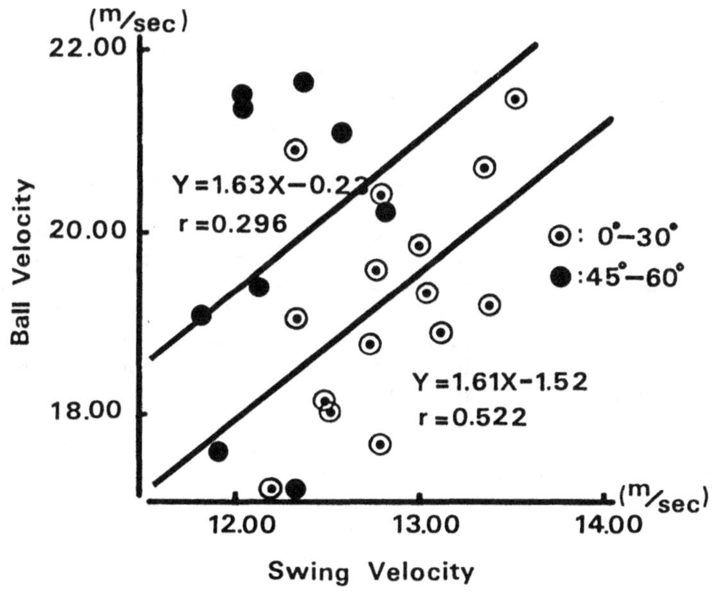

Figure 2. Relationship between swing velocity and ball velocity at 0-30 degrees, and 45-60 degrees approach angle

Fig. 2 shows the relationship between swing velocity and ball velocity at 0-30 and at 45-60 degrees. Ball velocity was significantly correlated with swing velocity at 0-30 degrees ($r = 0.522$, $P < 0.05$), but not significantly correlated at 45-60 degrees. Ball velocity at 45-60 degrees tended to be about 1.5 m s^{-1} larger than that at 0-30 degrees for the same swing velocity.

In this study although ankle velocity was lower at an approach angle of 45 than at 30 degrees, the ball velocity reached maximum at 45 degrees It is considered that the reason for this is due to the increased striking mass, depending on a greater fixation of knee and ankle joints. Shibukawa (1973) has demonstrated the effect of joint fixation on the ball velocity using a kinetic model, assuming that joints of man were linked at the joints of hip, knee and ankle. He has reported that the increase in striking mass depended on the fixation of joints and affects the ball velocity. From these results, it is considered that optimum approach angle for the instep kick with one step is about 45 degrees.

Kinetic analysis

The peak vertical force changed little as the approach angle increased. However, the peak frontal force showed a reduction, gradual at first and then marked, as the approach angle increased. The lateral force showed a reverse trend. These trends would be expected as the approach angle varied from 0 to 90 degrees as the applied frictional force of impact is orientated increasingly in the lateral direction. However, the change in direction of the applied horizontal friction force is not constant and this suggests that some weight shift from the lateral to the frontal direction takes place between the approach angles of 0 and 45 degrees to keep the latter component high. Beyond an approach angle of 45 degrees this weight shift cannot be effected and so the peak frontal force rapidly reduces.

The torque at impact is noted to reduce with increasing approach angle. The torque is a reflection of the vertical twist imparted to the body by the action of the swinging leg. In the straight approach no rotation of the leg about a vertical axis is required in order to kick the ball straight ahead. Therefore the torque measured is the positive resistance torque due to the assymetry of body movement. As the angle of approach increases the leg has to be actively rotated about a vertical axis in order to kick the ball straight ahead. This actively generated torque reduces the resistance torque supplied to the body via the ground contact. At an approach angle between 45 and 60 degrees the active torque completely balances the body motion. At 60 degrees and above the active torque applied to the leg is an excess of that required to perform the kick and a negative torque results. An angled approach would serve to reduce the torque applied to the foot and may be considered as a sound injury prevention technique.

Consistent with the peak forces, the time integrals of the forces to impact demonstrate similar trends. The vertical impulse showed a more marked increase as approach angle increased and this could be explained by the greater time it takes to make the kick from landing to impact. This is reflected in the increased values of swing time.

In conclusion it can be said that an approach angle of between 30 and 60 degrees will be likely to produce greatest ball velocity while minimising torque applied to the foot. The peak vertical forces and impulses will not be minimised but these change relatively little. The horizontal frictional forces are greatest within this range of approach angle.

References

Aitchison, I. and Lees, A. (1983) A biomechanical analysis of place-kicking in rugby union. In: Proceedings of Sport and Science (edited by D.A. Brodie, J. Burnie, R.G. Eston, F. Sanderson and J.J. Thornhill) pp. 1-7, University of Liverpool.

Asai, T., Kobayashi, K., and Oshima, Y. (1980) Biomechanical analysis of instep kick in soccer. In: Proceedings of Japanese Physical Education, pp.369.

Asami, T., and Togari, H. (1968) Study on kicking in soccer. Jap. J. Phys. Ed., 12-14, 267-272.

Bloomfield, J., Elliott, B.C., and Davies, C.M. (1979) Development of the soccer kick: A cinematographical analysis. J. Human Mov't. Stud., 5, 152-159.

Elliott, B.C., Bloomfield, J., and Davies, C.M. (1980) Development of the punt kick: A cinematographic analysis. J. of Human Mov't. Stud., 6, 142-150.

Hoshizaki, T.B. (1984) Strength and Coordination in the soccer kick. International Symposium of Biomechanics in Sports, Colorado Springs, pp.271-276.

Isokawa, M. (1981) Kinematic analysis of kicking in soccer. In: Proceedings of Japanese Physical Education, pp.444.

Kermond, J.K., and Kong, S.A. (1978) Support leg loading in puntkicking. Res. Quart., 49-1, 71-79.

Lindbeck, L. (1983) Impulse and moment of impulse in the leg joints by impact from kicking. J. Biomech. Eng., 105, 108-111.

Plagenhoef, S. (1971) Patterns of Human Motion. Englewood Cliffs, N.J.: Prentice Hall.

Roberts, E.M., and Metcalfe, A. (1968) Mechanical analysis of kicking. In: Biomechanics I, (edited by J. Wartenweiler, E. Jokl and M. Hebbelinck) pp. 315-319. Baltimore: University Park Press.

Roberts, E.M., Zernicke, R.F., Youm, Y., and Huang, T.C. (1974) Kinetic parameters of kicking. In: Biomechanics IV, (edited by R.C. Nelson and C.A. Morehouse) pp. 157-162, Baltimore University Park Press.

Shibukawa, K. (1973) Effect of joint fixing when kicking a soccer ball. Bulletin of the Institute of Sports Science, 11, 81-83.

Togari, H. (1972) Kinesiological study of soccer (1). Jap. J. Phys. Ed., 16-5, 259-264.

AN INVESTIGATION OF LINEAR AND ANGULAR KINEMATICS OF THE LEG DURING TWO TYPES OF SOCCER KICK

Pavle Opavsky
Faculty of Physical Education, University of Beograd, 11000 Beograd, Blagoja Parovica 156, Yugoslavia.

Introduction

The kicking action is a fundamental element of the game of soccer, but is relatively unresearched. The purpose of this research is to establish the linear and angular kinematic characteristics of a standing (A) and running (B) kick with the foot making contact with the ball on the dorsal surface in both cases.

Methods

High speed cine film was taken at 60 Hz of each of the standing and running kicks for six subjects. In both cases the ball was stationary. In the running start the player made six to eight steps into the kick. Five representative points were digitised from the film. These were the foot centre of gravity (C_p), the lower leg centre of gravity (C_s), the upper leg centre of gravity (C_f), the centre of gravity of foot and lower leg (C_{sp}), and the whole leg centre of gravity (C_{fsp}). From these points the loci of each point was identified and the linear circumferential velocity and acceleration were calculated. In addition the angle made by the upper and lower leg to the vertical, was measured from which the angular velocity and angular acceleration were calculated.

Results and Discussion

In the linear velocity data presented in Fig.1 three general phases can be identified. The first is where the velocity shows an increase, the second where a velocity peak is reached and the third phase where the velocity shows a reduction. Both sets of data are similar in appearance, although it is noted that the actual speed of each point (C_p, C_s, and C_f) is greater in the running kick. However, if the speed of movement of the body is accounted for the velocities of movement of each point relative to the body is greater for the standing kick. This suggests that muscular effort applied to the leg is greater in the standing kick. This is confirmed in general by the acceleration profiles in Fig.2, particularly of the lower leg and foot.

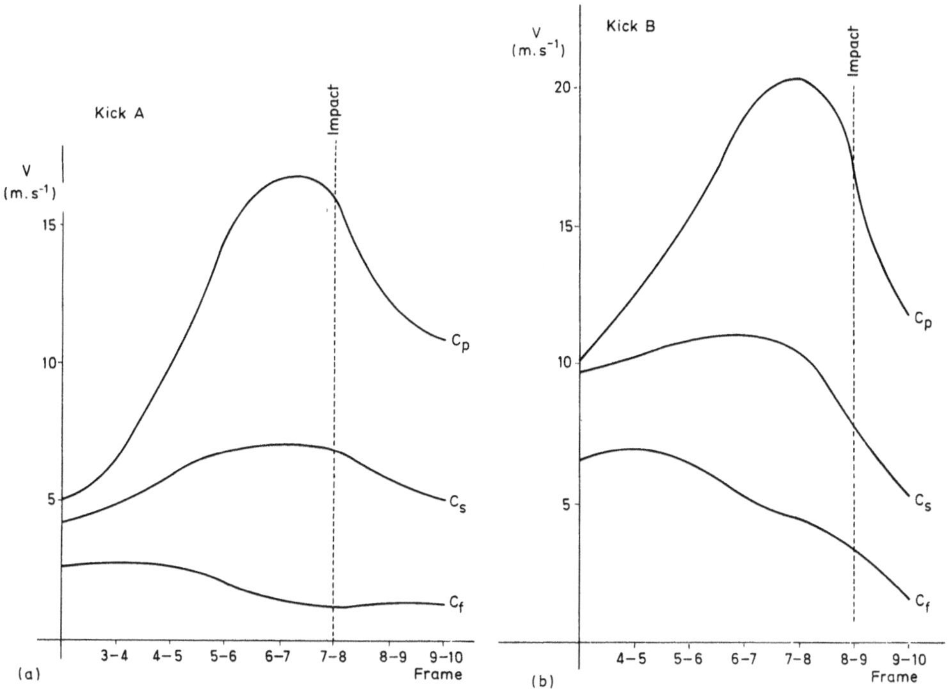

Figure 1. Velocities of the centres of gravity of the foot (C_p), lower leg (C_s) and upper leg (C_f) during a running kick (A) and static kick (B)

It should be noted, however, that the range between maximal and minimal acceleration values for each segment are about the same in each case.

Angular velocity profiles were similar for the foot for both types of kick reaching values in excess of 20 rad s^{-1}. However, the angular velocities of the lower and upper leg were greater in the running start. The angular acceleration profiles again showed greater values for the standing kick, confirming that more muscular effort was being applied during this type of kick (Fig. 3).

If the ratio 0 of the absolute velocities of the joint centres of the hip, the knee, the ankle and the ball centre are taken for each type of kick (Table 1) this ratio is seen to reduce in an hyperbolic way.

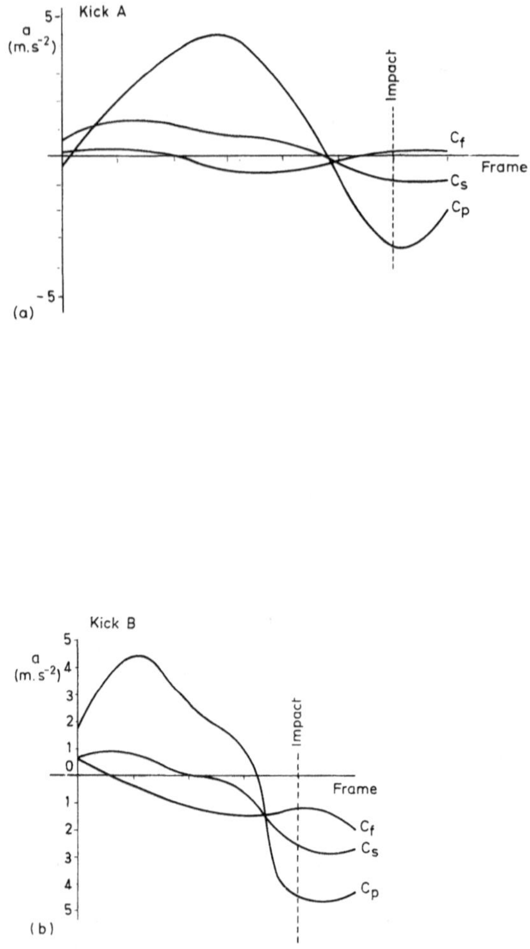

Figure 2. Accelerations of the centres of gravity of the foot (C_p), lower leg (C_s) and upper leg (C_f) during a running kick (A) and static kick (B)

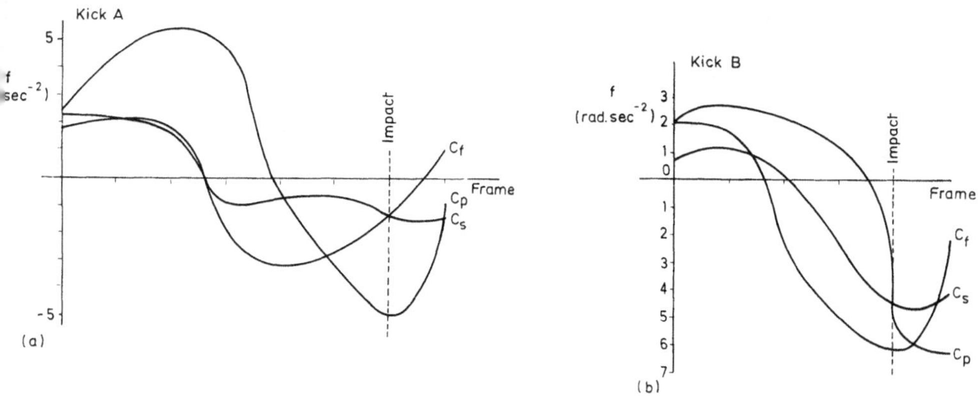

Figure 3. Angular accelerations of the centres of gravity of the foot (C_p), lower leg (C_s) and upper leg (C_f) during a running kick (A) and static kick (B)

Table 1. Joint centre and ball velocities and their ratio for two types of kick.

Joint	Velocities m s^{-1} Standing (A)	Running (B)	Ratio
hip	0.75	3.28	4.4
knee	4.10	8.20	2.0
ankle	9.69	13.42	1.38
ball	23.48	30.78	1.3

Conclusions

The running kick produces greater linear and angular velocities of the leg than the standing kick. However, the latter produces higher accelerations suggesting that greater muscular effort is being employed. Kicks made for maximum velocity should therefore be preceded by a run.

BIOMECHANICAL ANALYSIS OF THE SOCCER THROW-IN

Erich Kollath and Ansgar Schwirtz
Institut für Sportspiele, Institut für Biomechanik,
Deutsche Sporthochschule Köln, Carl-Diem Weg 6, D-5000 Köln 41,
West Germany.

Introduction

In soccer, kicking is a fundamental skill and has therefore often been investigated from a biomechanical point of view, for example by Stoner and Ben-Sira (1981), Roberts and Metcalfe (1967) and Putnam (1981).

The present study enters into the particulars of a so-called 'standard situation' in a soccer match - the throw-in. At first sight it might seem pointless to cast greater light on the precise nature of this movement because it is against the rules to score a goal directly with a throw-in. In recent years in national and international soccer matches, the number of players who are capable of throwing the ball over a considerable distance has increaseed. A close examination of the games during the World Cup in Mexico in 1986 showed that the number of throw-ins near the opponent's goal was similar to the number of free kicks in this area (Laux, 1986). Therefore it would seem important to have specialists in a team not only for penalties, corners and free-kicks but also for long throw-ins.

To get more quantitative information about the nature of long-range throw-ins, a combined kinematic-dynamic investigation has been carried out in order to give brief answers to the following questions:-

(i) what parameters and measured results characterize long throw-ins from both the standing position and after a run-up?
(ii) what relevant conclusions can be drawn from the results for the game itself?

Methods

This investigation took place at the Deutsche Sporthochschule Köln. Thirteen experienced students were the subjects of the study. At that time they were all active players in soccer teams, two playing in the first West-German amateur league. None were specialists in the long throw-in. After individual warming-up and several trial throws each player had to execute at least three maximum range throw-ins both from a standing position and after a run-up, in a match situation. In doing this the subjects contacted the surface of a force platform with both feet in the standing position and with one foot after their run-up. A black and white 60 Hz video shutter camera, exposure time 0.002 ms, with a 50 mm lens, was positioned perpendicular to the plane of motion. The trials were stored on magnetic tape with an U-matic video recorder. All dynamic test data were recorded directly by a HP-1000 F computer.

About 30 motion-pictures per trial with 18 xy-coordinates each were digitized by a Video-Position-Analyzer. Computer programs were written to calculate kinematic and statistical parameters as well as to produce graphical output. The following margins of error should be taken into consideration: for distances ±15 mm; for angles ±2 degrees, and for velocities ±0.2 m s^{-1}.

Results and Discussion

Throw-in distances

Twenty-six throw-ins from the standing position and 32 throw-ins after a run-up were included in the data evaluation. It should be noted that all the players achieved longer distances with their throw-in after a run-up, compared to those from a standing position. The differences in throw-in length between the two types of throw varied from individual to individual. For example, subject 7 improved only about 0.8 m, while for subject 5 an increment of 13 m was measured. As expected the average throw-in lengths of both types show highly significant differences.

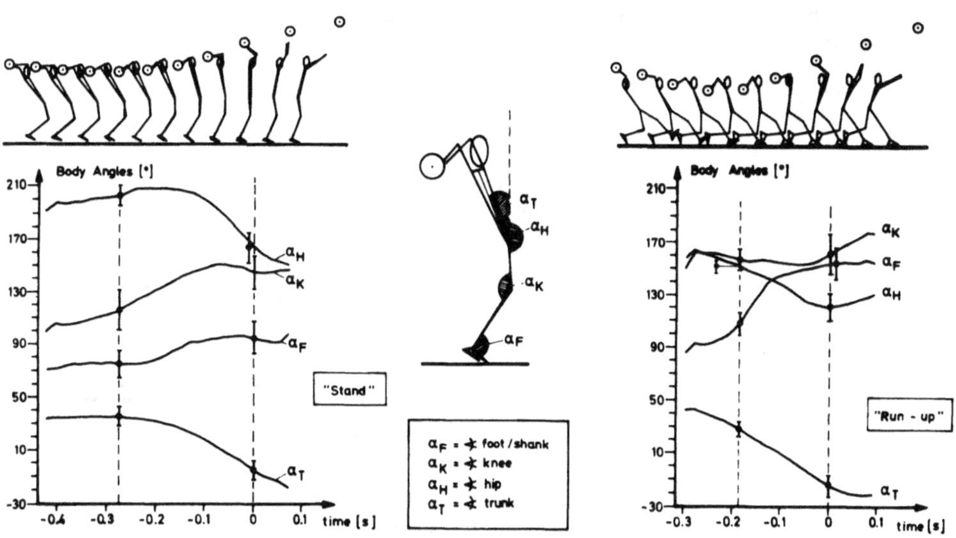

Figure 1. Typical curves of four body angles of the throw-in from a standing position and after a run-up

Body angles

In this study four angles representing the amount of flexion and extension between two parts of the body, or relative to a vertical axis were defined. Those angles involved only the movement of the trunk and the lower extremity (Fig. 1), and were calculated from the xy-coordinates of each joint axis.

In all the graphics, the essential throwing time is marked by interrupted vertical lines. Differences between the two types of movement can be seen by looking at the knee angle. During the throw-in from a standing position an ever-increasing extension can be noted. This points to the supporting effect of the concentrically active thigh muscles. During the final positioning of the foot in a run-up throw-in, the knee angle curve shows almost constant values. Therefore one can presume more static muscular activiy in the m.quadriceps femoris of the front leg.

Fig.1 provides further information about the disparity between the individual performances. Concerning the angles at the beginning and the end of the take-off interval, large standard deviations of the average values are evident. It seems that there was more variability in the throw-in from a standing position than during the course of movement following a run-up.

Ground reaction forces

By using a dynamometer it was possible to measure the ground reaction force in three orthogonal directions. A complete measurement of the body's accelerating force was only possible during the double stance phase of the throw-in from a standing position. From the other type of movement ground reaction forces were measured only between the foot of the front leg and the ground. Examples of both techniques can be seen in Fig.2.

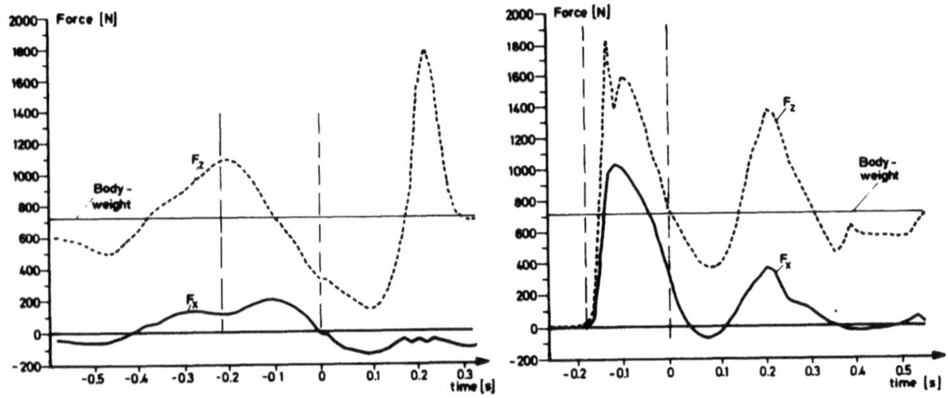

Figure 2. Ground reaction forces in the vertical (F_z) and horizontal (F_x) directions from both types of movement

The throw-in from a standing position was mainly characterized by vertical forces. The wave-like course of F_z with values above and below body-weight occurs because of the downward and upward movement of the player's centre of gravity. Compared with the vertical plane, forces in the horizontal plane were small. As a result of the initial impact of the front leg during the last step of the run-up throw-in, maximum vertical and horizontal ground reaction forces amounted to 2 and 3-times body weight. These external forces must be compensated by internal (muscle) forces.

Statistical, mechanical and individual considerations

In the present study statistical calculations were used only to establish interrelations between kinematic parameters and the throw-in length. As expected during the throw-in from a standing position, highest correlations occur between the velocity of the ball (r = 0.93) and the hand joint (r = 0.56) with the throw-in length at the moment of ball release. A lower but still significant correlation coefficient (r = 0.46) was found between the hip velocity when the ball was at its furthest point behind the player and the throw-in length. This points to the need for the initial phase of the throw-in to be performed quickly. Concerning the throw-in after a run-up the same variables closely correlated with the throw-in length, i.e. the velocity of the ball (r = 0.82) and the hand joint (r = 0.64) in the release position.

It is remarkable that in both types, no significant correlations between any body angles and the throw-in length could be found. Therefore observations from the body are unlikely to provide evidence for a positive or negative influence on the throw-in length.

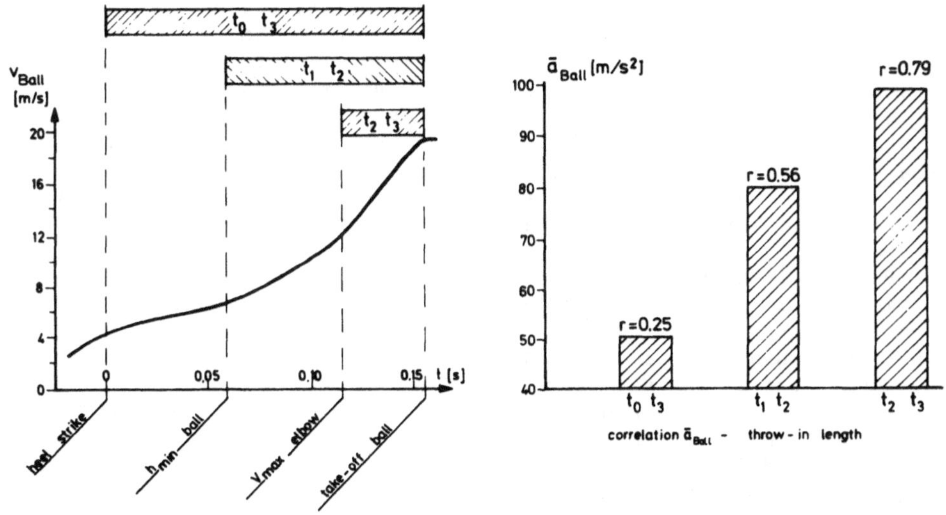

Figure 3. Average accelerations of the ball in three time intervals correlated to the throw-in length

A rather close correlation exists between the approach velocity of the player's centre of gravity at the moment of heel strike after the run-up (r = 0.82): this means that the throw-in length is very dependent on the subject's approach velocity. Whether high or low average accelerations of the ball would have a positive effect on the throw-in length was also investigated. For this purpose the throwing phase is divided into three time intervals:- from the moment of the heel strike of the front leg (t_o) to the ball's release (t_3), from the minimum height of the ball (t_1) to the ball's release (t_3) and from the moment of maximum elbow velocity (t_2) to the ball's release (t_3) (see Fig. 3, left side).

It was found that the shorter the defined time intervals, the higher were the corresponding changes in ball velocity. For this reason, the calculated average accelerations of the ball over these time intervals increase the closer the time intervals are to the ball's release. The correlation coefficients belonging to each time interval can be interpreted clearly: obviously it is advantageous when the ball is rapidly accelerated just before its release, rather than over a larger period (see Fig. 3, right side).

From a mechanical point of view the ball shows a parabolic flight curve. Since it was not the purpose of this study to determine air resistance, the effect of this on the ball has been neglected. As a consequence of this simplification, the throw-in length L_{cal} can be calculated only as a function of the constant acceleration by gravity ($g = 9.81$ m s^{-2}), the release height (h_o), the release velocity (v_o) and the release angle (α_o) of the ball at the moment of release. In order to reach a maximum throw-in distance an optimal release angle (α_{opt}) can also be determined mathematically in relation to a particular release height and release velocity. The following figure (Fig. 4) shows the flight parabola of the ball. The table below includes average values of the release velocity, the actual and the optimum release angle and the resulting throw-in length.

This table points out that in both types of movements the subjects reached take-off angles about 10° below the optimum. The average values for the loss in the possible throw-in distance are 1.6 m and 1.9 m respectively. Regarding all 58 trials only one player released the ball at a steeper angle than the optimum. In all the other cases the take-off angle was too flat. The highest individual losses in the possible throw-in length were more than 5 m in both types of movement.

How far it is possible to realize this mechanical optimum in a biomechanical way must be tested out in individual cases. In this connection the following note is important: the throw-in length was increased when the ball was released at a take-off angle near the optimum. But at the same time the flight time of the ball was increased, too. For example, there was an increase in the time the ball is in the air from 1.12 s to 1.95 s, when the release angle α_o was increased from 23° to $\alpha_{opt} = 43°$ with the values $v_o = 14$ m s^{-1} and $h_o = 2.0$ m. The gain in throw-in distance in this instance was 3.8 m.

With regard to the actual match it is possible that an extended flight time of the ball offers a better chance for defensive players to intercept the ball. Consequently the player who performs a long throw-in must consider the actual match situation before deciding on a flat or steeply released ball.

Finally, a comparison of two individual attempts using both throw-in techniques was made. By this, one can verify that it was possible for two almost identical throw-in distances to result from different

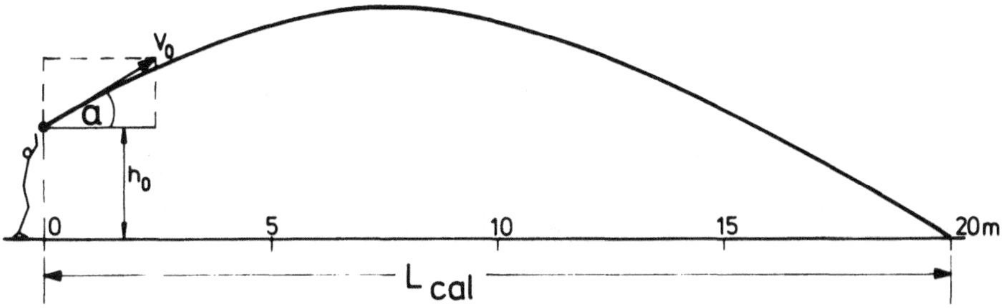

	Take-off velocity [m/s]	Angle of release [°]		Throw-in length [m]		Reduced length [m]
	calculated	calcul.	optim.	calcul.	optim.	calculated
"Stand" (n = 26)	14.2 ± 1.3	33.0 ± 6.9	42.3 ± 0.4	20.9 ± 2.9	22.5 ± 3.0	-1.6 ± 1.6
"Run-up" (n = 32)	15.3 ± 1.6	32.3 ± 5.7	42.8 ± 0.4	24.1 ± 4.7	26.0 ± 5.3	-1.9 ± 1.6

Figure 4. Flight parabola of the ball and table with calculated actual and optimum take-off angles (average values)

throw-in methods. For this purpose two players of approximately the same height and body weight were selected. Essential kinematic parameters for the throw-in from a standing position and after a run-up can be seen in Fig.5.

In both cases the take-off height of the ball was virtually the same. The salient points of the other parameters can be summed up quite simply: subject 7 achieved a low release velocity and a steep angle of release when his throwing action covered a longer distance and took a longer time. Both trials of subject 9 show opposite values. Also the defined body angles were quite different from each other, but the throw-in distances were nearly identical.

This example brings the heterogeneous appearance of the throw-in movement to light. In order to improve performance, a coach should not overaccentuate the geometry of particular parts of the player's body but rather he should concentrate on the size of the ball's release angle and velocity.

Summary and Conclusions

In a kinematic and dynamic investigation 13 subjects had to perform maximum range throw-ins from a standing position and after a run-up. In total 58 trials were evaluated. The most important results have been summarized below:

"Stand"	Throw-in Length [m]	Ball: take-off- height [m]	velocity [m/s]	angle [°]	Ball: acceleration- path [m]	time [s]
Sj. 7 (1.72m,65kp)	19.40	2.00	13.3	40.3	0.70	0.22
Sj. 9 (1.70m,63kp)	19.40	2.03	14.8	23.9	0.66	0.15

"Run-up"	Throw-in Length [m]	Ball: take-off- height [m]	velocity [m/s]	angle [°]	Ball: acceleration- path [m]	time [s]
Sj. 7	20.60	1.90	11.6	35.7	0.99	0.23
Sj. 9	21.20	1.91	13.1	28.0	0.87	0.11

Figure 5. Nearly identical throw-in distances resulting from different individual parameters concerning both techniques

(i) As expected all the subjects achieved longer throw-in distances after a run-up than from a standing position. The individual improvement was between 0.8 m and 13.0 m.

(ii) The consideration of four body angle curves showed that the players performed the particular movements in widely differing fashions. No relationships were found between the angles studied and the distance thrown.

(iii) The following variables were significantly correlated to the throw-in length:

(a) throw-in from a standing position: velocity of the ball and the hand at the moment of ball release and velocity of the hip when the ball was at its furthest point behind the player;

(b) throw-in after a run-up: approach velocity, velocity of the hand and the ball at the moment of ball release and average acceleration of the ball immediately before ball release.

(iv) Compared to the mechanical optimum, with one exception all the subjects threw the ball at too flat an angle of release. The calculated loss in the throw-in length was as high as 5 m+. In practice it must be taken into consideration that a more steeply released ball produces a longer flight time.

(v) Finally, an individual comparison of two trials with nearly identical throw-in distances verified again the diversity of individual performances.

(vi) In order to maximize the throw-in distance we recommend not overaccentuating details of the body position. One should emphasize a much faster run-up, a rapid final acceleration of the ball and a high release velocity of the ball close to the optimum angle of release.

References

Laux, D. (1986) Der Fussballeinwurf mit Anlauf - eine kinematische Bewegungsanalyse. Diplomarbeit Deutsche Sporthochschule Köln.

Putnam, C.A. (1983) Interaction between segments during a kicking motion. In: Biomechanics VIII-B (edited by H. Matsui and K. Kobayashi) p.258, Nagoya.

Roberts, E.M. and Metcalfe, A. (1967) Mechanical analysis of kicking. In: Biomechanics I (edited by J. Wartenweiter, E. Jold and M. Hebbelinck) pp. 315-319, Zurich.

Stoner, L.J. and Ben-Sira, D. (1981) Variation in movement patterns of professional soccer players when executing a long range and medium range in-step soccer kick. In: Biomechanics VII-B (edited by A. Morecki, K. Fidelus, K. Kedzior and A. Wit) pp. 337-341, Warszawa: Polish Scientific Publishers.

Tuna, E.S. (1986) Kinematische Untersuchung des Einwurfs aus dem Stand beim Fussballspiel. Diplomarbeit Deutsche Sporthochschule Köln.

ANALYSIS OF THE GOALKEEPER'S DIVING MOTION

Shigeru Suzuki[1], Haruhiko Togari[2], Masanori Isokawa[3], Jiroh Ohashi[2], Tetsuro Ohgushi[4]

[1] Department of Sport and Sciences, Seikei University, Musashino, Tokyo, Japan.
[2] Department of Sport and Sciences, University of Tokyo, Meguro, Tokyo, Japan.
[3] Department of Sport and Sciences, Tokyo Metropolitan University, Meguro, Tokyo, Japan.
[4] Department of Physical Education, Sophia University, Chiyoda, Tokyo, Japan.

Introduction

The goalkeeper is the last line of defence and he has a specialised role. Hughes (1980) stated that of all the eleven individuals in a soccer team the goalkeeper is the most important. If his performance is poor, he can and does lose matches on his own account. There have been several studies of the goalkeeper. From the point of view of goalkeeper's judgement, Eda (1969) studied the anticipation of a shooter's motion, and Kanamoto (1979) reported on the eye-fixation diffusion of the goalkeeper. Nakayashiki (1980) analysed the posture of the goalkeepr and Tamai (1979) and Masunaga (1984) reported on the effect of pre-jump on the jumping motion. However, there has only been one study (Asai, 1982) which has been concerned with the main motion of the Goalkeeper diving action. Therefore, the purpose of this study was to analyse the goalkeeper's diving motion by cinefilm analysis.

Methods

Four subjects, two upper class goalkeepers (KT and FK) from the Japan Soccer League (JSL) and two lower class goalkeepers (SK and TS) from the College Soccer League (CSL) participated in this investigation. Age and selected anthropometric characteristics are given in Table 1. All signed an informed consent form prior to participating in the study.

Table 1. Age and characteristics of subjects

	Subject	Age year	Height cm	Weight kg	Chest cm
JSL	KT	27	179.4	79.9	96.0
	FK	21	183.9	73.8	89.3
USL	SK	22	173.0	69.0	89.0
	TS	20	172.5	63.6	91.2

Subjects were instructed to perform a dive in order to contact the ball as fast as possible on the indication of a signal. The goalkeeper made a pre-jump and as soon as the goalkeeper landed on the forceplate, the direction of diving was randomly indicated by the signal. The signal was put 5.0 m in front of the forceplate. Balls suspended from the roof on both sides of the goalkeeper were spread 2.5 m apart from the middle of the forceplate, and were 0.3 m, 0.9 m and 1.5 m from the ground. Subjects performed about twenty dives at each ball height. In the low and middle ball height condition (0.3 m, 0.9 m), subjects had to catch the ball completely, and in the high ball condition (1.5 m) were permitted to deflect the ball.

High speed photography was performed using a Bolex 16 mm cine camera. The camera was position 12.5 m from the forceplace and the frame frequency was 60 frames per second. Locus, horizontal velocity, vertical velocity and absolute velocity of the body's centre of gravity were calculated using a motion analysis system SPORTIAS-300 (Nac.Co.). In the present study, only trials of which goalkeepers dived to their left side were used as data. The film analysis was made using the trial giving the shortest diving time, and was analysed at every three frames. The experimental dives of the present study are illustrated in Figure 1.

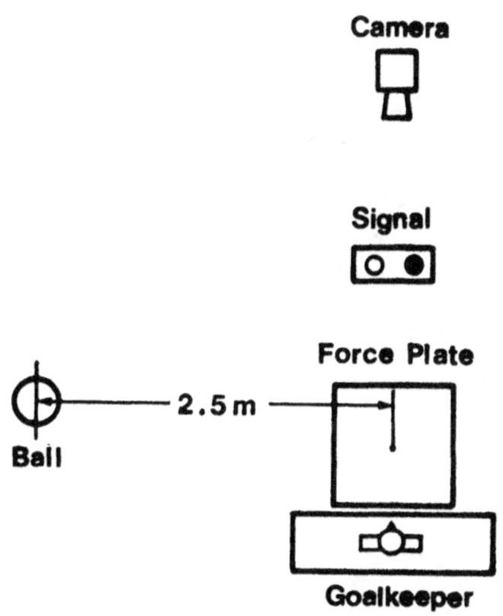

Figure 1. Experimental arrangement

Results

Locus of the body's centre of gravity

The locus of the body's centre of gravity of each subject at three ball heights from the beginning of motion is presented in Figure 2 to Figure 4.

In the ball height 0.3 m, subject SK made his centre of gravity move to the ball with little unpward movement and at take-off the height of centre of gravity reached a peak. After take-off the centre of gravity moved downward to the ball. Subject TS made his centre of gravity move to his lateral side downward. However, subject KT and subject FK made their centres of gravity move down noticeably after they landed on the forceplate. The centres of gravity of subject KT and FK were closer to the ball than subject SK and TS's at take-off. At the time of contact with the ball the JSL subjects' centres of gravity were also closer.

For the ball height of 0.9 m, all subjects made their centres of gravity move downward after landing on the forceplate, but JSL subjects' centres of gravity moved down more noticeably. Loci of the centre of gravities of JSL subjects followed a low gradient curve although, CSL subjects' loci followed a high gradient curve. The position of the centre of gravity at take-off and contact tended to be similar as at the ball height 0.3 m.

In the case of the ball height of 1.5 m, all the loci of centres of gravity followed a higher gradient curve than the other ball heights. However, the gradient of the JSL subjects' loci of centres of gravity were lower than the CSL subjects'.

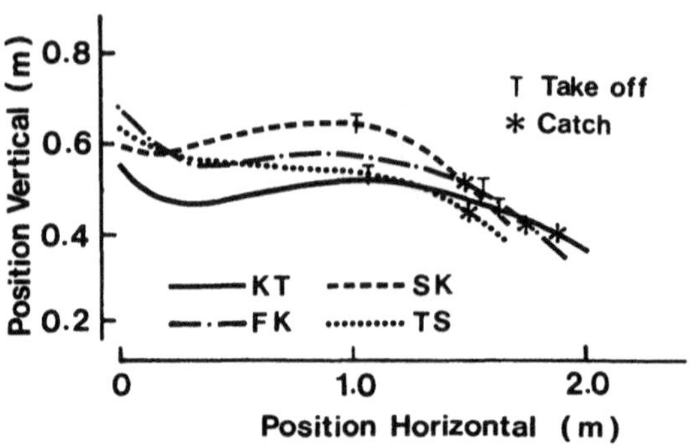

Figure 2. Locus of the body's centre of gravity (ball height = 0.3 m)

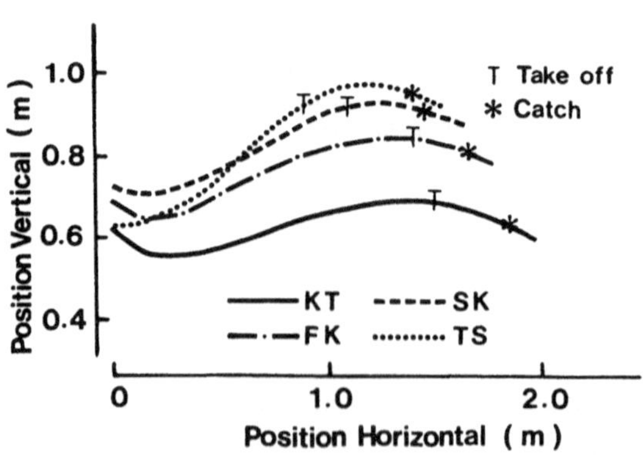

Figure 3. Locus of the body's centre of gravity (ball height = 0.9 m)

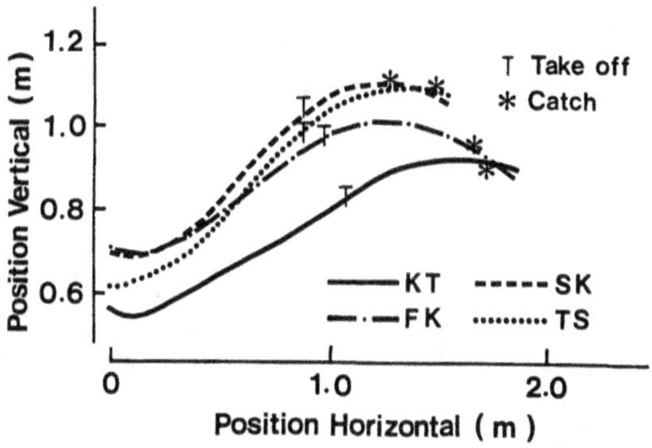

Figure 4. Locus of the body's centre of gravity (ball height = 1.5 m)

Velocity of centre of gravity at take-off

Horizontal velocity, vertical velocity and absolute velocity of the centres of gravity at take-off of subjects KT and SK are presented in Figure 5 to Figure 7 as typical cases.

In the ball height of 0.3 m, horizontal velocities were 4.74 m s^{-1}, 3.23 m s^{-1}, vertical velocities were -1.22 m s^{-1}, -0.11 m s^{-1} and absolute velocities were 4.90 m s^{-1} and 3.27 m s^{-1} for each of subjects KT and SK respectively. Therefore, the velocity of the centre of gravity of subject KT was greater and it was directed more downward.

In the ball height of 0.9 m, the horizontal velocities were 4.14 m s^{-1}, 3.24 m s^{-1}, vertical velocities were -0.33 m s^{-1}, -0.43 m s^{-1}, and absolute velocities were 4.14 m s^{-1}, 3.26 m s^{-1} respectively for subjects KT and SK. Subject KT's centre of gravity had greater velocity and the angle of velocity was directed more downward.

In the ball height of 1.5 m, subject KT's horizontal velocity was 3.78 m s^{-1}, vertical velocity was 1.21 m s^{-1}, and absolute velocity was 4.05 m s^{-1}. In subject SK the horizontal velocity was 2.91 m s^{-1}, vertical velocity was 1.30 m s^{-1}, and absolute velocity was 3.19 m s^{-1}. Subject KT's centre of gravity had greater velocity and was directed more downward than subject SK's.

Consequently, at all ball heights subject TK's centre of gravity had higher velocity and directed more downward than subject SK's.

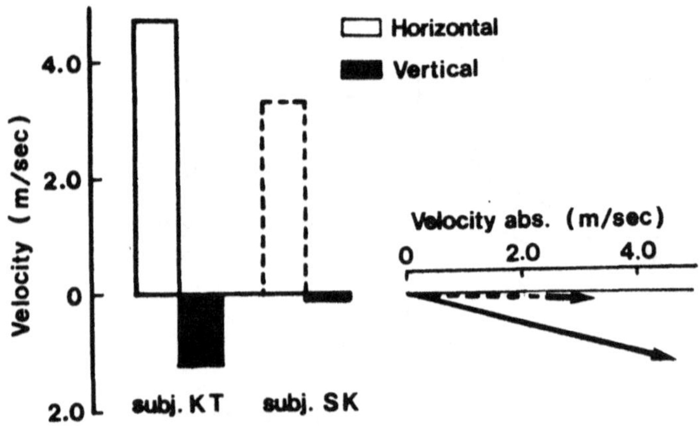

Figure 5. Velocity of the body's centre of gravity (ball height = 0.3 m)

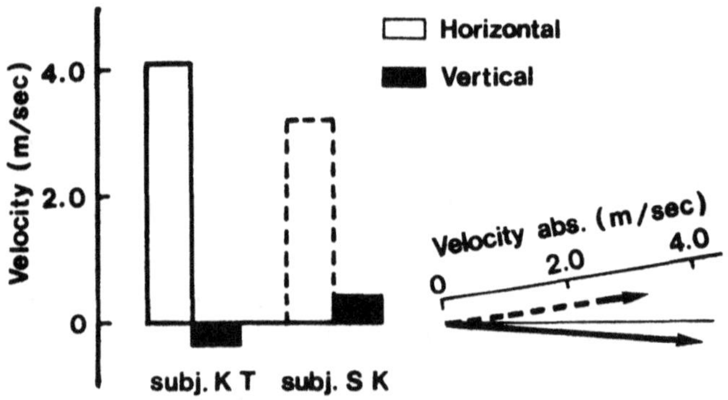

Figure 6. Velocity of the body's centre of gravity (ball height = 0.9 m)

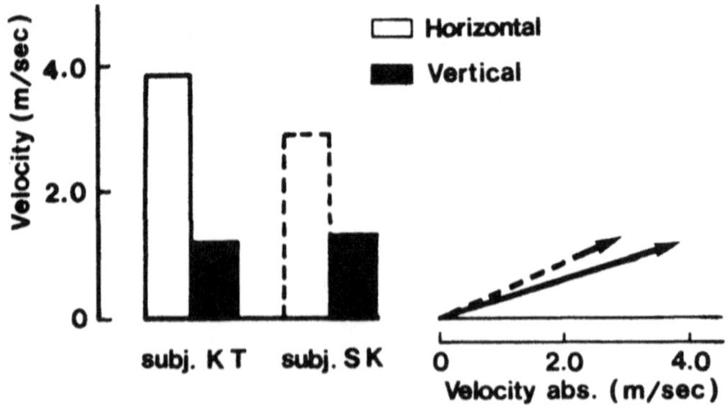

Figure 7. Velocity of the body's centre of gravity (ball height = 1.5 m)

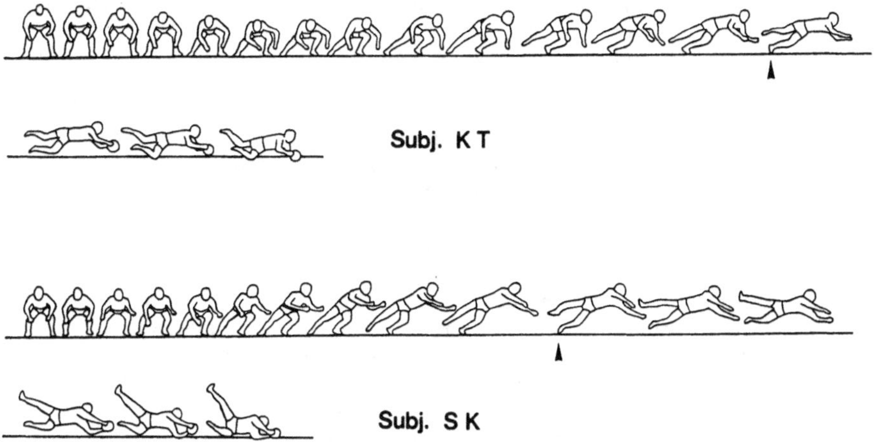

Figue 8. Trace of diving motion (ball height = 0.3 m)

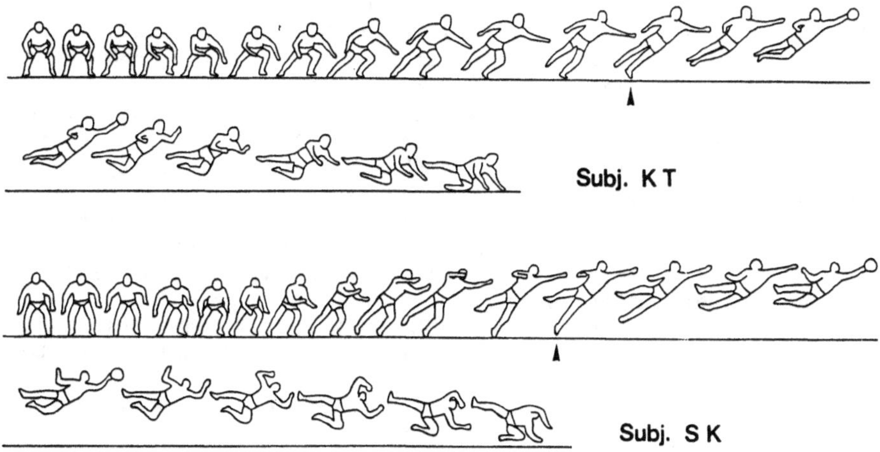

Figure 9. Trace of diving motion (ball height = 1.5 m)

Discussion

Diving is the most typical of all of goalkeeper's techniques. In this case, it is important that goalkeepers anticipate the direction, height and speed of the ball quickly (Eda, 1969). However, the performance of goalkeeping depends on the diving motion itself. Therefore, the key factor that makes good diving is the ability to throw the body faster and further. In other words, it is necessary to move the centre gravity quickly to the ball.

On the low-ball condition (0.3 m), JSL goalkeepers made their centre of gravity describe a low gradient locus and moved the centre of gravity more closely to the ball than CSL goalkeepers. That is, CSL goalkeepers took off shortly after beginning the motion; however, JSL goalkeepers took off after moving their centre of gravity to the ball.

After starting the motion, JSL goalkeepers had flexed hip and knee joints and then, turned upper body to the ball. On the contrary CSL goalkeepers had not flexed hip and knee joints and also did not turn their upper body to the ball (Figure 8). A key factor of the diving motion is the flexing of the hip and knee joints. Zagalo (1980) stated that for the lower ball, the goalkeeper must lower a body's centre of gravity.

For the higher ball, JSL goalkeepers' loci of the centre of gravity were lower than CSL goalkeepers'. Also, JSL goalkeepers flexed their hip and knee joints but did not turn the upper body to the ball. In this condition, flexing knee joints is a prior action to throwing the body with high velocity by accumulating energy (Figure 9). Nakayashiki (1980) reported there were motions of flexing hip and knee joints; this motion contributed to fast and strong dives.

Asai (1982) reported that with the lower ball goalkeepers rotated the body about their centre of gravity. In this study, there was no such motion of rotation. It is probable that this difference is due to the distance from the goalkeeper to the ball. In this study the ball distance was 2.5 m, but was 2.1 m in the study of Asai. Put in another way, using a body rotation is better with a ball near to the goalkeeper, but for the long distance ball it is necessary for the centre of gravity to approach the ball. It is clear that diving for long distance needs a higher velocity at take-off time. Centres of gravity of JSL goalkeepers had higher horizontal velocity than CSL goalkeepers' at all of ball heights. These data suggest that JSL goalkeepers threw their bodies with higher velocity to the lateral side. Vertical velocity indicates the angle of trajectory of the centre of gravity. At all three ball heights the angle of trajectory of JSL goalkeepers' centres of gravity were lower than CSL goalkeepers'. This suggests that JSL goalkeepers threw their bodies more directly while the CSL goalkeepers threw their bodies with too high a trajectory.

These results suggested that for a more effective diving motion, the velocities of the centre of gravity should be higher and it should be moved more directly to the ball.

References

Asai, T. (1982) A biomechanical study of diving technique of goal keeping in soccer. Tokyo Journal of Physical Education 12, 11-14.

Eda, M. (1969) A biomechanical study of goalkeeper's technique in soccer. Science of Physical Education, 19, 372-376.

Hughes, C. (1980) Soccer (The Football Association). London: British Broadcasting Co. and Oueen Anne Press.

Kanamoto, M. (1979) A study on the eye-fixation diffusion of the goal keeper. Journal of Sport Science of Tokyo Metropolitan University 12, 29-34.

Masunaga, M. (1984) A study of goal keeper's pre-motion in soccer. Journal of Sport Science of Kokugakuin University, 16, 45-49.
Nakayashiki, M. (1980) A study of goal keeper's posture in soccer. Journal of Sport Science of Sendai University, 12, 23-31.
Okano, S. (1976) Soccer, Tokyo: Fumaidoh Co.
Tamai, A. (1979) An experimental study of the effect of pre-jump in the soccer goalkeeper's diving. Journal of Sport Science of Tuskuba University, 83-85.
Zagalo, J. (1980) Soccer Coaching Association (special edition of Goalkeeper). Tokyo: Japan Football Association, Coaches Association.

A QUANTITATIVE ANALYSIS OF THRUST AND MOTOR COORDINATION IN A RUGBY SCRUM

Renato Rodano and Antonio Pedotti
Centro di Bioingegneria, Politecnico di Milano - Fondazione Pro Juventute don Gnocchi, Milano, Italy.

Introduction

Like any team sport, rugby requires individual skills, team skills and unit skills, one fundamental unit being the scrum. The main objective in the scrum is to win the ball. This is achieved by pushing the opposition pack backwards as a result of applying a powerful shove.

The pack thrust is applied through three front-row players who come in direct contact with their opposite numbers while, usually, five more players at their back shove and hold in the forwards in order to achieve the maximum thrust. The overall pack shove in a scrum depends on the strength of each player, but also on every man's correct position in the pack, correct grip on his team mates, proper binding and foot-placing and proper-coordination of individual shoves. Some criteria regulating these factors have emerged from the experience of coaches (Raper, 1964; Duthen, 1976). But they have no common quantitative standard measures and are affected by both the coaches' backgrounds and the players' own characteristics.

The present paper's aim was to achieve a quantitative evaluation of rugby players' thrust characteristics by a bioengineering approach. This should provide coaches with useful data and considerations for improving the pack's shove in scrummages.

Methods and Test Equipment

Procedure

The research was carried out on eight Italian junior athletes (BW(N):$\bar{x}$ = 940, SD = 69: height (m): $\bar{x}$ = 1.89, SD = 0.05). Each player was selected to represent one of the members of a traditional scrum pack. The athletes exerted their thrust against a solid mechanical structure simulating an opposing scrum pack. The choice was made in order to create experimental conditions simulating field conditions and easily repeatable in time. The test structure was designed to ensure a correct shoulder position and could be adjusted so as to allow the athletes to take the same position as in field scrum packing as required by the test protocol. According to their roles, they arranged the structure as if it were the front-row of a field scrum pack.

All, except the hooker, were required to apply a series of

thrusts, defined as follows:-

CTU: continuous thrust in usual position;

ITU: impulsive thrust in usual position.

The two props and the two second-row players were required to apply two more shoves, defined as follows:-

CTA: continuous thrust with one foot forward and one foot backward;

ITA: impulsive thrust with feet in above position.

The hooker performed the same actions as he would in an actual scrum.

For each series of shoves, the data relating to three trials which were approved as correct by a rugby team coach were recorded.

Test Equipment

Figure 1 shows a scheme of the test equipment used for measurements. Two Kistler force plates were used to measure the Rz, Ry and Rx components of ground reaction for each weight-bearing foot. Simultaneously, ELITE, a system for automatic analysis of TV images (Ferrigno and Pedotti, 1985), recorded the x, y coordinates of six markers fixed on the athlete's right side at the relevant anatomical points, viz. the axis of rotation of the shoulder, hip, knee, ankle, the iliac bone and the fifth metatarsal head.

Ground reaction forces and marker coordinates were acquired and recorded by a host computer, which also computed and visualized the following data:

- time course of Rz, Ry and Rx components of each foot ground reaction;
- the sum of each foot component Rz, Ry and Rx (Fig. 2);
- stick diagrams and curves of hip, knee and ankle angles (Fig. 3).

Theoretical Assumptions

In this study, the Ry component was used to quantify the thrust on the following grounds:

i) Ryt (Ry total) was assumed to be equal to the horizontal force Fy at shoulder level, since in equilibrium the inertial forces are negligible.

ii) The Rzt component was not taken into consideration because it acts directly to push onto the supporting surface. On the other hand, Rzt is used, particularly by the front-rowers, to force the opponents up, thus reducing the efficiency of their effort.

iii) The Rx component has much lower absolute values than Ry. Moreover, since the direction on the two feet is opposite, the overall Rxt reaction tends to stabilize around zero.

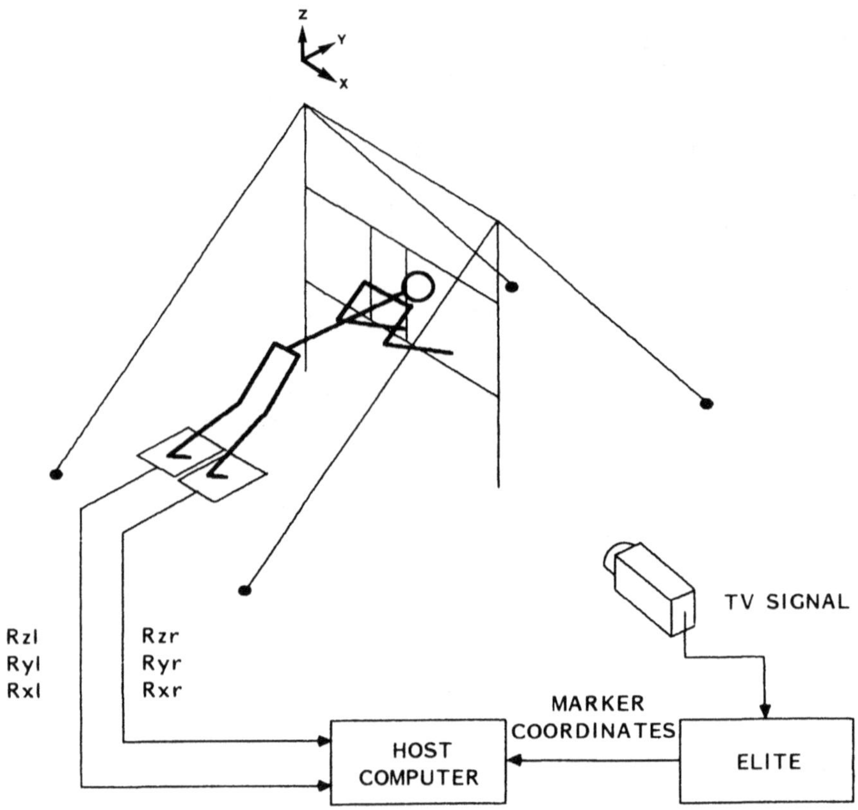

Figure 1. Scheme of the test equipment

Results and Discussion

The analysis of the reactions measured on the athletes (excluding the hooker) highlighted the two typical trends of Fyt for both continuous and impulsive action, as shown in Fig. 4. For continuous thrust (CT) there is a transient during which, in 0.5 s, Ryt grows steadily from the initial value recorded when the athlete rests against the structure to the steady-state value reached when he pushes at full vigour which is maintained at constant level till the end of the shove. Upward and downward variations of Ryt in this phase may be used to quantify the resistance to the athlete's thrust. The impulsive thrust (IT) is also characterised by a similar transient and steady state phase of Ryt. In this case the former, which lasts about 1 s, is of a fundamental importance since it determines the tactical purpose of the shove, i.e. causing disruption in the opposing pack to better exploit the steady-state phase of the shove.

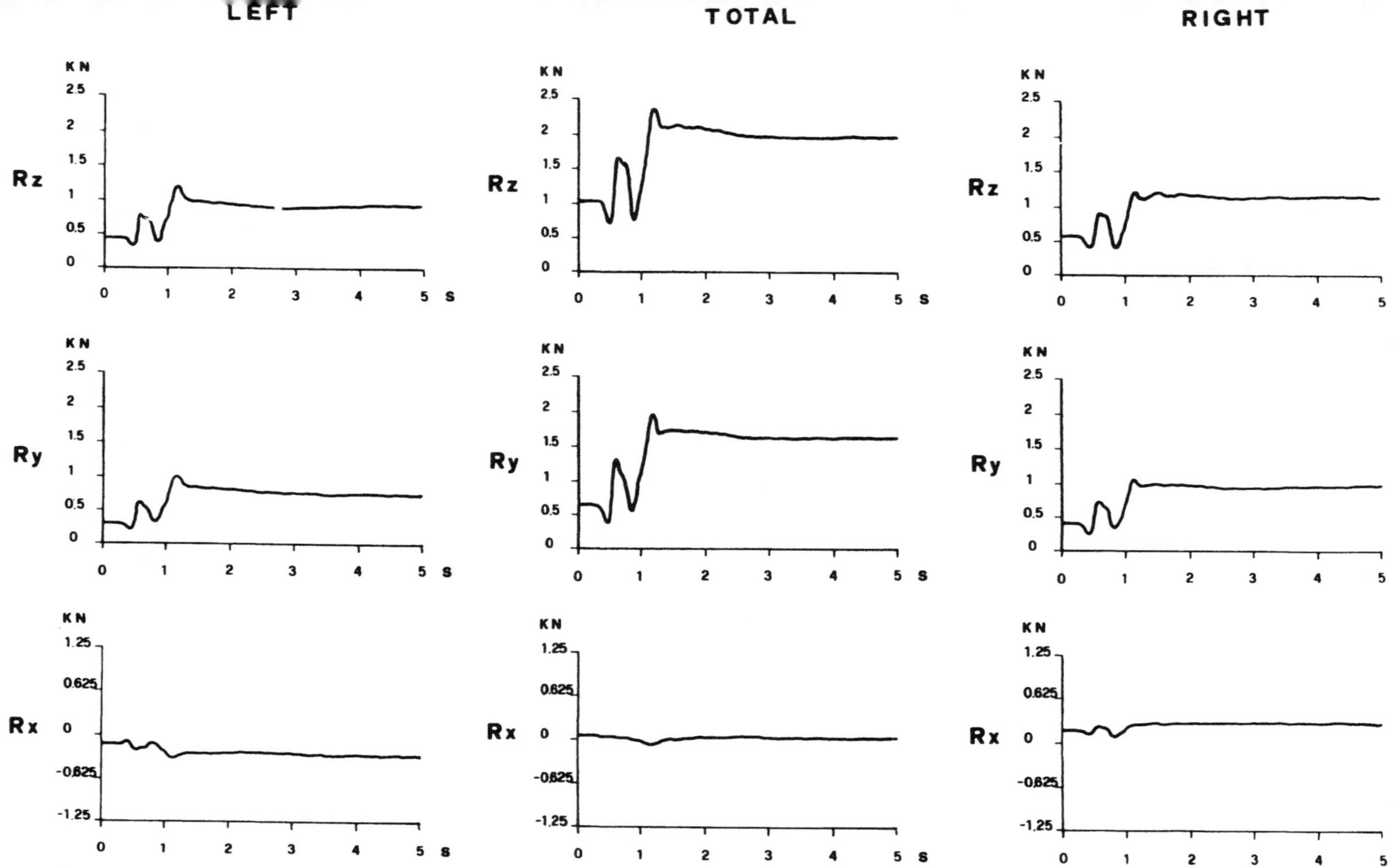

Figure 2. Curves of Rz, Ry and Rx components relating to right and left foot and sums of same data from an impulsive thrust trial

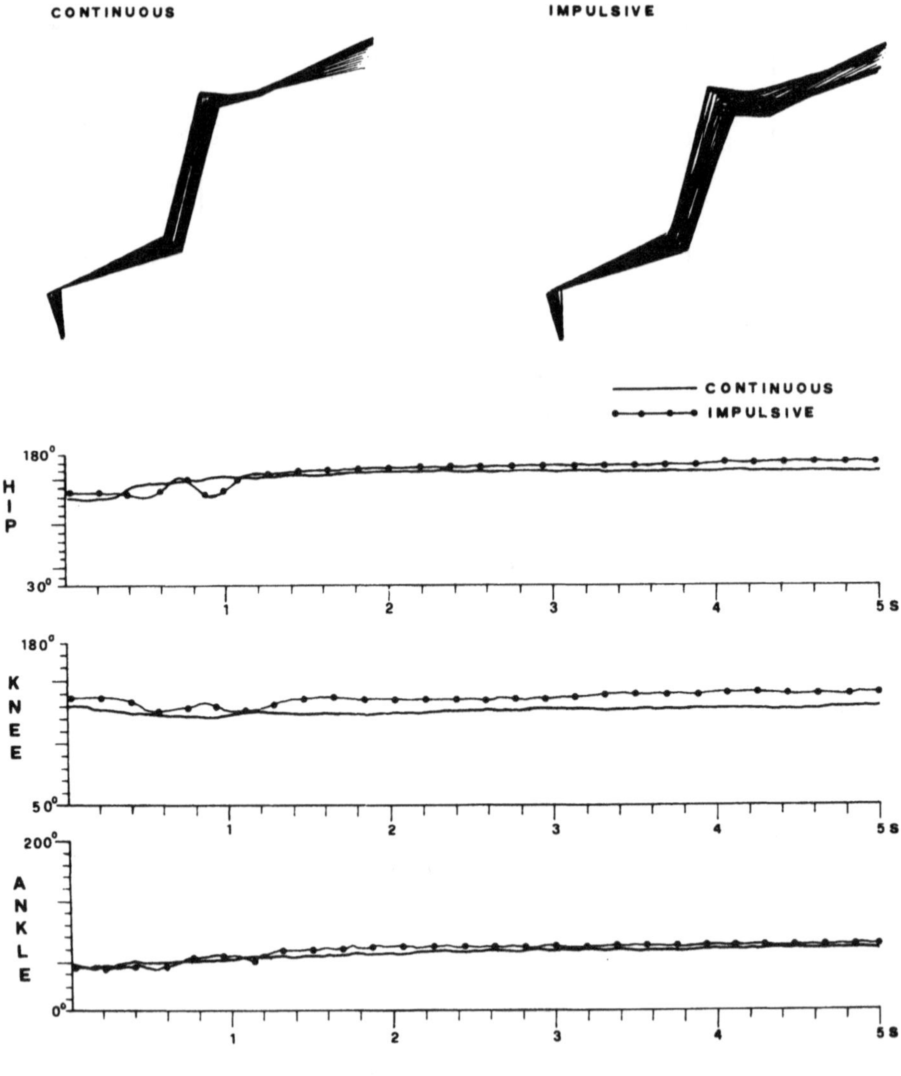

Figure 3. Stick diagrams and lower limb's angles of one athlete's right side. Data from continuous and impulsive thrust. Below average trends of Ryt for the two types of thrust

The transient is characterized by two peaks of growing amplitude with a minimum in between. During the steady-state phase, Ryt has a value which is 10% lower than the second peak on the average. Also in this case, upward and downward variations of Ryt are observed during the steady-state phase. Of course, there is a correspondence between the Ryt trend and the athletes' movements as described by the joint angles in Fig. 3. The CT transient corresponds to the change from the rest to the thrust phase which involves a quick contraction of leg extensors achieved by a slight opening of joint angles.

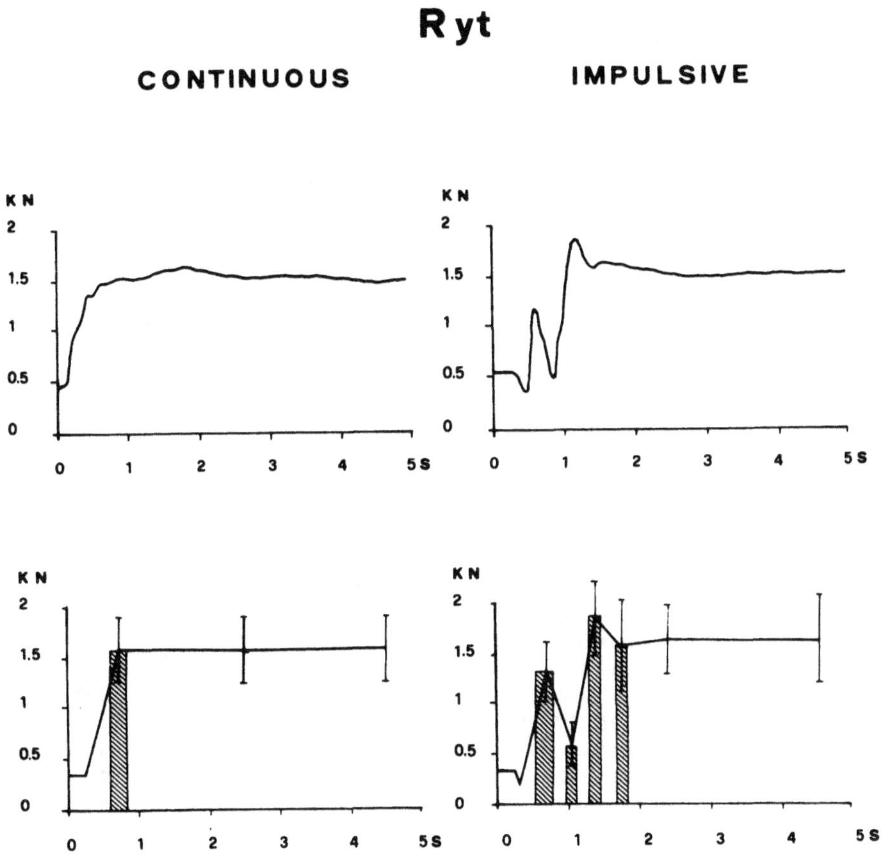

Figure 4. On the top typical trends of Ryt for continuous and impulsive thrust. Below average trends of Ryt for the two types of thrust

In IT, the contraction of leg extensors at sub-maximum levels produces a first peak, the controlled release of the thrust following a voluntary reduction of joint angles produces the minimum; then a second maximum extension (second peak) precedes the steady-state phase. The Ryt decrease during the latter is a result of the reduction of the inertial forces associated with the movements initiated during the transient phase.

The solid lines in Fig. 4 on the bottom, depict the average trends of Ryt for the two types of the thrust. The trends were matched with histograms whose height is proportionate to the mean of the values calculated in the transient significant points in all trials. The histograms were centred on the mean value of the time co-ordinate and their width is equal to the standard deviation. The Figure also shows Ryt mean values and standard deviations measured at 2.5 and 4.5 s from the beginning of the transient phase.

The IT shows the Ryt higher value which always shows up when the second peak is reached (1759 N). The two thrusts show no difference in the steady-state phase since, in both cases, Ryt reaches steady values between 1520 and 1529 N, which suggests that CT and IT are equivalent when the athlete's shove reaches a steady-state condition. But, IT affords the advantage of significantly higher force peaks which, if properly applied may win a pack a big gain. If one considers the limited time variability in the transient shown by athletes in IT, shove co-ordination seems to be a group rather than an individual issue.

Shove effectiveness may be quantitatively defined by a number of parameters, e.g. by peak Ry values (Ry max). It was, however, deemed convenient to select a parameter which would consider the possibility of applying a high power thrust for a reasonably long period of time. Such a parameter was identified as RyE, which is mathematically defined as the maximum of the function

$$\frac{\int_{t_0}^{t_1} R_y(t)\, dt}{(t_1 - t_0)}$$

where $(t_1 - t_0) = 1$ s is the time interval under consideration and to varies steadily along the duration of the thrust.

Ryt E defines the 1 s of the thrust when the highest average Ry is exerted. Ry E was calculated with reference to both feet in all trials. The interval was chosen on the grounds of the duration of the transients and overall shove. A comparison of Ryt E values between IT ($\bar{x}$ = 1648 N, SD = 225 N) and CT ($\bar{x}$ = 1540 N, SD = 255 N) shows that on the average IT is more effective than CT.

The results of a further mathematical processing of available data can quantitativly question the widespread opinion among team coaches that 'a scrum pack with the heaviest men produces the most powerful shove'.

This statement which sounds so reasonable deserves careful consideration since it strongly affects game strategies. It should not be forgotten that the men in the scrum pack are also involved in other phases of the match where the motor characteristics of too heavy men may prove to be a disadvantage. Thus the coefficient of linear correlation (r) between the athlete's body weight and Ryt max and Ryt E in both CTU and IPU were calculated. The coefficient values vary in all combinations between 0.24 and 0.33 which rejects any significant correlation between the athlete's body weight and thrust magnitude.

Table 1 gathers Ryt E mean values measured under the different test conditions and the mean values for the same parameters referring to the right and left foot. A comparison between CTU and ITU shows that all players display higher Ryt in the latter which once again indicates that at least at an individual level ITU is the most efficient thrust.

As far as the Ryt E distribution on the legs is concerned, in CTU the athletes display a fairly even distribution of thrust, one only among them showing differences higher than 10% between his two legs. In ITU, the number of athletes showing an uneven distribution of Ryt E on the lower limbs rises to three, which indicates a growing difficulty in motor coordination.

Table 1. Mean values of Ryt E, measured on each athlete under the different experimental conditions (in Newtons)

	CTU			CTA			ITU			ITA		
Player	RytE	RyrE	RyIE	RytE	RyrE	RyIE	RytE	RyrE	RyIE	RytE	RyrE	RyIE
PROP	1520	735	745	1422	706	1049	1569	902	676	1520	559	961
PROP	1844	1000	853	1648	981	706	1942	1059	892	1549	912	637
2nd ROW	1520	755	735	1746	1039	647	1844	922	804	1863	1108	598
2nd ROW	1137	608	500	1255	765	461	1599	814	568	1461	882	353
FLANKER	1667	705	873	-	-	-	1883	873	960	-	-	-
FLANKER	1746	882	902	-	-	-	1873	902	922	-	-	-
No. 8	1844	1079	774	-	-	-	1981	1157	676	-	-	-

A comparison of the data relating to CTU and CTA shows that two out of four players display higher Ryt E in the usual position, while the opposite is true for the remaining two. All four subjects show a marked increase in Ryt variability between the right and left leg (Ryr and Ryl respectively). Similar considerations arise from a comparison between ITU and ITA data. In this case, the increase in Ryt E variability is far more apparent in ITA and most probably due to two factors - firstly a change from the usual position disturbing the athletes' motor automatisms regulating the thrust, and secondly the different joint angles which may be better or worse for the

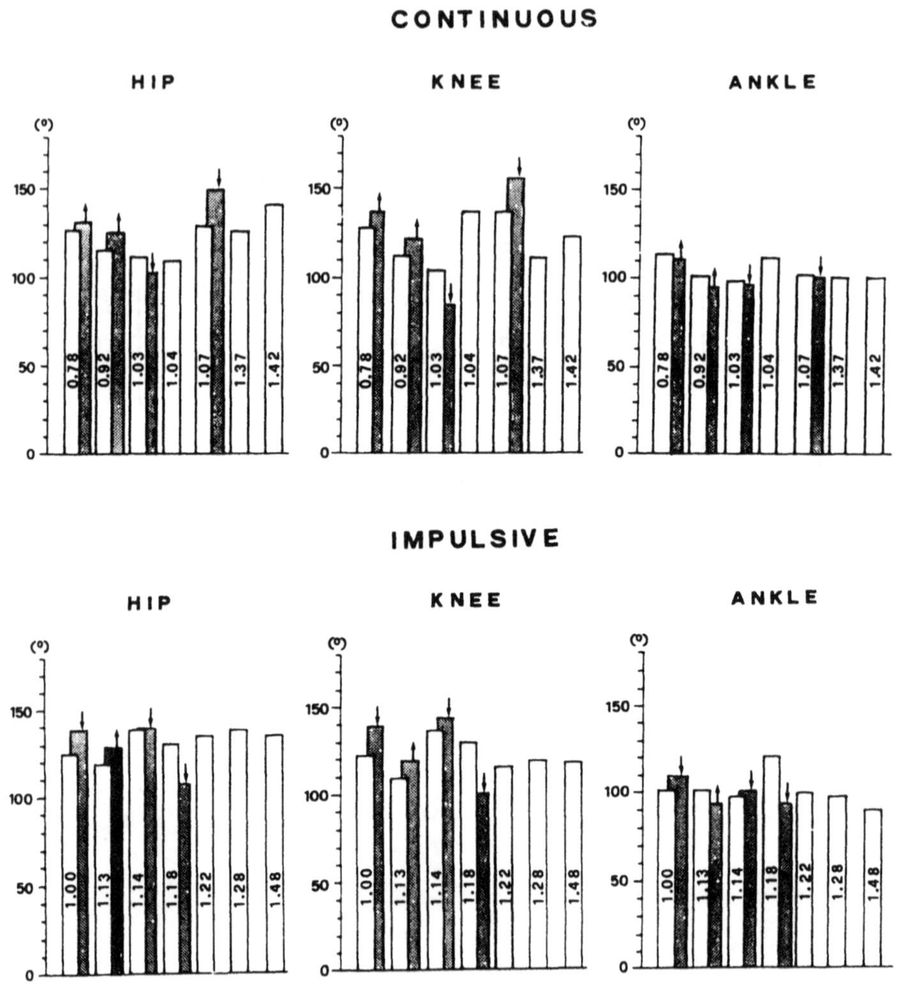

Figure 5. Histograms relating to the right lower limb joints. The data are those recorded when Ryt max was reached during the best performance, evaluated through Ryt E. The figures into the histograms indicate the Ryt max body weight ratio. Shaded histograms relate to alternative positions

muscular action required by IT. Therefore, the adoption of positions other than the standard ones requires further research.

Fig. 5 shows the histograms referring to the angles of the right leg joints of each athlete measured at the moment when the Ry max is deployed at the right foot level. The data refer to the next performance under the various test conditions. Each histogram includes the value of the Ryr max/body weight ratio. Dotted histograms refer to the joint angles measured when the athletes are in the alternative position required by the operator and the arrows indicate whether the Ryr max increases (upward) or decreases (downward) at the new angle.

When considering CTU, the ankle angle is shown to be very similar for all athletes (97 to 112 degrees) while the variations for the knee (104 to 138 degrees) and hip (110 to 140 degrees) angles are more marked. An analysis of data for joint angles in CTU in relation to the Ryr max/body weight ratio indicates that there is no best position for maximizing the thrust. Yet, it should be noted that the best and second best athletes tend to push with a rather open hip angle and a knee angle of 112 to 122 degrees. An analysis of angles in CTA, on the other hand, gives no more precise indications. It is not possible, in fact, to attribute the higher or lower thrust levels to either wider or narrower joint angles.

When considering ITU, there is a slight joint angle variability in the athletes with higher Ryr max/body weight ratios - ankle 90 to 100 degrees, knee 116-120 degrees, hip 40 to 43 degrees. For all other athletes, distribution seems to be random.

As for ITA, the same considerations as made for CTA hold good. Yet, it is worth emphasising that the only athlete who could supply a stronger thrust in the new position bent his angle and knee at angles similar to the best athletes' threshold values and his hip too tended to fall in line with the patterns of the latter.

The above considerations suggest that the link between thrust and position is more marked in ITU. Since an adoption of the ideal position not only depends on the structural needs of the scrum, but also on the players' anthropological characteristics, it will be convenient to further study the issue focusing on physical parameters more directly related to the display of force as a function of position, such as for instance joint moments, which can be obtained by working out appropriate mathematical models of the lower limbs (Cappozzo et al., 1976).

Conclusions

Results were obtained from a quantitative analysis of the thrust in a rugby scrum under two different actions, the continuous and impulsive thrust. At individual level, IT produces force peaks higher than CT. Higher IT effectiveness is confirmed by its greater value at time intervals of 1 s, but IT also requires greater motor coordination skills as compared to CT. It is thought that these skills would be easily acquirable by players. For individual IT force peaks to be properly exploited during the match, great coordination of scrum pack members is essential. The IT seems to better suit the attack or facing an opposing pack in lock position, i.e. when the risks resulting from bad co-ordination or a controlled reduction of the thrust in the transient phase are lower. The mathematical correlation between body weight and Ryt max and between the former and Ryt E rejects any significant correlation between the athlete's body weight and thrust.

No definite paradigm of optimum joint angle position has emerged, although available data show some preferential trends which are more apparent in IT. In this connection, tests on a wider sample of athletes and measurements of other biomechanical parameters are of a fundamental importance.

The study proved that the method has potential as an instrument to evaluate the athletes' individual thrust objectively with a view to maximizing it according to individual motor characteristics.

References

Duthen, G. and Spranghere, W. (1976) Le Rugby. Paris: Denoel.

Cappozzo, A., Figura, F., Marchetti, M. and Pedotti, A. (1976) The interplay of muscular and external forces in human ambulation. J. Biomech., 9, 35-43.

Ferrigno, G., Pedotti, A. (1985) ELITE: a digital dedicated hardware system for movement analysis via real-time TV signal processing. IEEE Trans. on Biomed. Eng., Vol. BME 32, No. 11, Nov.

Raper, J.W. (1964) The Jonny Raper Rugby. Rugby League Book. Sidney: K.G. Murray Publishing Company Pty Ltd.

Part XI

Psychological aspects of football skills

PENALTY-KICK STRATEGIES FOR SHOOTERS AND GOALKEEPERS

Werner Kuhn
Deutsche Sporthochschule, Carl Diem Weg 2, 5000 Köln 41, West Germany

Introduction

In this paper two exploratory studies are presented which focus on different control strategies for penalty kicks from the perspective of both shooter and goalkeeper. Penalty kicks play a decisive role in regular games but are especially important in cup competitions. A review of English and German soccer literature reveals some tactical advice on taking penalty kicks. For example, Cramer (1952) and Schmid et al., (1968) have identified two basic styles of executing penalty kicks, one emphasising power, the other accuracy. The kick for accuracy (position kick) is usually initiated with a fake. Cramer (1952) recommended the power kick as it can hardly be stopped even if lacking precision.

A lot more advice is given in the literature to goalkeepers. Maier and Pfaff (1984) rated as 0.50 the goalkeeper's probability of success in stopping the ball. They concluded that for the goalkeeper to be successful it was necessary to wrest the advantage from the shooter by clever positioning which could dictate the direction of the ensuing shot. A second strategy of advantage, outlined by coaches is careful analysis of pre-contact cues (e.g. angle of approach run and body orientation in addressing the ball) which could again provide valuable anticipatory signals on intended direction of ball flight. Other favourite strategies include the use of faked upper body movements and the use of detailed notes on favoured strategies gained from detailed observation of selected penalty takers.

Clearly what is necessary in this topic is a detailed observational analysis of penalties, which could aid in identifying successful strategies for both shooters and goalkeepers. In this way more meaning would be attached to the subjective opinions of coaches and expert goalkeepers in the coaching literature on this important aspect of play.

The restrictions on both takers and stoppers of penalties are outlined by FIFA in the laws of the game. Of significance are the sub-clauses which stress that the shooter must play the ball forward and shall not play the ball a second time until it has been touched by another player. A further restriction that the goalkeeper must not move his feet until after the ball has been played by the kicker.

The temporal and spatial structure of the penalty-kick may be divided into three phases for both types of player:- premotor, motor and postmotor. The motor phase is composed of the approach run and the shot. There are virtually no time constraints.

With these factors in mind it was decided to observe in detail and analyse the control strategies of both shooters and goalkeepers with the aim of identifying precisely the most successful in performance.

Methods

A sample of 83 penalty kicks from German Bundesliga and European Cup matches during two consecutive seasons (1981-2 and 1982-3) were videotaped. These were analysed with regard to success, duration of ball flight and types of control strategies.

Three categories were established to measure success:- goal, miss (hitting the woodwork or complete miss) and save. To determine the duration of ball flight a video timer was interfaced with a videorecorder. The time between contact of the ball and crossing the goal-line ranges approximately from 400 ms (100 km h^{-1}) to 800ms (50 km h^{-1}). Ball speed was classified as slow or medium when flight time lasted up to 600 ms (75 km h^{-1}) and as fast or very fast when flight speed was greater than this value. Perspective was a limiting factor in this study since in the case of saves or deflected shots, the passing of the goal-line had to be estimated. Twelve penalty kicks were eliminated as the recordings did not allow a refined determination of the duration of flight.

Results

Shooting

An analysis of 66 penalty kicks showed that 42 (63.6%) were successful with 24 (36.3%) unsuccessful. Fifty-three penalties (80.3%) were placed and only 13 (19.7%) were power kicks. Two main types of strategy were identified. The first (Strategy SA) could be termed open-loop in that the whole action appeared pre-programmed. Speed appears to be the dominant variable as the kicker shows little sign of careful aiming towards a particular area of the goal. The second type of strategy (Strategy SB) involves a closed-loop approach in that completion of the motor phase is dependent on the goalkeeper's actions. Simply, the shooter delays the completion of the shooting action until the last possible moment so as to process feedback from the positioning of the goalkeeper and to delay the presentation of his own body cues. This often results in a slow to medium preparatory phase for ball contact. Fifteen penalties from the total belonged to Strategy SA (22%) and 51 (78%) to Strategy B.

Goalkeeping

With regard to control strategies again, two types could be identified. In the first (Strategy GA) movement to one side or another occurs at the moment of ball contact or immediately afterwards. This strategy may imply either decision-making at ball contact or anticipation before ball contact. With the alternative strategy (GB), movement to one side or another occurs before the ball is contacted. This involves speculation or acute anticipatory processes.

Five penalties were eliminated from this analysis because a clear distinction between strategies GA and GB was not possible. Of interest here was the interaction of strategy GA and the penalties saved. The majority of experts at saving penalties used Strategy GA: they were successful in 9 out 15 cases (60%). Goalkeepers using Strategy GB had a much lower success rate, 4 saves out of 51 (7.8%). The data were not statistically treated because of the low number of cases in each cell. Although more data are needed on this issue, it can be concluded from this study that goalkeepers are capable of being successful when moving after contact of the ball in the case of ball velocities which are slow or medium paced.

Since most German professional penalty takers play the waiting game, Strategy GA seems to be most adequate. In the case of the use of strategy GB, the goalkeeper still need not resort to guessing which corner the ball will be blasted. Instead, there are important cues such as angle of approach and angle of foot contact on the ball which can aid the choice of diving direction. Knowledge of the preferred foot of the kicker, the predominance of team-mates standing on one particular side of the penalty area in anticipation of a knock-down and the eye movements of the kicker in placing the ball are others (Hoek, 1983; Kaipel, 1983; Tyldesley et al., 1983).

Discussion

In addition to the strategies outlined which were subjectively identified from the data, some players engaged in what may be termed 'psychoregulative' measures. Examples are deliberately delaying the execution of the kick by walking around the penalty area, telling the shooter which corner is his favourite or making allusions to the morality of the shooter's wife! The aim is to invoke a loss of concentration on the part of the shooter.

There are a number of practical considerations for the goalkeeper which may be developed in training. Improvements in specific reaction and movement times should be emphasised in practice. Initial practice could occur in 'underload' conditions (e.g. the use of distances such as 13 and 12 m), thereafter switching to "overload" values (e.g. 10 and 9 m). Priority should be given to specific game situations. Practice should be realistic and probability of shot direction must vary as it would under match conditions.

Finally, there is a clear need for more objective data in the realm of penalty strategies. These might be best obtained utilising computerised notational analysis to support the detailed observations from this study.

References

Cramer, D. (1952) Fußball-Taktik. Wuppertal: Berenbrock.

Hoek, F. (1983) Der Fußball-Torwart. Göttingen: Vandenhoek and Ruprecht.

Kaipel, W. (1983) Torwarttraining. Maria Enzersdorf: Verlag für Sportpublikationen.

Maier, S. and Pfaff, J.-M. (1984) Das Torwartbuch, Hamburg: Hoffmann and Campe.

Schmid, R.I., McKeen, J.L. and Schmid, M.R. (1968) Skills and strategies of successful soccer. Englewood Cliffs, N. Jersey: Prentice-Hall, Inc.

Tyldesley, D.A., Bootsma, R.J. and Bomhoff, G.T. (1983) Skill level and eye-movement patterns in a sports-oriented reaction time task. In Motorik-und Bewegungsforschung (edited by H. Rieder, K. Bös, H. Mechling and K. Reischle), pp.290-296. Schorndorf: Hofmann.

THE USE OF A SIMULATOR IN EVALUATION AND TRAINING OF TACTICAL SKILLS IN SOCCER

W. Helsen and J.M. Pauwels
Instituut voor Lichamelijke Opleiding, K.U. Leuven, Tervuursevest 101, 3030 Heverlee, Belgium.

Introduction

One striking aspect of soccer is the complex set of relations that arise as the player is confronted with team-mates, opponents, the ball, the goal, and the field of play. The player must continually perform tactical acts that place high demands on his perception, decision-making ability and motor output because of the rapidly changing environment. These acts can be expressed as individual or team tactics.

In this paper individual tactical skills are considered in relation to the conceptual capacity with which each player operates during the game. Constantly, in order to make appropriate decisions, players have to use their 'soccer brains'. According to Morris (1982 p94-99), analysis of an international soccer game between France and Argentina revealed that there were 2622 ball contacts, each preceded by a tactical decision.

Typical questions a player must face during the game include:- when to dribble, when to pass and to which team-mate; when to shoot at the goal and in which spot, how to solve an off-side situation? In addition, the player has to make such decisions in a fraction of a second. Any hesitation permits the opponents to anticipate the decision (Pauwels, 1980). Tactical skill thereby concerns the ability to make fast and appropriate decisions at the right moment.

In the present study, a real-game simulator is evaluated to establish the extent to which tactical game problems of varying complexity are solved by subjects of different skill level. The purposes of this study were to determine:- i) the reliability of the test set-up; ii) whether the simulator is sensitive enough to evaluate the tactical decisions of soccer players of different skill level. The main concerns mainly were the speed and the quality with which players perceive and solve these game problems by examining their motor output.

Methodology

Subjects

Subjects were 20 male soccer players, mean age being 21 years. Ten of them were seriously involved in soccer and had 10 years of active competition. The other ten players played soccer recreationally.

Simulation of tactical movement patterns
The simulator consisted of simulated game situations, presented dynamically by means of a 16-mm film display. Game situations were presented and had to be solved by means of a motor output.

Using video films, different tactical situations were selected from real soccer matches in European Cup and World Cup games. The six types of decision are listed in Table 1.

Table 1. Summary of the nature and the number of each of the tactical actions that were studied on video films

The type of decision required by one of the players in the total action	Total number of each
1 shooting at the goal	7
2 passing to a free team-mate	8
3 passing around the goalkeeper or an opponent	4
4 avoiding an off-side	4
5 taking a penalty kick	3
6 taking a free kick (direct and indirect)	4

For each situation, the actions of all the players (attackers, defenders, referees) were studied and carefully schematized. Thirty different situations were taken into account.

The simulation of these tactical actions is now described. These game situations were replaced 'live' on a real soccer field with all the relevant elements, including the advertising panels. The camera (16-mm film) replaced one of the players who was confronted at a specific moment with an important tactical decision. The actors (referee and players) were given clear instructions and then played the situation as recorded on video. Like the player from the actual match, the camera travelled on a track within the game and recorded what the player was confronted with during the real game situation. This can be called 'acted soccer', realistically played by experienced soccer players and with a camera taking the place of one of the athletes.

Test set-up
This 16-mm film was projected on a screen (Fig. 1). The pictures on the screen occupy a field of 10 m x 4 m. To achieve this realistic size, several special lenses were used. By using such lenses, the dimensions from the 'live' soccer game were well equated with the simulated actions on the screen. Team-mates and opponents on the screen, for example, were shown life size. The test set-up itself consisted of a film-projector, a screen (2), check-lights (3), a ball, a control unit (4), an Apple II microcomputer (5) and a printer (6).

The experimental set-up was explained individually to each subject by means of an introduction program on the film, and five subactions were used for familiarization. The distance between the screen and the subject (1) was 7 m so that the field of vision was completely filled with the projection. The trials were all conducted in the same room with the individual subject at the same distance from the screen.

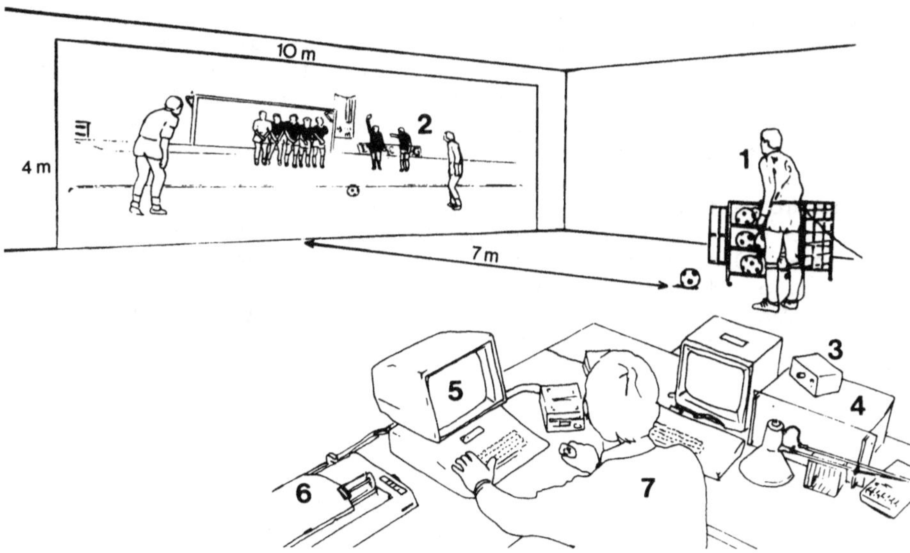

Figure 1. The experimental set-up showing the position of apparatus, subject and experimenter

Procedure

When the film started, the ball moved on the screen from one player to another. At that specific moment, the ball was played by one of the attackers in the direction of the subject who was instructed to perceive himself as an attacker. In response to a signal on the film he was required to perform a tactical decision with the ball which lay 2 m in front of him (see Fig. 1). Just like a real game situation the player can choose between shooting at goal on the screen, passing around an opponent just in front of him, or passing the ball to a free team-mate on the screen. Thus the subject was required to solve these game problems by motor output with the ball. This was important since output processes are integrated with perception and decision processes; attempts to isolate them experimentally fail to provide meaningful results unless they have been assembled in conditions reflecting real game imitations and reconstructions.

Dependent variables

Before the start of each game situation, the subject stood with both feet on electronic contacts. The ball was controlled by a microwave detector. A timer in the microcomputer was activated in response to the appearance of the signal and stopped automatically when the subject started his movement (initiation time), and when he touched the ball (response time).

This provided indications of the analytical time (how long it took to make the decision) and execution time (how long it took to kick the ball). The difference between initiation time and response time was called 'movement time'. The time indications were transmitted to the microcomputer, stored on a disk and printed out. The correctness of the decisions was also evaluated for each situation, since a number of soccer experts had previously agreed on the right solution for each situation. For example, for an indirect free-kick (situation 8) it is clear that subjects have to pass to their free team-mate instead of shooting at the goal.

Independent variables
Subjects were categorised according to experience by the following criteria:- i) extensive experience in soccer competition (at least 10 years), or ii) limited experience in soccer competition (only few years). Their decisions were one of the following:- i) shooting at the goal; ii) passing around the goalkeeper or an opponent; iii) passing to a free team-mate.

Results

Reliability
The reliability of the experiment was determined by the split-half method. The results of the even-numbered response times were compared to these of the odd-numbered response times by means of the Spearman-Brown formula and resulted in a coefficient of 0.99.

Initiation time - movement time - response time
An analysis of variance revealed that there was statistically no significant difference between both groups for the initiation times ($F_{1,19} = 0.76$ $P > 0.05$) However, differences in movement times ($F_{1,19} = 8.33$ $P < 0.01$) and response times ($F_{1,19} = 8.37$ $P < 0.01$) were noted. In order to evaluate the ability to make fast and appropriate decisions at the right moment, response times and the quality of the decision were combined by the following (Table 2). The 5 shortest right response times calculations were averaged, the mean being indicated by 5 SR. The mean of the 10 shortest right response times is expressed by 10 SR whilst 20 SR refers to the mean of the 20 shortest right response times.

Analyses of variance revealed that there were statistically significant differences between both groups for all the parameters $F_{1,19} = 26.08$, 5SR; 24.56, 10SR and 19.91, 20 SR respectively - all $P < 0.01$). Additional analyses revealed that soccer players with extensive experience in competition responded more accurately when shooting at goal or passing to a free team-mate, while there was no difference between the two groups in the number of wrong decisions.

Discussion

These results clearly indicate that soccer players with long experience in competition can make faster and more appropriate tactical decisions at the right moment than players with a limited experience in competition. This seemed to be particularly true for

Table 2. Mean ($\bar{X}$), standard deviation (SD), standard error (SE) and coefficient of variation (CV) of the mean of the 5, 10 and 20 shortest right response times (ms) for both groups

Group		5SR	10SR	20SR
Players with limited soccer experience	$\bar{X}$	1312.8	1381.8	1493.5
	SD	83.0	84.6	96.6
	SE	27.7	28.2	32.2
	CV	6.3	6.1	6.5
Players with long experience in soccer	$\bar{X}$	1119.7	1194.0	1306.7
	SD	77.3	75.9	80.3
	SE	25.8	25.3	26.8
	CV	6.9	6.4	6.1

passing-situations, indirect free kicks and off-side problems. Furthermore, there was a reasonable correlation for both groups between initiation times and response times. This suggested that they followed the same strategy to solve tactical situations. Firstly, the appropriate decision was taken, then the ball was kicked. Decisions were not changed during responses. The differences in solving these tactical game situations must therefore be mainly due to differences in response processes and response production.

The finding is strengthened by the fact that there was no difference between the groups in the quality of the decisions. Even players with a limited experience in soccer competition seemed to have enough knowledge to correctly solve tactical game problems. Perhaps the differences in quality of decision making would be greater if the levels of experience were wider apart. The suggestion here is that further research must occur if knowledge of the tactical understanding of players is to be advanced. For example, work comparing the decision-making performance of children of different age groups represents a useful issue for further investigation.

References

Morris, D. (1982) The Soccer Tribe. London: Jonathan Cape.
Pauwels, J.M. (1980) Tacticometry: a tool to improve the learning process of tactical skills. In: Psychology of Motor Behaviour and Sport 1979 (Conference of the American Society for the Psychology of Sport and Physical Activity Trois-Rivières, 1979, (edited by C.H. Nadeau, W.R. Halliwell, K.M. Newell and G.C. Roberts), pp690-701. Champaign (Illinois): Human Kinetics.

AGCO: THE CONSTRUCTION OF AN AGILITY-COORDINATION TEST

Sean O'Dwyer
CICE, University of Dublin, 96 Upper Rathmines Road, Dublin 6, Eire.

Introduction

In many sports, such as football, coordination may optimally drive performance when utilised in interaction with agility. Krus et al. (1981) identified two overall motor performance dimensions, one based on a 'speed-precision-strength' axis and the other on a 'balance-coordination' factor. Agility appeared to be strongly reflected in the former and coordination in the latter. Moroever, the interdependence of these two abilities has been recognised elsewhere (Kirkendall et al., 1980; Phillips and Hornak, 1979). Agility-coordination is defined in this paper as the integration of body parts and the interaction of movement qualities in the rapid and controlled execution of complex multidirectional motor tasks. The construction of a test to measure agility-coordination (AGCO), in a valid and reliable manner, was the primary purpose of the present study. A subsidiary aim was to test the hypothesis that AGCO would be significantly related to a general ('g') measure of motor performance according to qualified general classroom teachers' subjective rating of a pupil's motor ability in physical education.

Study I

Methods

Apparatus

An agility mat, common to most well-equipped gymnasia (dimensions 182.9 x 121.9 x 2.5 cm), was marked with sticky tape parallel to and 30 cm from one of the long sides (see Figure 1). The backs of 3 chairs were centred on the 2 m marks. Two foam rubber plates (20 x 20 x 5 cm), 20 cm apart, were placed parallel to each other as can be seen in Figure 1.

White tape (38 mm thickness) was used to mark two squares (30 cm^2) and the other circuit lines shown clearly in Figure 1. A stop-watch was used to time the speed of the subject negotiating the circuit area.

Procedure

The subject was required to start in the supine position on the mat outside the 30 cm taped line. On the presentation of an auditory signal the subject was required to elevate himself to his feet as

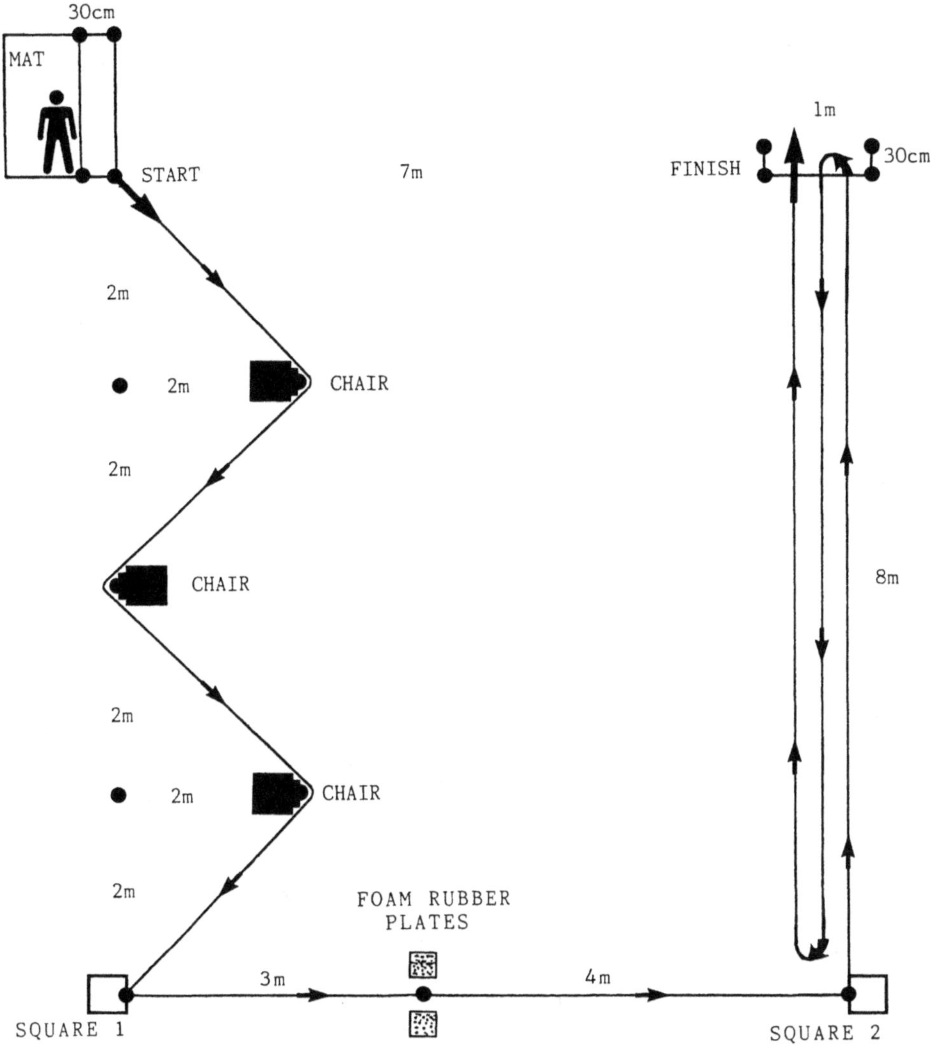

Figure 1. Layout for the AGCO test

quickly as possible and zig-zag left, right and left of three chairs and place any foot inside square one. Then the subject has to change direction, bend to pick up one foam rubber plate with each hand and must run to place them one on top of the other inside square two. The subject was then required to sprint and place any foot beyond the finish line, to return and collect both foam rubber plates from square two and, finally, to race to cross the finish line holding one foam rubber plate in each hand.

The circuit was demonstrated and explained to all subjects in each class at the same time in the interests of standardisation. There was one practice trial allowed and, thence two timed test trials. Subjects were tested in groups of four with each performing one trial in sequence to allow for recovery time between trials. Non-slip footwear and surfaces were utilized in the testing.

The score of the subject was defined as the time from the onset of the auditory signal to the crossing of the finish line at the end. Timing was to the nearest 0.1 s and the subject's score was the average of two valid trials. A penalty of 0.1 s was added for the following errors in performance:-

(i) touching any of the chairs;
(ii) not crossing the line of square one with a foot;
(iii) not placing the foam rubber plates in square two;
(iv) not placing the foam rubber plates on top of each other in square two;
(v) not fully crossing the finish line with the foot during the turn phase.

Subjects

The AGCO test was administered to physically able fifth grade boys (n = 53). All subjects were Caucasian with scores on the Culture Fair Intelligence Test (Cattell and Cattell, 1973) ranging from 69 to 132 and were approximately equally representative of blue and white collar socio-economic status (SES). Subjects were chosen at random and were tested in groups of four.

Results of Study I

Reliability

An intraclass correlation coefficient of 0.87 was obtained as an estimate of reliability (test-retest). Thirteen days separated the two testing sessions. Objectivity in testing was extremely high in that a correlation coefficient of 1.00 was obtained between the present author and a trained tester.

Validity

The AGCO test was deemed to have content validity because of the logical inclusion of acts of coordination in interaction with agility. Concurrent validity was examined by correlating AGCO scores with other criterion measures of high esteem. The validity coefficient found between AGCO and the shuttle run agility test (Latchaw, 1954) was r = 0.74 and when compared to the lateral moving coordination test (Schilling, 1974) r was -0.48. All criterion tests were administered within 13 days of the AGCO test.

Study II

Method

A larger sample (n = 112) was used to test the hypothesis that AGCO related significantly to the teacher's ratings of general ability in physical education. Again fifth grade males were used who were Caucasians, of similar intelligence range and were fairly equally divided into blue and white collar SES.

Procedure

The rating of general physical education ability by qualified general classroom teachers (n = 4) was obtained by converting to a T-score each teacher's rating of the subject's ability in physical education. T-scoring adjusts for possible percentage rating differences between the assessors involved.

Additionally, age of the subjects was calculated to the nearest month, height to the nearest 0.25 inch (0.6 cm) and weight to the nearest 0.5 pound (0.25 kg). As an estimate of body fat, readings were taken with a Harpenden skinfold caliper (to the nearest 0.1 mm) at three sites on the right side of the body - triceps, subscapular and abdominal area. The score was the sum of the mean of two readings per site.

Results of Study II

Results of the Pearson Product Moment correlation analysis appear in Table 1. As can be seen the hypothesis received significant support since AGCO scores correlated significantly with the assessments of qualified primary teachers. No significant relationship was found between AGCO scores and the anthropometric measures taken.

Table 1. Pearson Product Moment correlations (n = 112)

	PE Rating	Age
AGCO	-0.43^{a}	-0.03^{b}
($\bar{x}$ = 17.8; SD = 1.1)	($\bar{x}$ = 50.0; SD = 9.9)	($\bar{x}$ = 134.6; SD = 4.7)

	Height	Weight	Fat
AGCO	-0.11^{b}	0.04^{b}	0.21^{b}
	($\bar{x}$ = 56.1; SD = 2.6)	($\bar{x}$ = 75.4; SD = 12.8)	($\bar{x}$ = 25.0; SD = 9.6)

a: P 0.001, one-tailed

b: Not significant for two-tailed alpha set at 0.01

Discussion

In the administration of the test it was found that for subjects of this age and intelligence range a verbal explanation followed by a demonstration and a period for questions (Baumgartner, 1978), and finally, a practice trial provided sufficient understanding of the test. The motive for including penalties in the design of AGCO was to facilitate an alignment with sports, such as the football codes, where rules and penalties apply. In exploratory analyses AGCO was found to be unrelated to age, height, weight and body fat. The coefficient of 0.21 for the latter variable demonstrates to some extent a negative relationship with AGCO performance, but it failed marginally to reach significance.

With its logical content validity it was concluded from the results that the test is highly reliable (Kirkendall et al., 1980) and highly objective for fifth-grade boys. The test appears to reflect a greater degree of running agility than of coordination which is in line with its functional construct.

Further developments of AGCO could include:-

(i) testing for sport-predictive power;
(ii) the analysis of both genders in testing;
(iii) extending the age range of testees in both directions;
(iv) the examination of learning effects by administering more than two trials;
(v) the establishment of test norms.

The AGCO test was found to have a shared variance of 18.5% (- 0.43^2) with the subjective ratings of physical education ability by qualified elementary school teachers. The value of these ratings was that they were comprehensive and 'blind'.

Current reviews of the research evidence indicate that motor ability may be task specific (e.g., Singer, 1980; Baumgartner and Jackson, 1982; Safrit, 1986). While the present results may not be overwhelmingly supportive of a 'g' theory, the fact that a single one minute test can account for almost one-fifth of a general physical education score does offer a challenge to the theory of specificity in motor ability (Henry, 1958).

Since there have been clear difficulties in defining or even in separating agility and coordination in some previous tests (see Johnson and Nelson, 1986), the practical relevance of this defined interacting agility-coordination test is offered as a contribution to 'g' measurement in physical education. AGCO may possibly be found to make an important contribution in evaluating and selecting junior footballers for advanced competitive teams and for further coaching programmes. The empirical investigation of such a question would be a worthwhile project.

References

Baumgartner, T.A. (1978) Modified pull-up test. Res. Quart., 49, 80-84.

Baumgartner, T.A. and Jackson, A.S. (1982) Measurement for Evaluation in Physical Education. Boston: Houghton Mifflin.

Cattell, R.B. and Cattell, A.K.S. (1973) Manual for the Culture Fair Intelligence Test. Champaign, Il: Institute for Personality and Ability Testing,

Henry, F.M. (1958) Specificity versus generality in learning motor skills. Proceedings of the College Physical Education Association, 61, 127.

Johnson, B.L. and Nelson, J.K. (1986) Practical Measurements for Evaluation in Physical Education, 4th ed. Edina, Mn.: Burgess.

Kirkendall, D.R., Gruber, J.J. and Johnson, R.E. (1980) Measurement and Evaluation in Physical Education. Dubuque, Io.: W.C. Brown.

Krus, P.H., Bruininks, R.H. and Robertson, G. (1981) Structure of motor abilities in children. Percept. Motor Skills, 52, 119-129.

Latchaw, M. (1954) Measuring selected motor skills in fourth, fifth and sixth grades. Res. Quart., 25, 439-449.

Phillips, D.A. and Hornak, J.E. (1979) Measurement and Evaluation in Physical Education. New York: John Wiley.

Safrit, M.J. (1986) Introduction to Measurement in Physical Education and Exercise Science. St. Louis: Mosby Times Mirror.

Schilling, F. (1974) Manual for the Body Coordination Test for Children. Weinheim: Beltz Test GmbH.
Singer, R.A. (1980) Motor Learning and Human Performance. London: Collier Macmillan.

THE EFFECT OF POWER TRAINING ON THROW-IN VELOCITY AND RELEASE IN SOCCER

V. Stijnen, A. Noe and E. Willems
Institute of Physical Education, Catholic University of Leuven, Tervuursevest 101, 3030 Heverlee, Leuven, Belgium.

Introduction

The importance of a powerful and technically correct kicking action in free kicks and penalties is obvious. The relationship between these factors and the ability to create or score goals is clear. Unfortunately there has been no similar tradition of technical analysis into throw-in techniques. Until the early 1960s, players only used the short throw-in. From that period there occurred an additional interest in the role of the long throw-in to open space down the wing or directly to the front post in order to create scoring opportunities (Batty, 1980).

A long throw-in to the penalty area can be a very efficient attacking move which is difficult to defend against. To practise the long throw-in one must have knowledge of the movement patterns involved. In other words, the question for the athlete in practice is how the distance of the throw-in can be increased? The most important factors are those of a technical, physical, biomechanical and kinematic nature. A great deal of research on the technical performance of the throw-in has been carried out in the past few years (e.g. Dowell, 1978; Chang, 1979).

It has been clearly demonstrated that a run-up increases the initial velocity of the ball. For release angles between 35° and 45°, the initial velocity of the ball seems to be the most important factor. The influence of a higher angle of release appears negligible. Physical characteristics of the individual have little influence and of these only strength has some importance.

Initially, what is required is an understanding of the kind of strength needed in terms of the muscle groups to be used and the type of power training to be engaged in. If power training develops muscle hypertrophy, it is possible that movement velocity and flexibility could suffer. Training with sub-maximal weights (80 to 90% of maximum) brings the greatest increments in strength (Hay, 1983) as well as sustaining improvements in movement velocity (Bührle and Schmidtbleicher, 1981).

Didden (1984) argued that specific power training can be an outstanding aid to performance improvements in all forms of power-based activity. The implication is that the exercises must have the same timing in application of strength structure as does the movement itself (Schröder, 1969). In the throw-in technique, the muscles of the upper limbs, the pectorals, the dorsal muscles, the abdominals and hip flexors are utilised with appropriate timing and coordination. Independent development of the muscle groups via strength training is recommended. Movement specific exercises include pull-overs, hyperextensions of the spine and throws in a sitting position with a medicine ball.

A power training programme was set up to attempt to improve throwing performance. This was examined experimentally.

Method

A variation of the Bulgarian Contrast method was chosen to develop strength for the throw-in technique. This method consists of submaximal power exercises alternated with elastic strength exercises (4 series of 6 repetitions at 80% max and 4 series of 10 repetitions at 60% max).

In terms of analysing the effects of strength development on the throw-in, specific equipment was manufactured to measure ball velocities with a high degree of accuracy ($\pm$ 1% error). The apparatus consisted of two frames at a distance of 1.5m from each other (see Figure 1). In each frame infrared beams and receivers were built into the horizontal and vertical planes at a location of 0.07 m. The smaller frame contained 14 infrared transmitters (IT) and 14 receivers (R) and the larger version contained 34 of each. Each IT has a transmission angle of 16° emitting signals to three nearby receivers on both sides.

Therefore, in the largest frame there was an initial simultaneous emission of light beams. Each emission takes 30 ms (9 x 30 = 270 ms). The same occurred in the smaller frame but only for 7 transmitters (7 horizontal and 7 vertical)

When a ball passed through the frames at least two beams were broken in the vertical and horizontal planes. A microprocessor started a timer (Forth-single chip processor) when the ball broke the beam in the first frame. The timer was stopped when the ball was thrown through the second frame. Each beam interruption (time and location) in the first and second frame was stored in a computer memory. Ball speed was calculated by measuring the time taken for the ball to pass between the frames. The results were immediately displayed on a VDU for analysis.

Procedure

Eight amateur soccer players (age range 21-27 years) were divided into two groups. Four subjects were given specific power training for the throw-in and the rest of the group acted as controls. The pre- and post-test conditions for measurement of ball velocity were standardised as much as possible (i.e. location of testing: equipment throwing technique). After a guided warm up and five practice throws, the subject was required to throw the ball as powerfully as possible through the measurement apparatus. After each of five test trials immediate feedback was provided.

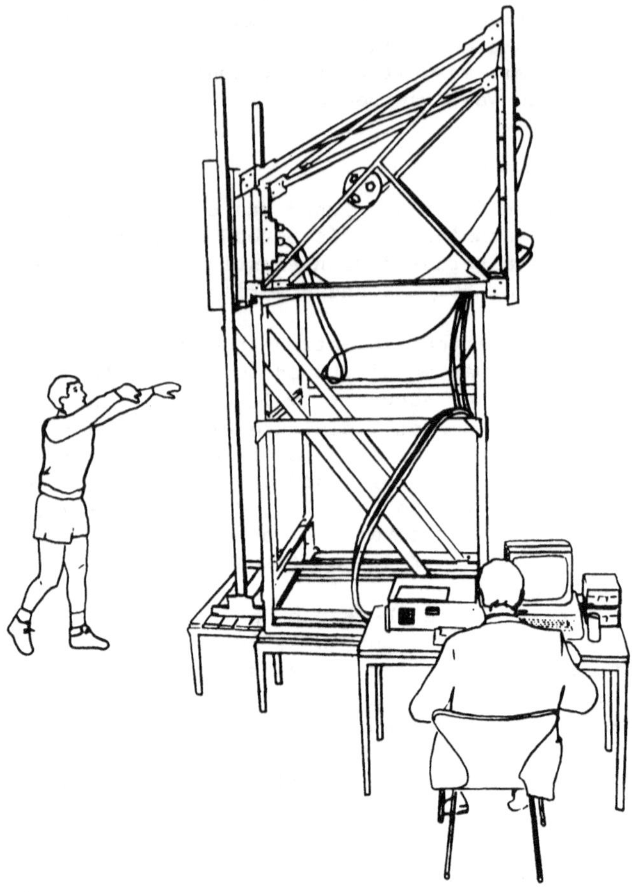

Figure 1. Apparatus for measurement of ball velocity

Results

For all trained muscle groups there was clearly an increase in strength due to specific power training. Maximum strength was measured on 4 different occasions: prior to the training programme and after 5, 10 and 15 sessions (Table 1).

Table 1. The increase in strength for the hyper-back extension, the sit-up and the pull-over (N = 4) for 4 measurement occasions

Subject	Hypa-Back extension Max.Force (N)	Increase (%)	Sit-up Max.Force (N)	Increase (%)	Pull-over Max.Force (N)	Increase (%)
1	32-36-38-42	31.3	18-22-24-24	33.3	36-38-40-43	19.5
2	32-36-40-42	31.3	20-22-24-28	40.0	38-41-45-48	26.3
3	24-32-38-38	58.6	12-16-18-20	60.0	36-38-43-44	22.2
4	30-36-42-42	40.0	16-20-24-24	50.0	34-38-41-44	30.0

The increase in ball velocity was not in proportion to the increase in strength obtained by power training (Table 2).

Table 2. Average ball velocities (m s^{-1}) in throw-ins (N = 8)

	Experimental Group (N = 4) 1	2	3	4	Control Group (N = 4) 1	2	3	4
Mean values of the pre-test (m s^{-1})	13.89	12.87	13.35	15.92	14.33	13.71	12.60	13.53
Mean values of the post-test (m s^{-1})	13.96	13.14	14.34	16.22	14.52	13.68	12.17	13.41
Increase	0.08	0.27	0.99	0.30	0.19	-0.03	-0.43	-0.12
t-value	.409	1.072	10.910	.500	.495	-.112	-2.576[a]	-.436

a, P 0.05; b, P 0.01

For the experimental group a positive trend was seen. The increase in velocity was only significant for one subject who also showed the greatest increment in strength (58.6% for hyper-extension of the spine and 60% for sit-ups). The controls actually decreased in strength. On analysing the results of the groups it seems that for the power training group there was a significant improvement in velocity (P 0.05). The results of the controls showed no significant changes.

Discussion

The apparatus in use appears to be a highly accurate measurement device since maximum error in determining ball position, due to slow interruption of the light beams or to distance between the infrared transmitters was calculated as approximately 1% in total for velocities under 16.6 m s^{-1}. The potential for use in research on other forms of physical activity e.g. shooting in soccer and quarter-back passing in American Football, is a topic for future research. This preliminary investigation provides limited evidence that specific power training for the throw-in positively affects the initial velocity of the ball. Obviously, before conclusions are firmly drawn it is necessary to use a larger sample and a more refined and wide-ranging training programme.

Another variable which requires careful analysis is the role of coordination in generating throw-in velocity since it has been clearly demonstrated that strength is an important but not over-riding factor in the development of a long throw-in soccer. In this sense, there is a clear need for an examination of different training methods and programmes in conjunction with the apparatus designed in this study.

References

Batty, E. (1980) Coaching Modern Soccer-Attack. London: Faber and Faber, 81-88p.

Bührle, M. and Schmidtbleicher, D. (1981) Maximalkraft-Schnell-kraft-Bewegungsschnelligkeit. In: Leichtatletiktraining im Spannungsveld von Wissenschaft und Praxis (edited by D. August and N. Müller), p.271. Niederhausen: Golling.

Chang, J. (1979) Biomechanical analysis of selected soccer throw-in techniques. Asian J. Phys. Ed., 2, 254-260.

Didden, R. (1984) Force and force training (Dutch: Kracht en krachttraining). Hermes (Leuven), 17, 265-271.

Dowell, L.J. (1978) Throwing for distance, air resistance, angle of projection and ball size and weight. Motor Skills: Theory into Practice, 3, 11-14.

Hay, J.G. (1983) Load, speed and equipment in strength-training exercises. In: Biomechanics VIII-B (edited by H. Matsui and K. Kobayashi), pp. 939-950. Champaign, Illinois: Human Kinetics Publishers.

Schröder, W. (1969) Merkmale einer sportartspecifische Krafttrainings. Theories und Praxis der Körpercultuur, 18, 992-1000.

Part XII

Stress and psychological attributes

STRESS REGULATION IN SOCCER

Laszlo Nadori
Hungarian University of Physical Education, Alkotas utca 44, H-1123 Budapest, Hungary.

Introduction

Because of the pressures experienced by present-day international soccer players, stress anxiety has become widely recognised as exercising a major influence on performance. For example, players experience the stress of heavy playing schedules, the competition for team places and the attentions of the communication media. These and other stressors have physical and psychological effects on players sometimes to a career-threatening degree. Accordingly, it is important that the modern player and his handlers become aware of the practical implication of the extensive knowledge which exists concerning stress and performance.

What is Stress?

There are many definitions of this concept but an internationally accepted interpretation is provided by Hans Selye, a Canadian researcher of Hungarian origin. He argued that stress is the psycho-physiological response of the individual to any influence which disturbs his homeostasis, or inner balance. Stress can be produced by a wide variety of stimuli such as physical injury, illness, surgical intervention, climatic influence, spectators, peers and nutritional factors. The stress response involving the somatic and autonomic nervous systems, the endocrine system and psyche, has three phases:- an initial mobilisation phase during which the individual's resistance to stressors is reduced, a compensation/resistance phase when adapation to one stressor is effected and, after long-standing exposure to the stressor, the phase of exhaustion. Collectively, these phases have been referred to by Selye (1976) as the General Adaptation Syndrome (GAS).

What is Anxiety?

There are numerous conceptions of anxiety, many of which state that it involves a feeling of fear or a perception of threat and which may be specific to a particular situation or 'free-floating'. For instance, a player's anxiety might be quite obviously connected with an imminent and important match or it may be impossible to determine its cause. Anxiety, of course, can be biologically functional in the sense that it can provide a warning or initiate a defence in threatening circumstances. The symptoms, often linked with increased sympathetic activity of the autonomic nervous system, include nausea, loss of composure, reduced motor coordination and excessive aggression, all contributing to a deterioration in tactical skill and increased incidence of errors.

From these observations, it should be self-evident that there is a reciprocal influence and interdependence between stress and anxiety.

Stress Effects in Sport

The sports participant is exposed to many potential stressors, some having their origin in the environment and others being internally produced. A number of examples can be itemised for illustrative purposes:-

i) Climatic variables such as air-temperature, humidity, wind direction are potential stressors which are experienced by every footballer on a frequent basis.

ii) Circadian rhythms are known to affect performance. For example, it has been found that the first 3-4 hours after awakening are not conducive to maximal effort or strenuous loading (Reilly, 1987).

iii) Related to the previous point is the problem of time-lag or jet-lag. When travelling through more than three time zones, a period of acclimatisation is essential. An interesting practical finding has been that a longer period of adaptation is required when travel is in an easterly direction.

iv) Potential stressors associated with the playing environment include the nature and dimensions of the playing surface, the visual impression of the stadium and the effects of spectators. The effects on the individual could be frightening, overwhelming, neutral or positive in character.

v) The game officials can cause stressful reactions, not only by their conduct of the game but by their reputation. In the European Cup semi-final between Bayern Munich and Real Madrid, this year, the referee's award of a dubious penalty to the German team triggered a furious reaction from the Spanish team with two of its players being sent off. Ironically, the Real Madrid manager admitted to a long-standing respect for the referee's ability.

vi) The potential stress created by opponents depends to some extent on the quality of players' attitudes if the opponents are known to them and on the quality of knowledge in cases where opponents are not known.

vii) Stress can also result from interpersonal communication, for example, between a player and his team-mate(s), between a player and his opponent(s) and between the players and the coaches.

All these objective and subjective influences are more or less stressful depending on the perception or inner experience of the player. The intensity and quality of the psycho-physiological changes induced is a function of the stress-tolerance of the player.

Reactions to Stress

The reaction to stress can take two quite different forms - aggression and anger versus inhibition, regression and fear. The two-kinds of responses were experimentally identified by Funkenstein (1955) and termed 'anger-in' and 'anger-out'. The anger-out response was found to be most functional, with the damaging anger-in response being regarded as 'the price we pay for civilisation.' The anger-in response is clearly a poor strategy in that the problem remains unresolved and assures a continuous tension within the individual which in turn interferes with performance. Although the anger-out response is psycho-physiologically more healthy, it is important in sport that the anger or aggression is controlled and instrumental (Alderman, 1974).

Inhibition or repression in the face of stress can be identified not only physiologically but also, for example, perceptually. Below are outlined two examples of how stress can negatively affect perception, together with suggestions as to how such problems could be resolved.

The first example is the anxiety-prone 'martyr' type, seeking sympathy and support as a reward for his suffering. This kind of player could be prone to perceptual 'blindness' under stress. For example, he may not see a ball moving towards him or he may not see the possibility to pass to a free player, even when it is obvious to everyone else. A filmed record of the events can help the player to appreciate the reality at a later time.

This phenomenon has been well explained by Easterbrook's (1959) cue utilisation theory and subsequently by Nideffer's (1976) work on attentional narrowing under stress. Under stress, the individual's attentional focus becomes narrower to the extent that, particularly in open-skill situations, important cues are not being processed. It is exemplified by tunnel vision but it also applies to the other senses, including kinaesthesis.

This so-called 'underinclusion' of information is believed to be a major cause of injury in soccer in that the player does not recognise the danger in particular situations. Consequently, the player is prone to repeated injury and most often the psychological antecedants are not appreciated or are ignored (e.g. Bramwell et al., 1975).

Research into injury-prone players at the Hungarian University for P.E. suggests that such players tend to be aggressive and hard-tackling but that the behaviour is determined by high levels of anxiety. There is a compulsive drive to perform which produces a vicious circle: anxiety → compulsive performance → injury → higher anxiety, greater fear of injury. The phenomenon has been described as counter-phobic (Moore, 1967) and Karen Horney described it as the process of 'ruthlessly marching over an anxiety.'

For this condition it is typical that the enforced rest occasioned by the injury is beneficial psychologically with the depleted psychic energy stores being restored. The problems associated with the actual tissue damage are often of secondary importance (Sanderson, 1981).

Repression via avoidance of responsibility for outcomes is the second example of stress negatively affecting perception. This kind of player has an accusatory personality, constantly finding fault with others. His social contacts are full of tension and his perception of situations and his decision-making are a function of the usefulness of those with whom he interacts. He is likely to make mistakes in critical situations, or if possible, he will 'hide', thus avoiding the responsibility for any negative outcome. He is what Weiner (1974) has described as an external attributor in that, in order to protect his self-esteem he attributes the causes for negative outcomes to external factors beyond his control. Thus the team's failure will be blamed on others and he might consider successful opponents as 'lucky'.

This type of player needs to be handled sympathetically and firmly. Unlike the first case described earlier in which the problems are intra-personal, the conflict weighs heavily on the interpersonal relations. Team discussions could be organised in such a way as to sensitively make him aware of his responsibility as a team member, thereby opening the way for empathy to be formed with team-mates. He can learn to listen to the viewpoints of others, giving them due consideration.

Factors Determining Behaviour in Soccer

At a general level, two factors determining behaviour can be identified. The first encompasses the learned conventions, motivations, roles and stress tolerance acquired during the development of the personality, i.e. the player involved is influenced by stressors, his previous experience and the will to win. The coach needs to understand these factors mainly to help him in team selection and secondarily, to help him deal with problems at the individual player level. Secondly, behaviour is determined by the team as a reference group. The team's components are relatively constant, it has a Captain and a Coach, the members have a common purpose, as well as individual functions and roles and the activity is performance-centred and goal-directed.

Insights into the team's function can be provided by sociometry. It can reveal emotional linkages: who likes whom, who would select whom as a training partner, who is able to substitute for the coach and so on. A mature group is indicated when there is a consensus selection for important functions which is independent of emotional criteria. For example, 'the captain should be my best friend' is an immature judgement at the 'nursery school' level. Sociometric techniques can also be used to identify the technically most advanced player, who are the fittest, the calmest and so on, thereby providing more objective criteria on which to base team selection. Research has demonstrated that team selection based on subjective emotional criteria is highly variable across squad members, but that selection based on objective performance-related criteria is highly consistent, i.e. almost every player would select the same other players (Carron, 1980).

Sociometry can provide valuable insights into the group structure, identifying the central and peripheral players, rivalries, cliques and the information channels. It emphasises the fact that there are two main group functions: the commonly accepted aspiration to winning and the establishment/development of the 'hidden network' - the interrelaionships amongst the group members, the team cohesion.

Poor performances, particularly when they are continuous, significantly affect team cohesion. Tension increases amongst team members and eventually a crisis develops (Jacobson, 1965). In this case, the usual problem-solving responses are not applicable. A solution may involve, at worst, the break-up of the team and at best, reorganisation.

However, there are some questions:-

i) Are there sufficient players in the team with an ability to solve problems?

ii) Is the team prepared for conflict situations in which unique problems need resolving in a systematic manner?

Traditional coaching conduct in most European countries attempts to improve team cohesiveness by organising, for instance, training camps, banquets and excursions. But such events rarely offer enough possibilities for relevant social learning and the fostering of team cohesion. The overriding concern is with winning the next game rather than developing cohesion per se.

The leadership style of the coach is critical in determining the extent of team cohesion. The authoritarian approach with its arbitrary commands, one-way communication, and extensive use of punishment makes for a seemingly well organised, well functioning team. However, such a regime frequently leads to exhibitionist and anti-social behaviour which, in turn, may lead to the break-up of the team.

Team cohesion can be affected by the professional or amateur status of the players. For the professional player, his contract defines his obligation and also offers him some protection. Obligations are less well defined at amateur level, causing less clear role definition with consequently reduced possibilities for tension reduction.

The development of the focal conflict in a team was described by Whitaker and Lieberman (1964). This conflict is unavoidable when winning is stressed too much in the group function. Actually, the hidden function becomes stronger, like the wish to speak out, ventilate the uneasy sentiments or hear other opinions. All these are not permitted by the authoritarian leader and even the problems cannot be identified because of the fear of punishment. Thus a conflict is established: the wish and the fear are dominating the psychic energies. Among the different solutions, the most successful will be the one promoted by most members of the group:- either the coach becomes more tolerant and democratic under the pressure or the players present a united front against him thereby creating a coach crisis.

The conflict and the crisis are avoidable when the coach has some familiarity with the dynamics of group function. Of course, he is not expected to be a psychotherapist but he should be a democratic leader with corresponding empathic ability. Most importantly, he should acknowledge the importance of communication and be able to interpret verbal and non-verbal communication signals.

Reduction of Anxiety: Some of the Psychotherapeutic Methods

The training sessions and games as well as the familiar existential influences are functioning as stressors, producing tensions, with one of their consequences being anxiety. The anxiety may have different intensities - it is not necessarily pathological - and can be identified in different forms. In soccer the most characteristic consequence of the anxiety is 'injury proneness'. As already mentioned, there are players who are repeatedly injured. However, we can often see the 'group anxiety' syndrome whereby a team begins a game with a defeatist mentality.

There are several psychological methods, which, when used consistently, are fairly efficient in promoting improved performance:-

i) autogenic training;
ii) transmitting information or lectures or organising theme-centred groups;
iii) T-groups, training groups, directed to the interpretation of behaviour;
iv) structured exercises, to solve topical problems (Lieberman, Yalom and Miles, 1967).

The aim of the sessions is to promote personality maturation through self-confrontation, problem solving, development of social perception and empathic ability.

Analysis

The analysis of the causal mechanisms may offer a key to the exploration of the stress present in soccer. Thus, for example, the conflicts and contradictions within the social environment may lead to stress. The stress is always a secondary effect, with its eliciting causes being worthy of our consideration. What are these environmental causes and factors?

A significant number of fans suffer frustration at their working place. Many belong to the lower working class, as confirmed by Eric Dunning at this Conference. Among the fans there are many unemployed young men. The soccer, the enjoyment of the game, the mingling with and the identification with the crowd may lead to uncontrollable emotional reactions. In this case the mayhem occurs on the terraces and perhaps on the field too.

Many authors discuss the emotional 'acting-out' function of sport. Both active participation and passive spectating may have a sublimating and balancing effect on the individual. It may reduce the frustrations temporarily. On the terraces of soccer stadia at international matches different ethnic groups may meet. The subjective identification with a team reinforces the consciousness of national identity. Thus the soccer stadium may become the scene of nationalist manifestations.

The soccer teams have greater responsibility. The behaviour of players during the game may create a social climate in which the personal identity of the spectator is absorbed by an undefined group psyche which causes the release of uncontrolled emotions and behaviours. The behaviour often becomes inarticulate.

Conclusion

In the framework of the activity of pressure groups within society soccer has become a powerful political force. With the strengthening of the professional nature of soccer, the best players should not need to train in any dehumanising system which requires uninhibited brutal behaviour in order to win. Although the success orientation in soccer has become intensive, fair play will predominate over uncontrolled aggression.

The mass media have created a close link between soccer and society. Through the modern mass media soccer has become a major influence. The publicity has become capable of qualitatively influencing the product and the consumers' custom through mass sport events. This process has transformed soccer, at the professional level, to a world-wide business.

Last but not least, it would be a matter of great regret if there was an eventual moral decline of soccer, a game causing joy for millions! What a pity if the soccer stadia become the arenas of brutality. This game is enjoyed and practised by millions of boys and nowaday of girls from Lapland to Tierra del Fuego, from America to Europe and Africa to Asia. Administrators and practitioners have to do their best to save the beauty of the game. The beneficiary will be the whole of humanity with enrichment of the quality of human life.

References

Alderman, R.R. (1974) Psychological Behaviour in Sport. Philadelphia: W.B. Saunders.

Bramwell, S.T., Masuda, M., Wagner, N.N. and Holmes, T.H. (1975) Psychosocial factors in athletic injuries. J. Human Stress, 1, 6-20.

Carron, A.V. (1980) Social Psychology and Sport. Ithaca, N.Y.: Mouvement.

Easterbrook, J.A. (1959) The effect of emotion on the utilization and organisation of behaviour. Psychol. Review, 66, 183-207.

Funkenstein, D.H. (1955) The physiology of fear and anger. Sci. Amer., 192, 74-80.

Jacobson, G.F. (1965) Crisis theory and treatment strategy: some sociocultural and psychodynamic considerations. J. Nerv. Ment. Disease, 141, 209-218.

Lieberman, M.A., Yalom, I.D. and Miles, M.B. (1967) Encounter Groups: First Facts. New York: Basic Bookes.

Moore, R.A. (1967) Injury in athletics. In: Motivations in Play, Games and Sports. (edited by R. Slovenko and J.A. Knight) Springfield, Illinois: Charles C. Thomas.

Nideffer, R.M. (1976) The Inner Athlete. New York: Thomas Crowell.

Reilly, T. (1987) Circadian rhythms and exercise In: Exercise: Benefits, Limits and Adaptations (edited by D. Macleod, R. Maughan, M. Nimmo, T. Reilly and C. Williams) pp. 346-366), London: E. and F.N. Spon Ltd.

Sanderson, F.H. (1981) The psychology of the injury-prone athlete. In: Sports Fitness and Sports Injuries (edited by T. Reilly) pp. 31-36. London: Faber and Faber.

Selye, H. (1976) The Stress of Life. New York: McGraw Hill.

Weiner, B. (1974) Achievement, Motivation and Attribution Theory. Morrison, N.J.: General Learning Press.

Whitaker, D.S. and Lieberman, M.A. (1964) Psychotherapy Through the Group Process. Chicago: Aldine.

PSYCHOLOGICAL ASSISTANCE FOR FOOTBALLERS

C.P. Davey
Physical Education Department, Victoria College, Rusden Campus, 662 Blackburn Road, Clayton 3168, Victoria, Australia.

Introduction

For a footballer to reach his maximum potential he needs the assistance of not only a coach, but a small team of sport scientists, including an exercise physiologist, biomechanist and a sports psychologist. Footballers, like most team game athletes, need a high level of skill and fitness if they are to be successful at the elite level of their particular code. This is not sufficient if they wish to reach the potential of which they are capable: most need psychological assistance to play at their peak particularly at the highest level of competition, e.g. as in finals.

In Australian Rules football it is possible for the coach to test the player's skills in kicking (left and right foot), handball (left and right), marking, bouncing the ball, and so on, to identify various strengths and weaknesses (Davey, 1977).

Similarly, the coach with his exercise physiologist can help the player's fitness in cardio-respiratory endurance, muscular strength, muscular power, speed, agility and flexibility, and again identify strengths and weaknesses. The competent exercise physiologist can improve each of these fitness components (Parkin et al., 1984).

In a similar way sports psychologists can now highlight weaknesses in the psychological make-up of an athlete and can provide counselling so that the footballer may produce his optimal level of performance. Indeed, it may be argued that at elite levels the mental attitude of the athlete may be the major focus of inter-player differences since conditioning and skills practices remain relatively standardised. To establish a profile of the psychological make-up of top footballers there has been a need to utilise a wide range of tests for this purpose. A brief summary of some of the psychological inventories that have been used in Australian Rules football is outlined in this paper.

Personality

Although many personality inventories have been used in the sporting situation, the most common are those by Eysenck, Spielberger, Martens' SCAT and the POMS (McNair et al., 1971).

Eysenck's Personality Questionnaire (Eysenck and Eysenck, 1975) measures personality in terms of two independent dimensions - extroversion-introversion and neuroticism-stability (neuroticism suggests a high level of anxiousness). Hence it is possible to classify·footballers into one of four categories - stable or anxious extroverts, stable or anxious introverts. Figure 1 shows the distribution of Australian Rules footballers into these four categories.

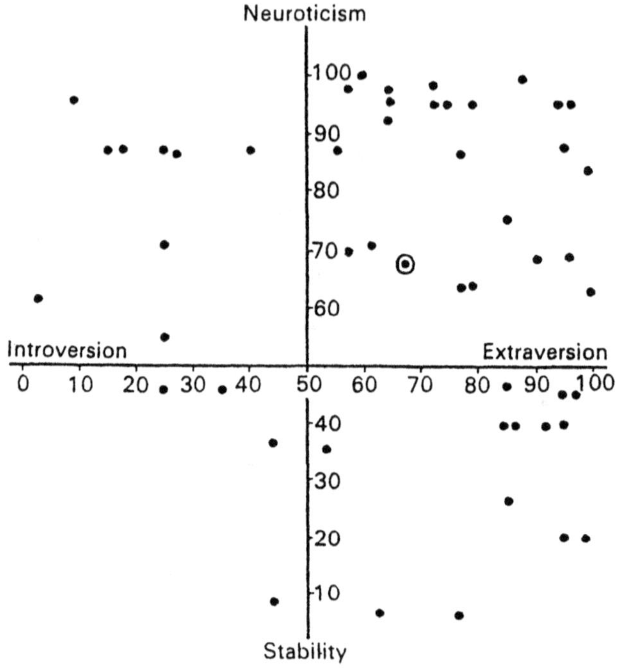

Figure 1. Eysenck Personality inventory profile of Australian football team

As can be seen footballers are drawn from each of the four categories with the average for this team being at the 70th percentile for anxiety and the 65th percentile for extroversion. Since the average of all footballers measured over 10 years is at the 60th percentile for extroversion and anxiety, it is no wonder that this team has a history of failure in finals with over-anxious players. The winners have been shown to have scores for anxiety between the 50th and 55th percentile. Such information can assist the coach with a knowledge of the individual differences among his players and how best they should be handled, particularly with respect to arousal levels.

The sport competition anxiety test (SCAT) (Martens, 1977) is a psychological tool that is sport specific. It measures a sport specific trait anxiety and is believed to be a superior predictor of state anxiety than most general trait anxiety inventories. This competitive anxiety trait is defined as a tendency to perceive competitive situations as threatening and to respond to these situations with feelings of apprehension or tension.

Of the many questionnaires that can be used, the SCAT would be the shortest and simplest to administer. It has the advantage of taking only 5 min to complete and less to score.

Research conducted recently with football teams revealed that some players were well above the 80th percentile for anxiety and, therefore, in need of some assistance to help calm them down. This was in contrast to a group of Australian Rules football umpires who scored well below the 50th percentile on the SCAT (Davey, 1985).

Although psychological tests should not be used to predict success, one that has been most highly predictive of athletic success in America is the POMS (McNair et al., 1971), and recent research shows similar trends in Australian Rules football (Davey, 1985). The results of a POMS test take the form of a 'mood profile', comparing the individual's combined scores on six general categories - tension, depression, anger, vigour, fatigue and confusion.

Figure 2 shows the POMS profile, the solid line representing the successful footballers and the dotted line representing the unsuccessful footballers. This 'iceberg' profile of successful footballers shows that they scored below the surface on tension, depression, anger, fatigue and confusion, but significantly above on vigour.

This shows that successful footballers possess superior mental and emotional health as well as identifying individuals who may be in need of counselling or psychological support (high on tension, depression).

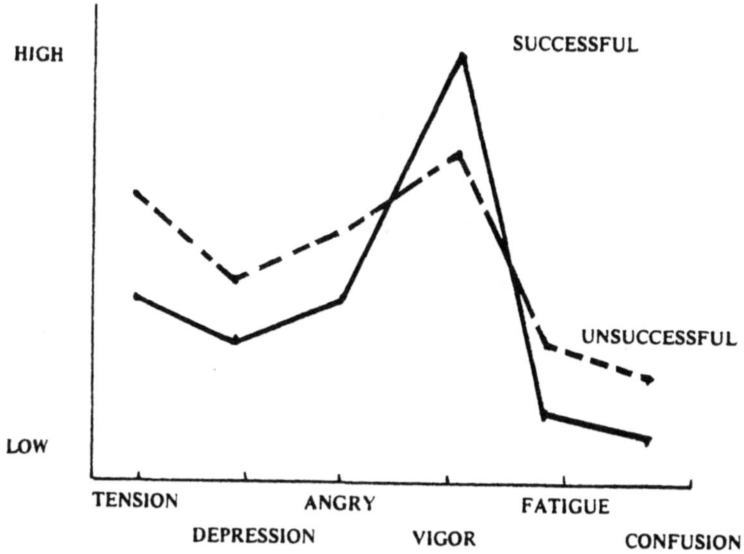

Figure 2. Psychological profiles of successful and unsuccessful footballers

Motivation

Similar to personality it is now possible to measure motivation as defined by a number of factors and obtain a score on each of these factors for each individual. Two such tests, the Athletic Motivation Inventory and the Incentive Motivation Inventory, will be discussed.

The Athletic Motivation Inventory (Tutko and Richards, 1972) measures five desire factors (drive, aggression, determination, conscientiousness and leadership) and six emotional factors (self-confidence, coachability, emotional maturity, trust, responsibility and mental toughness). The desire factors give an indication of an individual's willingness to work hard towards accomplishing desired goals while emotional factors reflect an athlete's personal attitudes and feelings about himself and his coach. A brief description of each of these factors is given in Table 1.

Table 1. Description of factors in the Athletic Motivation Inventory

* Drive - desire to be a successful competitor
* Self-confidence - sure of oneself
* Aggressiveness - finds it easy to be aggressive
* Coachability - accepts leadership
* Determination - willing to work hard
* Emotionally mature - mature and stable
* Conscientiousness - likes to do the correct thing
* Trust - accepts people
* Responsibility - accepts responsibility
* Leadership - likes making decisions
* Mental toughness - accepts strong criticism.

Figure 3 shows the profile of six Australian Rules football teams measured during a recent season. The higher-scoring profile represents the average of the three teams that finished first, second and third, while the lower profile represents the average of three teams which did not make the finals that year.

The Incentive Motivation Inventory (Wood, 1981) is a recent addition to motivation theory. He identified seven major incentive systems for sport - excellence, power, stress, independence, success, aggression and affiliation. An explanation of each incentive is presented in Table 2.

Fig. 4 shows the motivational profile of a football team. While the incentive motivation to achieve excellence and success is extremely high, stress, aggression and affiliation are above average, and power and independence low.

Arousal

One of the most frequently-used psychological constructs is arousal. Simply stated, arousal refers to the level of awakeness, alertness, attention or even emotional excitement of an individual, and it varies on a continuum from low to high. When we are at low

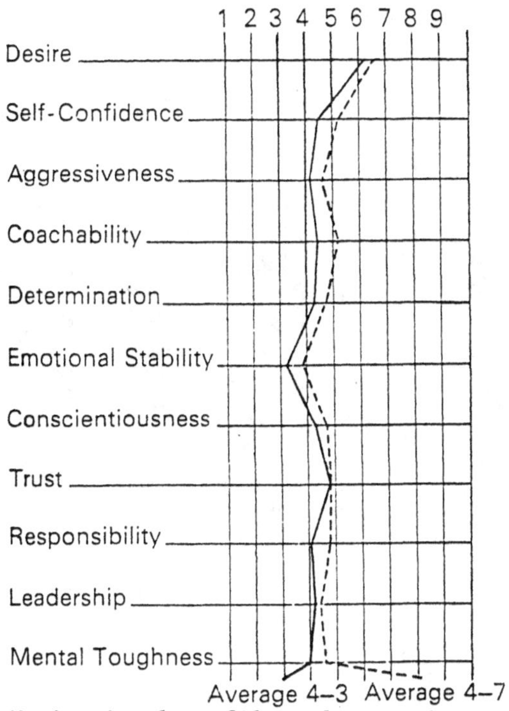

Figure 3. Motivational profiles of Australian Rules footballers

Table 2. Description of items in the Incentive Motivation Inventory

Excellence:	Incentives revolving around opportunities to do something well, for its own sake as better than others.
Power:	Incentives revolving around opportunities to influence and control others.
Stress:	Incentives revolving around opportunities for excitement, tension and pressures that sport can provide.
Independence:	Incentives revolving around opportunities to do things on one's own without help from others.
Success:	Incentives revolving around the opportunity to obtain extrinsic rewards that staff can provide: status, prestige, recognition and social approval.
Aggression:	Incentives revolving around opportunities to subdue, intimidate, dominate or even injure other people.
Affiliation:	Incentives revolving around opportunities for social intercourse, being socially reassured by making or maintaining friendships.

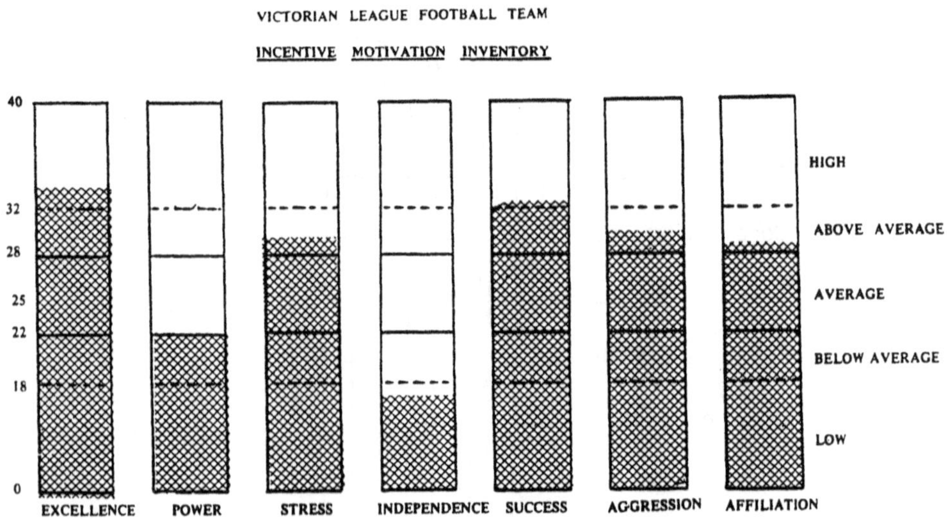

Figure 4. Motivational profile of football team

levels of arousal (rather drowsy) our performance, both cognitive and physical, is very poor, but as we increase our level of arousal our performance greatly improves. At the other extreme if we are very highly aroused, tense or overly excited, our performance is also very poor. Between these two extremes we reach an optimal level of arousal and at this point we appear to give our best performance. This is called the inverted-U function.

Obviously, one of the coach's tasks is to have all footballers at their optimal level of arousal so that they may give their best performance. The level of arousal can be affected by various means - drugs, shock, noisy music, or emotional outbursts by the coach - but a convenient method, and perhaps a more healthy way, is by a sub-maximal amount of physical exertion. A solid burst of 5-8 min of vigorous physical activity is enough for most footballers to reach their optimal level of arousal (Davey, 1980).

However, coaches should be warned that there are personality based variations between resting and optimal levels of arousal and arousability. For example, introverts are usually more highly aroused than extroverts, and reach their optimal levels of arousal earlier with a similar amount of stimulation. Similarly, more anxious personalities are more quickly aroused than stable personalities. Coaches should be prepared to experiment with individuals in order to find optimal levels of arousal, but they must also be aware of increasing a particular footballer's level of arousal too highly (whether by exertion or a fiery emotional speech) as too high a level of arousal is just as unsatisfactory as a low level.

Attentional Styles

The most recent test to appear in the sports psychology literature is Nideffer's (1976) 'Test of Attentional and Inter-personal Style'. Although the test has 17 scales, for the purpose of this article only the 6 attentional scales are considered. The aim of the test is to measure whether a footballer can develop the type of attention necessary under non-stressful conditions, and then see how he reacts physically and attentionally under conditions of competitive stress.

From the test it is possible to state whether the footballer can broaden or narrow his attention, whether he can direct it internally or externally, and whether he is capable of shifting from one focus to another whenever he needs. The six attentional scales are described in Table 3.

Table 3. The six attentional scales of Nidiffer (1978)

BET:	Broad external attentional focus - high scores means one is able to integrate effectively many internal stimuli at one time.
OET:	Overloaded by external stimuli - the higher the score, the more one makes mistakes because one becomes confused and overloaded by external stimuli.
BIT:	Broad internal attentional focus - high scores indicate an ability to integrate ideas and information from several different areas.
OIT:	Overloaded by internal stimuli - the higher the score, the more mistakes are made of confusion due to about too many things at once.
NAR:	Narrow attentional focus - the higher the score, the more one is able to narrow attention when needed.
RED:	Reduced attentional focus - a high score indicates that mistakes are made because of over-narrowed attention.

Figure 5 shows a most effective attentional profile of a footballer who won the best and fairest award in Australian Rules football. It is also interesting to note that there are high scores on self-esteem, extroversion, and there is a high positive affect. Figure 6 shows a footballer who is overloaded externally and internally and as a result is taking in too much information and missing the relevant cues needed to perform his skills at his optimal level.

Psychological Preparation

Having discovered the personality, motivational and attentional profiles of a group of footballers, the coach may wish to choose one of the intervention procedures in order to optimise performance. The following psychological methods are being used in Australia, although only some will be briefly described.

Visual Motor Behavioural Rehearsal (Suinn, 1980) is a method used successfully by American athletes and Australian footballers and is a combination of what coaches may know as mental practice and behaviour

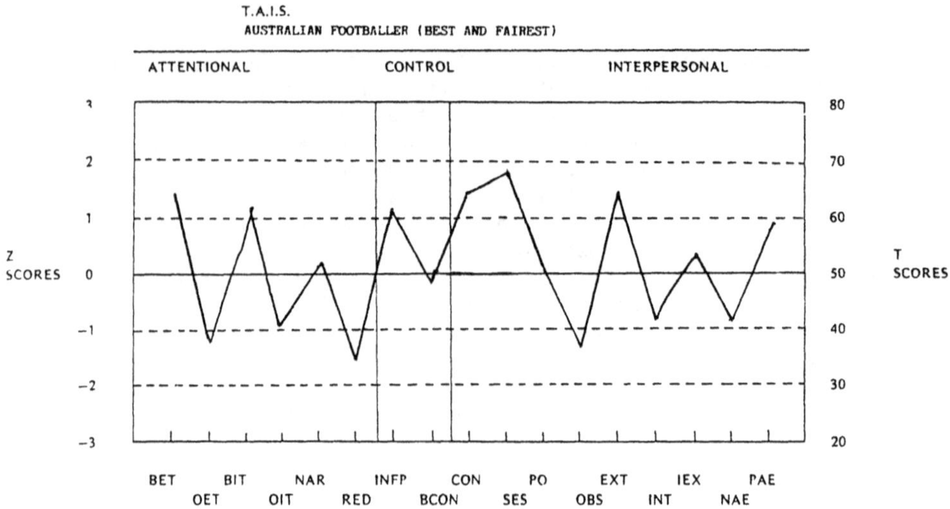

Figure 5. Effective attentional profile

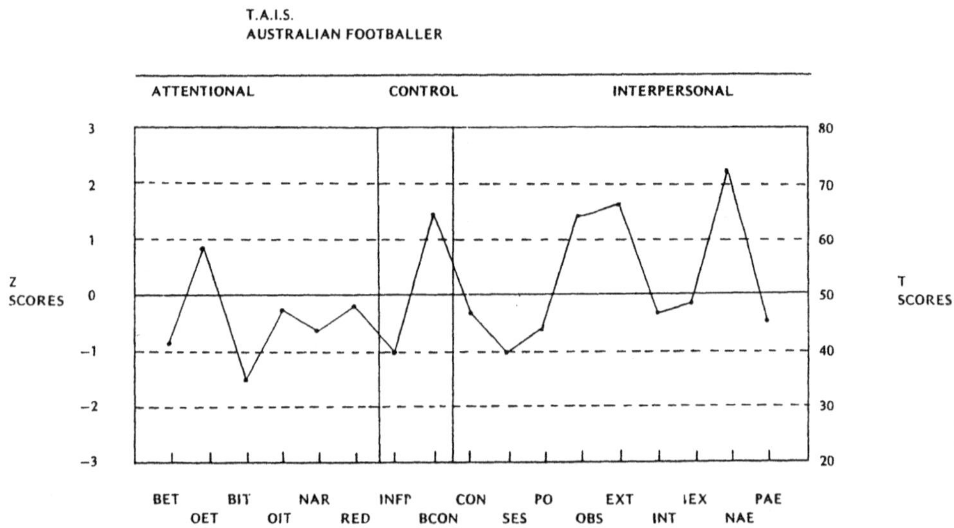

Figure 6. Ineffective attentional profile

modification techniques. The method has three steps - relaxation, the practice of imagery and the use of imagery for strengthening motor skills.

The method of relaxation is identical with that suggested for progressive relaxation (Jacobsen, 1938). After relaxation the footballers practice mental imagery of themselves performing particular skills used during the game. This imagery of behaviour rehearsal is more than sheer imagination. It is a well-controlled copy of a previous experience, a practising in the brain of specific muscle movements.

The final step is to use this imagery in the actual playing of the game or preparing for the event and, if possible, visualising opponents (or team-mates) so that when the time comes for the actual event the situation has been rehearsed many times.

Sports Psyching (Tutko, 1976) is a method that uses some of the material already described. It consists of a three-step routine called preparation, practice and play and takes many weeks to learn.

The preparation stage consists of relaxation, which puts the footballer in the state of mind and body most conducive to achieving his best. Having learnt to relax at will, with his mind clear, he needs to learn how to focus and concentrate on the particular skill required so that he can cut out distractions. This state of relaxed concentration can be achieved by breathing easily and repeating a word or phrase that has meaning for the athlete in his sport (e.g. ball). Having learnt the art of relaxing and concentrating in a non-stressful situation, the athlete is able to apply the same procedures in competition.

In the practice state the footballer goes over skill techniques by mental rehearsal so that the most desirable patterns become automatic. For example, in kicking for goal the player rehearses the grip of the ball, swinging the foot through, and generally goes through the physical actions of the skill to get the feeling of them.

With the third play stage the footballer practises the sports psyching techniques by going through the preparation and practice stages very quickly so that he can relax and let go and commit himself fully to the action of his sport. This gradually builds up positive experiences which reinforce confidence so that he can use the technique in competition. Once learnt, this sports psyching technique becomes the footballer's private ritual, to be used at the start of each game or portion of the game. This helps to counteract pressure, focuses his attention and prepares him for successful play.

Sybervision (De Vore and De Vore, 1981) is a most recent innovation as a method of psychological preparation. It is a form of muscle memory programming whereby a previously perfectly-performed skill is imprinted (tattooed) on the brain.

The coach or photographer takes a film or videotape of the footballer performing all the skills required for his particular game (this, of course, may require many hundreds of metres of film). Then the film is computer-analysed and is edited for perfection, and may be duplicated many times.

Sybervision then consists of the performer watching himself perform perfected skills for many hours. It is believed that this watching of perfection imprints the technique on the brain so that these skills may be reproduced in the pressure of competition. The sport that has been used to pioneer this method most successfully is tennis, but it has been also used in Australian Rules football.

Attention control training (Nideffer and Sharpe, 1978) occurs after having identified the strengths and weaknesses in an athlete's profile. Attention control training (ACT) is especially useful for footballers who are overloaded either externally or internally. Tension, anxiety and pressure may inhibit the footballer causing confusion and hence cognitive overload.

This method involves 'centreing' where the attention is directed to the stomach area about the level of the navel. The athlete adopts a balanced body position where they feel steady. As they physically relax (chest, neck and shoulders) and concentrate on their breathing, the footballers should be able to redirect their attention to the relevant football cues. It is then suggested that the footballers mentally rehearse, narrowing their attention to the right cues and seeing themselves being successful. In advanced stages of ACT the footballer might place himself in a losing situation, feel the anxiety, and begin centreing, relaxing, breathing, mentally rehearsing.

Inner mental training (Unestahl, 1983) is a method similar to that of Nideffer and of Tutko. It is a programme which requires approximately 20 min daily for 5 days a week, lasting 12 weeks. The most important aims of the first six weeks are to lower basic tension, to increase tension-regulative ability whereby situational control is replaced by increased self-control, and learning alternate or altered states of consciousness. The content of the programme is summarised in Table 4.

In the ideo-motor training in Week 8 the footballer, through imagery, can focus on kinaesthetic and proprioceptive feedback which is essential to good performance. The purpose of Weeks 9 and 10 is to break vicious circles caused by previous failures and to create the 'ideal performance feeling'. The self-confidence training concerns itself with the self-concept which in turn gives rise to specific and automatic expectations of success.

Table 4. Outline of inner mental training programme

Week 1	Muscular relaxation 1	Week 7	Goal-programming training
Week 2	Muscular relaxation 2	Week 8	Ideo-motor training
Week 3	Mental relaxation 1	Week 9	Systematic desensitisation
Week 4	Mental relaxation 2	Week 10	Problem-solving
Week 5	Dissociation training	Week 11	Self-confidence training
Week 6	Detachment training	Week 12	Concentration training

Finally the concentration training begins in Week 12. Concentration varies not only from person to person, but also in intensity and duration. Unestahl uses post-hypnotic suggestions so that concentration can be changed from external mechanisms, to an internal one, e.g. a breathing rhythm.

According to Unestahl the greatest effects of mental training cannot be expected until the footballer has not only learned the training but has automated it. It becomes a way of thinking, a way of goal-programming, a way of behaving, which comes quite naturally and automatically.

Conclusion

In the introduction it was stated that in order for a team to reach the potential of which it is capable it was necessary to examine three important areas, namely skill, fitness and the psychological aspects. In most sports we can objectively measure skill and obtain a skill score. In all sports we can measure the various components of fitness and obtain a fitness score. We have now reached the stage where we can measure personality, motivation, attention, moods and so on, and hopefully should be able to obtain a psychological score, with positive loadings on those characteristics that are felt desirable for success, and negative loadings on those felt undesirable. It should then be possible to predict ability to play football by adding together, with appropriate weightings, a footballer's score in skill, fitness and psychological aspects for example. These would be employed to formulate a multiple regression equation which could permit a limited element of prediction.

Although such a view must be regarded as speculative at our present level of knowledge, sport psychology is moving closer to estimating ability to play football. This would prove to be a valuable service to the coach in helping our teams reach the potential of which they are capable.

Also, it was earlier stated that the sports psychologist is only one of a small team of sports scientists whose assistance is required by both the coach and footballer if they wish to reach peak performance. However, although various psychological methods have been used with varying degrees of success, it is clear that no one method is the panacea for all footballers, coaches or teams. One of the greatest difficulties for the sports psychologist is to know which method will best assist each player or team to reach their potential in skill and fitness in crucial final games. Obviously a great deal of research is still required to answer these questions.

References

Davey, C.P. (1977) Skill Tests in Australian Football. In: Coaches Manual, National Football League of Australia.

Davey, C.P. (1980) Exercise and mental performance. Patient Management, New Zealand.

Davey, C.P. (1985) What makes a good footballer - psychologically? Australian and New Zealand Association for the Advancement of Science, Melbourne, August.

De Vore, S., and De Vore, G. (1981) Sybervision. Chicago, Illinois: Chicago Review Press.

Eysenck, H.J. and Eysenck, S.B. (1975) Eysenck Personality Questionnaire. London: Hodder and Stoughton.

Jacobson, E. (1938) Progressive Relaxation. Chicago: University of Chicago Press.

McNair, D.M., Lorr, M. and Droppleman, L.F. (1971) Edits Manual for Profile of Mood States. San Diego, California.

Martens, R. (1977) Sport Competition Anxiety Test. Champaign, Illinois: Human Kinetics.

Nideffer, R. (1976) Test of attention and inter-personal style. J. Person., Soc. Psychol., 34, 394-404.

Nideffer, R. and Sharpe, R.C. (1978) Attention Control Training. New York: Wideview.

Parkin, D., Smith, R. and Schokman, P. (1984) Premiership Football. Melbourne: Hargreen Publishing Company.

Suinn, R.M. (1980) Psychology in Sports. Minneapolis: Burgess.
Tutko, T.A. and Richards, J.W. (1972) Coaches Practical Guide to Athletic Motivation. Boston: Allyn and Bacon.
Unestahl, L.E. (1983) The Mental Aspects of Gymnastics. Orebro: Veje Publications.
Wood, N.L. (1981) Improving the Motivation of Your Athletes. Ottawa: Coaching Science Update.

ANXIETY IN RECREATIONAL AND COMPETITIVE 4-A-SIDE SOCCER

K. Davids and F.H. Sanderson
Department of Sport and Recreation Studies, Liverpool Polytechnic, Byrom Street, Liverpool L3 3AF, England.

Introduction

The effects of anxiety in sport have been well documented in previous research (e.g. Power, 1982; Cox, 1986). It is clear that anxiety appears to pervade the highest levels of structured competition and there are numerous anecdotal examples of athletes 'choking' in important games. As a consequence, many performers and coaches recognise the need to utilise pre-competition relaxation strategies that minimise the detrimental effects of anxiety. In the sport of soccer there is an apparent paradox in that the performer typically requires high levels of arousal to cope with the substantial element of physical contact and yet there is the danger that this may be superceded by anxiety which may eventually impair perceptual awareness, speed and flexibility of decision-making and the precision of movement coordination (Landers, 1980).

Interestingly, despite the need to balance the level of arousal with calmness, very little research has been conducted on the patterning of anxiety prior to and following competitive soccer. Indeed that which has been completed has been fraught with methodological difficulties. For example, in the study of Dowthwaite and Armstrong (1984) preliminary data were presented suggesting that anxiety levels in soccer players may be differentiated according to the perceived level of competitive intensity of forthcoming matches. The main findings indicated that soccer players are more anxious immediately prior to matches than after and that this is a function of perceived competitive intensity of the impending event. In other words, the higher the level of competition the greater the level of anxiety. However, this study of full-sided soccer only utilised 11 subjects and did not categorise level of competition in a formal and structured manner. The three matches studied were categorised subjectively as 'easy' or 'crucial' based on past results with the same opposition. Similarly, Scanlan and Passer (1978), also utilising the CSAI, found that winning soccer players, in full-sided competition, were lower in post-game A-State than losing players. The implications for coaches and teachers of soccer are obvious but there is little known about the manner in which competitive intensity affects the player in small-sided soccer. Assumptions that it may be similar have not been directly verified and neglect the point that there is far more frequent ball contact in the small-sided version of the game, which does not allow the peformer opportunity to 'hide' during the match to regain steadiness.

Small-sided Soccer and Anxiety

Recently small-sided soccer (e.g. 4 vs 4; 5 vs 5) has been recognised as a popular and exciting activity played at recreational, competitive, amateur and professional level. There has been a significant increase in professional competition in many countries (e.g. U.K. and U.S.A.), where the growth of indoor soccer leagues and national knock-out competitions has been well received; this has been mirrored by the rise of participation rates at recreational and competitive levels. This is due to several factors. Initially, small-sided sport has developed an entrenched position in the educational philosophy of many western countries due to an increased frequency of contact with the ball. As a consequence soccer skills develop more rapidly. Similarly, the current ethos of health education, with the emphasis on exercise as a means of improving the quality of life, has signalled an important role for recreational soccer because it is inexpensive, easy to learn and predominantly aerobic in make-up (Reilly and Thomas, 1976). The nature of the game demands speed of thought and movement, precision in the skill performance and agility. It is possible that high levels of anxiety would have detrimental effects on performance

It is argued here that there has been a general tendency among coaches and physical educationists to view small-sided soccer as either a purely recreational activity played for fun and leisure or as a training device for full-sided soccer. This would appear to be at odds with the recent growth in competitive levels of play.

The aim of this study was to analyse anxiety levels in 4-a-side soccer under three levels of competitive intensity. The main questions concerned the patterning of pre-game and post-game anxiety states in relation to the level of competition and the presumed effects of specific match results. Trait measures of anxiety were also examined in the analysis.

Method

In order to assess these questions seven teams were studied during a collegiate 4-a-side soccer programme over two consecutive seasons. The adapted version of Spielberger's Competitive State Anxiety Inventory (Martens et al., 1979) was administered in short form to subjects (n=27; mean age = 25 years) to measure state anxiety levels pre- and post-event. A repeated measures design was utilised to study anxiety reactions of each subject in each of the three different treatments. This yielded 81 measures of A-State across three different conditions.

Results

Table 1 shows the summarised data from all three conditions of structured competition, displaying means and standard deviations for A-State and A-Trait scores.

Table 1. Means (± SD) of A-Trait (SCAT) and A-State measures in each of three different levels of competition

Level of Competition	SCAT		A-State Pre-game		A-State Post-game	
Friendly	29.8	3.65	14.7	3.9	20.2	5.5
League	29.8	3.65	17.4	5.4	20.5	4.7
Knock-out	29.8	3.65	22.2	4.6	21.6	5.6

A one-way ANOVA was performed on the A-Trait scores of subjects in each condition to ascertain if they differed prior to treatments. The results indicated no significant differences between subjects in terms of trait anxiety ($F_{2,79} = 2.94$; $P > 0.05$). Next, correlation analysis was used to investigate how indicative A-Trait measures were of anxiety levels, prior to and preceding matches in the three different competitive spheres.

Table 2. Pearson Product Moment coefficients relating SCAT measures to pre- and post-game A-State levels

Level of Competition	A-State Pre-game		A-State Post-game	
Friendly	-.26	N.S.	-.03	N.S.
League	.36	N.S.	.32	N.S.
Knock-out	.01	N.S.	.08	N.S.

As can be seen in Table 2, the results show that anxiety levels may be specific to perceived levels of competitive intensity in any given match. The A-State data were initially pooled and a comparison was made of pre- and post-game levels across all three conditions. Paired t-test revealed a highly significant difference between these scores ($P < 0.001$).

A two-way repeated measures ANOVA on pre- and post-game A-state levels within each competitive sphere (2 x 3) indicated highly significant differences ($F_{5,76} = 17.65$; $P < 0.001$). Tukey HSD post-hoc testing indicated that pre-and post-game A-State differed highly in the friendly and league conditions alone. There was no such difference in the knock-out condition (see Table 1).

Correlation analysis of the relationship between A-Trait and match outcome (win/loss) suggested no significant links ($r = -0.12$). A-State data were pooled into pre- and post-game totals and correlated with match outcome. The results indicated a significant relationship only with the post-game measures ($r = 0.31$; $P < 0.05$). This was then categorised according to competitive conditions in order to isolate exactly where the relationship lay. The results indicated significant relationships between post-game A-State and match outcome in the friendly ($r = 0.44$; $P < 0.05$) and the knock-out ($r = 0.43$; $P < 0.05$) conditions.

At first sight this appears puzzling but, as will be seen in the discussion section, current state anxiety questionnaires have difficulty in differentiating how much CNS energisation is excitement and how much is due to anxiety. The former is a pleasant reaction to desired stimulation and the latter an unpleasant reaction to social or physical threat.

Discussion

Previous research on the relation between anxiety and soccer performance has failed to examine the nature of this personality variable in the context of small-sided structured competition. It was the aim of this study to evaluate and examine A-Trait and A-State levels in different competitive settings in the small-sided game. Three distinct levels of structured competitive intensity as well as match outcomes were examined.

The results indicated clearly that SCAT measures were not significant predictors of pre-game A-State levels. Hence, there seems to be some specificity in the context of small-sided competition which influences the perception of the athlete before competing. Partial support is provided for the notion that many soccer players who join a small-sided competitive programme do so because of the view that it is useful training for the full-sided version of the game or because it is an exciting way of keeping fit. Indeed match outcome significantly predicted post-game A-States which suggests that the impending result of a particular game may play an important part in elevating anxiousness of the individual during competition. The complexity of this issue is apparent because this is the case in both the friendly and knock-out conditions. Previous research on adult soccer players (e.g. Dowthwaite and Armstrong, 1984) failed to analyse the relationships between SCAT and CSAI measures. Although it has been shown that, generally, subjects with higher A-Trait measures show greater increases in A-State close to competition (e.g. Scanlan and Passer, 1978), there has been little previous work on the small-sided game with adult subjects. It is feasible that, in general, subjects high in trait anxiety may not have perceived the small-sided competition as threatening as the full-sided game due to reasons outlined previously. Interestingly, A-Trait scores did not correlate well with match outcome which again suggests, amongst other things, that performers who generally find sport competition anxiety-provoking may succeed in small-sided competition and actually enjoy the high levels of stimulation in such fast, continuous physical activities.

A significant feature of the data is the variation in pre-game state anxiety levels as a function of competitive intensity. From Figure 1 it is clear that pre-game anxiety levels are highest in the knock-out condition.

Pre-game anxiety levels were higher than the post-game measures in the knock-out condition, which reverses the findings in the other two conditions. Clearly, in the latter stages of a small-sided cup competition subjects consider it highly important to succeed. Hence, the lack of differences between pre- and post-game A-State in the knock-out condition may be due to the elevated states of anxiety

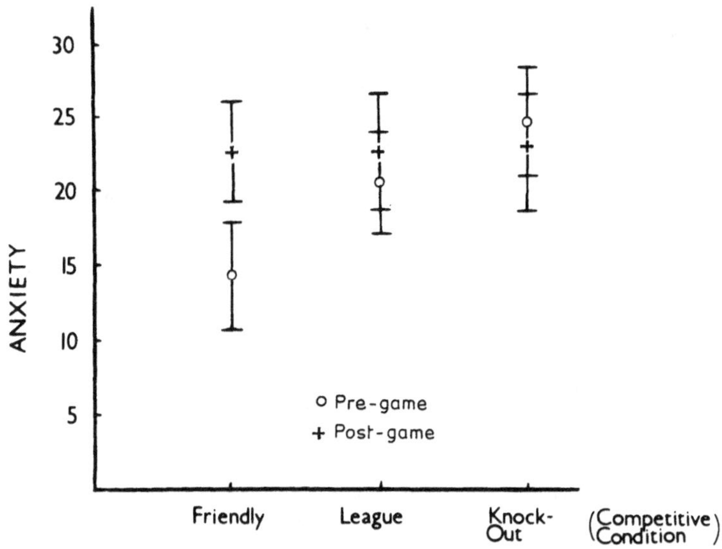

Figure 1. Mean A-State score (± standard deviations) in each competitive condition

experienced prior to competition. In the other two conditions the clear differences may be due to much lower pre-game anxiety levels since post-game A-States remained remarkably constant across all conditions.

Clearly, there is a need for more research in the area of small-sided sport, given the increasing levels of participation for leisure. A possible reason for elevated post-game A-States in some conditions is provided by reversal theory (Apter, 1982; Murgatroyd, 1981). Reversal theory has been proposed as a new approach to the study of arousal and anxiety in sport (Kerr, 1985). The suggestion is that previous attempts to measure high levels of arousal in sport performance have neglected a subject-oriented approach in that some athletes seek high levels of stimulation (i.e. actually finding low levels anxiety-provoking due to boredom) whereas others are happiest in a state of low arousal. Indeed, the current measurement tools for assessing anxiety levels in written form (e.g. SCAT and CSAI) fail to differentiate clearly when a subject is in a state of pleasant excitation or is experiencing an unpleasant amount of anxiety. The Telic Dominance Scale (TDS) has been proposed as a means of estimating the preferred level of sensation-seeking for each subject so that A-State may then be deduced (Murgatroyd et al., 1978). Although this idea is intuitively appealing, at present, there are difficulties with its application. Initially, the TDS is not sport-specific whereas SCAT and CSAI have a record of reliability and validity in sport contexts (Martens, 1977; Martens et al., 1979). Since reversal theory argues that sudden psychological reversals or immediate changes in emotional state may occur, it would be difficult to ascertain the exact nature of the emotional state of a performer without recourse to immediate match analysis and for subjective interpretation of mood. An alternative approach to the adaptation of the TDS to the sport context would be to use it in conjunction with the CSAI and perhaps the POMS (McNair et al., 1971) in order to validate levels of extreme arousal as either excitement or anxiety.

In the present study, it is possible that the significant relationship between post-game A-State and match outcome in the friendly condition may have been due to perceived inadequacy of performance or frustration due to contingent events for subjects who were anxious, and perceived levels of satisfaction and exhiliration for subjects who were excited through enjoyment of a thrilling match. There is no denying that some participants may find recreational soccer anxiety-provoking, in that the need to succeed may be strong even in this unstructured context. This distinction may be fundamental to physical educationists and exercise tutors who are becoming increasingly aware of the detrimental effects of stress in every-day life. Clearly, a psycho-physiological approach is necessary. Measurement of catecholoamine and cortisol levels, if correlated with concomitant questionnaire data, from the CSAI and the TDS, could help to validate the notion that anxiety and excitement are being confused in current research methodology. Preliminary work on this issue by McLaren et al., reported elsewhere in this volume, has provided initial support for this approach.

A much more refined picture of match outcome in which the results of games were scaled from close victories to heavy defeats, might reveal a more detailed perspective of the relation with excitement and anxiety. Indeed the utilisation of a number of psychological tests together may provide a much needed overview of the mental side of small-sided sport. Evaluation of attributions amongst successful and unsuccessful teams, along with a detailed psycho-physiological picture of the emotions involved may help the coach in preparing for competition. Finally, whether this is also the case for full-sided soccer remains to be seen since there is a clear need for such an eclectic form of pychological profiling in this area. Whatever the case the primary question to be raised by the present study concerns the validity of conducting future research into the complexity of emotions in the sport context without due consideration of many wide-ranging modes of investigation. In this way a much clearer and refined picture of the emotions and cognitions of the sport performer under different levels of structured competition may emerge.

In summary, the findings of the present investigation of small-sided soccer fail to support the results of previous research on the full-sided game (e.g. Scanlan and Passer, 1978; Dowthwaite and Armstrong, 1984) that A-Trait was a significant predictor of pre-game A-State. Also the data suggest that post-game A-States are consistently higher than pre-game measures which may be due to the extent of the stimulation experienced in small-sided sport. This differed from previous research and whether this may be due to the greater speed of the game and higher frequency of ball contact in the adapted version of the game is a question for future research.

References

Apter, M.J. (1982) The Experience of Motivation: The theory of Pyschological Reversals. London, New York: Academic Press.

Cox, R, (1986) Relationship between skill performance in women's volleyball and competitive state anxiety. Int. J. Sport Psychol., 17, 183-190.

Dowthwaite, P. and Armstrong M. (1984) An investigation into the anxiety levels of soccer players. Int. J. Sport Psychol., 15, 149-59.

Kerr, J. (1985) The experience of arousal: a new basis for studying arousal effects in sport. J. Sports Sci., 3, 169-79.

Landers, D. (1980) The arousal-performance relationship revisited. Res. Quart., 51, 77-90.

Martens, R. (1977) Sport Competition Anxiety Test. Champaign, IL: Human Kinetics.

Martens, R. Burton, D. Rivkin, F. and Simon, J. (1979) Reliability and Validity of the Competition. Unpublished Manuscript, Univ. of Illinois.

McLaren, D. Davids, K. Isokawa, M. Mellor, S. and Reilly, T. (1987) Physiological strain in 4-a-side soccer. This volume.

McNair, D. Lorr, M. and Droppleman, L. (1971) Profile of Mood States Manual. San Diego: Educational and Industrial Testing Services.

Murgatroyd, D. (1981) Reversal theory: a new perspective on crisis counselling. Brit. J. Guidance and Couns., 9, 180-93.

Murgatroyd, S. Rushton, C. Apter, M. Ray, C. (1978) The development of the Telic Dominance Scale. J. Pers. Assess., 42, 519-28.

Power, S. (1982) An analysis of anxiety levels in track and field athletes of varying ages and abilities. Int. J. Sport Psychol., 13, 258-267.

Reilly, T. and Thomas, V. (1976) A motion analysis of work-rate in different positional roles in professional football match-play. J. Human Mov't. Stud., 2, 87-97.

Scanlan, T. and Passer, M. (1978) Factors related to competitive stress among male youth sports participants. Med. Sci. Sports, 10, 103-108.

SOURCES OF STRESS IN SOCCER OFFICIATING: AN EMPIRICAL STUDY

A.H. Taylor and J.V. Daniel
School of Physical and Health Education, University of Toronto.
320 Huron Street, Toronto, Ontario, Canada.

Introduction

Sports officiating has been recognised as a potentially stressful activity (Conti and McClintock, 1983; Quinn et al., 1986). Officials are in a highly evaluative position in which their integrity is often questioned. Reports of verbal, and instances of physical abuse of soccer officials are on the increase according to the Director of The Ontario Referee Development Programme (Agnew, J. personal communication 1986). Numerous psycho-social stressors have been identified in the occupational stress literature (Cooper and Marshall, 1976). These appear to be associated with various psychological, behavioural, and physiological stress reactions.

In a study of Saskatchewan ice hockey officials, Fry and Sefton (1982) reported that criticism and attitudes of others towards officials were major factors affecting continuation or retention of the officials in the sport. Given the nature of the experiences an official may face, it is hardly surprising that a variety of sports officiating administrators in Ontario, (e.g. rugby union, baseball and soccer) have reported a shortage of experienced officials. Of those taking the initial 15 hour soccer referee course in Ontario only about 10% continue as registered officials (Agnew, J. personal communication, 1986). The excessive drain on the resources of sports governing bodies, due to high turnover of officials, is a financial concern. The shortage may also serve to reduce overall standards of officiating.

The game of soccer requires that an official is physically fit, possesses technical knowledge concerning the rules, and has the necessary psychological attributes to deal with a broad range of situations and experiences. For the sports of American Football, and Rugby League, Conti and McClintock (1983) and Quinn et al. (1986) respectively, proposed that psycho-social stressors played a major role in unexpectedly high heart rates while officiating. It seems that physical training alone was not adequately preparing officials for the demands of officiating. This placed some individuals at risk of serious health problems.

If officials' training programmes are to consider psychological aspects (e.g. stress management techniques), it is initially important to identify the main sources of perceived stress. The present study involved the development of a reliable instrument to assess perceived officiating stress. High levels of perceived stress may be associated with an intent to discontinue officiating, which was also investigated.

Method

The Soccer Officials' Stress Survey (SOSS) was constructed following conventional procedures to provide content and face validity. Extensive interviews with officials across all levels of certification in Ontario led to a 90-item pool of potential officiating stressors. A 12-member panel with experience in either psychometric construction, stress research or soccer officiating, reduced these to a final 53 items. Items were selected to minimize ambiguity and overlap whilst spanning a broad range of potential acute and chronic stressors.

Subjects responded on a 4-point Likert-type scale (0=Did Not, to 3=Strongly) how much each item contributed to the stress they felt during the past season. In addition, 39 of the 53 items with an anticipated high variability in frequency occurrence required officials to rate, on a 4-point scale (0=Never, to 3=Often), how often they had experienced the item.

At the end of the outdoor season, 400 randomly selected male soccer officials from all levels of certification in Ontario (Youth to FIFA), were mailed a copy of the SOSS with a stamped addressed envelope. Selected demographic data from the 215 officials who returned the survey are summarized in Table 1.

Table 1. Demographic characteristics of a sample of Ontario soccer officials

	% of sample		% of sample
1. Age (years)		4. Certification level	
20	7.4	Youth (probation	12.6
20-30	9.3	Three (probation)	13.9
31-40	32.6	Three	26.5
41-50	39.1	Two	21.9
50	11.6	One	18.1
		National	5.1
		FIFA	1.9
2. Occupation			
White collar		5. Hours per week as an official last season	
-Professional	42.3		
-Technical	19.3	2-6	24.7
Blue collar	25.8	7-12	30.4
Primary	0.9	13-18	24.3
Student	11.7	18	20.6
3. Marital status		6. Years as an official	
Divorced/separated	7.5	5	24.7
Single	15.9	6-10	30.4
Married	76.7	11-15	24.3
		15	11.1

Results

The 14 most stressful items perceived by the subjects are shown in Table 2. The most stressful event was 'Having a 'bad' game' (Mean $\pm$SD=1.72 $\pm$0.93). The last two columns in Table 2 indicate the percentage of the sample reporting 'sometimes' or 'often' for frequency, and 'moderate' or 'strong' for intensity (the two highest points on each scale). Clearly the most frequently experienced potential stressor was a lack of understanding of the rules by players and coaches. This belief is probably not shared by players or coaches to the same extent.

Table 2. Major psycho-social stressors for Ontario soccer officials

Rank	Situations/Events	How Stressful Mean	SD	Often (a)	Much (b)
1	Having a 'bad' game	1.72	0.93	NA	61.0
2.	Working with poor officials	1.41	1.05	52.2	49.8
3.	Making a 'bad' call	1.40	0.87	NA	44.2
4.	Players or coaches who don't understand the laws	1.36	0.98	87.4	40.9
5.	Dismissing players	1.33	0.92	NA	43.2
6.	Dealing with over-excited or hostile coaches	1.28	0.85	59.0	37.7
7.	Dealing with abusive players	1.21	0.84	54.9	33.6
8.	Very important games to one or both teams	1.15	0.92	76.6	36.1
9.	Little recognition for officials	1.15	1.03	NA	34.4
10.	Critical decisions during a game	1.13	0.83	NA	32.7
11.	Aggressive game	1.13	0.82	73.2	33.0
12.	Spectators - close to field	1.08	0.88	75.0	27.1
13.	Violence/fighting in a game	1.01	0.99	19.1	30.8
14.	Conflict between officiating and daily family demands	1.00	1.01	39.5	32.9

(a) Percent of sample indicating 'sometimes' or 'often' for 'How Often'

(b) Percent of sample indicating 'moderate' or 'strong' for 'How Much'

NA 'How Often' not assessed

The Pearson Product-Moment correlation coefficient for the relationship between the frequency and intensity scales was found to be 0.59 ($P < 0.0001$). This correlation supports the contention of Lazarus and Launier (1978) that in the assessment of stress greater importance should be placed on how events are perceived rather than merely how often they are experienced.

A principal components factor analysis with varimax rotation produced a 15 factor solution using the eigenvalue of 1.00 as criterion. Those items with a factor loading of at least 0.40 on only one factor were retained. One purpose of the study was to establish conceptually meaningful sub-scales with a minimum of 3 items for each factor. These criteria resulted in the 6 factors shown in Table 3 and accounted for 35.4% of the intensity variance. Factor loadings below 0.40 are not given in the Table.

Table 3. Factor analysis of intensity responses to potential soccer officiating stressors

Stressor	Factor Loading					
	I	II	III	IV	V	VI
Personality clash with player(s)	.70	-	-	-	-	-
Very important games	.64	-	-	-	-	-
Personality clash with coach or club official	.60	-	-	-		
Aggressive game	.60	-	-	-	-	-
Dealing with abusive players	.59	-	-	-	-	-
Spectators - noisy	.58	-	-	-	-	-
Dealing with over-excited or hostile coaches	.55	-	-	-	-	-
Being accused of bias towards one team	.51	-	-	-	-	-
Violence/fighting in a game	.48	-	-	-	-	-
Physical assault from player	-	.77	-	-	-	-
Threat of assault from spectator	-	.75	-	-	-	-
Physical assault from spectator	-	72	-	-	-	-
Threat of assault from player	-	61	-	-	-	-
Spectators - post-match personal security problems	-	.48	-	-	-	-
Conflict between officiating and occupational demands	-	-	.75	-	-	-
Conflict between officiating and family demands	-	-	.67	-	-	-
Too many game assignments	-	-	60	-	-	-
Arrive late at a game	-	-	.49	-	-	-
Competition and jealousy between officials	-	-	-	.77	-	-
Personality clash with co-official	-	-	-	.55	-	-
Not selected for important games	-	-	-	.52	-	-
Working with poor officials	-	-	-	.42	-	-
Little recognition for officials in soccer	-	-	-	-	.81	-
Lack of recognition for good officiating	-		-	-	.67	-
Players or coaches who don't understand the laws	-	-	-	-	.49	-
Making a 'bad' call	-	-	-	-	-	.79
Having a 'bad' game	-	-	-	-	-	.69
Critical decisions during a game	-	-	-	-	-	.60
Percent of variance accounted by factor	9.32	6.09	5.39	5.14	5.12	4.49

Hoyt's estimate of reliability for the 6 sub-scales ranged from 0.67 to 0.87. This showed internal consistency was acceptable.

Sub-scale labelling was primarily determined from those items with the highest factor loading. Sub-scale I (mean item score=0.95) was labelled 'interpersonal conflicts'. Poor relations would appear to originate from abusive or hostile behaviour towards officials and personality clashes. Important, aggressive and violent games also appear to involve inter-personal conflict.

Sub-scale II (mean item score=0.49) was called 'fear of physical harm'. It reflected the degree of stress associated with threat of, or actual assault.

Sub-scale III (mean item score=0.69) was labelled 'time pressures', insofar as the items reflect feelings that officiating may be conflicting with other time demanding interests.

Sub-scale IV (mean item score=0.78) was labelled 'peer conflicts'. It represents items reflecting strained relations, perhaps due to competition for assignments or advancement of one's officiating career.

Sub-scale V (mean item score=1.03), labelled 'role-culture conflict', is best explained by lack of appreciation and support that an official appears to perceive.

Sub-scale VI (mean item score=1.42) was termed 'fear of failure'. The items reflect situations in which officials may perceive others to be particularly critical of their officiating ability.

No significant differences in the total perceived stress score (or any of the sub-scale scores) were found between those who intended to officiate in the next season (N=181) and those who did not (N=7) or were undecided (N=27). The latter two groups were combined for t-tests with unequal group size.

Discussion

The top ten stressors were all rated as at least moderately stressful by over 33% of the sample, providing a good indication of the major stressors for the sample as a whole. Interestingly, the four most stressful items appear to involve a subjective assessment of the ability of those in the game to understand or administer its laws. This concern may well reflect a recent rapid growth period for Ontario soccer during which technical knowledge concerning the rules has advanced more slowly. One may speculate that in countries where soccer is more established other stressors may have a potentially greater impact.

One of the main purposes of the study was to develop conceptually sound sub-scales reflecting major sources of officiating stress. Future empirical work should examine possible causal relationships between sources of stress, retention and performance.

Based on the mean item score for each factor, officials regarded fear of failure or evaluative incidents to be most stressful. Officials are placed in a competitive environment involving social evaluation of an ability. This can be threatening if they anticipate failure or negative appraisal from others. Increased introspection on the part of an official may well reduce the ability to maintain an appropriate broad external focus of attention. This has important implications for applying techniques of stress management and attention control.

The second most important group of stressors is related to recognition and gratitude. There would appear to be a discrepancy or misfit between the expectations of some officials and the expressed appreciation of their work, in terms of the person-environment fit model of French et al. (1982). While 61% of the present sample experienced a lack of recognition for good officiating at least 'sometimes', only 23% reported this item as at least 'moderately' stressful. Most officials appear to have developed a coping mechanism for this lack of recognition. However, those who perceive an imbalance between their needs and rewards, in terms of social facilitation, may be more vulnerable to consequences of stress, such as turnover.

During an intensely competitive soccer match, officials may have to deal with inter-personal emotional conflicts. Failure to remain calm when faced with such stressors is likely to result in an inappropriately narrow attentional focus while officiating. Nelson (1979) suggested that antagonistic behaviour towards officials has become increasingly acceptable in certain sports. When such conflict does not fit an official's expectations, then stress reactions are likely.

Local refereeing associations have a tradition of weak support in Ontario. There are currently plans to encourage the development of more active social networks. This may not only help to reduce peer conflicts but also attract officials and retain others frustrated by the lack of social support.

Considerable responsibility rests upon an official to fulfill a commitment to officiate a match. It is often impossible to find a replacement and providing an excuse may not encourage further requests for the services of that official. Almost half the sample in this study reported spending at least 13 hours a week, including travel and preparation, as an official. Such demand on his time is very likely to be a source of pressure. Officials who begin a match with thoughts of concurrent occupational or social demands are unlikely to provide an optimum service to the game. Techniques to enhance mental preparation before a match, particularly in such 'time-pressured' situations, should be made available to officials.

The low mean score on the 'fear of physical harm' items may be explained by the fact that less than 5% of the present sample experienced these stressors. However, those who did reported considerable stress, as one would anticipate.

It was surprising to find that those not intending to officiate the next season perceived their role as no more stressful than those who suggested they would continue. However, the former group largely consisted of subjects uncertain of their future involvement as officials; besides, intentions are probably not perfect predictors of behaviour. Further research to examine the dynamic relationship between the various facets of stress identified in this study and actual turnover is under way.

The Soccer Officiating Stress Survey, with reliable sub-scales, will also have practical utility as an aid to identifying areas of concern for the individual. Techniques to facilitate management of time, people, and stress may then be recommended to enhance officiating performance, satisfaction and the likelihood of retention.

Acknowledgements

This research is supported by a grant from the Ministry of Tourism and Recreation, Ontario (Wintario 86-80-0034).
Appreciation is also expressed to Joe Agnew, Director of The Referee Development Programme of The Ontario Soccer Association, and Drs. Peter Klavora and Larry Leith for their assistance.

References

Conti, D.J. and McClintock, S.L. (1983) Heart rate responses of a head referee during a football game. Physician Sportsmed., 11, 108-114.

Cooper, C.L. and Marshall, J. (1976) Occupational sources of stress: A review of the literature relating to coronary heart disease and mental ill health. J. Occup. Psychol., 49, 11-28.

French, J.R.P., Caplan, R.D. and Van Harrison, R. (1982) The Mechanisms of Job Stress and Strain. New York: John Wiley.

Fry, D.A.P. and Sefton, J.M. (1982) Retention of game officials for ice hockey. Unpublished paper, University of Saskatchewan, Saskatoon.

Lazarus, R.S. and Launier, R. (1978) Stress related transactions between person and environment. In: Perspectives in Interactional Psychology. (edited by L.A. Pervin and M. Lewis). New York: Plenum Press.

Nelson, K.H. (1979) Study of the relationship between support for political authority, support for sports officials, and disrespectful behaviour towards sports officials. Doctoral Dissertation, University of North Colorado.

Quinn, G., Pilkington, R., and Smiley, N. (1986) Relationships between laboratory, league matches, and occupational performance of a selected group of senior rugby league referees. Sport and Medicine Volume, Proceedings of the VIII Commonwealth and International Conference on Sport, Physical Education, Dance, Recreation and Health. London: E. and F.N. Spon.

ATTRIBUTIONAL RESPONSES OF 4-A-SIDE SOCCER PLAYERS

F.H. Sanderson and S.K. Kneale
Department of Sport and Recreation Studies, Liverpool Polytechnic, Byrom Street, Liverpool L3 3AF, England.

Introduction

Since the work of Heider (1958) on inter-personal relations, causal attribution has become a popular area of social psychological inquiry. In particular, Weiner and colleagues (1971) have postulated an attributional model of achievement behaviour which maintains that individuals assume more personal responsibility for success than failure. Specifically, people appear more inclined to ascribe success to ability (stable) and effort (unstable), whereas failure is attributed, when possible, to external factors of task difficulty (stable) and luck (unstable). These attributions have been explained in terms of a self-serving bias in which the individual attempts to protect or enhance his self-esteem. The uniqueness of the sport environment has suggested that other attributions, such as unstable ability, i.e. a player's 'form', team function, playing conditions and match officials are important considerations (Roberts and Pascuzzi, 1979).

Much of the original research on attribution theory was conducted by means of artificially contrived laboratory-based 'games' in which outcome could be manipulated, but it has increasingly been acknowledged that sport offers an ecologically-valid testing ground for the various theoretical perspectives. For example, Sanderson and Gilchrist (1982) examined attributional responses of competitive squash players and found that, although winners were more internal and less external than losers, the latter still assessed internal attributes to be the most important determinants of match outcome. It was argued that social norms or constraints associated with squash tend to limit the acceptability of external attributions. This finding is not untypical in the sport literature, notwithstanding the fact that most field studies are concerned with team sports (Rejeski and Brawley, 1983).

The team-sport research has generally not included a neutral outcome condition, a fact which has prevented precise explanation for attributional differences between winners and losers. With this in mind, Scanlan and Passer (1980) investigated the attributional responses of young female soccer players after winning, tying (drawing) and losing. They found that a game was not a neutral experience in the sense that response pattern of players when drawing tended to resemble that of winners more clearly than that of losers. Winners and players were more internal than losers and no evidence was found of an external bias amongst losers. In terms of self versus team attribution, there was some evidence of self-protective behaviour by tying and losing players, i.e. 'I'm okay, but the team's so-so', but more solid evidence of winners thinking 'I'm good but the team's great.'

It can be argued that one versus one competition, as in squash, provides a more meaningful setting for attribution research in that the fewer degrees of freedom allow more precise examination of the relationship between attribution and outcome. Indeed, Scanlan and Passer (1980) acknowledged this problem by not considering the impact of self-attribution on team outcome. However, in small sided-soccer, each player is heavily involved in the action and is likely to make a significant 'impact' on the outcome. It was thus seen as a useful setting for a team attribution investigation with the added advantage of a tying outcome.

On the basis of previous research, it was hypothesised that:
i) winning and tying players would be more internal in their attributions than losing players;
ii) losing players would show no significant externality bias:
iii) self versus team attributions would show evidence of a) self-protective behaviour by tying and losing players; b) team aggrandisement by winning players.

Method

Subjects

The subjects were participants in the Liverpool Polytechnic 4-a-side soccer leagues: there are 8 leagues and 8 teams per league. The league winners progress to a knockout competition with the overall winners and runners-up receiving trophies and medals. Data were collected from 52 teams, giving 208 subjects. All were male and either undergraduates or staff with an age range from 18 to approximately 40 years.

The Questionnaire

A 19-item post-match questionnaire included statements on self versus team attributions in relation to ability, effort, confidence, mistakes, will to win and match importance, together with miscellaneous items concerning the referee, the equipment, degree of concentration, fitness, fairness of outcome and luck. Statements were responded to on a 4-point Likert-type scale ranging from 'Not at all' to 'Very much so'. The questionnaire was designed to provide a comprehensive and ecologically valid range of attributional statements and which could be completed relatively quickly and without difficulty by respondents.

Procedure

Subjects who had previously agreed to participate in an investigation, completed the questionnaire immediately after each 10-min match and before showering and in the presence of the experimenter. Responses were thus obtained while the meaning of the match was still vivid, and conferring amongst subjects was avoided.

Subjects were assured that their responses would remain confidential. The results of all the matches were checked with the referee.

Results

For the analysis, the independent variable was match outcome, i.e. win, draw (tie), loss, with the dependent variables being the responses to the 19 statements.

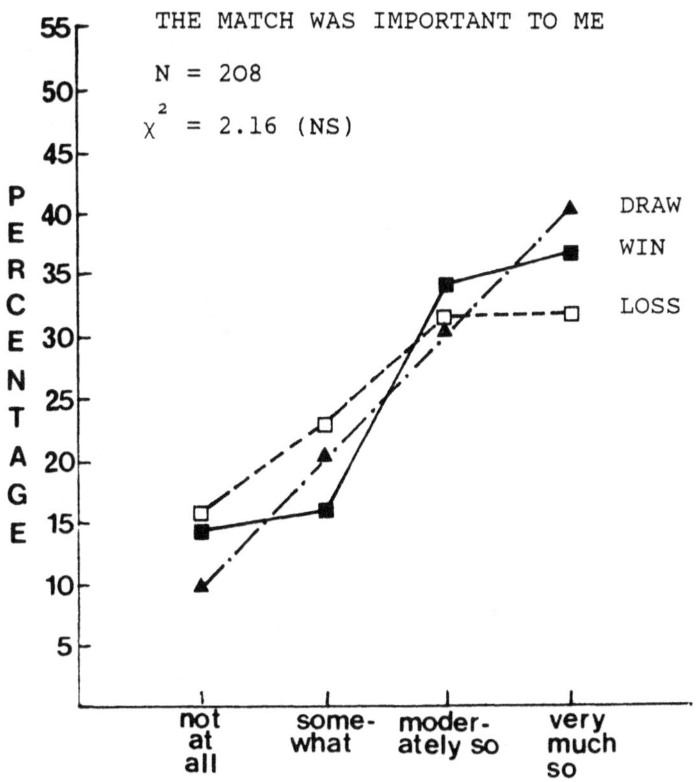

Figure 1. Perceived match importance for winning, losing and tying players

The univariate ANOVAs performed on the individual dependent variables revealed no significant win-tie-loss differences in estimation of fitness, self-ability, self-concentration, self and team estimates of match importance, self and team will-to-win, self-mistakes, self and team effort and luck. Significant differences were found for team ability ($F = 18.70$; $P < 0.01$) with a post-hoc test revealing that winners and tying players rated team ability significantly higher than losers, the attitude to the referee ($F = 8.45$; $P < 0.05$) with winners and tying players being significantly more positive, fairness of outcome ($F = 31.88$: $P < 0.01$), with winners being significantly more convinced of the fairness than losing or tying players, pre-match confidence ($F = 14.53$: $P < 0.01$) with tying and winning players being significantly more confident than losers, and team mistakes ($F = 9.92$: $P < 0.05$) with tying and losing players being significantly more critical of the team than winners.

A more detailed examination of these trends was undertaken using outcome x response category contingency tables for selected statements. Winning, losing and tying players did not differ in perceived match importance ($\chi^2 = 2.16$; Fig. 1) which suggests that the matches were similarly ego-involving for all three groups. Fig. 2 illustrates no differences in self mistakes ($\chi^2 = 8.80$) and significant differences in team mistakes across the three groups ($\chi^2 = 24.04$; $P < 0.01$). Outcome groups were assigned to 'lower' and 'higher' internality categories on the basis of composite scores.

Fig. 3a shows close similarities between winning and tying players

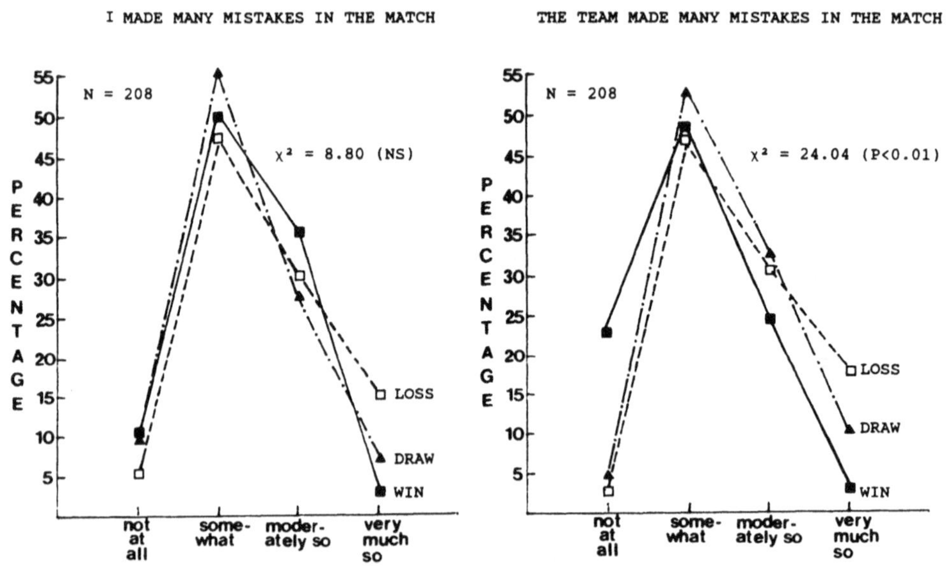

Figure 2. Self and team mistakes for wins, losses and draws

with losers exhibiting a marked inclination to lower internality, thus confirming the first hypothesis. None of the groups exhibited evidence of high externality (Fig. 3b), although winners and tying players who had similar patterns of responses were less external than losers, giving some support to the second hypothesis.

Figs 4a and 4b illustrate group differences concerning opinion of self versus team ability. A similar pattern is apparent for tying players with the majority of tying players having a relatively high opinion of self and team ability. Concerning self-ability, winners and losers are similar in that a majority hold a relatively low opinion, but the pattern markedly changes for team ability. The negative opinion is accentuated for the losing players, whereas the

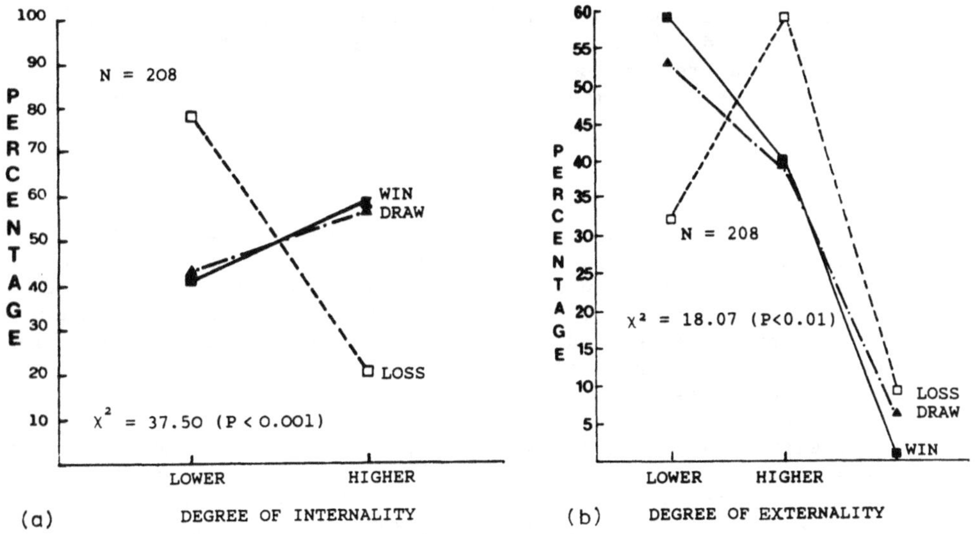

Figure 3. Internality (a) and externality (b) for winning, losing and drawing

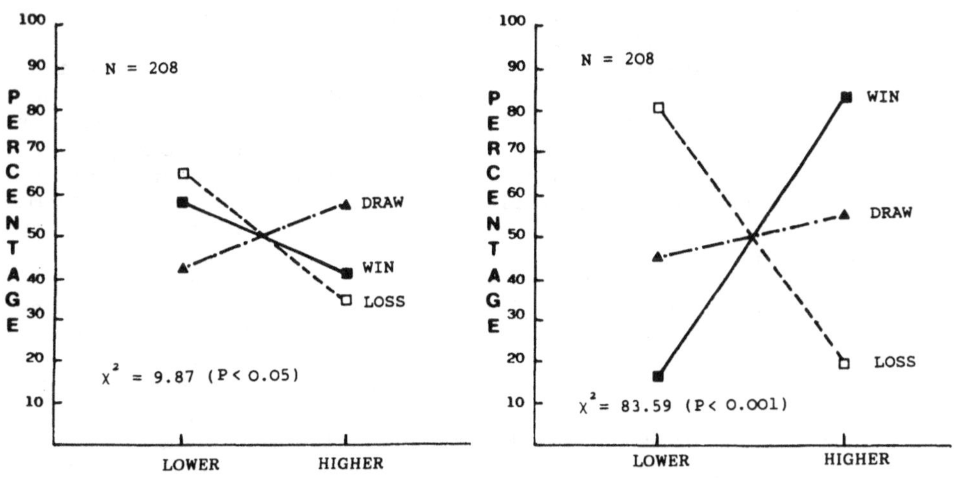

Figure 4. Self (a) and team (b) ability for winning, losing and drawing

winners exhibit a pronounced high opinion of their team's ability. As hypothesised, there was evidence of self-protective attributions by losing players but the prediction of such attribution by tying players was not confirmed. The hypothesis that there would be team aggrandisement by winning players was supported.

Discussion

When examining differences between the causal ascriptions of individuals as a function of game outcome, it is important that ego-involvement is not a confounding factor. Hence, the fact that the statement 'the match was important to me' was responded to similarly by the winning, tying and losing groups provided a basis for making direct comparisons across groups with regard to the other attributional statements.

Several non-significant differences between outcome groups were found with regard to self-ascription, i.e. effort, fitness, ability, concentration, will to win and mistakes. This is illustrated by responses to the statement 'I made many mistakes in the match' (Fig. 2). However, it is not clear from this evidence alone whether response patterns are similar because of a self-protective strategy of losing and drawing players or self-deprecation on the part of winners. Examination of Fig. 2 on team mistakes which mainly differs from self-mistakes in the response pattern of winners suggests that the self-deprecation strategy and/or the team aggrandisement strategy are being used by winners.

More dramatic evidence in relation to attributional strategies is provided by a comparison of Figs. 4a and 4b. Concerning opinions of self-ability, similar somewhat negative opinions were evidenced by winners and losers. In the context of the opinion of team ability it would appear that losers are using a self-protective strategy: they are only moderately self-critical but highly critical of the team. Winners on the other hand combine self-criticism with high opinions of team ability, which suggests the aggrandisement hypothesis. Scanlan and Passer's (1980) evidence that winners observed the 'competitive norm' of aggrandising the team rather than themselves after victory is supported. They found support for an 'I'm good but the team's great' response by winners, whereas the present study suggests a modest 'I'm so-so, but the team's great' response. Unlike Scanlan and Passer (1980) who found no evidence of the 'I'm okay but the team's so-so' response identified by Bird and Brame (1978), this study found clear evidence of such a response amongst losers who were much more critical of team ability than self-ability.

It was interesting that tying players exhibited similar response patterns regarding self and team ability suggesting an 'I'm okay and the team's okay' response. The tying players' responses appeared neutral and more 'honest' in the sense that a draw outcome is neither ego-threatening like losing nor encouraging of self-deprecation, like winning.

The composite internality scores revealed an internality bias amongst tying and winning players and much less internality amongst losers (Fig. 3), results which broadly support previous research findings. Tying and winning players were also similar in their relatively low incidence of causal ascriptions to external factors (Fig 3b). Although there was little evidence of high externality across all outcome groups, which was in line with previous research (Scanlan and Passer, 1980), losing players did show greater evidence of moderate external attributions. Therefore, it appears that losers were to some extent using a self-protective strategy in this respect.

This investigation has been useful in demonstrating the potential of small-sided soccer as a focus for field research in relation to attribution theory in sport. It has confirmed that winning players demonstrate an internality bias and has produced evidence of a subtle externality bias amongst losers. Moreover the neutrality of the draw condition has been questioned in the sense that results have generally approximated to winning rather than losing response patterns. There is the possibility that the tying responses are indeed neutral in that 'honest' responses have been elicited as opposed to the various attributional strategies which are adopted by winners and losers. Further research could usefully investigate this idea, perhaps using tying conditions in which the payoffs or penalties for tying were varied. More sensitive investigation of attributional strategies would also be possible if the closeness of defeat or victory was taken into account.

References

Bird, A.M., and Brame, J.M. (1978) Self versus team attributions: A test of the 'I'm OK, but the team's so-so phenomenon'. Res. Quart., 49, 260-268.

Heider, F. (1958) The Psychology of Interpersonal Relations. New York: Wiley.

Rejeski, W.J. and Brawley, L.R. (1983) Attribution theory in sport: current status and new perspectives. J. Sport Psychol., 5, 77-99.

Roberts, G.C. and Pascuzzi, D. (1979) Causal attributions in sport: some theoretical implications. J. Sport Psychol., 1, 203-211.

Sanderson, F.H. and Gilchrist, J. (1982) Anxiety and attributional responses of competitive squash players. Brit. J. Sports Med., 16, 115.

Scanlan, T.K. and Passer, M.W. (1980) The attributional responses of young female athletes after winning, tying and losing. Res. Quart. Exerc. Sport, 51, 675-685.

Weiner, B., Frieze, I., Kukla, A., Reed, L., Rest, S. and Rosenbaum, R.M. (1971) Perceiving the causes of success and failure. In: Attribution: Perceiving the Causes of Behaviour. (edited by E.E. Jones, D.E. Kanouse, H.H. Kelley, R.E. Nisbett, S. Valins and B. Weiner. Morristown, N.J.: General Learning Press.

AN INVESTIGATION INTO THE RELATIONSHIP BETWEEN FIELD INDEPENDENCE AND DECISION MAKING IN SOCCER

T. McMorris and W.W. MacGillivary
Faculty of Physical Education and Recreation, University of New Brunswick, Fredericton, New Brunswick, Canada.

Introduction

Skill in soccer has been categorised in terms of technique and decision making (Hughes, 1980). Knapp (1963) described technique as the ability to carry out the necessary motor act, for example, kicking a ball. While she described decision making as knowing what to do in a given situation. The skilful player is the one who can quickly assess when to pass, dribble or shoot. Furthermore he knows which technique to use in order to maximise his chances of successfully carrying out a chosen plan of action.

Making decisions in soccer places great demands on the individual's information processing ability. The display facing the soccer player is complex, ever-changing, and contains much irrelevant information. The skilful player must be able to extract relevant cues from the display for analysis, and put into action a chosen motor plan. A player in a good shooting position, for example, must ignore colleagues in poorer scoring positions. He should concentrate on the position of the goalkeeper and the defenders. Based on this information he will then decide which shooting technique to use and where to place his shot.

The ability to extract information from a complex display and to handle perceptual cues in an analytical manner has been shown to be indicative of individuals who possess a field independent (FI) cognitive style. Witkin et al. (1954) claimed that the way in which individuals process perceptual information can be placed in a continuum from FI to field dependent (FD). People possessing an FD cognitive style have relative difficulty in disembedding objects from their background and are less analytical of perceptual information than FI individuals.

It would appear logical to hypothesize that an FI cognitive style would be an advantage to sportsmen in a number of activities e.g. team ball games. There has been much previous research attempting to verify the existence of such a relationship. The results have been somewhat equivocal and, according to MacGillivary (1980), there is, as yet, no conclusive evidence of a relationship between FI and successful sports performance.

MacGillivary (1980) claimed that the contradictory findings may be due to the methods used to ascertain the individual's cognitive style. This claim has been supported by other research. Williams

(1975), examining the relation between fencing ability and FI, found no significant correlation. In this research she used an embedded figures test to determine cognitive style. However, when using the portable rod-and-frame test (PRFT) (Oltman, 1968) to ascertain cognitive style, she demonstrated a significant relationship (Williams, 1980). She concluded that the contradictory results may have been due to the inclusion of a visual-kinaesthetic cue articulation factor which is present in PRFT but not in embedded figures tests. Consequently, it was decided to use both PRFT and a hidden figures test [HFT] (Engel and Lowe, 1982) in the present study.

The research directly concerned with soccer performance and FI (Bard, 1972; Barrell and Trippe, 1975), utilized the PRFT, and found no significant correlation. However, the findings of Read (1983), examining the relationship between FI and decision making in field hockey, a game very similar to soccer in its perceptual demands, adds weight to the hypothesis that there may be a relation between FI and decision making in soccer. This hypothesis was examined in the present study utilising the HFT test.

Method

The cognitive style of varsity soccer players (N = 22), was determined by the administration of HFT (Engel and Lowe, 1982) and PRFT (Oltman, 1968). Decision making in soccer was assessed by two coaches, based on observations of the players in practices and games throughout one season (1985-86). The coaches rated the players on a 1 to 5 Likert-type scale where 1 = 'poor' decision-making and 5 = 'excellent' performance. The rating was based on a guideline which was developed following a review of the literature and discussion with experienced coaches. Overall soccer playing ability was assessed in a similar manner.

Decision making ability was also assessed using an objective test. Following a review of the literature, discussion with experienced coaches and a pilot study, 16 situations testing the decision making ability of varsity players, were identified. These were set up in a static display so that they could be photographed. Player figures (6.4 cm high) were placed on a table tennis table (2.74 m by 1.52 m), which was marked for soccer using white tape. Photographs of the situations were taken using a Nikon 35 mm camera with a lens size of 50 mm and colour slides were produced.

Each slide was tachistoscopically presented to the subject at exposure times of 0.5 s, 1 s, and 2 s. Order of presentation and exposure times were randomized and the slides were shown in a darkened room. With only one correct response for each situation, the subject had to indicate his choice of action before or immediately after exposure had ceased. The slides tested the subject's ability to make decisions for the player in possession of the ball and for those without the ball. The number of correct responses represented the individual's performance in the test.

Results

The objective test of decision making claimed face validity as it had been based on the literature and on expert opinion. Concurrent validity was determined by comparing the results of the test with coaches' assessments. A Pearson Product Moment correlation showed that performance on the tachistoscopic test concurred significantly with the coaches' assessments of decision making ($r = 0.74$; $P < 0.001$) and with the coaches' assessment of overall playing ability ($r = 0.75$; $P < 0.001$). Reliability of the tachistostopic test was determined by the Cronbach Alpha formula using SPSS - X. An alpha value of 0.71 was obtained.

Table 1. Differences in scores in HFT and PRFT of the top and bottom 5 performers on the tachistoscopic test of decision-making

Test	Top 5 Mean ± SD	Bottom 5 Mean ± SD
HFT	5.6 ± 2.15	8 ± 0.63[a]
PRFT	39.3 ± 4.93	19.2 ± 2.63

a denotes $P < 0.001$

A 't' test was used to determine whether or not there was a significant difference in the cognitive styles of those assessed as the top five and bottom five in decision making and overall playing ability, and the top five and bottom five performers on the tachistoscopic test. Significant differences were obtained when HFT was used as the criterion for determining cognitive style but not when PRFT was used. When HFT scores were used to ascertain cognitive style, the players assessed as the top five decision makers were more FD than those assessed as the bottom five, ($P < 0.05$). Similar results were obtained for those assesed as the top and bottom five players ($P < 0.05$) and the top and bottom five performers on the tachistoscopic test ($P < 0.001$) (see Tables 1, 2 and 3).

Table 2. Differences in scores in HFT and PRFT of the players assessed by the coaches as being the Top and Bottom 5 in decision-making

Test	Top 5 Mean ± SD	Bottom 5 Mean ± SD
HFT	4.5 ± 1.36	7.14 ± 1.06[a]
PRFT	38.2 ± 4.97	18.5 ± 2.53

a: $P < 0.05$

Table 3. Differences in scores on HFT and PRFT of the players assessed by the coaches as being the Top and Bottom 5 in playing ability

Test	Top 5 Mean ± SD	Bottom 5 Mean ± SD
HFT	4.2 ± 1.11	7.0 ± 1.41[a]
PRFT	33.083 ± 4.72	18.7 ± 2.78

[a] denotes $P < 0.05$

An intercorrelation matrix (Table 4) was calculated to compare scores on the HFT, PRFT, tachistoscopic test of decision making and overall playing ability. Application of the Omnibus Null Formula revealed that the chance of the matrix producing an alpha error was low ($P < 0.001$)); therefore, further examination of the Pearson Product Moment correlations was relevant. There was a significant negative correlation between FI as assessed by HFT and the coaches' assessment of playing ability ($r = -0.69$; $P < 0.001$). The coaches' assessment of decision making and their assessment of playing ability correlated significantly ($r = 0.72$; $P < 0.001$). As stated already, the performance on the tachistoscopic test correlated significantly with both of the coaches' assessments.

Table 4. Intercorrelation matrix

Test	Coaches' Assessment Decision-Making	Coaches' Assessment Playing-ability	Tachistoscopic Test Decision-Making	HFT	PRFT
Coaches' assessment decision-making		0.72[a]	0.74[a]	-0.35	0.28
Coaches' assessment playing ability			0.75[a]	-0.69[a]	0.19
Tachistoscopic test decision-making 3				-0.41	0.27
HFT					-0.24

[a] indicates significant $P < 0.001$

Discussion

Evidence was provided for the long held belief that decision making is an essential part of overall playing ability in soccer. It was also demonstrated that a reliable, objective and valid tachistoscopic test of decision making in soccer has the potential for development. Such a test could provide the coach with objective evidence to complement his own subjective evaluations. Similarly a test of this kind could be used to test students taking soccer courses. Furthermore the process could be adapted to be used as an aid to coaching. This has previously been shown to be effective in ice-hockey (Thiffault, 1978).

The failure to demonstrate a significant correlation between PRFT results and soccer playing ability is in essential agreement with previous findings (Bard, 1972; Barrell and Trippe, 1975). The failure to show a relationship between HFT results and decision making is in contrast with previous research in field hockey (Read, 1983).

The HFT results would suggest the possibility of significant relation between FD and soccer playing ability. However all the HFT results did not demonstrate such a relationship. Furthermore the PRFT results failed to show any significant relationship between cognitive style and performance in soccer. These add to the contradictory results found for other sports and FI (MacGillivary, 1980) and supply further evidence for the disparity between HFT and PRFT results. The only definite statement that can be made, is that no evidence for a correlation between FI and soccer performance was obtained.

The failure to demonstrate a significant relation between FI and soccer playing ability could be due to a number of factors. The HFT and PRFT examine perceptual style in static situations. Information processing in soccer, however, occurs in a moving environment. It is possible that movement adds another variable to cognitive style, one that is not measured by HFT or PRFT. The work of Herkowitz (1972), who found no significant correlation between performance on a static and moving version of a hidden figures test, adds some support to such a claim. Furthermore she discovered that movement increased the difficulty of some items, yet facilitated the problem solution in others. Unfortunately, Herkowitz's (1972) research was with children but it may well apply also to adults.

Another possible reason for failure to find a correlation between FI and decision making in soccer, could be the factor of time. In the HFT and PRFT the subject has time to solve the problem whereas the soccer player is often under temporal stress to make an instant decision. To some extent this may be offset by the fact that the experienced soccer player can see play developing and can anticipate likely alternatives.

Nevertheless neither of these hypotheses can explain why, in this study, the analytical quality of the FI players, did not prove to be an advantage in decision making. It is possible that when making a decision a player uses set response patterns i.e. he searches the display for situations for which he has a predetermined response and he ignores all other possibilities. In other words, he does not analyze the situation but acts in a pre-programmed manner. He uses his analytical capacities only in novel situations and this will normally take place during training or after a game when he has time to analyze the play. Often this analysis will be undertaken by the coach who will then produce a new pre-set response for the player. As a result the FI player would have little or no advantage over the FD player.

In conclusion the absence of a relation between FI and performance in soccer may well be due to one or all of the following factors:- (i) that players use set response patterns rather than analyzing the situation; (ii) that the disembedding processes in soccer are not as complex as those facing the subject in the HFT and PRFT; and (iii) that movement adds a dimension that is not measured by the tests of cognitive style. More research, preferably with a larger sample, is needed before the position can be clarified. The development of an adult version of Herkowitz's (1972) moving embedded figures test may be a significant development in research on the possible effects of movement on cognitive style.

References

Bard, C. (1972) The relation between perceptual style and physical activities. Int. J. Sport Psychol., 3, 107-113.

Barrell, G.V. and Trippe, H.R. (1975) Field dependence and physical ability. Percept. Motor Skills, 41, 216-218.

Engel, E. and Lowe, D. (1982) Gottschaldt Hidden Figures Test. University of Kentucky.

Herkowitz, J. (1972) Moving embedded figures test. Res. Ouart., 43, 479-488.

Hughes, C.F.C. (1980) Soccer Tactics and Skills. London: BBC.

Knapp, B. (1963) Skill in Sport. London: Routledge and Kegan Paul.

MacGillivary, W.W. (1980) The contribution of perceptual style to human performance. Int. J. Sport Psychol., 11, 132-141.

Oltman, P.K. (1968) A portable rod-and-frame apparatus. Percept. Motor Skills, 26, 503-506.

Read, B. (1983) Reading the game. Hockey Field, 71, 90-91.

Thiffault, C. (1978) Tachistoscopic training: an aid to improve hockey players' visual perception of tactical situations. Paper presented to the C.I.A.U. Hockey Seminar, Moncton, N.B., Canada.

Williams, J.M. (1975) Perceptual style and fencing skill. Percept. Motor Skills, 40, 282.

Williams, J.M. (1980) Differential figure-ground perception in classified and un-classified fencers. Sports Psychol., 2, 74-78.

Witkin, H.A., Lewis, H.B., Hertzman, M., Machover, K., Meissner, P.B. and Wapner, S. (1954) Personality through Perception: An Experimental and Clinical Study. Westport Ct.: Greenwood Press.

Part XIII

Sociological aspects of football violence

WHY 'CORE' SOCCER HOOLIGANS FIGHT: ASPECTS OF A SOCIOLOGICAL DIAGNOSIS

E. Dunning, P. Murphy and J. Williams
Sir Norman Chester Centre for Football Research, University of Leicester, Leicester, LE1 7RH, England.

Introduction

The argument in this paper is that soccer hooliganism as a social phenomenon is deeply rooted in the sense that, for 'core' soccer hooligans, those who nowadays engage most persistently in its more violent and disruptive aspects, hooliganism at and in conjunction with soccer forms part of a way of life to which they are deeply committed. Why should that be so? In order to arrive at a sociological diagnosis, some statements by 'core' soccer hooligans which shed light on aspects of their typical motivation will be considered. Following that, data on the social origins of soccer hooligans from the 1960's through to the 1980's will be examined. Then, some popular explanations will be critically looked at. Finally, aspects of a sociological diagnosis will be offered.

Some Statements by 'Core' Soccer Hooligans

Reminiscing about the emotions he experienced in the 1960's during his days of hooligan involvement, Taylor (1984) wrote:-

'...the excitement of battle, the danger, the heightened activity of body and mind as the adrenaline raced, the fear and the triumph of overcoming it. To this day, when trouble starts at a game I come alive and close to getting involved. I may not forget the dangers of physical injury and criminal proceedings but I do ignore them.'

Basically similar sentiments were expressed by a 26 year old lorry driver and self-confessed soccer hooligan who was interviewed by Harrison (1974) in conjunction with the 1974 Cardiff City - Manchester United game. The subject is reported to have said:-

'I go to a match for one reason only: the aggio. It's an obsession. I can't give it up. I get so much pleasure when I'm having aggro that I nearly wet my pants....I go all over the country looking for it ... every night during the week we go around town looking for trouble. Before a match we go round looking respectable ... then if we see someone who looks like the enemy we ask him the time; if he answers in a foreign accent, we do him over; and if he's got any money on him we'll roll him as well.'

Here is how one of the informants in the first Leicester University project on soccer hooliganism put it in 1981. His words illustrate the sort of rationality that tends to be involved in soccer hooliganism:

'If you can baffle the coppers, you'll win. You've just gotta think how they're gonna think. And you know, half the time you know what they're gonna do 'cos they're gonna take the same route every week, week in, week out. If you can figure out a way to beat 'em, you're fuckin' laughin'; you'll have a good fuckin' raut.' (Raut is Leicester slang for a 'fight').

Finally, when interviewed for the Thames TV programme, 'Hooligan', in 1985, a member of West Ham's 'Inter City Firm' said:-

'We don't - we don't go - well, we do go with the intention of fighting, you know what I mean .... We look forward to it .... It's great. You know, if you've got, say, 500 kids coming for you, like, and you know they're going to be waiting for you, it's - it's good to know, like. Like being a tennis player, you know. You get all geed up to play, like. We get geed up to fight ....

I think I fight, like, so I can make a name for meself and that, you know. Hope people, like, respect me for what I did, like.'

Despite the fact that they cover a period of more than twenty years, these statements are remarkably consistent. Moreover, although there might be minor variations of emphasis - for example, some might lay greater stress on loyalty to mates in a confrontation than on fighting *per se* - similar statements could be replicated by 'core' soccer hooligans up and down the country. Sociologically, they are illuminating. What they reveal are the underlying motives that tend to govern soccer hooligan behaviour. More particularly, they reveal that 'core' soccer hooligans are engaged in a 'quest for excitement' or emotional arousal; that, for them, fighting is a central source of meaning and gratification in life; and that hooligan activity provides a source of status for the males involved. Thus the lorry driver spoke of 'aggro' as a pleasurable, almost erotically arousing obsession; Taylor talked of 'battle excitement' and 'the adrenaline racing'; and the member of the "Inter City Firm" referred, not only to the excitement generated in a fight, but also to the respect among his peers that he hoped his involvement would bring. A quest for pleasurable excitement, of course, is a common feature of leisure activities, a counter to the emotional staleness engendered by the routines of non-leisure life (Elias and Dunning, 1986). Furthermore, ours is a patriarchal society in which, under certain circumstances, males generally are expected to fight. Moreover, high status can legitimately be accorded to good fighters in particular situations, for example in the military. However, the dominant norms demand that males should not be the initiators of fights and require them to confine their fighting to self-defence, 'defence of the realm' and to sports such as boxing. The 'core' soccer hooligans contravene these norms. They are more liable to initiate and plan attacks, and to fight publicly in situations where, according to the dominant norms, fighting is taboo. For them, a quest for status and the pleasurable 'battle excitement' engendered in soccer hooligan confrontations forms a central leisure interest. Sociologically, the point is to explain why. Who are the 'core' soccer hooligans and what in their social circumstances and experiences explains their deep interest in fighting and the fact that they deviate from the dominant norms of British society in this regard?

The Social Origins of Soccer Hooligans

Knowledge of the social origins and experiences of soccer hooligans is crucial for developing an explanation of their behaviour because it is only by exploring the social backgrounds and circumstances of people that it is possible to discover how and why their life-experiences have led them to acquire the values, attitudes and motives that are expressed in what they do. Put in slightly different terms, for persistent soccer hooligans a quest for a kind of battle excitement in a soccer or soccer-related context is a shared and socially constructed quest. It follows that, at least in the first instance, it has to be explained *sociologically*, that is, by reference to social rather than simply individual causation. To say this is not to imply that psychological explanations are irrelevant in this context but simply to say that psychological explanations of social phenomena are not meaningful *on their own*. In establishing what the social origins of the persistent soccer hooligans are, it will be useful to start by comparing them with the social profile of the 'typical' soccer crowd.

In the Leicester University research, we have established that between 2% and 6% of any soccer crowd is likely to consist of professional, or the Registrar General's Social Class 1, personnel. A not dissimilar proportion - between 13% and 15% - is likely to fall into the 'intermediate' occupational category, that is to come from the Registrar General's Social Class 2. The overwhelming majority, however, around two-thirds (65%), are likely to be skilled non-manual and manual workers, that is to belong to the Registrar General's Social Class 3. By contrast, attendance by semi-skilled and unskilled manual workers, that is by people from Social Classes 4 and 5, tends to be considerably lower, ranging, according to our data, between 11% and 13% for the semi-skilled, Social Class 4 category, and between 2% and 4% for unskilled workers, members of the Registrar General's Social Class 5.

The available data on soccer hooligans contrast markedly with these. Harrington (1968) was the first to undertake a systematic study of this issue. His data are summarized in Table 1.

As one can see, 318 (around 64%) of Harrington's sample of 497 belonged to the Registrar General's Social Classes 4 and 5. However, even as early as 1968, some soccer hooligans came from higher up the social scale. Thus, 50, or just over 10% of Harrington's sample were skilled manual workers and a further 19, just under 4% were salesmen or clerical workers. That is to say, around 14% of Harrington's sample belonged to the Registrar General's Social Class 3. Two were even employed in a professional or managerial capacity and so qualify for membership of the Registrar General's Social Classes 1 or 2.

Table 1. Occupations of convicted soccer hooligans

Occupation	Number
School or apprentice	79
Unskilled/labourer	206
Semi-skilled	112
Skilled	50
Salesman/clerical	19
Professional and managerial	2
Not known or unemployed	29
Total	497

The findings of Trivizas (1980) were broadly similar. More particularly, on the basis of data about 520 offences committed in 'football crowd events' in the Metropolitan Police Area during the years 1974-1976, he found that 68.1% of those charged with soccer-related offences were manual workers, the majority being apprentices: 12% of football offences were committed by unemployed persons and 10% by schoolboys. Only 8 soccer-related offences were committed by people in 'intermediate occupations', 6 by students, 3 by individuals in professional occupations and 3 by members of the armed forces.

Table 2. Social class membership of West Ham's 'Inter City Firm' (Registrar General's classification)

Class	No's	%
1. Professional, etc.	0	0.0
2. Intermediate	8*	5.6
3. Skilled non-manual	2	1.4
Skilled manual	34	23.8
4. Partly skilled	10	7.0
5. Unskilled	25**	22.4
Unemployed	32	22.4
Unclassifiable	32***	22.4
Total	143	

* Includes a bank manager and the manager of a clothing store.

** Includes 14 bouncers.

*** Includes 10 rock musicians, all of whom were non-professional, 12 ticket touts and 6 members of the armed forces.

That the kind of occupational and social class distribution of soccer hooligans discovered by Harrington in 1968 and by Trivizas for

1974-1976 continues, broadly speaking, to hold good is suggested by the analysis of the social origins of 143 members of West Ham United's 'Inter City Firm' that we carried out in 1985 (Table 2).

It is interesting to note that 32 (22.4%) of our ICF sample were unemployed at the time of the research. This compares with the 29, or just under 6%, of Harrington's sample who were classified as 'not known or unemployed', and with the 12% of the soccer-related offences reported by Trivizas as committed by persons who were unemployed. These figures provide a clear reflection of the generally increasing rate of unemployment since the 1960's.

The Registrar General's classification, of course, is neither precise nor unproblematic as a measure of social class. However, more qualitative assessments of the social origins of soccer hooligans point broadly in the same direction. Harrington, for example, concluded that 'the present evidence suggests that they are mainly from a working class background with the special problems inherent in large industrial cities and ports where violent and delinquent sub-cultures are known to exist. Some youths behave on the terraces in ways which are not unfamiliar to them in the streets around their slum houses.' Harrison's (1974) account of Cardiff City's 'committed rowdies' paints a similar picture. He had them coming from ' '... Canton and Grangetown, rows of terraced houses with few open spaces, and from Llanrumney, a massive council estate with an appalling record of vandalism.' Although Marsh and his colleagues (1978) did not directly address the issue of class background in their study of Oxford fans, some of their informants did provide relevant comments. For example, one of them is reported as having said:-

'If you live up on the Leys (a local council estate), then you have to fight or else people piss you about and think you're a bit soft or something.'

In fact, over half the large contingent of Oxford fans arrested during serious disturbances at the Coventry City-Oxford United FA Cup match in January, 1981, came from the estate in question (Oxford Mail, 9 January, 1981). Evidence from Leicester supports this general picture. Of the 428 local persons arrested at Filbert Street between January, 1976 and April, 1980, 200 (46.7%) came from eight Leicester council estates and 87 (43.5%) of these came from one estate alone - 'West Kingsley'. This was the estate where we conducted the fieldwork part of our original research in 1980 and 1981. Of the 23 'Kingsley lads' - chosen because they were in the 18-30 age group and into 'the football action' - 5 were skilled manual workers (Social Class 3); 7 were partly skilled (Social Class 4), 3 were unskilled (Social Class 5), and 8, at the time of the research, were unemployed.

The currently available data thus suggest that, whilst soccer hooligans are recruited from all levels in the class hierarchy, the overwhelming majority come from the manual sections of Social Class 3 and from Classes 4 and 5. The data also suggest that this sort of distribution has remained remarkably stable since the problem of soccer hooliganism first began to reach its current levels in the late 1960's. Within this stable pattern, only the proportion of soccer hooligans who are unemployed has shown a steady tendency to rise. More particularly, the data of Harrington in the 1960's, of Trivizas for the 1970's and our own for the 1980's, all suggest that the majority of soccer hooligans come from towards the bottom of the social scale. A much smaller and relatively stable proportion is recruited from around the middle and an even smaller, equally stable one from the top. This suggests that popular ideas about the causes of soccer hooliganism, particularly the contradictory ideas that it is caused, on the one hand, by unemployment, and on the other hand, by affluence, are pretty wide of the mark.

A Critique of Some Popular Explanations of Soccer Hooliganism

On its own, the fact that soccer hooliganism in England began to reach its current levels in the 1960's, a time when unemployment rates, including rates of male youth unemployment, were, by current standards, very low, is enough to show that there is no simple relationship between soccer hooliganism and unemployment. Similarly, the evidence suggests that, throughout the 1960's, 70's and 80's a small but relatively stable proportion of football hooligans have come from affluent, middle-class backgrounds. Perhaps the idea that the 'affluent' or 'bourgeois' hooligan is now general is based on a superficial and erroneous response to the replacement of the 'soccer skinheads' by the 'soccer casuals'? Perhaps it is bolstered, too, by the apparent affluence of fans who are able to engage in hooliganism abroad (Williams *et al*., 1984). All the systematic evidence, however, suggests that the majority of soccer hooligans come from Social Classes 4 and 5 and that a smaller but nonetheless sizeable proportion come from the manual sections of Social Class 3. What is it about the experience of being working class, especially of coming from the lower levels of that class, that has made fighting at soccer an attractive proposition over the last twenty years? This issue raises complex problems of sociological interpretation and only a few of them are touched on in this paper. Of necessity, the present discussion will have, to a degree, to be abstract and schematic.

The Sociogenesis of Soccer Hooliganism

At the outset, it is important to repeat that the fighting propensities of males from the lower levels of the working class express a variant of the masculinity norms that remain dominant in British society and many others besides. That is to say, British males *generally* are expected to fight and show physical courage in specific situations. However, whilst the dominant norms lay stress on defensive fighting and the display of aggressive prowess in socially legitimate contexts such as sport, the military and the police, the soccer hooligans have norms which involve, to a far greater extent, the granting of prestige to males who initiate fights in public. That is to say, 'hard men', males who adhere to what one might call an 'aggressive masculine style', tend to be accorded respect, sometimes tinged with a degree of fear and awe, in the social circles from which the soccer hooligans principally come. That tends to be especially the case when they show courage and fighting prowess on behalf either of their mates or, as they see it, the local community. This helps to explain why they often see themselves as 'battling', for example, for Liverpool or Leicester and, when they are abroad, for England. It also helps to explain why they sometimes find it difficult to understand the local and national opprobrium that is heaped upon their exploits.

The prestige that accrues to such males from their peers on account of their fighting helps to explain why fighting is enjoyable for them. Because it receives peer-group support, fighting is, for them, a source of positive self-regard and it tends not to be associated with the arousal of guilt-feelings to the extent that tends to be characteristic of the members of higher social classes. Why is that the case? What is it about the lower levels of the working class and the way they are integrated into the wider society that explains the recurrent generation among them of aggressive masculinity as a dominant characteristic?

The first thing to note in this connection is that, because their norms and standards tend to deviate in certain ways from those that are dominant in society at large, the sections of the working class from which the soccer hooligans are principally recruited can be described as 'relatively unincorporated.' Another term for describing them would be the 'rougher working class.' Such a term is appropriate because it captures the pattern of aggressive masculinity that tends to be characteristic of their dominant males.

The pattern of aggressive masculinity of the 'rougher', relatively unincorporated sections of the working class appears to have two fundamental social sources. It appears to derive from:- i) specific aspects of a culture and pattern of social organization that tend to be found most frequently and in their clearest forms in lower working class communities. (One of the manifestations of this is the recurrent formation of male adolescent 'streetcorner gangs'); (ii) from certain consequences that tend to flow from the relative poverty of the lower working class and from their occupancy of positions at or near the bottom of the social scale.

As Suttles (1968) has noted, one of the dominant features of most lower working class communities is the single-sex male peer group or 'streetcorner gang'. Such gangs tend to develop out of the high levels of age-group segregation and segregation of the sexes that tend to characterise lower working class communities. Their formation is reinforced by the strong, narrow bonds of local identification usually formed by lower working class people. This works in the following way. Age-group segregation tends to involve, as one of its components, a pattern of sending children into the streets to play, unsupervised by adults, at an early age. Such a pattern is exacerbated by poverty, cramped living conditions and a variety of domestic pressures. For its part, segregation of the sexes is conducive to a higher than usual level of objectification of each other by the sexes, particularly on the part of males. It also involves a tendency for girls, by adolescence, to be drawn into the home. Some, however, form aggressive gangs of their own or, to the extent that they are tolerated, simply 'hang around' the groups of boys. One of the consequences of this overall pattern is that adolescent males in such communities are left largely to their own devices. As a result, they tend to band into groups that are determined, on the one hand, by ties of kinship and close or common residence, and on the other, by the threat posed by the development of parallel gangs in adjacent communities. But why do such gangs fight and what part do they play in the production and reproduction of aggressive masculinity?

One of the crucial social structural determinants of the aggressive masculinity of the 'rougher', relatively unincorporated sections of the working class is the comparative freedom from adult control experienced by such working class children and adolescents. More particularly, the fact that so much of their early socialization takes place on the street in the company mainly of their age peers means that such children and adolescents tend to interact roughly with each other and to develop dominance hierarchies in which age, strength and physical prowess are crucial determinants. Such a pattern seems to emerge, in part, because children generally are dependent on adult controls for the chance to develop stable internalized restraints over aggressive behaviour. Where adult controls are lacking or applied only intermittently, there are few direct and immediate checks on the emergence of dominance hierarchies of this kind.

Such dominance hierarchies do not only operate in lower working class neighbourhoods but also in the informal life of schools. Above all, they are operative in the playground where ability to fight is one of the crucial determinants of relative prestige and power. In the formal life of schools, of course, such tendencies are a source of perpetual tension and conflict with the school authorities (Willis, 1977).

The socialization into relatively aggressive norms and standards that takes place in the streets and schools of lower working class communities, especially among males, also tends to be reinforced by the socialization many children in such communities receive at home. At that level in the social hierarchy, parental controls are more likely to take what Bernstein (1971) called a 'positional' than a 'personal' form. That is, they are likely to involve invocation of the status of parent and to be punitive and violent as opposed to nominally egalitarian, persuasive and discursive. Lower working class male children are also likely to be presented with local adult role models that involve more violent behaviour than is sanctioned in the wider society and perhaps to be more receptive than most children higher up the social scale to the violent role models depicted by the media. But why is that the case? In particular, what is it about the culture and social structure of lower working class communities that leads many of their adult males to continue the relatively aggressive patterns of behaviour that are instilled in them from an early age?

In approaching this aspect of the problem, reference has crucially to be made to the position of the lower working class in the wider society. Several aspects of this position lead to the production and reproduction over time of a sub-culture which is in many respects more violent than the parent culture from which it stems. For example, the relative poverty and economic insecurity of the lower working class are conducive to violence because of the frustration they engender and because, especially in more disorganized lower working class neighbourhoods, they contribute to a reduction in people's capacity to identify with others (Parker, 1974). The relatively low levels of formal education that their members typically achieve are conducive to a greater degree of violence and aggressiveness, too. For most of them, school is an alien environment and relatively few learn in that setting to defer gratification and to strive continuously in order to reach long-term educational and occupational goals. Their values tend to be inimical to education and characterised by what one might call a 'present-centred fatalism'. As a result, they experience formal organizations such as schools as threatening and hostile. The contrast between the relative freedom of the streets and the restrictive controls and regulations of the school is particularly significant in this regard. They also react against schools on account of the educational stress on the abstract and intellectual as opposed to the immediate, the concrete and the physical, regarding the former as 'effeminate' and only the latter as in strict conformity with the ideals of masculinity they espouse.

If they manage to find employment on leaving school, they tend to be employed in unskilled and partly skilled manual jobs that do not demand for their performance a high level of intellectually and emotionally demanding self-control. That is, the occupations they tend to be employed in are usually routinized and repetitive, and do not demand high levels of skill, initiative, judgement and responsibility. They usually stand at or near the bottom of the authority hierarchies of these occupations, too. Moreover, cultures that lay stress on *macho* masculinity have usually developed in conjunction with such occupations and, to the extent that they participate in them, the aggressive tendencies of lower working class males will tend to be reinforced.

Such tendencies will be further reinforced by the pattern of male-female segregation and the general male dominance that tend to characterize lower working class communities. Under such conditions, males will not be systematically subject to 'softening' female pressure. Indeed, to the extent that lower working class females grow up to be relatively violent themselves and to expect such behaviour from their men, the violent tendencies of the latter will be reinforced. Further reinforcement comes from the relative frequency of feuds and vendettas between families, neighbourhoods and, above all, streetcorner gangs.

It is easy in a theoretical characterization such as this to convey the idea that lower working class males are violent all the time. That, of course, is not the case. They are, however, more liable to resort to violence and physical intimidation more openly and frequently than males from higher up the social scale. That is largely because they are typically faced from early in life with higher levels of violence and have to learn how to 'handle themselves'. More particularly, they are faced with the regular erruption of violence from a variety of sources: when they are children, from their parents; as they grow up, from their peers in the street and at school; as adolescents, from gangs in their own and from neighbouring communities; as young adults, in *macho* sub-cultures at work and from prowling gangs on their nights 'downtown'; and on

Saturdays, from invading 'fighting crews' who support a visiting soccer team. Of course, in most of these settings, because they tend to deviate in public from dominant social standards, they are liable to experience rough treatment at the hands of the police.

Sociologically, one can say that these relatively unincorporated, 'rougher' working class communities are characterized by feedback processes which result in the regular production of aggressive masculinity. The fact that people have to adapt to a higher than usual level of violence is reflected in their norms and values. These lay stress on being able to 'handle oneself' and have as one of their effects, the conferral of prestige on males who can fight. Correlatively, because it is associated with the conferral of ego-enhancing prestige from their peers, there is a tendency for such males to develop a deep interest in fighting, to see it as a central source of meaning, gratification and exciting emotional arousal. A central difference between these 'rougher' sections of the working class and their more 'respectable' counterparts in the upper, middle and working classes appears to be that, whilst in the latter violence in face-to-face relations tends to be normatively condemned, in the former it tends to a greater degree to be normatively sanctioned and rewarded. A further difference is that there is a tendency in the 'respectable' classes for violence to be 'pushed behind the scenes', to take, on balance, a 'rational' or 'instrumental' form and to be associated with the arousal of guilt. By contrast, among members of the 'rougher' working class, violence tends to occur to a greater extent in public and to take, on balance, an 'expressive' or 'affectual' form. As such, it tends to be associated to a greater extent with pleasurable feelings and to be sought after on that account. Finally, the aggressive tendencies of males from the more 'respectable' classes tend to find expression in avenues such as formal sport which are legitimate in terms of currently dominant values. Alternatively, they tend to be sublimated by being channelled into competition in the educational and occupational spheres. Members of the 'rougher' working class, however, tend to reject formal sport as too regulated and tame. Or, if and when they do take part, they tend to be castigated for being overly rough.

References

Bernstein, B. (1971) Class, Codes and Control: Theoretical Studies towards a Sociology of Language. Vol. 1, London: Routledge and Kegan Paul.

Elias, N. and Dunning, E. (1986) Quest for Excitement: Sport and Leisure in the Civilizing Process. Oxford: Basil Blackwell.

Harrington, J., (1968): Soccer Hooliganism. Bristol, John Wright.

Harrison, P. (1974) Soccer's tribal wars. New Soc.,29, 602-4.

Marsh, P., Rosser, E. and Harre, R., (1978) The Rules of Disorder. London: Routledge and Kegan Paul.

Parker, H.J. (1974) View from the Boys: a Sociology of Downtown Adolescents. Newton Abbot: David and Charles.

Suttles, G. (1968) The Social Order of the Slum. Chicago: University of Chicago Press.

Taylor, E. (1984) I was a soccer hooligan, class of '64. The

Guardian, 28 March.
Trivizas, E. (1980) Offences and offenders in football crowd disorders, Brit. J. Crim., 20, 276-88.
Williams, J., Dunning, E. and Murphy, P. (1984) Hooligans Abroad: The Behaviour and Control of English Fans in Continental Europe. London: Routledge and Kegan Paul.
Willis, P. (1977) Learning to Labour. London: Routledge and Kegan Paul.

SECTARIANISM AND SOCCER HOOLIGANISM IN NORTHERN IRELAND

J. Sugden and A. Bairner
University of Ulster, Jordanstown, Shore Road, Newtownabbey, Co. Antrim, Northern Ireland.

Introduction

Soccer is played and watched with passion throughout the world. While English soccer supporters tend to hold the headlines, incidents involving crowd disorder seem to occur wherever the game is played and patronised. In continental Europe, particularly in the North, forms of spectator violence similar to the English experience are on the increase. In the last few years in the Soviet Union and China popular disturbances at soccer matches have led to punitive government intervention (Williams, 1986). Likewise, Latin America has a long history of soccer-centred civil unrest. In the emergent countries of black Africa the development of the game has been hindered by tribal rivalries manifesting themselves through violent confrontation in and around soccer stadia (Monnington, 1986). While examples of soccer violence can be found throughout the world the forms it takes and the conditions which generate it tend to vary from region to region and from culture to culture. To verify this proposition we can look to Northern Irleand where patterns of football support and soccer hooliganism are bound up with the same social and political conditions which continue to fuel the province's sectarian divisions (Sugden and Bairner, 1986).

In February 1985 both of the authors stood in the rain on the terraces of Windsor Park in Belfast and watched England gain a narrow victory over Northern Ireland by 1-0 in a World Cup qualifier. The Northern Irish team lined up in green and white but it was the Union Flag, the Cross of St. George and the Red Hand of Ulster which dominated the favours of home supporters. Not that this indicated a warm welcome for the English visitors. On the contrary, the emergence of the Anglo-Irish Agreement, a treaty giving the Eire government in Dublin limited say in the institutional arrangements of government in the province, had incensed the local Protestant population whose flags and emblems were more a testimony of loyalty to the crown of King William III than a sign of fidelity to the current British government. Before the match began, dressed as John Bull, England's self-appointed mascot and cheer leader met with a torrent of abuse and a hail of missiles as he approached the enclosure dominated by the Ulster supporters. No doubt had they been there in numbers local Catholics might have joined in the abuse of a revered British symbol, albeit for different reasons. But, despite being only a walking distance away from the predominantly Catholic west Belfast area, there was little evidence of Catholic support in the ground. This is hardly surprising since Windsor Park is sited in the heart of a staunchly loyalist Protestant community and is itself the home stadium of Linfield, the city's only exclusively Protestant soccer organisation. Shortly before the final whistle a bomb planted by the Irish National Liberation Army exploded in a nearby street, delaying the departure of the disgruntled crowd. This scene was repeated 18 months later in April 1987 when the two sides met in a European Nations Cup qualifier. Threats of rocket attacks, sectarian violence on the terraces and an IRA car-bomb reinforced the message to the English soccer authorities and the British government that sporting encounters are not immune from the 'Troubles' in Northern Ireland.

The Setting

For those who are not familiar with the complexities of Northern Irish social and political culture it is necessary to make a few introductory remarks. After more than a century of political and armed struggle, culminating in the Easter Rising in Dublin in 1916, the British government was pressured into granting independence to most of Ireland. Despite extreme resistance from Irish nationalists an exception was made for the six counties of Northern Ireland, of which two thirds of the population were Protestant and vehemently loyal to the British Crown. In 1921 the Irish Free State was established as the country was partitioned, leaving most of Ulster as a province of the United Kingdom and holding within its borders a large minority population of Irish nationalists, most easily identified by their affiliation to Catholicism.

Since Partition, while the Free State, albeit with one eye on Ulster, has gradually settled down to the business of self-government, Northern Ireland has become increasingly divided. Simmering resentments exploded in the late 1960s after a series of pro-Catholic civil rights marches in Belfast and Londonderry. Organised peaceful protest against discrimination in jobs and housing soon gave way to widespread inter-community conflict as Loyalists mobilised themselves against what they identified as a renewed struggle for Irish nationalism in the North. This prompted the introduction of British troops into Ulster and at the same time stimulated the return and growth of para-military and terrorist organisations on both sides of the divide. Increasingly, through the 1970s and the 1980s the sticks and stones of the mobs have given way to bombs, snipers' bullets and high profile state security. Thus we have the current situation in Northern Ireland where civil unrest has become institutionalised as the 'Troubles'; two communities, for the most part sharing the same social and commercial space, endeavouring to live out routine lives in the face of an undercurrent of deep mutual mistrust and deadly sectarian violence. It is in this context that soccer is played and supported in Northern Ireland.

Soccer in Northern Ireland

There are three forms of football played in Ireland as a whole, Gaelic, Rugby Union and soccer. Of these only Gaelic football can claim to be native to Ireland. Both rugby football and soccer came to the country in the nineteenth century through British influence. Centred around Belfast the Irish League was formed in 1890 and only gradually did the game expand into other parts of Ireland, most notably in Leinster, the second most anglophile province in the country. For a time, at least, the game was organised nationally and was open to all, regardless of regional, cultural or political affiliations. This harmony, however, was short lived.

Partition in 1921 and the setting up of an Irish Free State prompted the Leinster FA to break from the parent body. From then on, soccer was organised separately in Ireland with the League of Ireland and the Football Association of Ireland (FAI) responsible for the sport in the Republic and the Irish League and the Irish Football Association (IFA) as governing bodies north of the border (Brodie, 1980). While relations between the IFA and the FAI are now more cordial than at any time since 1922, the political division remains and despite, or because of, the Anglo-Irish Agreement the pooling of resources for international competition, whilst regularly discussed, appears unlikely to mature in the present political climate.

For the Record - Belfast Celtic

Belfast Celtic, established in 1891, was closely modelled on its namesake in Glasgow which has traditionally held strong Irish-Catholic affiliations. In fact its first game was on a relined Gaelic Football pitch. The early history of Belfast Celtic is littered with instances of crowd disturbance particularly during games with the city's leading 'unionist' sides, Linfield and Glentoran. As its name suggests, despite an open recruitment policy, there was no denying the nationalist orientation of Celtic and the volatile political situation in the province before the First World War led club officials to consider withdrawing from the Irish League. Further trouble followed in the wake of the 1916 Easter Rising and in the charged atmosphere leading up to Partition. In 1920 over eighty people were injured when shots were fired into the crowd by security forces at a cup replay between Glentoran and Celtic after the latter team's supporters waved banners and sang songs in support of an independent and united Ireland. As Tuohy (1978) observed 'this stupid outburst left a huge stain on Celtic's reputation since they were held responsible'. The club withdrew from league competition for four seasons but returned in 1924 after approaches by influential members of the Irish soccer fraternity whose action helped to sustain in the short term the League's apolitical image.

Partition meant that, in the long term, Celtic would be the side looked to by many whose loyalties were directed towards the Irish Free State and would be increasingly perceived by the Unionist population as a sporting symbol of the enemy within. This came to a head in 1948 when during the Boxing Day fixture between Linfield and

Celtic at Windsor Park an accidental clash between Jimmy Jones (Celtic) and Bob Bryson (Linfield) resulted in the latter being stretchered off with a broken ankle. At the end of the game Linfield supporters invaded the pitch and in the ensuing violence Jones' leg was broken. As Tuohy reported 'a mob stampeded across the Park thirsting for the blood of Celtic players'. Celtic officials decided that under such circumstances they could no longer continue to function and the club went out of existence in 1949.

Soccer and the 'Troubles'

The impact of sectarianism on professional soccer has been exaggerated during the current "Troubles". In 1972, at the height of the civil unrest, Distillery Football Club, was obliged to abandon its home ground, Grosvenor Park, because of its sensitive location on the dividing line between two communities in west Belfast. In the same year for security reasons Derry City was forced to withdraw from the Irish League. Derry's misfortunes began with the first riots in the city. The violence which attended the team's matches at the Brandywell on the fringe of the predominantly republican Bogside area, particularly against those from clearly Protestant communities, added to the security forces' difficulties. Escorting thousands of loyalist supporters through the nationalist controlled streets of 'Free Derry' developed as a major military operation for the RUC (Royal Ulster Constabulary) and the army. The matter came to a head in 1971 in events surrounding a fixture with Ballymena United. As Edmund Curran reported in the Belfast Telegraph:

> 'The now customary riot went on nearby to such an extent that there was more noise from the Army's rubber bullets than from the referee's whistle. Ballymena United scored the only goal of the match but lost their coach which was towed off and given a Bogside burning.'

Three days after this incident the club's directors announced that they were moving out of the Brandywell and would play the rest of their home matches in 'neutral' Coleraine. Although Londonderry's 'no-go' areas were theoretically brought to an end by the British Army's 'Operation Motorman', practical considerations by other Irish League clubs and security forces meant that, within the present political environment, there could be no return for senior soccer to the Brandywell. Crippling debts incurred while playing home fixtures elsewhere persuaded the club's officials to suspend operations completely.

Recently senior soccer in Northern Ireland's second city has been revived, but only through an unprecedented arrangement whereby Derry City has been admitted to the Dublin based League of Ireland. Currently playing in the second division, Derry's home crowds of 10000-15000 are the envy of the major clubs both north and south of the border. Despite attracting relatively large numbers of supporters, to date Derry's games have been free from any serious crowd trouble. Significantly the RUC does not maintain a presence during matches at the Brandywell. Crowd control is effected by club officials and it is widely believed that a record of good behaviour is encouraged by the various nationalist organisations who have a stake in maintaining an image of Irish autonomy in certain quarters of the city. According to the RUC, who are observing the situation closely, the real test of this experiment in community self-control will come next season when Derry City, having been promoted to the League of Ireland's Premier division, meet the representative clubs of the Republic's main cities which, unlike Derry's current opponents, have large numbers of supporters.

More recently, in the absence of other clubs with obviously Catholic roots, most of the nationalist soccer support has been directed towards the north Belfast team, Cliftonville. In terms of ownership, administration and players, Cliftonville would appear to be neither Catholic or Protestant. However, because its ground, Solitude, is located close to a predominantly Catholic area the club has been appropriated by the locals as the symbolically Catholic team: so much so that, reminiscent of the days of Belfast Celtic and Derry City, on the insistence of the Irish League and the RUC, for a decade or more, Cliftonville has had to play its home fixtures against rivals Linfield at that club's own ground, Windsor Park. This is done, even though it is roundly acknowledged that a hard core of Linfield supporters is responsible for most of the crowd trouble. It is the prospect of droves of Protestant supporters trekking through nationalist north Belfast on route to Solitude which renders such encounters unacceptable in terms of security and not the violent reputation of the Cliftonville fans.

In fact, serious trouble has attended only a few of Cliftonville's games, including one at Seaview against Crusaders after loyalist supporters disrupted the match. In the 1978 IFA Cup Final, once more trouble broke out between Cliftonville fans and loyalists purporting to support opponents, Portadown, necessitating the intervention of the police in full riot gear. Off the field, as reported in the Belfast Telegraph, Unionist politicians have protested at the behaviour of the Cliftonville supporters who, they allege, act as cover for politically motivated Republican troublemakers who intimidate Protestant residents by shouting pro-IRA slogans.

In 1984, during a home 'friendly' against Glasgow Celtic, confrontations between sections of the crowds and the Royal Ulster Constabulary led to violent clashes. On the Sunday before the match, Sean Downes had been killed by a plastic bullet fired by a member of the RUC at a Republican rally attended by Martin Galvin, spokesman for the American fund-raising organisation, NORAID. Only a few days later, in the wake of this incident, the presence of a large contingent of the RUC at a soccer fixture which inevitably attracted an almost exclusively Catholic support acted as a focus for rage and retribution for nationalist elements in the crowd.

While a history of confronting civil unrest and terrorism means that the RUC is better equipped, better informed and more experienced in techniques of crowd control than its English counterparts, the generally unstable situation in the provinces forces them to adopt a 'softly-softly' approach through which serious disturbances at football matches are largely played down. Indeed with the emergence of the Anglo-Irish Agreement and the role the RUC has played in quelling loyalist resistance to it, the police are increasingly becoming the focus of rage and retribution for elements of both communities. Recently, during encounters between Linfield and Cliftonville, the RUC has come under attack from both sets of supporters who remain otherwise bitterly divided. The problems faced by the police are clearly illustrated by disturbances which took place during the last encounter between these two teams (24.1.87). As reported in the Sunday News the following day, a larger than usual crowd of home supporters taunted both the Cliftonville players and the RUC throughout the game. Missiles were thrown and ball-bearings catapulted, one of which struck and felled the Cliftonville keeper who finished the game in a dazed condition. According to the police such attacks are organised and carried out by a cadre of no more than 150 dedicated Linfield hooligans, most of whom are known to them. However, because of the sensitive position of the police within the current webbing of Northern Irish politics, it was calculated that the risks to general security would have increased dramatically if officers had been dispatched into the crowd to arrest the culprits. Instead, they chose to contain the crowd at arm's length even though it meant sustaining several injuries within their own ranks.

While it would be a mistake to draw from all this that the affiliations which surround certain clubs and the crowd problems which beset senior soccer in the province can be explained simply and exclusively in terms of sectarian division, for the most part it is impossible to understand even inter-Protestant soccer rivalry without reference to the wider political context. For example, following a pattern established throughout British soccer, the most serious crowd trouble at any match held in Northern Ireland in the 1980s took place on April 30, 1983 during and after the cup final between two staunchly Protestant clubs - Glentoran of east Belfast and Linfield in the west of the city. In this particular case regionalism and sectarianism are interwoven as the 'Blue Men' of Linfield at every opportunity stress their sectarian purity as supporters of a club with an exclusively Protestant playing and administrative staff. For their part the Glentoran supporters, even though most are in all other respects loyalist and Protestant, are prepared to invert this image and goad their rivals during football confrontations by mimicking Catholic rituals. This sort of behaviour by loyalists can be understood only in terms of the special relationship between Linfield and Glentoran. The peculiar position of the latter is underlined by the threats of certain Protestant paramilitary organisations concerned with this "Protestant" club's willingness to play Catholics and employ Catholic officials.

Conclusion

Northern Ireland is beset by industrial decline, inner-city decay, massive youth unemployment and a range of social problems which are held in common with depressed regions of the British mainland and are theorised as being germane to the root causes of soccer hooliganism. However, while divisions based on class, region, age and opportunity are important, the most potent force of group solidarity is religious labelling and it is this, more than anything else, which determines the patterns of football support and crowd trouble in the province. The fact that crowd trouble at Windsor Park does not grab as much media attention as it does at Old Trafford does not mean soccer hooliganism is ignored in Northern Ireland. It is simply that on a scale from mortar bombs to assassinations, a skirmish at a soccer match hardly registers.

Acknowledgement

The authors acknowledge the achives of the following newspapers which provided soccer material for this work: Belfast Telegraph; Fortnight; Irish Times; Newsletter; Sunday News.

References

Brodie, M. (1980) 100 Years of Irish Football. Belfast: Blackstaff.

Monnington, T. (1986) The politics of black African sport. In: The Politics of Sport (edited by L. Allison). Manchester: Manchester University Press.

Sugden, J. and Bairner, A. (1986) Observe the sons of Ulster. In: Off the Ball (edited by A. Tomlinson and G. Whannel). London: Pluto.

Tuohy, M. (1978) Belfast Celtic. Belfast: Blackstaff.

Williams, J. (1986) White riot. In: Off the Ball (edited by A. Tomlinson and G. Whannel). London: Pluto.

AGGRESSIVE PLAY AND AGGRESSIVE BEHAVIOUR IN PROFESSIONAL SOCCER

G. Gerisch and A. Kosel
Deutsche Sporthochschule Köln, Institut für Sportspiele, Carl-Diem-Weg 2, D-5000 Köln 41, West Germany.

Introduction

In spite of extensive research into aggression in sporting contexts knowledge is still lacking in this area. In particular this is the case with soccer, where the phenomenon of aggression occurs in various forms and at different levels of competition. The lack of a theoretical frame of reference has resulted in a variety of definitions of the concept of aggression and multitude of methodological approaches. In previous research differing views on the origins and the amplifying circumstances of aggressive behaviour have been well documented (Dennert et al., 1976; Gabler, 1976; Pilz and Trebels, 1976). Theories based on instinctual and ethological concepts or social-learning at first glance seem incompatible, although the viewpoint of integrative learning (based on socialization and hereditary dispositions) may possibly supply a powerful explanatory model. Such a model must be based on a clear definition of the concept of aggression.

The present study has two main aims. Firstly, an attempt to understand what 'aggressive play' means to professional players, coaches and referees is presented. Secondly, an investigation is undertaken which purports to examine how these groups associated with professional soccer perceive behaviour during competition. The hypothesis is that due to differing interests, needs and roles within the three groups, rule interpretation will significantly differ, reflecting an inability to maintain an objective outlook on Rule 12 of the FIFA book of laws governing aggressive behaviour in soccer.

The methodology of the study used as a base a definition of aggressive behaviour which encompasses any action in which a person intends to harm another in a physical or psychological way such that pain or insult may result (Gabler, 1976). It is clear that the media and coaches often use the term 'aggressive play' in a positive sense signifying high drive or willingness to fight hard for a result. Therefore, it is necessary to differentiate between instrumental and destructive aggression (the former a means to an end and the latter gratuitous violence) and a third type of behaviour which may be defined as aggressive on the basis of a bellicose, dynamic form of competitive, albeit rule-conforming, action.

Method

Subjects belonged to three different groups associated with professional soccer in West Germany: players of the Bundesliga Divisions 1 and 2 (n = 64), coaches with DFB-licences for the 1st Division level (n = 47) and referees qualified to arbitrate at the level of Divisions 1 and 2 (n = 46).

A standardised interview with 133 questions was given to all subjects.

Results and Discussion

A factor matrix was provided for the groups of players and the coaches which resulted in four factors being significantly differentiated. These were sport-specific tactical and physical competitive actions, sport-specific physical actions, unfair competitive actions and approved competitive actions. For referees, differentiation on only three factors was significant - sport-specific competitive actions, unfair competitive actions and approved competitive actions (Table 1).

Table 1. Definitions of aggressive play in professional soccer by players, coaches and referees

Factors	Players	Coaches	Referees
Sport-specific tactical-physical competitive actions	(4.47) Rule-conforming hard physical actions to pressurize opponent	(3.60) (as players)	-
Unfair Competitive Actions	(4.15) Psychologically-based disorderly strategies to provoke or intimidate opponent	(4.27) (as players)	(5.15) (as players)
Sport-specific physical competitive actions	(2.06) Harsh physical challenges (rule conforming) to dominate opponent	(2.96) (as players)	(5.35) (as players)
Approved competitive actions	(1.91) Regular measures and strategies to emphasise dominance of opponent (Psycholigically-based)	(2.06) (as players)	(2.07) (as players)

Factor loadings are given in parentheses

There are clear distinctions in the hierarchy of importance attached to factors which were significantly differentiated in the interview data. In all three groups there was a clear-cut crystallisation between rule-conforming and rule-offending means and strategies in competitive action. For coaches aggressive play was best characterised by pressurising the opposition as a team, although they are more likely to condone behaviour seen as aggressive by referees if an important goal is to be achieved.

Challenging for the ball and concentrating on attacking the opposition are key features of this type of instrumental aggression. With the exception of one item, the opinion of the referees on aggressive play differed considerably from those of the players and coaches. Behaviour such as provocation, threats and foul play did not meet the criteria for aggressive play, especially by the players. Players and coaches are more likely to see fouling as an acceptable form of 'discouraging' the opposition than referees (Table 2).

A high percentage of the 24 items were considered as aggressive or very aggressive by all three groups (n = 13). The items mainly described physical actions which are painful and harmful to an opponent and also include harsh unsporting behaviour such as spitting, threatening and verbally insulting. High grade aggression was agreed upon by all three groups as kicking, hitting and spitting. Bumping into an opponent did not merit a definition as aggressive and it is interesting that other actions which did not involve direct physical contact were not merited as aggressive. For example, the act of faking a foul in order to gain advantage was not considered as aggressive. The indication is that the danger of injury is a primary motivating factor in estimating the element of aggression in any action in soccer. It is possibly for this reason

Table 2. Significant differences in median factor values for players, coaches and referees in estimating 'aggressive play'

Types of Behaviour	Player(G1)	Coach(G2)	Referee(G3)	Significant differences
1.Great physical action	1.94	1.79	2.50	G1,G2*G3
2.Disguised foul play	4.84	4.70	3.85	G1,G2*G3
3.Obstruction	1.66	1.74	2.63	G1,G2*G3
4.Retaliation	4.17	4.13	5.11	G1,G2*G3
5.Discouraging the opponent through fouls	4.22	4.30	3.33	G1,G2*G3
6.Not giving up the ball	2.25	2.32	3.13	G1,G2*G3
7.Harsh defensive play	2.14	1.98	2.80	G1,G2*G3
8.Wanting to fight down the opponent	2.11	2.15	2.87	G1,G2*G3
9.Not letting the opponent get into the game	2.27	2.36	2.98	G1*G3

that referees generally evaluate most actions in soccer as higher in aggression than do players and coaches. In fact it appears that the role assigned to various groups associated with professional soccer plays an important part in shaping perspectives on action during competitive matches.

References

Dennert, B., Pilz, G. and Trebels, A. (1976). Zur Problematik der Aggressions-forschung. Sportunterricht, 8, 252-262.

Gabler, H. (1976). Aggressive Handlungen im Sport. Ein Beitrag zur theoretischen und empirischen Aggressions forschung. Schorndorf. Hoffman:

Pilz, G., Trebels, A. (1976) Aggression und Konflikt im Sport. Ahrensburg: Cwalina.

PLAYERS' ATTITUDES TO VIOLENCE AND FOUL PLAY IN AMATEUR RUGBY LEAGUE

S. Mellor and W.J. Murphy
Department of Sport and Recreation Studies, Liverpool Polytechnic, Byrom Street, Liverpool L3 3AF, England.

Introduction

In recent years there has been a growing tendency towards over-aggressive and violent play in many sports (Crawford, 1976). This trend may be related to the dominant ethic in many areas of contemporary competitive sport. The ethic is preoccupied with winning and is exemplified in the so-called Lombardian ethic. This product-oriented stance emphasises the importance of winning irrespective of the means or methods used to achieve victory. Players view the opposition as a mere obstacle in the way of victory. As McIntosh (1979, p.102-103) has suggested:

> 'One of the most disturbing features of modern sport, especially contact sports at top level is the permission and even encouragement of behaviour verging on the psychopathic. This is particularly the case in failing to control or reverse the increase in violence in various codes of football.'

Aggression, especially when it generates violent conduct, results in increased injuries in Rugby Union (Hardiker et al., 1981). One of the major problems with both codes of rugby is that the essence of the game is based on physical contact and the aim is to physically dominate the opposition. According to Laidlaw (1973, p.134) 'Rugby is a series of physical confrontations which may be extremely provocative. Nevertheless, if there is discipline the high degree of tension will have an outlet through proper channels'.

The governing bodies of rugby attempt to ensure that the sport is played according to the norms and principles which they as legislators find acceptable. They may try to achieve this objective by compiling appropriate rules, issuing instructions to referees on how to interpret those rules and by giving advice to players concerning behaviour not necessarily covered by specific rules (McIntosh, 1979). An alternative contention is that rugby is not more violent than in previous eras. It appears to be so due to the attention given to certain aspects of the sport by the mass media.

Milgram (1974) has demonstrated experimentally that many people will perform acts which are normally abhorrent to them and which they know to be wrong in obedience to an accepted authority. In the context of sport a coach who encourages foul and violent play is one stage removed from the action. The players who commit offences in these circumstances may regard themselves as mere instruments for carrying out another person's wishes and thus free of responsibility for their own actions.

The current investigation attempted to discover something of the attitudes of the players towards foul play and violence in Rugby League football. Players from a top-class amateur club were chosen as the subjects of the study. It was hoped that the research would give a valuable insight into the attitudes and values of players regarding foul play and violence in Rugby league and that the findings might have certain implications for the prevention of such offences.

Methods

All the subjects were or had been (within the previous two years) players for the 1st and 'A' teams. These teams play in the Premier and First Divisions, respectively, of the North West Counties Amateur Rugby League. The subjects ranged in age from 19 to 45 years old.

A simple questionnaire of ten questions was administered to members of one club on one afternoon during the playing season. The questions were concerned mainly with the players' reaction to certain match situations. They were also concerned with the attitudes of players towards the possibility of on-field outbreaks of violence, the size of suspensions currently imposed for foul play and fighting. They also sought to ascertain whether players had ever been sent off, and if so, for which offence(s). Fifty questionnaires were distributed; forty-two were retrieved for analysis. Two questions attempted to determine whether the players were willing to carry out illegal and violent acts on the orders of a coach.

Results

Responses by the players to each question are expressed in Table 1 and Table 2 as a percentage of the sample, with the total number of responses in parenthesis. The results show a significant trend amongst the players towards foul play and violent conduct, especially when these actions are instrumental (Table 1), that is with the primary goal being the attainment of victory. Consequently, 64% of the players indicated that they would foul an opponent in an obvious scoring position if there was no other way to stop him. Also they may decide to "knock" a dangerous opponent out of the game, while 58% would conceivably start a fight with the opposition if they thought it would help them to win the game. Half of the subjects (50%) said they would injure an opponent or start a fight with the opposition if instructed to do so by the coach (Table 1). Thus, in this instance, Milgram's (1974) suggested transfer of responsibility for such orders to the coach, does not seem to be applicable. This may be due to the fact that the players' own acceptance of the inevitable existence of on-field violence is overwhelming.

Table 1. Attitudes towards violent behaviour and foul play: Questions 1-6

Question/Statement	Response Yes	No	Don't Know
1. An opponent who is in an obvious scoring position must be brought down by a foul tackle (i.e. high tackle or trip) if there is no other way to stop him. Do you agree?	64% (27)	31% (13)	5% (2)
2. Would you ever attempt to get an opponent sent off?	48% (20)	50% (21)	2% (1)
3. Would you ever decide to "knock" a dangerous opponent out of the game (i.e. get him carried off)?	64% (27)	29% (12)	7% (3)
4. If you were instructed by the coach to attempt to injure an opponent would you do so?	50% (21)	36% (15)	14% (6)
5. Would you ever decide to start a fight with the opposition if you thought it would help you to win the game?	58% (24)	31% (13)	11% (5)
6. If you were instructed to start a fight with the oppositon would you do so?	50% (21)	40% (17)	10% (4)

Violence is seen as a means to an end rather than an end in itself as is evidenced by the players' responses, since none of the players considered the possibility of outbreaks of violence to be one of the attractions of Rugby League. Altogether 79% considered it to be an acceptable and inevitable part of the sport, while the remainder regarded it as one of the worst features of the game (Table 2). However, there seemed to be a predominant 'fight fire with fire' attitude amongst the players. Only 10% would appeal to the referee; 14% would ignore the incident if they were the victim of undetected foul or dangerous play while 64% would wait for the next opportunity to 'get even'. A 'hot headed' 12% would seek revenge immediately at the risk of being penalised.

Such attitudes suggest that many of the players adhere to an unwritten code of conduct whereby it is seen to be less acceptable to seek justice via the referee than to apply retribution oneself. This attitude is further supported by comparing the responses to questions 2 and 3. While 48% of players would attempt to get an opponent sent off, a further 64% would try to accomplish the same end by a distinctly more 'macho' method of injuring the player so that he is unable to continue.

Table 2. Attitudes towards violent behaviour and foul play. Questions 7–10

Question/Statement	Response
7. If you were the victim of foul or dangerous play which went undetected by the referee would you:	
(a) appeal to the referee	10% (4)
(b) seek revenge immediately at the risk of being penalised	12% (5)
(c) ignore the incident	14% (6)
(d) wait for the next opportunity to 'get even'	64% (27)
8. Do you consider the possibility of outbreaks of violence during the game to be:	
(a) one of the attractions of Rugby League	0% (0)
(b) an acceptable and inevitable part of Rugby League	79% (33)
(c) one of the worst feature of Rugby League	21% (9)
9. Do you feel that the suspensions currently imposed for foul play and fighting are:	
(a) about right	52% (22)
(b) too harsh	21% (9)
(c) inadequate (should be tougher)	26% (11)
10. Have you ever been sent off:	
(a) no	40% (17)
If yes:	
(b) for foul play	10% (4)
(c) for fighting	14% (6)
(d) for both (b) and (c)	31% (13)
(e) for technical offences	5% (2)

Of the 55% who admitted to being sent off, only 21% regarded the suspensions imposed for such actions as too harsh. The indications are that many players are prepared to accept the consequences of their 'crimes' imposed on them by their governing body, in this case the British Amateur Rugby League Association. Furthermore, many of the players were well aware that their answers would not have been acceptable to anyone in an official capacity as they indicated that they would never be able to play again if the questionnaire "fell into the wrong hands".

Discussion

The individual goals of the players in this club may have led to their attitudes regarding the use of instrumental violence. They may have hoped to maintain their team place or gain promotion to the first team or else attract the attention of professional scouts and may feel, rightly or wrongly, that such conduct can help them fulfil their ambitions.

There are a number of reasons which may help explain why many players are prepared to use foul play and violence as a means of securing victory. It is likely that at some stage in the players' development similar behaviour has resulted in positive reinforcement either by being instrumental in winning or by receiving approval from a peer group (team-mates), coach or spectators. This reinforcement encourages the reoccurrence of such behaviour (Skinner, 1969). Bandura (1969) suggested that aggression can be learnt by observing the appropriate models. Since Rugby League is presented as a hostile, aggressive sport, part of the socialisation process for the game may be to learn to act aggressively and even violently. The players may thus display violent, goal-oriented tendencies because they are expected to do so. It is possible also that many players completed the questionnaire in the way that they felt they were expected to, substituting 'model' answers for their own, possibly more sensitive attitudes.

In the highly competitive rugby environment to which these players belong, it would appear that instrumental violence and foul play may have a function in satisfying their primary objectives of winning. For such players this type of behaviour would, and often does, cease to perform the correct function if it is punished to the extent that it ultimately jeopardises the chances of victory. It would appear that administrators and the match officials are able to eliminate much of this product-oriented violence and foul play by awarding penalties and suspensions of a sufficient magnitude. It must be stressed that the population used may not be indicative of amateur Rugby League as a whole and that players of different standards may well have different attitudes regarding violence and foul play.

The high levels of aggression and often violence generated in sports may have a cathartic effect on providing the participant with a means of releasing tension built up by the frustrations of daily life (Alderman, 1974). However, it would seem that contact sports such as Rugby League provide many opportunities for legalised aggression and 'letting off steam'. The first coaches with whom young players come into contact have a chance to stress the functional, non-violent aggression requirements of the game. By punishing foul and dangerous play and positively reinforcing fair play from an early age the coach may be able to socialize beginners away from the current 'win at all costs' ethic. Unfortunately, the current trend in many areas of contemporary organised children's sport is towards a highly competitive and success-oriented system which encourages such Lombardian values.

Future studies of this type could include the comparison of attitudes to violence and foul play amongst rugby players of different standards, codes, ages and between amateur players and professionals. Any information which can be obtained to explain why players resort to such behaviour may be valuable in helping to understand, analyse and perhaps even solve the problem of on-field violence.

References

Alderman, R. (1974) Psychological Behaviour in Sport. New York: Saunders.

Bandura, A. (1969) Principles of Behaviour Modification. Toronto; Holt, Reinhard and Wilson.

Crawford, S.A.G.M. (1978) New Zealand rugby: vigorous, violent and vicious. Review of Sport and Leisure, 1, 64-84.

Hardiker, R.J., Murphy, W.J. and Shuttleworth, J.J. (1981) Injuries in Rugby Union football. In: Sports Fitness and Sports Injuries (edited by T. Reilly), pp. 115-126. London: Faber and Faber.

Laidlaw, C. (1973) Mud in Your Eye. Wellington: Read.

McIntosh, P. (1979) Fair Play: Ethics in Sport and Education. London: Heinemann.

Milgram, S. (1974) Obedience to Authority: An Experimental View. New York: Harper and Row.

Reilly, T. (1981) Sports Fitness and Sport Injuries. London: Faber and Faber.

Skinner, B.F. (1969) Contingencies of Reinforcement: A Theoretical Analysis. New York: Appleton-Century-Craft.

Part XIV

Management and coaching

SPONSORSHIP: THE DOUBLE EDGED SWORD

Alan Clarke The Faculty of Social Sciences, The Open University, Walton Hall, Milton Keynes, England.
Lawrie Madden Sheffield Wednesday FC., Hillsborough, Sheffield S6 1SW, England.

Introduction

The idea of sponsorship predates the organisation of sports into professional competitions but it has now been developed to the point where it is difficult to think of major events without also naming a leading company who have attached their name to the event. In this country, the only footballing event which does not bear the name of the sponsor is soccer's FA Cup. All the others are covered by new and changing names(Simkins, 1986). This paper seeks to account for the different types of sponsorships found in the different codes of football played in this country, by looking at the national situation and by concentrating on the local experience of South Yorkshire where all the codes are played.

The problem of sponsorship has in the past been addressed in terms of the difficulty experienced in raising increasing amounts of money. We want to approach the issue from a rather different angle and suggest that sponsorship may increase some of the financial problems faced by clubs rather than ease them. Sponsorship provides a welcome source of income to the clubs, but the distribution of this income reinforces some of the differences between the clubs rather than overcoming them. Moreover as an additional form of income, there is a possibility that clubs will become dependent upon that income for the development of the clubs and we see a real danger in that as the clubs and we see a real danger in that as the sponsorship income cannot be guaranteed. This danger is reinforced by the way that most clubs live from week to week, season to season, rather than developing a long term strategy at club level.

The clubs included in this study were from the Budweiser League the Steel City Giants, from the Rugby League Sheffield Eagles and from the Football League Sheffield Wednesday, Sheffield United, Barnsley, Rotherham United and Doncaster Rovers. We would like to thank them for their assistance and have observed their request not to reveal confidential financial information. More detailed figures are available in the clubs' annual reports but often in forms which are quite difficult to unpack. We have, therefore, presented the argument in terms of general principals rather detailed financial analysis of a particular club.

National Sponsorship

The introduction of sponsorship at national level has grown at a rapid rate and the injection of money into the sports has been generally welcomed (Howell, 1983). There has been an interesting difference in the types of company which have secured the national leagues between soccer and the other codes. The Football League has been sponsored by 'Canon' and is currently being sponsored by 'Today'. Canon have said explicitly that their sponsorship was designed to increase the public awareness of Canon goods and to develop that awareness to the full range of products beyond their cameras. As a national newspaper, priding itself on the quality of its soccer coverage Today have similar hopes for their sponsorship. Both codes of Rugby and the more recently established American Football have attracted sponsorship from breweries. The other major sponsors of Rugby League are drawn from the tobacco industry. The growth areas of sponsorship seem increasingly to be the service sector, especially financial services and this is already being felt with the presence of 'Save and Prosper' in the Rugby Union field.

The links between the products and the sport appear to be quite straightforward, especially when the restrictions on the other forms of promoting tobacco are considered. However, the position of breweries in soccer has been complicated by the problem of hooliganism. Not only were the breweries disappointed by the Government's decision to ban the sale of alcohol inside football grounds but they were also deeply concerned at the implications of the argument which blamed much of the hooliganism on the effects of alcohol. Although there was little evidence which would support this hypothesis, there was a collective decision to maintain a low profile at least until the atmosphere was calmer. As a result the breweries did not negotiate any new sponsorships within soccer for the season 1985-86, although Wimbledon attracted sponsorship from Trumans in 1986-87.

It is interesting to note that the larger national deals are usually presented as three or five year packages, allowing some stability to both the sport and the sponsor. This time is particularly important if product identification is the main reason for undertaking the sponsorship as the constant repetition of the sponsor's name reinforces the public profile of the company.

There is also an interesting difference between the uses to which the money which has been raised is then put. Rugby League is a good example of where the money is used to protect all aspects of the game. The sponsorship money is divided between the clubs after prize money has been deducted and approximately 50% is set aside for the completion of specific projects. This Capital Development Fund identifies particular areas where improvements are necessary and makes the resources available to the clubs to enable them to complete the work. Although recently these have been largely in response to the demands of the Safety at Sports Grounds legislation, previous examples demonstrate the importance of the project idea as they have promoted toilet facilities for women, the provision of press boxes and the extension/introduction of seating. This allocation of funds for the development of the game contrasts starkly with the debates around the Super League in soccer where the heart of the argument is the amount of money which is diverted away from the largest clubs to the smaller ones. Again with the Budweiser sponsorship of the American Football League, we see a concern for establishing the grassroots of the sport through the provision of scoreboards - a very important element in following the state of play and which would otherwise not have been generally available - as well as through the financial support of the game. It may be that these sports have not reached the point at which the pressures on the top teams to succeed match those in the Football League, although the Rugby League is beginning to show the signs of the development which characterised soccer ten or fifteen years ago. The pressure on transfer fees and the introduction of overseas players may produce pressure on the League itself to change the distribution of income.

The history and state of development of the sport are important factors both in attracting sponsors and in deciding the reallocation of those funds by the national associations. From this brief survey, it would appear that the more secure a sport becomes the less attention is given to the maintenance of the structures which support its growth. It is also beginning to appear that the larger companies may be adopting a strategy of sponsoring the competition rather than a single team competing within that competition. Although the sums involved are probably greater, the risks of being associated with failure are greatly diminished. Sponsorship of the league rules out the danger of regulation and may actually make the publicity surrounding the struggle against relegation a positive bonus to the company. The fear is that companies making this decision may also go a stage further and arrange their own competitions which will detract from the significance and position of the established tournaments. This has to be seen in parallel with another issue facing these sports in relation to television and the amount of change which the national organisations are willing to allow in the basic formats in order to encourage television coverage. It is interesting to look at the decisions which must now be taken by the administrators about whether the priority for the sport is to attract sponsors or television, with one eye constantly on the range of 'new' sports competing for the television contracts (Esomar, 1985).

Local Sponsorships

The whole area of non-gate income has become increasingly important at a local level and much effort is being put into maximising the amount of money made through these activities. One of the big incentives for the clubs is that most of the sponsorship packages can be achieved with the addition of very few extra costs to the clubs themselves. Obviously this will vary from club to club, but where there are empty seats in a stadium, for instance, the offer of a package which includes seats does not necessarily cost the club the full price of those tickets offered. The overall picture may become clearer after a brief consideration of the types of sponsorship packages offered by the clubs in South Yorkshire.

Main sponsorships
These sponsorships are the club sponsorships which offer the sponsor the opportunity of seeing their name on the front of the club shirt. The cost to the clubs of putting a name on a shirt is virtually nothing, but the package often includes other rights for the sponsor - such as hospitality and seats - which do incur costs for the clubs. This makes the evaluation of the sponsorship gained by clubs almost impossible. There is a degree of secrecy surrounding the exact figures provided by the companies to the clubs which is understandable but not helpful. There can be clashes of interest and initially the Budweiser League explicitly rejected sponsorship from other breweries. The commercial logic of this is apparent for the League, but the rule denied a major form of sponsorship from a still profitable industry to clubs which were desperately attempting to establish a new sport in a very competitive environment. The restriction has now been modified to allow brewery sponsorship as long as it does not involve the changing of the club name. This allowed the Sheffield American Football Team, the Steel City Giants, to approach the Stones Brewery and to obtain sponsorship from Carling Black Label - a direct rival to Budweiser in the growing Lager market. However, it does mean that the club cannot become the Black Label Giants and does stop the conflict of brand names becoming too direct. Deals with the breweries will usually include a franchise to provide the drinks for the ground or a part of the ground, limiting the choice to their own products. This will be particularly interesting with the juxtaposition of Budweiser and Carling.

Match sponsorships
This type of sponsorship allows people to use certain of the facilities at the clubs before and after the game. These packages usually involve catering, seats and a chance to meet some of the players. All of the South Yorkshire clubs have developed separate lounges for the sponsors and their guests, although these vary in standard due to the age and scale of the grounds they have been fitted into, creating an aura of exclusivity. There will also be concessions in terms of ground advertising and advertising space in the matchday programme. These packages have become very closely attuned to the demands of the sponsors, especially where there are problems in obtaining sponsors for every game. Reduced rates will be offered where there are particular problems about an unattractive fixture and there are frequent cases where the sponsorship is undertaken as part of a wider set of negotiations with the club.

Amongst the football clubs, it was generally seen that Sheffield Wednesday enjoyed a distinct advantage over their neighbours not because of their ground but because of their First Division status. The fact that First Division football is played at Hillsborough attracts a different type of sponsor as well as permitting the club to charge more for its package. The other clubs deal predominantly with local business people or people with strong connections with the visiting team. Hillsborough can attract regional clients and national clients where there is the possibility of television as an added bonus.

With the Sheffield Eagles Rugby League side, the aim of attracting sponsorship for match days is to cover as large a part of the costs of staging the event as possible. Ironically for one of the youngest clubs, the Eagles enjoy one of the best facilities in the county, with a glass fronted lounge and restaurant permitting excellent viewing and hospitality accomodation. This in a stadium which is owned by the City Council although leased to a Stadium Company, who are responsible for all bookings. The Giants will be playing in the same stadium and will be facing the same rental charges and it will be interesting to see what approach they take to offsetting match day costs.

The sponsors should obtain a greater sense of awareness for their product from their sponsorship and improve their corporate image. This improvement can focus on key themes within the organisation or a particular promotion. There is also a sense of status for the company in being involved with the club and for the guests who are invited to share the benefits of the sponsorship, whether these are prospective clients or members of the company possibly being rewarded for their work (Head, 1981). The clubs which pay the greatest heed to these needs of their customers and are most successful in meeting them are the ones which will maximise their revenue. These are not necessarily the largest clubs where clients will be fitted in to existing packages but smaller clubs offering tailor made options can compete effectively (ISBA, 1980).

Other income

Other sources of income for the clubs come through the selling of ground boards for perimeter advertising and programme advertising. The costs for these services will also vary between the clubs in the different divisions of the Football League and on the presence of television. This also means that certain sites within the ground are more advantageous than others and that certain sports are more suitable for board advertising than others. The classic examples come from ice hockey where the sheer pace of the game makes reading the boards on television very difficult and from snooker, where the cameras are often in close focus. This income is not open to the Eagles and the Giants as the Stadium Company take the revenue from advertising within the arena, except for that sold on the scoreboard. The Company also takes the profits from the catering facilities, which again marks these two clubs off from their soccer rivals. The difference between the soccer clubs revolves around the decision of whether or not to franchise out the catering, replacing the hard work and fluctuating profit of doing it yourself with the steady, although probably lower, return from the franchise. Franchises are also available for operating the club shops and selling the team merchandise.

The harsh realities of life mean that all the clubs except Wednesday and the Giants have established a form of lifeline scheme, where in return for £ 2 a week supporters are eligible for raffle prizes culminating in a large prize at the end of the season. This can generate income in the region of £80000 a year and many clubs have shown the practical benefits they have received from the schemes by identifying where the money has been spent on a specific development or the signing of a new player. The cost of the membership has led the Eagles to introduce a 50p a week 'Cashline' with the tickets sold through newsagents as a way of attracting a broader range of people to the scheme. The Giants did not feel it was appropriate to ask the public for support until they had had the opportunity to see the team in action and were already taking weekly 'subs' from the players.

The Dangers of Sponsorship

The creation of a strong identity between a product or a company and the team can be mutually beneficial but it can also be mutually hazardous. A slump in form during the renegotiation of a sponsorship package could lose a club much needed income. We would argue for including a 'success' clause into the sponsorship contract, which could have major implications for lower division clubs especially if this flexibility encourages longer term contracts between clubs and sponsors. The broader context in which the sport is viewed may also deter sponsors, with the impact of the soccer disasters impacting on the local clubs who were not directly involved and who have relatively good records of crowd behaviour. The reluctance of companies to be associated with the game could have had damaging consequences for the development plans of the teams. Ironically it might have strengthened the position of the newer sports in the county, who had positive images to portray to would be sponsors. There was also a gap in the market in relation to television coverage and sports bodies actively lobbied the television companies in order to fill the perceived gap. It is not just the link in market segments which makes American Football interesting to lager brewers and Rugby League attractive to beer brewers. There was a co-incidence of local products with local sporting developments which came together at a time when the traditionally dominant sport was experiencing a hard time nationally. Equally there was also the chance to put your product in the public eye in front of one of your rivals and this competitive area should not be ignored.

It is difficult to compartmentalise the sources of income within a football club with any accuracy. For instance the traditional distinction has been between football and non-football income. However, football income has included payments for the use of executive suites and membership of the equivalent of Vice-Presidents clubs. In a sense these are extensions of the season ticket principle, but they are also part of the marketing drive for sponsorship. However, it is possible to draw up general figures which suggest that sponsorship accounts for approximately a third of all income and that proportion increases the more humble the league position of the club, there are exceptions at the very top of the Football League where the clubs can guarantee contracts for overseas television coverage and major international sponsors where their sponsorship revenue exceeds the total raised by the lower clubs.

It is increasingly becoming the case that the distinction between football income, i.e. gate receipts, and non-football income is being broken down. In the past, gate monies have been used for paying wages and everything else was met by the other monies coming into the club. The falling gates have put ever increasing pressure on that decision and there are now many clubs which are dependent on the sponsorship income.

The unfortunate position they face is that success attracts success, making it easier for the bigger clubs to pick up relatively lucrative deals. This will tend to reinforce the differences between the large and the small clubs rather than identifying a source of funds which could be used to close the gap between the clubs. What makes matters worse for the less successful clubs is that not only are they scouring the lower end of the sponsorship market, where the margins are narrower but they must also face up to the consequences of failure. For just as success attracts success, so failure repels. In the past, the concern for an unsuccessful side has been the tide of disappearing fans but that move is now compounded by the disappearance of the sponsors as well. This produces a pincer movement on the clubs income at the time when the club is least able to resist such pressure. Not only does sponsorship serve to increase the gap between the rich and poor but it can underline that divide by transferring across to the successful away from the poor.

Sponsorship is necessary for the clubs to progress but the evidence suggests that they must be very careful about how it is developed. Packages must be developed which maximise the attraction of the clubs and minimise the costs actually borne by the clubs. Thus the Sheffield clubs all have seats in abundance for the majority of their home games and they all have something different to offer. The important lesson to be taken from their current experiences is that it is the perceptions of the public about what they have to offer which is as important as what is actually provided. The most obvious example is the First Division imprimatur emblazoned across Hillsborough but Rotherham have developed close links with their local community and have produced a package which is flexible enough to meet those demands. Sheffield United make the best possible use of the facilities built into their new stand, making an impressive site for business meetings.

The clubs must look to extend these links over different time periods to avoid the situation where the different levels of sponsorship all run out at the same time. One problem for the clubs in spreading the packages in this way is that it makes it harder to respond to success in the short term as the prices have a fixity which they would not have in the day to day situation. However, as we have argued elsewhere success is enjoyed by only a small minority of clubs each season and a note of commercial caution could prevent problems from going from bad to worse. Nor would we want to denigrate the importance of the sponsors own input to the game as it has been and will continue to be of considerable importance. However, we think that the longer term links could be mutually beneficial to both the club and the sponsors.

Local contacts cannot be ignored, whether these be grassroots contacts in the schools and supporters clubs or in the local boardrooms. A high level of interest in which the club is doing generates business interest as well. The shortsignted pursuit of commercial goals at the cost of neglecting wider interests is likely to have serious consequences in the long and not so long term.

Finally clubs should look to consolidate developments made with sponsorship income with money from other sources wherever possible. The less recurrent expenditure which is met from sponsorship, the less dangerous the sword.

References

ESOMAR (1985) Below the Line and Sponsoring: The Use of Promotion and Sponsorship in the Marketing Mix. Amsterdam: European Society for Opinion and Marketing Research.

Head, V. (1981) Sponsorship: The Newest Marketing Skill. Cambridge U.K.: Woodhead-Faulkner.

Howell, D. (1983) The Committee of Enquiry into Sports Sponsorship. London: Central Council of Physical Recreation.

ISBA (1980) Sponsorship. London: Incorporated Society of British Advertisers.

Simkins, J. (1986) The State of Sponsorship Business in Britain. London: The Economist Intelligence Unit Special Report No. 1064.

THE REALITY OF SUCCESS IN PROFESSIONAL SOCCER

Alan Clarke : The Faculty of Social Sciences,
The Open University, Walton Hall, Milton Keynes.
Lawrie Madden : Sheffield Wednesday F.C.
Hillsborough, Sheffield S6 1SW, England.

Introduction

Traditionally soccer success has been judged in terms of winning and losing but increasingly winning has become more important than the style in which the result has been achieved. This concentration on success is understandable in an overtly competitive environment and not surprisingly is shared by the majority of supporters, players, managers, and directors. This paper considers the various ways success can be measured and the weaknesses with many of the approaches which produce mechanistic statements about falling crowds, poor spectator conditions, high wages of professional soccer players and high transfer fees, linking these into a causative account, either independently or cumulatively, for footballing failure. Those involved wish to be associated with a successful club. Moreover they know which the successful clubs are - they are the ones with their names on the League title, the F.A. Cup and the European championships. This footballing Roll of Honour establishes the criteria by which those in the Football League live and by which their performances are judged, creating extra pressure on the players, managers and administrators of the clubs.

The Nature of Success

The fact that these criteria are by definition unachievable to all but a minority of teams does not prevent them from being widely applied. For every team that wins, there will be one that loses. By the end of the season the odds against success are even greater. Only one team will win the League title, denying success to the 21 or 23 other teams in that League. In the F.A. Cup, the odds are even worse as one winner emerges at the end of the competition which has seen all 92 professional league clubs take part, plus the non-league sides as well. Absolute success in soccer is therefore very elusive.

However, the inclusion of the non-league sides in the F.A. Cup points to an argument for 'relative success' which can be seen in the way that 'giant killing' clubs are welcomed by the national media if not by the managers of some larger clubs. Allan Clarke, the manager of Barnsley F.C. was reported to have said that the third round F.A. Cup tie against non-league Caernarfon in 1987 could have cost him his job but his team won and he survived to be cast in the role of potential giant killer himself when his team were drawn against first division Arsenal in the fifth round. For the minnows the 'Cup Final' may be the reward of a game against one of the top teams and, win or lose, they will have been 'successful' because they have progressed that far in the tournament. It will be argued that there is a need to extend this notion of 'relative success' to all clubs to generate a realistic set of expectations for the game. It will also be argued that the definition of this 'success' may not appear purely in playing terms and may be achieved off the field as well as by results on it. Problems of developing an approach to soccer which deals adequately with the diverse factors affecting the viability of clubs will be considered without reducing the account to a simple formula.

Attendances

One measure of success is the level of attendances, and as the figures for the seasonal attendances show, the trend since world war two is indisputable. Crowds have more than halved from 41.27 million in 1948-9 to 17.38 million in 1986-7, having fallen to a low of 16.49 million in the season 1985-6. Many reasons have been offered for this decline, but one of the constant complaints centres on the loss of entertainment. This argument has tended to be related to the number of goals scored and there have been many attempts to link the decline to the number of goals scored during the season. Skinner (1982) observed that

> 'Since 1958, when the Third and Fourth Divisions were created, the number of goals scored each season has fallen by about twenty-seven percent against a shortfall in attendances of approximately thirty-five percent.' (p.36)

He was forced to conclude, however, that

> 'there is no correlation between the two sets of figures' (p.36)

It is possible that the lack of correlation arises from the failure to consider the stubborn nature of the supporter who may not be so quick to condemn negative tactics which Skinner blamed for the lack of goals, if they produce an improvement in their team's results.

The development of an economic approach to professional sports has been gaining ground in the U.K. in recent years. Also concern with the economic problems of professional clubs has helped to produce a very narrow definition of the factors involved when studying the viability of the sport. Put simply, the supply and demand argument poses the problem of admission prices to soccer stadia and concludes that the prices are not high enough to maximise gate revenue (Jennett and Sloane, 1985). The economic logic of this position is that clubs should charge higher admission prices to maximise gate receipts, despite the decline in numbers actually attending the games.

Revenue vs Atmosphere

To extend the terrain of the economist, there is an important question about the nature of the game which appears when the pricing policy is considered. If revenue is maximised with a gate of 10000 paying £10 per person, what effect does this have on the team which has to play in front of an empty terrace in a ground devoid of atmosphere? There are considerable problems for the manager in motivating the team and himself for games played in front of small crowds. Smaller crowds may also influence attitudes of supporters when the enjoyment of being part of a large partisan crowd is denied to them in the interests of economic rationality. One current experience which lends weight to this argument is the loss of atmosphere supporters complain of when they watch live matches on television.

Ticket money is only the beginning for the club as it creates a captive and motivated audience, since it then has the opportunity to take additional money from these consumers. This additional income is regularly ignored in surveys of successful clubs and may partly reflect the failure of many clubs to consider this aspect of their marketing with any degree of thoroughness. It will be interesting to see whether the new emphasis on financial management which is discernible at so many clubs will lead to developments in this area. There is certainly scope for improvement on the market research undertaken by soccer clubs, both of their own supporters and of the clients who sponsor the clubs. Yet in the economic analysis of the clubs, it is almost as if they should not be allowed to earn money from other sources as their success is usually only measured through the gate receipts. Aston Villa and Sheffield Wednesday's recent balance sheets show a figure of around 40% of total income coming from other sources and reveal that percentage has been increasing despite two very successful seasons for Sheffield Wednesday which saw attendances increased. It should also be remembered that these figures are calculated against overall club income, so that transfer dealings are also included. In the last two seasons this has represented a loss on the accounts as Sheffield Wednesday has spent more on players coming in to the club than it has received for those leaving. This loss has been met by non-gate revenues.

Uncertainty of Outcome

It may be argued that if the issues are posed within the wrong parameters, there will always be shortcomings in the findings of research programmes. One of the central tenets of this form of research is the principle of the "uncertainty of outcome" and an examination of this principle will serve to demonstrate problems with the general approach. El-Hodiri and Quirk (1971) argue that:

> 'As the probability of either team winning approaches one, gate receipts fall substantially, consequently, every team has an economic motive for not becoming too superior in playing talent compared to other teams in the league.'

In the United States, this has been built into the structures of the American Football Leagues to prevent one team becoming too dominant. The regulations for transfer in the professional league allow the weakest teams of the season to have first choice of players available for the following season.

In a review of empirical studies in this field, Cairns (1983a) concluded that uncertainty of outcome included two types of variables - closeness of competition and relative quality. Closeness of competition can be seen as the difference between the two teams' league standings (Cairns, 1983b) and relative quality as the percentage of games won during a season (Noll, 1974). Undoubtedly there is some merit in the thesis but it appears to fall far short of the explanatory power assumed by many of the studies. Even Cairns' review concluded that the evidence only offered moderate support for the argument.

Relative Success

One of the most fundamental weaknesses comes in the consideration of success. There seems little evidence from the Football League to bear out the previously mentioned assertion that as the probability of winning nears one, gate receipts fall substantially. The experience of teams maintaining long unbeaten runs and teams who achieve most success over a season seems to indicate the opposite. Although not maintaining 100% records, Liverpool's recent history of unrivalled success provides the most interesting test of the case. Despite the effects of the recession on Merseyside, the attendance at Anfield has matched the national trends.

Another area where the definition of uncertainty seems to be weak is in the assumption that the relative strengths of teams can be assessed by their overall performance. Considering whether the success of teams affects the attendance patterns, it would seem that home records would be the most significant factor. If the team only has a 50% success rate during a season but has won every game at home, it would seem reasonable to assume the impact on demand would differ from a seasonal record of 50% which is made up of a mixture of home defeats and away successes. To the home supporters, the probability of success will be an added attraction rather than a deterrent.

Tradition and Significance

A further factor which will affect the level of attendance is the stage of the competition at which a particular game takes place. This issue is partially acknowledged in the 'uncertainty of outcome' literature in discussing attendances at games where championships or cups are at stake. It has been recognised that gates increase for these games and yet the theory would seem to suggest if the champions elect are due to win the title against the bottom of the league, then the gate should diminish. In practice the gate increases and theory is adapted to fit the empirical evidence however uncomfortably. The situation denies the logic of the market because the game has a significance to the supporters far beyond any simple economic calculation focused on the cost of the ticket.

It appears that unless the significance of the game can be formulated within the economic equation used to estimate the attendance figures, those estimates are always going to vary from the actual attendances. By quantifying the known variables it is all too easy to produce a formula which excludes those dimensions which are the most difficult to put into hard figures. That is precisely those aspects which make football into more than just another market.

An example of the importance of these factors can be found in the experience of the Freight Rover Trophy introduced in 1984 as an additional knockout tournament for clubs in the Third and Fourth Divisions of the English League. Attendances during the tournament led to some scepticism as to whether the extra games would actually help those clubs revenues. However, when the first Final was played at Wembley between Wigan and Brentford the gate was nearly 40000. It seems that part of this attendance was due to the rare privilege of seeing the team compete at Wembley Stadium. Roy Tunks, the player-coach of the winners Wigan, estimated that the Trophy was worth £100000 to his club, including the £4500 prize money for winning the competition itself. The total prize money of £47000 divided between the last 32 teams in the competition should be viewed in the light of this multiplier effect.

This assertion is based not simply on the League attendances for the two clubs but on the determination with which Manchester City and Chelsea struggled to hold the first final of the Full Members Trophy at Wembley in 1986. Both teams have adopted policies of sound economic management having been near bankruptcy, yet decided to underwrite the costs of staging the match at Wembley because they felt they would still profit from the advantages that a Wembley appearance offered. Appearing at Wembley is an important incentive for clubs and their supporters and it is interesting to compare the experience of the Freight Rover Trophy with some of its predecessors such as the Anglo-Scottish Cup, the Watneys Cup and the Texaco Cup in this respect. The status of the Football League Cup was transformed when the policy of a two-leg final was abandoned in favour of a Wembley final. The further reward of a place in European competition also helped to make the competition more of a serious venture but this should not blind us to the importance of Wembley as a symbolic arena.

Unfortunately for the administrators at the Football League, the very traditions that can appear to be the salvation of clubs can also be the ruin of a competition. If the scheme seems too artificial, there is a chance that the new competition will be rejected by the very supporters that it is designed to attract. In fact, memory and tradition are far more important than any passing reminiscence in soccer because they are an integral part of the meaning of soccer to its supporters. It is this collective memory which gives significance to such competitions as the F.A. Cup and the First Division championship. Teams which win these are seen to have achieved something worth winning, not only because of their own endeavours but because of the history which surrounds the two competitions.

Profit or Commitment

Sloane (1980) advocated harsh economic rationalisation of the Football League with teams moving to new centres of population or going out of existence altogether if they were not economically viable. The experience of Charlton Athletic F.C., who decided to leave its home ground and enter a ground-sharing agreement with near neighbours Crystal Palace during the 1985-86 season is being closely studied by many people in the game. The most recent suggestion of a merger involved Wimbledon and Crystal Palace and has again caused major protests from directors, fans and players.

An account of the future of soccer which ignores these historical legacies will never come to terms with the complexities of what seem to be illogical economic decisions. The question continues to be posed about why people will invest money in a soccer club with no apparent hope of any footballing success, let alone financial prosperity. Even where there is discussion of the financial management of the club, it is likely to follow the public service route of seeking 'efficiency' rather than focussing nakedly on profit. The reason why this question seems to be such an imponderable one is because the economist's approach looks in the wrong place for the answer. In many cases the directors and the supporters are not looking for an economic return on their investments but are seeking an affiliation with a cultural institution - their soccer club and their game. Just as the traditional loyalties of the supporters may be waning, so the loyalties of the directors may be waning also and there may be fewer people willing to support an investment in their local club when a more viable alternative is available elsewhere in the League. The economic rationale for investment is important but it is not a sufficient explanation for such decisions. We need to know more about why and in what context affiliation is declining and how it can be remobilised to benefit clubs.

The Costs of Success

Headlines about an international player earning £2000 a week fuel the argument about players' wages and the danger these salaries pose to the game. Even assuming that the figures quoted in such stories are accurate, the sums involved come to very few players over a very short playing career. Figures published in Labour Research (September, 1983) indicate that more than half the players in the First Division were earning less than £15000 per anumm. In the Fourth Division, only 36 players - out of a total of 497 - were earning more than £10000 and only one of them was earning more than £15000. Recent enquiries to the PFA suggest that the overall position of footballers has not improved, with some 70% of all footballers earning less than £15000 in 1985. Gordon Taylor, the Chairman of the PFA, has likened bonus schemes to the incentives paid for productivity in industry. However, in soccer they are linked only to success which by its very nature is a scarce commodity. For every team receiving a winning bonus, there is one team which is not and when the number of draws is added to this total, it can be seen that most players are not benefitting from bonuses most of the time.

Emphasis on success has affected the relationship between the clubs and the players. Clubs are under pressure to obtain the best players possible, which creates a scarcity as the top clubs secure the services of the top players. What has been more problematic is the way that transfers have been financed in the recent past, with clubs accumulating substantial debts in the form of unpaid transfer fees. The tightening of the restrictions, with a greater proportion of the fee having to be paid initially should help to overcome this situation. Indeed the PFA has commented that if such regulations had been in force in 1978, some of the financial difficulties which clubs have faced as a result of the increase in transfer fees would never have arisen. The lack of financial realism would seem to be applicable to the clubs who enter the inflated transfer market, rather than to the players who are bought and sold on it. It is the clubs themselves who hold the power to alter the situation.

Conclusion

Soccer clubs are victims of a false logic. At most twelve or thirteen clubs will be successful in the domestic competitions each year; the rest are doomed to middle table positions, early cup exits and possibly relegation. More reasonable definitions of success may stem the flood of sacked managers - already more than 1000 since world war two. Redefinition may help to restore some credibility to the game and motivation to the players more quickly than the introduction of new competitions. Current financial hardship and economic recession requires that broader criteria should be used in evaluating a club's financial future and viability, and a club's performance. Playing success will always be important but it should be only one of the factors in deciding the fate of a manager who is guilty of finishing without honours but has stopped the club from slipping into bankruptcy and receivership. Clubs could adopt three or five year plans, flexible enough to include unforeseen variations in playing strength caused by transfer activity or other changes within the club, based on an incremental improvement in performances and economic viability rather than immediate success.

References

Cairns, J. (1983a) Economic Analysis of League Sports - a critical review of the literature. University of Aberdeen, Department of Political Economy Discussion Paper 83 - 01.

Cairns, J. (1983b) The Demand for Scottish Football 1971-1980. University of Aberdeen, Department of Political Economy Discussion Paper 83 - 05.

El-Hodiri, M. and Quirk, J. (1971) An economic model of a professional sports league. J. Political Economy, 79, 1302-1319.

Jennett, N. and Sloane, P.J. (1985) The future of league football. Leisure Studies, 4, 39-56.

Noll, R.G. (Ed.) (1974) Government and the Sports Business. Washington: The Brookings Institution.

Skinner, W.E. (1982) The Football Industry. Sheffield City Polytechnic, Department of Management Studies.

Sloane, P.J. (1980) Sport in the Market? London: Institute of Economic Affairs.

INEQUALITY IN THE ENGLISH FOOTBALL LEAGUE

B.J. Webb, School of Accountancy and Applied Economics, Leeds Polytechnic, Lees LS2 8BW
A.J. Arnold, Department of Economics, University of Essex
I. Benveniste, Levy Gee Training Ltd.

Introduction

The objectives of this paper are to consider competition policies in the English Football League and to assess their effect on competition dominance and the income distribution of member clubs. The role of competition equalisation measures and the attendant schemes designed to redistribute income are outlined and discussed. The effect thereof on clubs' competition performance and on their financial position are assessed. The paper concludes by warning that recent policy changes are likely to lead to reductions in public interest, joint revenue and membership of the English Football League.

Competition Equalisation and Income Distribution

Sporting Leagues in general

It is the very nature of the product that differentiates sporting leagues from most other industries: member clubs must co-operate in order to produce the product, matches. These matches are not standard and vary in importance according to the league rankings of the participating sides.

Economic analysis of professional sport has identified the importance of uncertainty of outcome, wherein it is assumed that both public interest and club revenues will be larger if match results are uncertain. Uncertainty of outcome in the result of the games is the key to the economic analysis of professional team sports according to Sloane (1980). To Neale (1964), and others, the control of sporting competition is likely to maximise collective profits.

The English Football League

The English Football League has, since its formation in the 1880's, fixed the size of the League, increasing it so as to extend the scope of its labour constraints and in response to growing public interest. Membership had, until 1987, depended on the outcome of an annual choice by the members between the least successful clubs and would-be new entrants. The maximum wage and the retain and transfer system restrained both players' wages and their mobility until the 1960's, reducing the influence of market strength in the competition between clubs for playing talent. A minimum admission price was stipulated until 1982, while the sharing of gate money and other income has been practised since 1920. The management of the Football League also handles negotiations with television companies and with the pools promoters for the benefit of all league members. It is clear from this, and from the recent tensions between individual and collective interests, that the League has many of the features of a cartel.

Total gate receipts of the industry increased during the post-war period because admission prices rose faster than League attendances fell, even after allowance is made for inflation (Bird, 1982). Revenues were also increased by receipts from new cup competitions. The decline in attendances and the increase in receipts has not, however, been uniform. First Division match receipts nearly doubled in real terms between 1958-59 and 1984-85 while Fourth Division match receipts fell by a third during the same period of time (Arnold and Benveniste, 1987). Clubs also faced increasing player costs and public demand for improved stadium facilities. Accordingly they sought further sources of finance; some were club-specific such as ground advertising and lotteries, while others were joint, such as the increased fixture copyright payments negotiated with the football pools promoters.

Income Distribution

There has been some form of income sharing since 1920, increasing in both complexity and importance in recent years. Post-war, clubs have paid a proportion of gate receipts (net of certain costs) from all matches into a pool to meet the League's administrative expenses and other joint costs. Other forms of gate-money redistribution exist for cup competitions. Television fees have been shared relatively equally, in spite of the preference of television companies to show matches featuring top clubs, and sums paid by the pools promoters for the use of fixtures have also been shared equally. On the other hand cup and league sponsorship has generally been related to the level of performance with the successful clubs receiving a higher share.

Each club has in consequence received a substantial sum (approximately 98,000 in 1984-85 season) against which clubs have offset their own contributions. The net effect has varied between clubs; the contributions of lower division clubs are smaller and the annual sum received larger as a proportion of total turnover.

In the 1980s, however, larger clubs became impatient with the extent of financial support given to less successful clubs through these income-sharing schemes. Under the threat by the elite clubs to form a 'Super League' the schemes were modified. In particular, contributions to the FA Cup and League Cup match pools were reduced, and the pool shares and television fees were redistributed in favour of First Division clubs.

League Dominance and Club Income

Assumptions and methodology

If measures designed to encourage uncertainty of outcome are to be deemed successful one should be able to observe a substantial degree of fluidity in league rankings and a wide dispersion of 'success' in league and cup competition. We therefore analysed the results of league and cup competitions for the 25 seasons to 1985-86 both in terms of 'success' (defined as an FA Cup Final appearance or a top-three League placing) and First Division membership.

Income redistribution measures might reasonably be expected to maintain a level of financial viability commensurate with the support of a competitive team. In order to establish whether this had been successful we analysed the financial statements for the season 1984-85 of 64 Football League clubs (the remainder not having filed their accounts), using a standardised cash flow format. The cash flow approach was selected because it yields a measure of return which is less vulnerable to distortion than measures of income obtained through the use of conventional accounting techniques.

Results and Discussion

League dominance

In the 25 years to 1985-86, as few as 10 clubs took 87% of League 'honours'. Over the same period the same ten clubs accounted for 62% of FA Cup Final appearances and 34% of League Cup Final appearances (60% in the last 10 years). Findings are slightly lower for the previous 25 year period (ten clubs sharing 80% of league honours and 44% of Cup Final appearances), although only three clubs were elite sides during both time periods.

Table 1 summarises the findings on First Division membership. It can be seen that 73% of possible First Division places were taken by just 20 clubs, whereas the least successful 64% of League clubs in the period took only 4% of the First Divison places. The observations indicate that competition equalisation measures have occasioned neither a dispersal of 'success' nor a variable pattern of First Division membership.

Table 1. First Division membership, 1961-62 to 1985-86

Number of Seasons in First Division	Number of Clubs	% of Clubs	% total of possible seasons in First Division
20-25	11	11.6	44.9
15-19	9	9.4	28.4
10-14	7	7.4	14.6
5-9	7	7.4	7.9
0-4	61	64.2	4.2
TOTAL	95	100	100

Note: The total number of clubs includes late entrants and exits from the League.

Table 2. Average cash flows by Division 1984-85

	DIV.1	DIV.2	DIV.3	DIV.4
Turnover	2590200	852900	527300	340400
Wages	-1239600	-643000	-386500	-270800
Net Transfer Fees	- 190700	86500	27600	4400
Other Expenses	- 870000	-378500	-220300	- 83700
Funds from operations	289900	- 82100	- 51900	- 9700
Working capital Adjustment	134500	31400	16900	- 10700
Cash flow from operations	424400	-50700	- 35000	- 20400
Other sources:				
Share capital	2100	3100	35300	16700
New debt	200	30700	6500	13800
Grants	31700	81900	24800	9800
Sundry	11700	9000	3500	0
Total other sources	45700	124700	70100	40300
Total cash generated	470100	74000	35100	19900
Applications:				
Long term investment	-250300	-96600	-8000	-2900
Dividends	-18500	0	0	0
Tax	- 6600	-700	-400	-100
Other	- 9700	-1700	-2900	-4900
Total applications	-285100	-99000	-11300	-7900
Net liquid change	185000	-25000	23800	12000

Income distribution

Table 2 details the average cash flows of clubs in each division. Turnover in Division Two was 33% of that in Division One (Division Three 21%, Division Four 13%), and in each case wages were a much higher percentage of turnover than in Division One, (48%), varying from 73% (Division Three) to 80% (Division Four).

Clubs in the three lower divisions generated negative cash flows on operations. The position was worst in Division Two partly because nearly 10% of turnover was spent on transfer fees to buy in new players, compared with 5% in Division Three and 1% in Division Four. By contrast an average First Division club generated positive cash flows on operations of £425,000.

It was also found that First Division clubs paid 1.7% of their turnover into the pools administered by the Football League. For Division Two, the schemes provided a benefit equal to 4.5% of turnover (Division Three 10%, Division Four 18%).

The new income-sharing arrangements agreed by the members of the Football League in 1986 will reduce the receipts of small clubs significantly. For every million pounds of income previously redistributed by the Football League on an equal sharing basis, there will be a fall in the amount paid to each lower division club of approximately £5500. As a result of these new arrangements, clubs in the Third and Fourth Division will each lose about £40000 a year.

These changes in income-sharing will have one of two effects. They will either promote better management (see Chester, 1983) or, alternatively clubs faced with substantially reduced income will be forced to leave the Football League.

Conclusions

The English Football League has long been based upon the concept of mutual interdependence and adopted policies to encourage some degree of performance equalisation. Income sharing and other equalising measures have, however, gradually been reduced in the face of pressure from elite clubs whose individual corporate objectives are at variance with the policy of maximising collective revenues.

We have shown that attempts to achieve performance equalisation have not been successful. While some clubs have undoubtedly achieved outstanding success from humble beginnings - Wimbledon and Oxford United are good examples - league and cup honours remain vested for the most part in an elite core of less than a dozen clubs. Membership of this elite core changes only slowly, and changes to the income sharing arrangements implemented in 1986 are likely to reduce still further the opportunity for smaller clubs to alter the success polarisation which we have observed.

References

Arnold, A.J. and Benveniste, I. (1987) Wealth and poverty in the English Football League, Accounting and Business Research, Summer, 1987.

Bird, P. (1982) The demand for league football. Appl. Econ., 14, 1982.

Chester, N. (1983) Report of the Committee of Enquiry into Structure and Finance; Royal Lytham St. Annes: The Football League.

Neale, W.C. (1964) The peculiar economics of professional sport: a contribution to the theory of the firm in sporting competition and in market competition. Quart. J. Econ., February, 1964.

Sloane, P. (1980) Sport in the Market, Hobart Paper No. 85, Institute of Economic Affairs, p.25.

PERSPECTIVES OF THE RETAIN AND TRANSFER SYSTEM IN PROFESSIONAL SOCCER IN ENGLAND AND WALES

R.J. Sutherland and G. Stewart
Department of Economics and Public Policy, Faculty of Business, Leeds Polytechnic, 43 Woodhouse Lane, Leeds LS2 8BW, England.

Introduction

This paper examines the retain and transfer system in professional soccer as operated in the Football League in England and Wales. A pluralist perspective is adopted to recognise the distinct and possibly conflicting objectives and strategies of the principal actors, namely the Football League, the soccer club and the soccer player.

Three data sets were used in the statistical examination. Player registration data were obtained from the Football League, Royal Lytham St. Annes. Transfer data were obtained from both Rothman's Yearbooks and the Football Trust (1985). Data relating to appeals made to the Appeals Committee of the Football League were also obtained from the Football League. The paper is divided into two sections. In the first, data pertaining to transfer activity are examined and in the second, the retain and transfer system is analysed from the perspective of each of the actors identified.

History of the Retain and Transfer System

Professional soccer was legalised in 1888 when players were required to sign with a club a one year contract which was registered with the Football League and which bound players to play only for that club. At the end of the contract clubs could either retain the player and negotiate a new contract, retain him but offer his registration for sale or cancel the registration and allow him to become a free agent. Where mobility between clubs occurred during the contract the player's registration could be transferred only with the consent of all parties.

These arrangements came to be described as the retain and transfer system. The system restricted labour mobility in a manner uncharacteristic of other labour markets and in 1907 a players' union, the Professional Footballers Association (P.F.A.) was formed to combat this and indeed another unilateral policy decision of the Football League the imposition of a maximum wage. Despite repeated attempts to remove these restrictions, it was 1962 before the P.F.A. succeeded in having the maximum wage abolished. Further success followed in 1963 when the retain and transfer system was modified as a result of the Eastham v. Newcastle Utd law case.

The modifications were two-fold. First, an option period was included in the contract. It was exercisable only by the club, for a period similar to that of the original and on no less favourable terms. Second, formal procedures were instituted which allowed the player a right of appeal against the terms offerred or the transfer fee requested.

Despite these changes, the question of contract renewal remained the prerogative of the club. Following continued agitation by the P.F.A., an alternative system was negotiated and implemented in 1977. Contract renewal became a matter of mutual agreement and regulations state that 'a player shall be free at the end of his contractual engagement to seek registration with any club of his choice.' (Football League Handbook, 1986). Should a club wish to re-engage a player and have its new terms declined that club is entitled to compensation should the player sign for another club. The level of compensation may be negotiated by the clubs or arbitrated upon by a Football League Appeals Committee. The regulations still allow transfers during the contractual period whereby compensation is automatically payable.

The data in Table 1 assist examination of the effects of these most recent changes and in conjunction with a more detailed disaggregated set, only the results of which are reported here, reveal that the continued decline in the number of contract professionals accelerated post-1979; the percentage of free transfers was similar to the 1960's (except for 1981-83) but were more prevalent with movement down the divisions; transfer activity was higher than in the 1960's and whilst there was no discernible change in the level of activity before and after 1978, contract renewal procedures have led to more transfers being negotiated during the end of season months post-1978 than previously. The changed appeals procedure was seen to have little effect on the number of players utilising this option.

Table 2 on transfer activity for the period 1973-74 to 1984-85 demonstrates that First Division clubs sell more players than they buy and generally spend more than they receive. Second Division clubs sell more players than they buy and generally receive more than they spend. Third Division clubs buy more players than they sell and generally receive more than they spend. Fourth Division clubs buy more players than they sell and generally receive more than they spend.

Three Perspectives of the Retain and Transfer System

The Football League as governing body of professional soccer, the clubs as the employers and the players as their employees together, constitute the 'actors' in professional soccer's 'industrial relations system'. In this section the retain and transfer system is examined from the perspective of each.

The Perspective of the Football League

The Football League is concerned with the collective welfare of its constituent member clubs. To facilitate this it establishes rules to constrain the competitive behaviour of such, the intention being to

Table 1. Number of registered players, transfers and free transfers

Season	No. of contract professionals	No. of free transfers[1]	% of contract professionals	No. of transfers[2]	% of contract professionals
1972-73	2155	292	13.5	238	11.0
1973-74	2144	294	13.9	260	12.3
1974-75	2050	323	15.8	233	11.4
1975-76	2066	331	16.0	170	8.2
1976-77	2041	304	14.9	229	11.2
1977-78	2068	222	10.7	278	13.4
1978-79	2236	211	9.4	289	12.9
1979-80	2368	325	13.7	336	14.2
1980-81	2249	357	15.9	194	8.6
1981-82	2101	435	20.7	199	9.5
1982-83	1930	371	19.2	181	9.4
1983-84	1919	300	15.6	247	12.9
1984-85	1941	293	15.1	255	13.1

1. Source: Football League data
2. Source: Rothman's Football Yearbooks

Table 2. Transfer Data 1973-74 to 1984-85

	Players bought[2] (Transfer expenditure) ('000)[1]	Players sold[2] (Transfer Income) ('000)	Net movement of players (and money) ('000)
Season 1973-74 (260 Transfers)			
DIV 1	46 (3710)	85 (3523)	-39 (- 187)
DIV 2	60 (2034)	71 (1748)	-11 (- 286)
DIV 3	87 (850)	64 (1061)	23 (211)
DIV 4	67 (291)	40 (553)	27 (262)
Season 1974-75 (233 Transfers)			
DIV 1	51 (4233)	79 (3600)	-28 (- 632)
DIV 2	44 (1778)	63 (2009)	-19 (230)
DIV 3	89 (791)	58 (1085)	31 (295)
DIV 4	49 (185)	33 (292)	16 (107)
Season 1975-76 (170 Transfers)			
DIV 1	33 (2238)	70 (1493)	-37 (- 745)
DIV 2	29 (524)	50 (1177)	-21 (652)
DIV 3	61 (542)	30 (581)	31 (38)
DIV 4	47 (200)	20 (253)	27 (54)
Season 1976-77 (229 Transfers)			
DIV 1	56 (4650)	85 (4120)	-29 (- 531)
DIV 2	61 (1527)	58 (1559)	3 (32)
DIV 3	64 (555)	46 (821)	18 (266)
DIV 4	48 (205)	40 (438)	8 (233)
Season 1977-78 (278 Transfers)			
DIV 1	65 (7,566)	92 (5776)	-27 (- 1,790)
DIV 2	70 (2,554)	77 (3614)	- 7 (1,060)
DIV 3	71 (1,145)	64 (1677)	7 (531)
DIV 4	72 (372)	45 (571)	27 (199)
Season 1978-79 (289 Transfers)			
DIV 1	51 (9,051)	89 (8851)	-38 (- 200)
DIV 2	61 (4,765)	91 (5403)	-30 (638)
DIV 3	95 (2,542)	65 (2264)	30 (- 278)
DIV 4	82 (825)	44 (665)	38 (- 161)
Season 1979-80 (336 Transfers)			
DIV 1	67 (18,303)	98 (17686)	-31 (- 617)
DIV 2	79 (9,331)	87 (8707)	- 8 (- 624)
DIV 3	103 (3,654)	97 (4386)	6 (733)
DIV 4	87 (1,516)	54 (2024)	33 (509)
Season 1980-81 (194 Transfers)			
DIV 1	40 (11,872)	74 (12786)	-34 (914)
DIV 2	51 (6,316)	54 (5807)	- 3 (509)
DIV 3	71 (2,664)	47 (2108)	24 (- 556)
DIV 4	32 (320)	19 (471)	13 (151)
Season 1981-82 (199 Transfers)			
DIV 1	58 (17,926)	85 (15481)	-27 (- 2,444)
DIV 2	48 (2,555)	47 (4408)	1 (1,853)
DIV 3	51 (1,278)	37 (1618)	14 (341)
DIV 4	42 (515)	30 (765)	12 (250)
Season 1982-83 (181 Transfers)			
DIV 1	49 (6253)	71 (5811)	-22 (- 442)
DIV 2	50 (2321)	51 (2688)	- 1 (367)
DIV 3	52 (1498)	39 (1033)	13 (- 465)
DIV 4	30 (123)	20 (664)	10 (541)
Season 1983-84 (247 Transfers)			
DIV 1	66 (8370)	68 (6213)	- 2 (- 2157)
DIV 2	55 (2717)	82 (4006)	-27 (1289)
DIV 3	77 (1459)	63 (1917)	14 (458)
DIV 4	49 (380)	34 (790)	15 (410)
Season 1984-85 (255 Transfers)			
DIV 1	68 (9467)	88 (7304)	-20 (- 2163)
DIV 2	73 (3283)	79 (4450)	- 6 (1168)
DIV 3	67 (1108)	57 (2009)	10 (902)
DIV 4	47 (344)	31 (438)	16 (94)

1. Source: Football Trust
2. Source: Rothmans

produce sustained competition. The retain and transfer system like the maximum wage was seen to act as an integral component of this system of rules such that a fundamental diminution of either constraint was perceived as detrimental to competition and the general well being.

Research has shown that inequalities within the Football League are tending to increase with time (Webb et al., 1987). However, attempts to ascertain the extent to which this is attributable to changes to the retain and transfer system are made difficult because of other changes made during the same period, including structural alterations to the leagues, modification of the rules relating to promotion and relegation and adjustments to cross-subsidisation policies.

The Perspective of the Football Club

The Commission on Industrial Relations (C.I.R.) referred to the functional aspects of the retain and transfer system from the clubs' perspective. Firstly, acting as a 'redistributive mechanism enabling smaller clubs......to survive' (Commission on Industrial Relations, 1974) the system sustained economic viability. Although little supported by the data then, the argument is substantiated by Table 2 and whilst this table presents aggregate data such that not all clubs can be deemed to have been beneficiaries, circumstances do not appear to have changed subsequent to the further removal of restrictions on player mobility in 1978.

The C.I.R. also suggested that the restrictions reduced labour turnover and created team stability. The extent to which stability is the most appropriate strategy is questionable applying, if at all, only to those few clubs which are successful in any given season. For most a more appropriate strategy is flexibility to adjust to changing circumstances. Thus transfers into a club may be seen as a form of reactive recruitment which compensates for shortfalls in prospective recruitment with transfers out and free transfers the means whereby clubs adjust to skill redundancies (Sutherland, 1986).

The adjustment pattern changes as one moves down the Divisions. For example, although clubs in all Divisions participate in transfer activity as buyers, only clubs in the First Division consistently appear as net sellers. Lower Division clubs make greater numerical use of reactive recruitment. Their principal source of recruitment tends to be players freed by higher Division clubs (Sutherland, 1986). As Table 2 illustrates, this pattern of transfer activity has not changed radically since 1978.

The third functional role of the retain and transfer system identified by the C.I.R. was that it was conducive to the promotion of youth policies. A detailed examination of apprenticeship statistics, only the results of which are reported here, shows that their number has declined throughout the period most probably because of the market context of the industry. Furthermore, the decline has been greater in the lowest division. In season 1972-73, 514 apprentices were registered (a ratio of apprentices to contract professionals of approximately 1:4). Of these, 12.5% were registered to Fourth Division clubs. In season 1984-85, 260 apprentices were registered (a decrease in the apprentices to contract professionals ratio to approximately 1:8). Of these, 8% were registered with Fourth Division Clubs. That lower Division clubs do not undertake youth policies to the same extent as higher Division clubs further strengthens the conclusion that reactive recruitment is more prevalent among such clubs.

The Perspective of the Player

Whereas the analysis so far suggests that the retain and transfer system is functional to the goals of the Football League and the club, conventionally it is assumed to be dysfunctional to the player. Despite 'freedom of contract', however, and the negotiating advantages which this appears to offer players whose contract has expired, the ratio of mid-contract to end of contract transfers is still 5:1 (Dabscheck, 1986). These findings are partly explained by players' experiences in an occupation fraught with insecurities (Stewart, 1986). Such insecurities are important determinants of players' attitudes. To reap the not inconsiderable rewards associated with a successful career, players must attain a first team place at the earliest opportunity and retain it for as long as possible. If frustrated in this apparently limited though crucial objective, they are likely to become discontented at their present club and seek some means of resolving the situation.

In general, discontented employees seek a resolution to their difficulties by resort to one of two adjustment mechanisms. First, they may adjust by means of 'exit' behaviour (Hirschman, 1976). This involves employee-induced separation i.e. quitting. Secondly, discontent may be brought to the employer's attention by means of a 'voice' mechanism. This involves an attempt to bargain away the difficulties.

The choice of mechanism will reflect the nexus of costs, returns and constraints associated with each. These also help determine whether the adjustment processes will involve individual or collective action. Generally, 'exit' behaviour is associated with individual action and 'voice' behaviour with collective action.

A 'voice' mechanism exists in soccer and the P.F.A. has successfully negotiated a number of improvements to players' conditions. Such negotiations take place almost exclusively at national level, however, and focus upon issues of general applicability. Collective bargaining at club level on issues of concern to specific players is not a common feature of the industry. At this level, almost all cases of actual or potential player discontent result in an individual response either because players prefer it or because collective action is not feasible (Stewart, 1986) or because grievance procedures require this of them. The latter, for example, requires players to take up grievances, informally in the first instance with the team manager, and subsequently formally with the club secretary and directors. If still unresolved, the player has a final right of appeal to the Football League Management Committee, at which he may be represented by a union official. Evidence from the Commission on Industrial Relations (1974) suggested that many players were neither satisfied with the handling of individual grievances at club level nor did they regularly appeal formally. The principal reason for this was the feeling that 'to complain might be to jeopardise the complainant's future prospects in the club'.

Deprived of the opportunities for utilising the 'voice' mechanism and reluctant to invoke the disputes and grievance procedures, player discontent may be resolved by resort to an 'exit' mechanism. The transfer system provides such a mechanism and offers several benefits to the player. It offers a quicker and more definite resolution to the conflict at his present club. It enables him to negotiate a new contract (inclusive of signing-on-fee), thereby allowing him to exploit any favourable change in his market situation. It also enables him to establish new and important links between himself and the manager who purchases his registration. Nothwithstanding their collective antagonisms towards it, the retain and transfer system acts as an important adjustment mechanism for individual players.

Conclusion

This paper has examined the retain and transfer system from the perspective of the Football League, the soccer club and the soccer player. It has shown that each perceives the system differently, sometimes facilitating sometimes constraining the attainment of their distinct goals. Traditionally, the system has been assumed to be functional to the objectives of the Football League and soccer club, but dysfunctional to the player. This paper has identified occassions when the system can be perceived to be functional also to the player.

More significantly, the paper has illustrated that it is not possible to undertake a comprehensive analysis of the retain and transfer system without adopting a pluralist perspective. To the extent that this perspective identifies the multi-faceted nature of the retain and transfer system, it is important that all concerned with problem identification and problem analysis in the industry be aware of the need for such an approach.

Acknowledgement

The authors gratefully acknowledge the cooperation of the Football League and in particular, Mike Foster, for providing access to some of the data reported in this paper.

References

Commission on Industrial Relations (1974) Report No. 87. Professional Football. London: H.M.S.O.

Dabscheck, B. (1986) Beating the off-side trap: the case of the PFA. Industrial Relations J.. 17, 350-361.

Football Trust (1985) Digest of Football Statistics. London: The Football Trust.

Hirschman, A.D. (1976) Exit, Voice and Loyalty. Cambridge (Mass): Harvard University Press.

Stewart, G. (1986) The retain and transfer system: an alternative perspective. Managerial Finance, 12, 25-28.

Sutherland, R.J. (1896) Hiring as an investment decision. The

recruitment policies of the professional football club. Managerial Finance, 12, 20-24.
Webb, B.J., Arnold, A.J. and Benveniste, I. (1987) Inequality in the English Football League. Paper presented at the First World Congress of Science and Football (Liverpool).

CAREER STRUCTURES AND CAREER OPTIONS IN SCOTTISH PROFESSIONAL SOCCER: AN EXPLORATORY ANALYSIS

S. McNeish
University of Glasgow, Department of Physical Education and Recreation, 77 Oakfield Avenue, Glasgow G12 8LT, Scotland

Introduction

This paper is concerned with Scottish professional soccer. It offers a summary of recent work on career structures in the professional game in Scotland.

Many people pursue occupations in sport and physical recreation, but there has been a relative neglect of social science research on sporting careers, particularly in Scotland. It was this apparent lack of information in this arena which prompted initial interest in Scotland's leading professional sport, soccer.

Methods

A review of the literature on careers and on careers in sport, showed the diversity of approaches used in understanding and explaining careers; yet no one single approach offered an adequate conceptual framework for the analysis of Scottish professional soccer careers, nor an integrated analysis of processes of career entry and progression. A grounded theory strategy as outlined by Glaser and Strauss (1968) was adopted. This approach involves the researcher going into the field of study to gather first-hand data. From these data and through continual update and reassessment, an appropriate framework for investigation is generated. Therefore, those directly involved in careers in soccer were asked for career contingengies which they felt were crucial to career options and opportunities. Initial investigations showed that a multi-disciplinary approach was required; personal experiences and details, together with structural and cultural issues, were of concern.

Inter-personal data came from full-time, first team, Premier League players, as they represented those earning a full-time living at the top end of the game. Their managers provided data on the club and on management. Subjects came from Celtic FC, Dundee United FC and Motherwell FC, with managers Billy McNeill, Jim McLean and Jock Wallace. Supplementary interviews were also held with a few Aberdeen players and manager, Alex Ferguson, and with pilot study manager, Mr. Alex Smith. In total 28 players and five managers were interviewed.

The players' schedule had 11 sections: it examined the pre-professional and professional career stages. The post-playing professional career stage was also covered but is not discussed in this paper.

The managers' schedule had six sections. This looked at managerial styles and strategic planning of the managers within different club contexts.

These data were supplemented by an examination of agencies which influenced the career structure such as the Scottish Football Association (SFA), the Scottish Football League (SFL), and the Scottish Professional Footballers' Association (SPFA). Cultural factors were also examined.

Results

The pre-professional stage

There is a cluster of pre-entry career factors which have been drawn together from the players' data. The first is that players, at a very young age, must have some personal degree of interest and skill to play with a football, to practise and develop skills. One subject stated:

> 'I have got pictures when I was just two of me just kicking a ball.'

The data suggest the need for support and encouragement from immediate family; an active family interest best allows the realisation of potential talent. One player, for example, was taken by his father to the Continent (of Europe) when he was four years of age to watch his father's favourite team.

Other relationships seemed to play their part in developing and sustaining interest. One player illustrated this, saying:

> 'Just the usual...playing up the park with your mates... maybe from six onwards'.

Competitive experience is a vital factor. In particular, the school soccer team with its structure, providing regular organised and sometimes coached soccer, helps the young player gain and develop the necessary skills and experience. Organisations such as Boys' Clubs also create these opportunities:

> 'I don't think I would have been playing football if I hadn't come to Celtic's Boys' Club'.

Equally important to actually playing is the support young players receive from enthusiastic adults who protect, discipline and develop the players' skills for competition.

> 'I was lucky that I went to a good club, there was good people around giving good advice, good coaching and I was really lucky I went to Aberdeen'.

As organised and competitive playing opportunities expand, the most skilful players become visible to clubs. The best qualifications appear to be basic skill, pace, the willingness to learn, commitment and a flair for competitive success. There are, however, others, as one manager explained:

> 'You can learn a lot from the background of the player, as to his habits, his living habits and the way he behaves...at school and the standards he sets himself as a person...it doesn't always follow that you should have a team of nice people. You've got to have some kind of aggression and some kind of flair about you'.

Professional career stage

During the pre-entry career stage, players are immersed in and influenced by the informal social network. When the career reaches the entry stage, professional controls start to impinge.

The manager

The starting point of this part of the analysis is the extent of control of employers over employees. The most potent form of organisational control in the professional soccer career lies in the authority invested in the employing club and in particular the manager. The single most important assessment of managerial success lies in the development and management of a team capable of winning. Towards this end, the manager has responsibility for the selection and employment of professional players, making his role in controlling professional careers one of immense importance.

One manager highlighted this:

> 'I cleaned out the first keen guys that I felt had no future in the club...If you get a young guy and train him, he gets to thinking your way and he grows up that way, but he's to think the same as the next guy...and the guy in front of him...and the guy behind him'.

Eager recruits and selective contracting give power to managers. But the security of the career depends upon the successful interplay of the player's personal commitment and structural approval. Throughout the early entry stage, negotiation of these factors continues.

Managerial style

The actual process of selection and employment is inevitably linked to the personal preference and style of managers. From the data, a typology of managerial styles could be described:

The first is the 'roustabout'. He delegates the jobs of club organisation and financial business to others, and sees himself purely in the business of selecting, dropping, recruiting and putting together a winning side. He is immediately concerned about results and the match-to-match performance of his team. Ultimately, therefore, he controls the day-to-day career of players and has no sense of future concern for his players' careers:

> 'I have learnt very, very quickly in my experience that the first thing you do is learn to handle the Directors, then the players and then the press and then the staff. There's job delegation for these people but the main thing is football - 95% of it is football.'

Next is the 'middle-man'. He is both a player's man and a gentleman in the boardroom. He is mediator between directors and players, and his players' careers and his directors' wishes are continually in a state of compromise.

> 'I know that a manager's got a dual role, because he's got a responsibility to his Directors who are his employers, but equally he's got a responsibility to players'.

Then there is the 'orchestrator'. One kind of orchestrator sees both sides of the job - club management and player management - but gives primary attention to what is happening on the playing side and with his players. He therefore plays an important role in the career development of his players. Another orchestrator overviews the total operation. He works within a clearly defined division of labour in his club and acts as a central figure in both the performance and revenue generating sides:

> 'I am totally in charge of doing everything here...there has got to be someone in overall authority of all the staff'.

The manager is clear in his own mind about exactly what success is and who is best to play for him. His single-minded approach can have great influence, therefore, on his players' careers.

Clearly, therefore, managerial style is a contributory factor in career structures and opportunities.

Managerial strategies and club context

The way in which the manager structures the environment of professional players' careers is inextricably linked to the context of the club. Various factors are important in determining the form of club strategy the manager can adopt and consequently the types of careers the club can offer.

The first factor covers former success and traditions, and League position. Stirling Albion, as a Second Division club, had a very different interpretation of success than the top Premier League and European Cup winner club, Aberdeen. In one case the club offered part-time career experience; in the other international career opportunities. One manager showed his view of success, but revealed the added problem of convincing the public of realistic expectations:

> 'If we win one trophy each season that is...successful...we are still and we will always remain a provincial club. We do not have the resources...as far as I'm concerned it will be easy for me to keep my feet on the ground, but I would hope that the people on the terraces do the same.'

Clearly, this manager knew the limitations of his club and consequent career opportunities.

The second factor concerned with finance or resources (as is expressed in the last quote) is closely linked to the club's location and the base of support, and is arguably the strongest force in influencing managerial scope and choice of strategies. Careers are obviously affected if it is possible for managers to buy success or opt for a comprehensive youth policy. The contractual demands of players are also important in determining the manager's need to buy or sell labour both to maintain financial security, and team and club success.

Structural factors

Two major agencies have influence upon career structures and options in Scottish professional soccer. They are:- (i) the SFA, by governing all levels of soccer and ultimately overviewing domestic employment and developing international careers; and (ii) the SEL, by operating a labour market in which employers have strict control over employees, their contracts and mobility. The SPFA tends, largely due to its lack of support, to be rather ineffectual in influencing career structures and options for the average professional player.

Cultural factors

Two main issues are of importance. There is a general complacency by Scottish clubs to run professional soccer on thoroughly commercial lines and therefore promote and advance career possibilities. There is also an acceptance of the urban working-class tradition that Scotland is the place for breeding and grooming talent to be exported, which simply prevents a concerted effort to develop a Scottish professional soccer career structure which will attract interest and fulfil player ambitions.

Discussion

Players are able to point to key factors such as skill and commitment in their analysis of career influences. They also identify their relationship with, and the opinion of, the manager as a key factor in their career development. In their day-to-day immediate view of their careers, however, players fail to recognise that managerial strategy is set by factors such as club context, finance, support and traditions, and that each of these will play a part in how their careers are structured.

Day-to-day careers are highly influenced by manager and club, but professional careers are structured and controlled by the SFA and the SPL. The latter is most crucial because it is the League which has formed an employer-biased labour market in which terms professional employment of players are highly controlled. The Union has little bearing on the average player; and conditions within the system suit and encourage individual rather than collective bargaining. In a wider sense, it can also be said that a certain Scottish cultural hold besets professional careers and influences their possible development.

Unlike most other careers, professional sporting careers are not laid out in graduating stages, with clear qualifications of entry and stable career progression. It is possible to discern pattern and order in the structuring of soccer careers, but extremely difficult to predict the specific form which an individual career is likely to take. This is because career progression is contingent upon a wide range of factors. These include broad cultural and structural factors, aspects of the wider club situation, the contractual situation, inter-personal and personal factors. From this exploratory study, the most obvious and crucial factors for success seem to be the player's exceptional ability and commitment matched with a manager's long-term commitment and leadership, and clear strategic thinking.

References

Glaser, B.G. and Strauss, A.L. (1968) The Discovery of Grounded Theory. London: Weidenfeld and Nicolson.

THE FUTURE OF SOCCER - A FINNISH PERSPECTIVE

S. Salminen
Department of Social Psychology, University of Helsinki, Fabianinkatu 28A, SF-00100 Helsinki, Finland.

Introduction

In this paper the future of soccer is examined up to the year 2020. The premise of this paper is that the so-called 'information society' will obviously change the status of soccer. These changes are analysed both theoretically and empirically.

This paper is part of the research project "Sport 2020" (Salminen, 1986). The purpose of that project is to examine the status of sport, as Finland moves to the 'information society'.

It is apparent that developed industrial countries are becoming what is known as information societies. Computers and information technology will be the driving force for the development of society (Masuda, 1980). Development to an advanced information society, it has been estimated, will take place before the next century (Barron and Curnow, 1979; Tiuri, 1984).

However, we know very little about the consequences of moving to the information society. The process may influence soccer in three different ways:

i) An indirect influence may be most important but it is difficult to observe. Information technology requires different skills from traditional industrial work. The worker needs a broader general education and he has a greater personal responsibility. At the same time hazards, previous experience and physical effort in the work are diminished (Allardt, 1985; Adler, 1986). This kind of worker is obviously interested in physical effort related to fast skilful play, which requires co-operation with others.

ii) Information technology also directly influences sport spectating. Satellite television will considerably increase sports programmes in that medium and local cable networks offer direct transmissions to the home (Wiio and Kulha, 1985). The stadia may be rather empty.

iii) The consequence of this development may be that players will perform for the cameras rather than for the live audience. If soccer has to compete with other sports to impress television audiences, show or exhibitionist elements in the play might increase (Sewart, 1986).

The status of soccer as the most popular sport in the world may no longer be taken for granted. This situation is due to two factors. Firstly, working-class communities, where most of the fans come from, are being broken down (Holt, 1986; Salminen, 1987). Secondly, television introduces youngsters to new sports which are now more available than in recent years.

Method

The opinions of 14 Finnish soccer experts were examined using a delphi questionnaire (Linstone and Turoff, 1975). The selected experts were surveyed using a mailed questionnaire. The following is an example of one of the questions:

Soccer is considered to be the most popular sport in the world.

How do you estimate the number of soccer players will change up to the year 2020? (Circle the answer which you choose.)

The number of players will:
1. decrease a lot
2. decrease a little
3. remain at the present level
4. increase a little
5. increase a lot.

Respondents returned their completed questionnaires to the researcher, who summarised the results. The questions were then sent back to the respondents for re-evaluation. The second questionnaire contained the respondents' previous answer together with the general opinion of the group (median). If the opinion of the respondent deviated from the general opinion, he was asked to give reasons for his opinion. Ten respondents returned the questionnaire.

In the third phase of the research respondents were informed of the rationale offered by the others. Finally they were asked to express their opinion once again. Ten respondents contributed to this final phase. The purpose of the delphi process is to identify consensus among the respondents.

Results

The number of soccer players

Soccer is probably the most popular sport in the world. There are about 40 million registered players around the world (FIFA, 1982). In Finland there were 54159 registered players and 1145 clubs in 1985.

The subjects were asked to estimate changes in the number of players both worldwide and in Finland by the year 2020. The median of the answers concerning the whole world is 'increasing a little'. The respondents tended to be unanimous, because the standard deviation of the answers on the third round was 0.7. The number of players in Finland was also expected to increase little.

The rationalisation of opinions in the second phase showed that girls' and women's participation was expected to increase. This was reinforced by the opinion that the status of soccer in girls' physical education was estimated to improve more than in boys' physical education.

Professional soccer

Soccer at the highest level is professional work. Perhaps the major problem facing professional soccer is the economic viability of the clubs. This is at least partly due to the decrease in the number of spectators. For example attendances in the English Football League have fallen by 50 percent since the Second World War (Wagg, 1984).

In spite of this problem the respondents were optimistic about the future of professional soccer. They believed that it would 'increase a little'. The replies were in general agreement, with a standard deviation of 0.5.

In Finland there is no professional league. In some top level clubs the players are semi-professionals who train twice a week. The respondents did not anticipate the establishment of a professional league before the year 2020.

Hooliganism

One of the worst problems in soccer is violence among spectators, which is called hooliganism. Sociologists and social psychologists have studied the phenomenon extensively in recent years. The explanations have varied from the changing status of the working-class (Clarke, 1978; Moorhouse, 1984) and defective 'civilizing process' (Dunning, 1986; Dunning et al., 1986) to the understanding of hooliganism as a means of competence within the marginal groups (Marsh et al., 1978). A tragic example of hooliganism was at the Heysel stadium in May 1985. Dunand (1986) has suggested that the events were due to false attributions. A complete explanation of hooliganism has not yet been presented. Government reaction has been to increase police control at stadia, which may result in hooliganism being relocated in the streets and railway stations (Weis, 1986).

Respondents to the questionnaire considered that hooliganism would remain at its present level up to the year 2020. The experts were in agreement, the standard deviation of their answers being 1.1.

In Finland there has not yet been violence among spectators. The experts were unanimous in considering that hooliganism is unlikely to increase in Finland (SD = 1.1).

Doping

Many athletes especially in strength sports use drugs in order to improve their performance. The process may be referred to as 'doping'. There is little scientific evidence to suggest that medicinal drugs positively enhance performance but they do provide a health risk (Ryan, 1981). Soccer players have rarely been caught using drugs although the German goalkeeper Harald Schumacher confessed that players in his team had tried out doping.

The respondents estimated that doping in soccer is likely to increase (SD = 1.0).

Overview

Respondents' views concerning the future of soccer were rather optimistic. They believed that the number of soccer players would increase mainly due to increased participation of women and girls. Professionalism would continue to expand, although not in Finland.

The problems of soccer would be kept under control and the impact of hooliganism would remain at the present level. Doping would not become widely used, although it would spread to soccer.

The results demonstrated two methodologically interesting points. First, experts were reaching consensus during the delphi process, although it was not complete after the third phase. Second, leaders and coaches who are more committed to soccer believed that professionalism would soon arrive in Finland ($\bar{x}$ = 2005, SD = 2.1). Less committed players, physical educators and researchers disagreed significantly ($P < 0.01$) on this point ($\bar{x}$ = 2020, SD = 1.8) Commitment to the organisation seems to increase the observer's need to look at the future in an optimistic way.

References

Adler, P.S. (1986) Rethinking the skill requirements of new technologies. In: High Hopes for High Tech (edited D. Whittington) pp.85-112., Chapel Hill, NC: University of North Carolina Press.

Allardt, E. (1985) Social impacts of the new information technology. University of Helsinki, Department of Sociology, Working Papers No. 36.

Barron, I. and Curnow, R. (1979) The Future with Microelectronics. London: Pinter.

Clarke, J. (1978) Football and working class fans: tradition and change. In: Football Hooliganism: the Wider Context (edited by R. Ingham) pp.37-60. London: Inter-Action Imprint.

Dunand, M.A. (1986) Violence et panique dans le stade de football de Bruxelles en 1985: Approche psychosociale des evenements. Cahiers de Psychologie Cognitive, 6, 235-266.

Dunning, E. (1986) Sport as a male preserve: notes on the social sources of masculine identity and its transformations. In: Quest for Excitement: Sport and Leisure in the Civilizing Process (N. Elias and E. Dunning) pp.267-283. Oxford: Blackwell.

Dunning, E., Murphy, P. and Williams, J. (1986) Spectator violence at football matches: towards a sociological explanation. Brit. J. Sociol., 38, 221-244.

FIFA (Federation Internationale de Football Association) (1982) National Associations of FIFA, 1982 edition. Zurich: FIFA.

Holt, R. (1986) Working class football and the city: the problem of continuity. Brit. J. Sports History, 3, 5-17.

Linstone, H.A. and Turoff, M. (eds.) (1975) The Delphi Method. Reading, MA: Addison-Wesley.

Marsh, P., Rosser, E. and Harre, R. (1978) The Rules of Disorder. London: Routledge and Kegan Paul.

Masuda, Y. (1980) The Information Society as Post-industrial Society. Tokyo: Institute for the Information Society.

Moorhouse, H.F. (1984) Professional football and working class culture: English theories and Scottish evidence. Sociol. Rev., 32, 285-315.

Ryan, A.J. (1981) Anabolic steroids are fool's gold. Fed. Proc., 40, 2682-2688.

Salminen, S. (1986) The future of sport: a research program. Paper presented at the 11th World Congress of Sociology, New Delhi, India, August 18-24.

Salminen, S. (1987) Helsingin Jyry vuonna 2020: Kaksi skenaariota (Helsingin Jyry in 2020: Two scenarios). In: Liikkeelle! (Start Moving!) (edited J. Salminen) pp.10-12. Helsinki: Yhteistyo.

Sewart, J.L. (1986) The commodification of sport. In: Media, Audience, and Social Structure (edited by S.J. Ball-Rokeach and M.G. Cantor) pp.174-188. Newbury Park: Sage.

Tiuri, M. (1984) Tulevaisuus Alkaa Nyt (The Future Starts Now). Keuruu: Otava.

Wagg, S. (1984) The Football World. A Contemporary Social History. Whitstable, Kent: Harvester Press.

Weis, K. (1986) Spectator violence at and around football matches. Lecture given at the Department of Sociology, University of Helsinki.

Wiio, O.A. and Kulha, K.K. (1985) Urheilu siirtyy tietoaikaan (Sport is Moving to the Information Society). In: Urheilun Tulevaisuus (The Future of Sport) (edited by A.O. Arponen and O. Pekkanen) pp.11-17. Helsinki: SVUL.

FEMALE SOCCER COACHES' SOCIALIZATION, ATTITUDES TOWARDS SOCCER, AND THEIR ASSESSMENT OF TRAINING AS LICENSED COACHES

R. Naul
University of Essen, FRG, Fb 2, Sportpedagogy, Gladbecker Str. 180, D 4300, Essen, West Germany.

Introduction

In 1970 the German Football Association (DFB) allowed girls and women to play soccer as members of and within the leagues of their association. At that time, nearly 75000 girls and women were already organized in 1100 club teams (Ratzeburg, 1983). In 1984, 13 years later, there were more than 437 000 females engaged in soccer in more than 3400 teams. There are no other sports for women in which figures of club membership have increased so rapidly during the last decade in Germany. Although thousands of girls and women were playing, there were only 102 licensed female soccer coaches in 1984 (N = 100 License B, N = 2 License A). They are the subject of the present investigation.

Procedures

Only a limited amount of research concerned with coaching in soccer and soccer coaches has been done (Reilly, 1979). Investigations about female soccer coaches, their personal traits, psychological profiles, assessment of soccer for women and so on, are not cited in articles or books about 'women in sports' (e.g. Boutilier and Giovanni, 1983). Thus a lack of scientifically derived data related to female coaches prompted this research. There were no suitable inventories available and so a questionnaire was constructed in three different parts. The first part was concerned with the soccer engagement and socialization of the female coaches; the second part was related to their attitudes towards soccer and the last part investigated their assessment of formal training as licensed coaches, provided by the Football Asociation. A pilot-study indicated that there was a greater interest in qualitative than in quantitative data. Furthermore it was intended to evaluate the training instruction by the Association.

It was expected that female soccer coaches would attribute soccer with similar characteristics as men do, especially the physical characteristics. All the social and psychological aspects of the game were expected to be ranked similarly. The questionnaire was sent to 87 licensed female coaches and was completed by 57 (65.2%) of them. All the data were computerized using SPSS.

Results and Discussion

Soccer engagement

Most of the female coaches only became members of a soccer club as a player after the age of 18 years. Before turning to soccer many of them had been handball players or track and field athletes. A few women had joined soccer clubs as girls and had played in youth-teams at the age of 10-14. Reasons for their soccer club membership are very different. Fun, pleasure, and sociability were the most popular motives expressed. A small percent offered reasons such as acquisition of soccer techniques or competing in matches.

Table 1. Playing soccer

Highest class of division/league	Sub-district	District	County	Regional	MV
	2 4%	19 33%	16 28%	17 30%	3 5%

Hours of training as player (per week)	0-2	3-4	5-6	MV
	7 12%	40 70%	9 16%	1 2%

Member of team (selection level)	Town	District	Regional	National	MV
	6 11%	11 19%	12 21%	0 0%	28 47%

*denotes missing values

At the time of investigation almost 90% of the female coaches were still active players. About half of the group were playing in the first and second leagues. Some women (18%) trained more than 4 h, more than twice a week.

There were no real differences in the amount of time spent training between subjects from the four leagues. On the one hand about 50% of the sample did not play in a team at any level of selection. On the other hand about 20% played in a district team and another 20% played in a regional selection.

A total of 21% of the female soccer coaches did not use their licenses for training and coaching teams. Another 23% coached for 1 or 2 h a week but more than 44% trained or coached teams for 5 h a week or more. This group of female coaches may train not only one team but several, regular boy and/or girl teams in the age ranges of 6-12 and 13-16. Only a few female coaches trained and coached older boy-teams or senior female-teams.

Table 2. Coaching soccer

Occupation as coach (hours per week)	0	1-2	3-4	5-6	7-8	Over 8	MV
	12 21%	13 23%	9 16%	7 17%	9 16%	6 11%	1 2%

Sex and age of trained teams: (multiple answers)	N	%
boys and girls, 6-12 years	28	49
boys and girls, 13-16 years	29	51
boys 17-18 years, seniors	5	9
no comment	14	25
Division/league of trained teams (multiple answers)		
mixed leisure-teams/youth teams up to district level	30	53
youth-teams up to regional-level/ senior teams up to district level	19	33
senior-teams on district-level up to county-level	8	14
no comment	14	25

Attributes of soccer

The female coaches were given suggested attributes of soccer players and they had to assess which are typical of male (M) and female (W) soccer. They were also required to identify those attributes which have nothing to do with soccer (No) or which applied to both men and women (M+W). A mean of approproximately 2 is typical for male soccer, a mean of approximately 1 for both, and a mean near 0 is right for female soccer.

Some motor and psychophysical attributes were considered to be typically masculine: these included power, roughness, athleticism, speed and also strength (Figure 1). One physical item, endurance, is also applicable to female soccer. Social items such as self-control and fairness were thought to be more attributable to female soccer. Also aggression was considered to be more masculine. The results suggested that a soccer player's profile is divided by coaches into motor-physical and social control parameters. This motor-physical sub-profile was attributed to men, the social sub-profile to women. Three of the categories - creativity, coolness and grace - were deemed to have little to do with soccer. It is remarkable that the majority of subjects failed to attribute creativity to soccer.

About 50% of the coaches had been members of team selections. Members of the best selection (regional) considered power and aggression to be more relevant to the masculine sport stereotype, with athleticism attributed to both sexes. The best players now also assessed self-control and fairness more to soccer. An interesting observation was that the majority of the best soccer players did not

attribute	no	m	m&w	w	s	mv	mean
power	2	35	15	1	51	4	1.66
roughness	4	33	16	0	49	4	1.66
athleticism	4	21	26	2	49	4	1.38
speed	0	21	31	1	53	4	1.37
aggression	8	12	27	4	43	6	1.18
self-control	18	4	12	15	31	8	0.64
fairness	2	2	23	24	49	6	0.55
tactics	0	7	41	5	53	4	1.04
endurance	0	7	37	8	52	5	0.98
ingenuity	3	8	35	6	47	5	1.08
strength	5	24	18	5	47	5	1.40
impulsiveness	5	11	25	8	44	8	1.07
self-confid.	10	8	29	4	41	6	1.09
intelligence	11	3	29	6	38	8	0.92
elegance	19	4	21	6	31	7	0.93
creativeness	30	1	13	6	20	7	0.75
coolness	31	5	7	5	17	9	1.00
grace	42	1	4	4	9	6	0.66

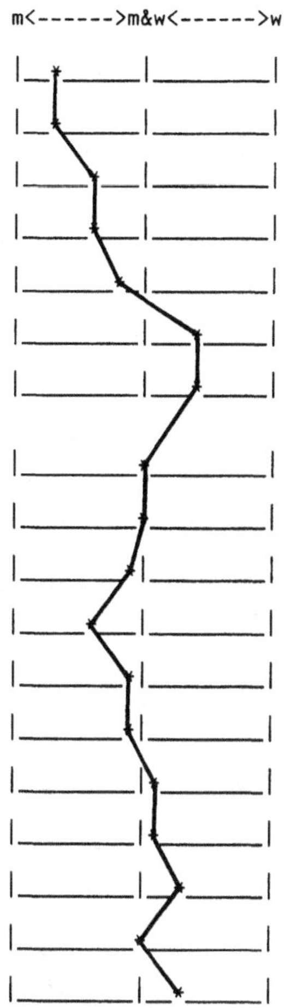

Figure 1. Motor, psychophysical and social attributes given to soccer by female coaches

attribute self-control to soccer. The women players of the highest level of selection considered the motor-physical and the social profile of soccer to be highly masculine traits,except for fairness. There seems to be an accord between high soccer performance of female coaches and masculine attribution of the game.

Probably coaches as members of the highest level of selection assessed soccer also on its highest level (professional, Bundesliga). That could be the reason why power and aggression were attributed much more to men and fairness at any competitive level more to women.

Assessment of training as licensed coaches

All the coaches were asked to evaluate their training course. The

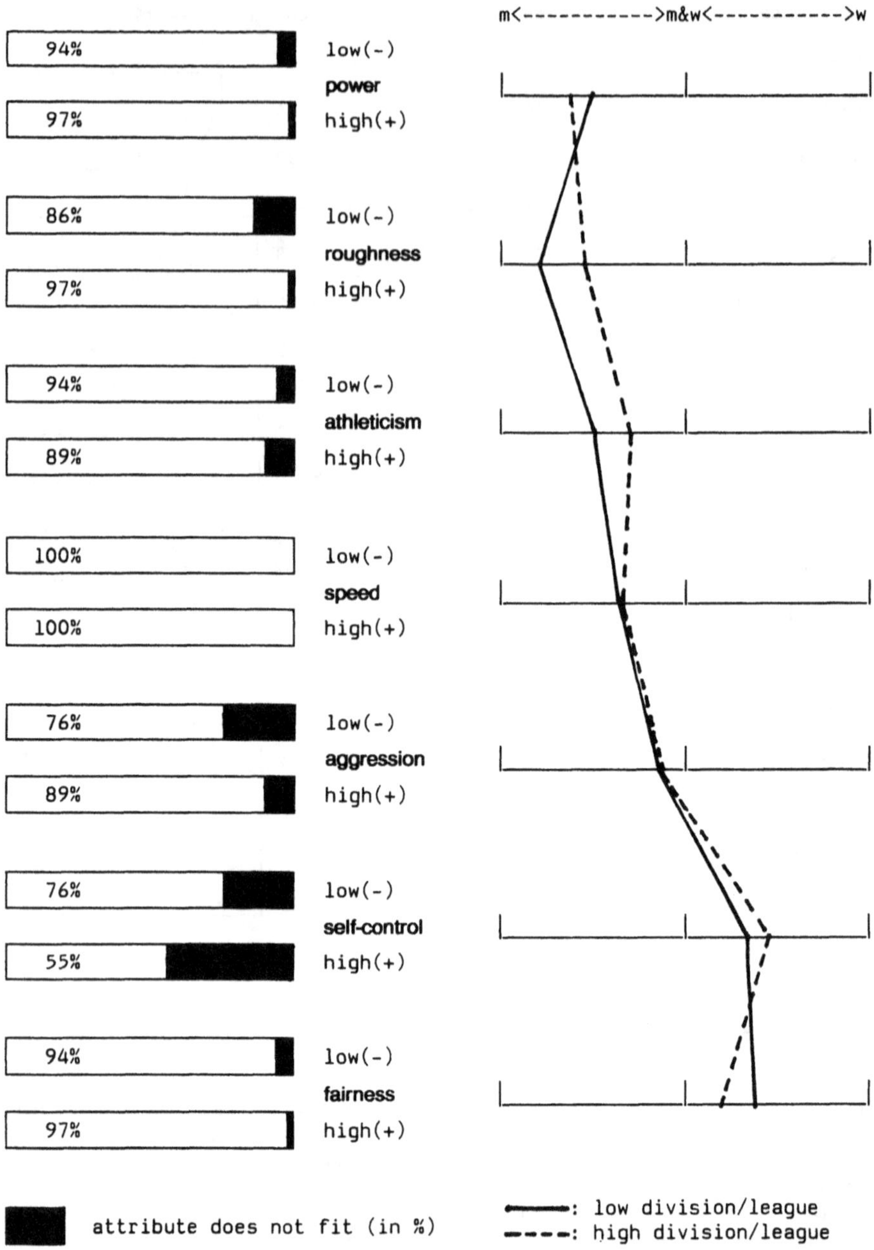

Figure 2. Selected attributes given to soccer by female coaches belonging to high or low selection-teams

subjects were asked to indicate the number of hours spent on each component of their curriculum. They indicated if they would prefer more or less instruction in particular components.

themes	hrs.	+	+/-	-	n	mean
administration, law	4.0	9	41	5	55	1.07
code of rules	7.2	5	44	5	54	1.00
anatomy, physiology	3.6	25	24	2	51	1.45
medicine, first aid	4.7	31	22	-	53	1.58
general methods of training	13.5	8	46	-	54	1.12
pedagogy, methods of instruction	5.1	27	26	1	54	1.48
psychology, coaching and counselling	5.7	32	22	0	54	1.59
soccer, techniques (p)	17.6	13	39	2	54	1.20
soccer, tactics (p)	11.7	18	33	3	54	1.28
soccer, techniques (t)	8.0	12	37	5	54	1.13
soccer, tactics (t)	8.7	12	39	4	55	1.14
teaching tests	8.3	13	41	3	54	1.24
preparations for examinations	15.5	1	48	4	53	0.90

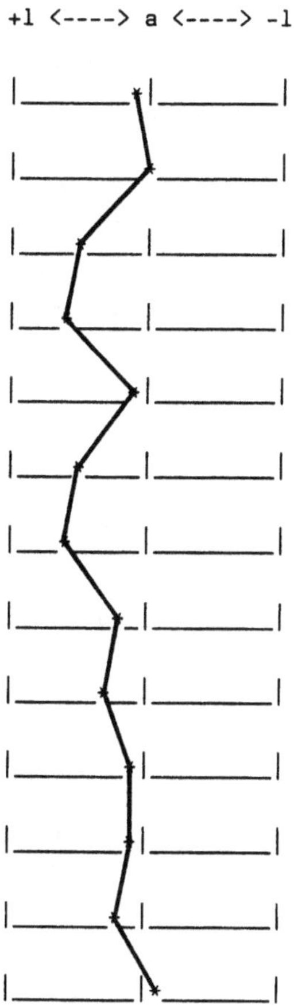

% of persons, who wanted more (+1) or less (-1) of one of these themes (a: adequate), divided by the number of valid answers

Figure 3. Estimation of time invested in various themes of the curriculum and their adequacy

With the exception of the topic 'preparation for examinations' there was no theme which they believed should be reduced. Most of the themes were evaluated as 'adequate'. The female coaches would have liked more information about anatomy, physiology, medicine and first aid and especially pedagogy, about coaching and counselling. Compared with administration, law, code of rules and methods of training there were fewer hours of instruction devoted to medical care and health and dealing with athletes. It was felt that lessons in soccer techniques and tactics also could be increased. These critical remarks were often supported by coaches who trained older youth teams and senior teams. Most of the coaches were dissatisfied with the lack of guidelines for girls' and women's soccer.

The findings lead to the following points of view about female soccer and female coaches licensed training courses. First, traditional methods of preparing physical education teachers are relevant to female participation in soccer. Traditional barriers need to be removed in order to encourage girls and women to participate in soccer and to learn the techniques and tactics of the game.

Second, soccer was evaluated by female coaches with both a low and high level of personal soccer performance. Both groups assessed soccer as a typical masculine sport in a physical terms. Only endurance and athleticism - by the best players - were ascribed as belonging to female soccer. Women with a low level of soccer performance attributed the social and psychological items such as aggression and self-control to both sexes. Female coaches with a high level of soccer performance attributed the physiological and the social sub-profile more to men, the exception being fairness. Therefore the results of the study were as predicted for coaches with a low level of soccer performance. Female coaches who had been players in the best teams assessed soccer as a masculine sport in general. This was contrary to expectations.

Third, training of licensed coaches by the Football Association should not be concentrated merely on the physical differences between males and females. Psychological and social aspects should also be considered. More emphasis should be placed on less powerful and more technical ways of playing to reinforce the spirit of fairness. Fairness and self-control should become educational aims. Specially designed programmes for girls and women and special curricula for instruction of female coaches should be developed. These should include instruction on how to coach and to counsel youth teams of boths sexes at different ages.

It is possible that the findings of the study merely reflect national outlines of German soccer, demonstrating a 'Teutonic' view. The results should have broader implications. Attempts to achieve more self-control and less aggression, more fairness and less roughness in soccer would meet with general support. That would not change the essential nature of soccer but would merely introduce a more humanistic approach to the game.

References

Boutilier, M.A. and Giovanni, L. (1983) The Sporting Woman. Champaign, Illinois: Human Kinetics.

DFB (1985) Mitglieder-Statistik. Franfurt: DFB.

Ratzeburg, H. (1983) Damenfussball-Grundlagen und Entwicklung. Frankfurt: DFB.

Reilly, T. (1979) What Research Tells the Coach about Soccer. Washington, D.C.: AAHPERD.

RELATIONSHIPS BETWEEN COACHES AND REGULAR AND SUBSTITUTE PLAYERS IN SOCCER

D. Teipel, Deutsche Sporthochschule, Carl Diem Weg 2, Köln 41, West Germany.

Introduction

Interactive sport teams are substantially dependent on the group orientation and cohesiveness of all members (Martens and Peterson, 1971; Carron, 1982; Landers et al., 1982). In the organisational structure of the club, relatively firmly established roles are assigned to such figures as the coach, team captain, regular players, substitutes, senior and junior players.

According to Tutko and Richards (1971) at least five different leadership styles can be differentiated amongst coaches. Obviously, the type of leadership and characteristic forms of coach behaviour can either negatively or positively affect the attitudes and actions of the team players. Hence the formal and informal team structure (performance and socio-emotional orientation) may be directly influenced. Within the team structure, the relationship between the coaches and regular and substitute players is of central importance. Generally, regular players are those who play in more than half of the season's games while substitutes often and over longer periods of time sit on the bench and play less than half of the games in a season. Bergmann (1978) differentiated three types of substitute or reserve players:- younger players without extensive game experience; players out of condition due to injury, illness or personal reasons and older players past the peak of their career.

Obviously, there are differences between the three types based on physical, technical, tactical and motivational capacities. Ueberle (1971) has argued that the coach is required to handle substitute players carefully since they are valuable members of the squad.

Detailed investigations of the relationship between regular and substitute players have been conducted elsewhere (e.g. Essing, 1977; Allmer, 1979). In fact, Essing (1977) investigated the relationship between 121 regular and 62 substitute players using a sociometric analysis concerning performance and emotional leadership. Regular players obtained higher ranking than substitutes in both performance-oriented and socio-emotional oriented hierarchy. In general, regular players selected other regular players for performance and emotional interaction rather than substitute players. On the other hand, substitutes tended to select regular players in respect of performance interaction, but not in respect of emotional interaction. However, Allmer (1979) utilising a cluster analysis technique failed to clearly differentiate between regular and substitute players in terms of performance satisfaction. Since there was only partial agreement between the findings of the previous two studies, it was the aim of this paper to analyse the following aspects of the relationship between regular and substitute players:-

i) differences in the distribution of regular players and substitutes during their last season;

ii) characteristics of performance and socio-emotional oriented interactions between regular players and substitutes by means of factor analysis of questionnaire data;

iii) differences in inter-subjective evaluations between regular players and substitutes

Method

Subjects

Seventy one male footballers (age range:18 - 33 years) were investigated. The average age of regular players was 24.02 years and the substitutes 22.65 years. They were asked whether they sat on the reserve bench at the end of the first season: 36 regular and 35 substitute players were identified. Twenty-six players were from the highest amateur level, 25 from the division below and 20 from the next level of play. There were 37 defenders and 34 attackers sampled.

Questionnaire

The initial phase in constructing the questionnaire was based on collecting items on the relations between coaches and regular and substitute players. Two pilot studies resulted in the revised form of the questionnaire consisting of 80 items along with personal data on each subject. All items required answering on a five-point Likert-type scale ranging from '1 = very true' to '5 = not true'.

Procedure

The final version of the questionnaire was given to 120 footballers of which 71 (56.6%) returned the completed forms. When questions arose concerning its content, additional information was provided for the subject. The data were collected between December, 1981 and January, 1982. This period, at the beginning of the mid-season, was chosen deliberately so that only established teams were used, thus avoiding instability due to early or late season competitive influences.

Statistical treatment of data

Data were stored in a computer and programs providing frequency distributions, factor analysis and analysis of variance were used in processing (Beutel et al., 1980)

Results

In this study only those 32 items which yielded significant differences between regular and substitute players are presented. Three distinct aspects of the results readily lent themselves for analysis and interpretation.

Nine players of the sample came from youth teams, 1 of whom became a regular, but 8 of whom became substitutes (See Table 1).

Table 1. Differences in the distribution of regular and substitute players in comparison to their previous level of experience

Last league		Contemporary status			
		Regular players (36)		Substitute players (35)	
	Fr.	Abs. Fr.	Rel. Fr.	Abs. Fr.	Rel. Fr.
Youth team	(9)	1	11.1%	8	88.9%
Lower league	(18)	9	50.0%	9	50.0%
Same league	(32)	17	53.1%	15	46.9%
Higher league	(12)	9	75.0%	3	25.0%

Eighteen of the players had arrived from clubs in lower divisions, 9 gained regular places and 9 became substitutes. There were 32 players from the same level, 17 were regulars and 15 were substitutes. Players arriving from a higher level were distributed in the following way:- 9 regulars and 3 substitutes. A χ^2 square value (8.52) for equal cell frequencies (df = 3) was significantly different ($P < 0.05$) from expected cell frequencies. This was because almost all of the youth players became substitutes, whereas most of the more experienced players took regular places in the teams. There is also further tentative support for this notion that experience appears to be an essential ingredient in high level amateur leagues, since the regular players were on average 1.5 years older than the substitutes.

A main axis factor analysis with iterations of communalities (Beutel et al., 1980) was computed on the basis of the 32 items presented (Tables 2 and 3). Four factors were selected for the following statistical reasons:- eigenvalue > 5% per factor, scree-test, sum of marking items > 1 ($\Sigma a^2 > 1$) and at least 3 marking items <0.50. In Tables 2 and 3 those items which show only a low loading on a factor (< 0.30) are in parentheses and, therefore, are not considered to offer significant contribution to the variance explained. Four different factors were identified in the factor analysis. The first factor (Table 2) is characterised by 9 significant items concerning performance satisfaction and concordance of personal and the coaches' evaluation of performance. Items 1,5 and 7 (Table 2) show evidence of a good relationship between coach and player. Other items which emphasise this high degree of uniformity of performance estimation are items 2,4 and 6.

Factor 2 may be regarded as an ambivalent factor with 4 items of a positive emotional relationship and 4 items of a fundamental discrepancy in performance evaluation between coach and players. Items 12 and 13 support the positive emotional relationship

Table 2. Analysis of performance and socio-emotional oriented aspects of the sample

Item	Factor Loading
Factor 1: Performance satisfaction and accordance of personal and coach's performance evaluation	
1 I am satisfied with the frequency of my games during the season.	.70
2 My chances are good to remain or become a regular player under this coach.	.65
3 I can definitely develop my abilities under this coach.	.61
4 I am satisfied with the duration of my play in the games.	.60
5 My performance is sufficiently appreciated.	.59
6 The coach often talks to me about my performance.	.55
7 In my opinion the coach arranges the team adequately.	.52
8 If I am on the team, I play because of my performance.	.42
9 As I wish to play, I don't criticise the coach.	.37
10 It means stress for me to be substituted for insufficient performance.	.27
11 I am satisfied with my results.	.23
(Whole summarised variance	4.21)
Factor 2: Positive emotional relation and discrepancy of performance evaluation between player and coach	
12 I am on good terms with the coach.	.73
13 The coach is liked by the team.	.72
14 The coach should try to motivate players more intensively during practice.	.67
15 Also after the games I have good personal contact with the coach.	.64
16 The coach favours more liked players on the team.	.60
17 The coach seems credible in his evaluation of my performance.	.53
18 The coach does not always arrange the team according to actual performance.	.45
19 The coach frequently leaves routined players on the team despite worse performance over a longer period.	.44
20 If I cannot become a regular player, I am willing to play on the lower team over a longer period.	.23
(Whole summarised variance	3.93)

extensively and items 14, 18 and 19 show clear evidence of differences in opinion (Table 2).

Factor 3 (Table 3) may also be viewed as an ambivalent factor with 2 items of dissatisfaction with the coach's evaluation and 2 items of competitive cognitions. For example, items 21 and 22 display a high loading showing individual performance evaluation as different from that of the coach. Items 24 and 25 clearly support the notion of intra-squad competition for places.

Table 3. Differences in inter-subjective evaluations between regular and substitute players

Item	Factor Loading
Factor 3: Discrepancy of performance evaluation between player and coach and competitive cognitions	
21 I feel myself reinforced by other persons (e.g. president, spectators) that my performance is better than the coach evaluates it.	.71
22 Sometimes I am substituted though I didn't play insufficiently.	.58
23 In order to avoid trouble on the team the coach mostly substitutes younger players without safe position.	.56
24 Sometimes I wish my team played insufficiently in order to provide my abilities more affirmatively.	.39
25 I would welcome, if the rival on my position left the team.	.36
(Whole summarised variance	2.78)
Factor 4: Positive personal performance evaluation	
26 At this time my performance is sufficient to be a regular player.	.70
27 I think I can remain or become a regular player for the next time.	.69
28 I think I am a good player in this league.	.64
29 The coach thinks highly of me.	.53
30 I like to play in front of many spectators.	.46
31 It means stress for me to get in play as a substitute.	.37
32 I'll change clubs, because I believe I am capable of a higher league.	.30
(Whole summarised variance	2.71)

In factor 4 (Table 3) a positive self-concept and performance evaluation can be detected in all 7 items. The three items with the highest loadings, 26, 27 and 28, all show firm conviction to become and remain a regular player and a valuable team member. Items 29 and 30 support the notion of high evaluation of the players' abilities by the coach and the motivational effect of the home crowd.

The factor analysis indicates clearly two rather homogeneous (factors 1 and 2) and two heterogeneous (factors 2 and 3) aspects of the questionnaire data. In this sense the questionnaire has received validation in the evaluation and analysis of coach and regular and substitute relations and cognitions.

The differences in evaluations can be described on the basis of the four empirically established factors, two of which exemplify this data characteristic.

Factor 1 was deemed as: 'Performance satisfaction and accordance of personal and coach's performance evaluation'. The regular players appeared significantly more satisfied with their status, the number of games played and the results than the substitutes. This is especially evident in item 1 in which the regular players have an evaluation mean of 1.97 versus 4.08 on the part of the substitutes. The regular players manifest an evidently higher degree of concordance with the coach's performance evaluation than the substitutes. This is clear in items 3 and 11. Indeed, there appears to be significantly greater communication between the coach and the regular players than the substitutes, the latter also experiencing considerably more stress than regular players when substituted for poor performance (items 6 and 10).

Factor 2 was deemed: 'Positive emotional relations and discrepancy of performance evaluation between player and coach.' The regular players generally have significantly better relations with coaches than substitutes as suggested by the indications that regulars are usually on better terms with the coach, are more sure that the coach is liked by the team and are more sure that the coach is credible in his performance evaluations (items 12, 13 and 17).

Factor 3 was called Discrepancy of performance evaluation between player and coach and competitive cognitions. The substitute players feel dissatisfied with the way of her substitution by the coach (items 22 and 23). They feel themselves reinforced by other persons that their performance is better than the coach evaluates it (item 21). Furthermore, they display competitive cognitions more emphatically than the regulars that the team plays insufficiently and the rival leaves the team (items 24 and 25).

Factor 4 was called 'Positive personal performance evaluation.' The regular players are more convinced than the substitutes that their performance is sufficient, they remain regulars, they have sufficient abilities and they are capable to play on higher leagues (items 26, 27, 29, 32). Thus, the regulars manifest a higher degree of self-confidence than the substitute players.

Discussion

The results of this exploratory study on the relationship between coaches and regular and substitute players can be summarised in 3 main directions. First, past experience is clearly influential in deciding whether a player is a regular or substitute, since most youth team players became substitutes on reaching a more senior level of play, whereas older players arriving from higher divisions tended to become regulars.

Second, the relationship between coaches and players can be grouped around four factors. Two of the factors expressed concordance between the views of the coach and the player, whilst the other two could be labelled as ambivalent. This clear distinction tended to support the factorial validity of the instrument.

Third, there were obvious discrepancies in the views of regular and substitute players, the former being more satisfied with number of games played, status, results and individual performance than the latter. This led to a closer and more positive relationship with the coach.

The results provide evidence of differences in attributions between the two groups of players and support previous work by Allmer (1979) of differences in performance evaluation. It is feasible that such differences may be even more extensive at professional levels of play. The results provide support for the implications that coaches must remain aware of the small group dynamics at work in their squads, such that problems and difficulties with specific players may be recognised and dealt with before deeper conflicts result.

References

Allmer, H. (1979) Leistungszufriedenheit und Leistungsperspektive bei Stammspielern und Ersatzspielern im Fußballsport. In: D. Albrecht, Fußballsport. Ergebnisse sportwissenschaftlicher Forschung. Berlin: Bartels & Wernitz, pp 65-85.

Bergmann, W. (1978) Probleme der Bank-und Kaderspieler. Leistungssport, 2, 124-129.

Beutel, A., Küffner, H. and Schubö, W. (1980) SPSS 8. Statistikprogramm-System für die Sozialwissenschaften. Stuttgart: Fischer.

Carron, A.C. (1982). Cohesiveness in sport groups: interpretations and considerations. J. Sport Psychol., 4, 123-138.

Essing, W. (1977). Sozialpsychologische Aspekte der Beziehungen zwischen Stamm- und Ersatzspielern in Fußballmannschaften. In: Das Sammelbuch der Arbeiten. v4. Prague: Weltkongreß für Sportpsychologie. (Edited by M. Vanek) Prague: pp148-151.

Landers, D.M., Wilkinson, M.O., Hatfield, B.D. and Barber, H. (1982). Causality and the cohesion-performance relationship. J. Sport Psychol., 4, 170-183.

Martens, R. and Peterson, J.A. (1971). Group cohesiveness as a determinant of success and member satisfaction in team performance. Int. Rev. Sport Sociol., 6, 49-61.

Tutko, T.A. and Richards, J.W. (1971). Psychology of coaching. Boston: Allyn and Bacon.

Ueberle, H. (1971). Trainingsleitung und Mannschaftsführung in den Sportspielen. Schorndorf: Hofmann.

Veit, H. (1971) Untersuchungen zur Gruppendynamik von Ballspielmannschaften. Schorndorf: Hofmann.

A COACH'S PERSPECTIVE ON MOTIVATION

Rex Hazeldine
National Coaching Foundation, 4 College Close, Beckett Park, Leeds LS6 3QH, England.

Introduction

Perspective is defined as a way of regarding situations and judging their relative importance. As each coaching 'situation' is unique, this paper is based on one particular Rugby Union football club. It considers strategies used by the coach to understand, evaluate and enhance the motivation of the players involved.

Players participate in the game of rugby football for a variety of reasons. These can be quite complex and are often inter-related. For purposes of simplification in this paper the factors are classified under three headings - affiliation, achievement and sensation. Each of these is considered from the basis of practical experience and related to one club - Loughborough University Rugby Football Club.

The club has a membership of one hundred players in any one season with a time span of three to four years for each player. It is an educational environment with a strong physical education influence and the club has a prestigious position within student rugby football. The experience with this club that is described covers seventeen years, which in total amounts to the coaching of approximately one thousand players.

Structuring the Situation

In order to enhance the motivation of players, one of the first strategies adopted was to structure the situation in order to provide the best environment for each player in terms of affiliation, achievement and sensation. Whenever one coaches there are always positive and negative aspects. On the positive side, the physical education influence meant that many of the players were professionally concerned with technical performance, fitness and other related factors. The prestigious nature of the club provided social esteem on the campus and a degree of recognition outside in the world of Rugby Union football. This prestige factor meant that students felt privileged to play for the club, but inevitably it also created the problem that all members wanted to play for the first team. Keeping lower sides motivated and preventing players from becoming disheartened, feeling failures and losing self-esteem was vital. This, of course, is a common experience with many top clubs with large squads of players.

To overcome this problem the structure was altered from five teams on a 1st to 5th basis to a five-squad system - three senior and two freshmen. A coach was employed with direct responsibility for each of the five squads. The squad had an identity, the twenty players within it had a sense of belonging and a chance to achieve. For example, any player entering the club in his first year would have recognition within a freshmen squad before moving to a senior squad in his second and subsequent years. There was, of course, movement between the squads during the playing season. Each squad had an inter-University championship or a particular challenge to aim for. The competitive programme included two matches per week, allowing ample opportunity to employ all players within a squad. This use of a squad system ensured that all players had an opportunity to play.

Affiliation

Once every four weeks there was a training session for the whole club. This was aimed at developing a total club identity and to give the opportunity for interaction between senior and junior players. In addition, the coach held regular sessions with each of the squads to keep in contact, to help with the development of individual players and to maintain a sense of belonging within the total structure. Strategies were also developed to create a club identity including overt signs such as sweaters, ties, tracksuits and certain dress requirements for away matches. An important criterion of success for the coach was that the players felt part of a club and did not necessarily judge success solely on winning a championship. This affiliation factor, the desire for friendly association with others, has often been judged in hindsight by players as very significant as they review their playing careers and lives as members of the club.

Achievement

Player development

Within this club structure various approaches were developed by the coach as part of his function to enhance and maintain the motivation of players. These were based on sound coaching practices and the creation of a caring environment.

One noticeable change in emphasis was the shift from the role of 1st Team coach to a Club coach, in other words a move from a traditional view of coaching a 1st team exclusively to a coach responsible for the development of all the players within the club. Considerable emphasis was placed on the development of the player over the three or four years and a search for individual improvement, with the objective of becoming a more complete player in terms of a complete range of individual skills, athleticism and fitness, together with a real tactical understanding of game strategies.

In summary the central theme was development of the individual as a rugby footballer and of the individual through rugby football. This required the combination of a subject-centred and individual-centred approach. The basis for this modus operandi was a consciousness of the players as individuals, i.e. the need to be aware of how they saw themselves and thereby attempt to meet their needs. Players have different motives for participating in Rugby Union Football and the exercise was to establish what they wanted to achieve as individuals. For example, certain players wished to attain achievements on the playing side by improving techniques and performance, and progressing to a higher level of competitive play. Others took on administrative responsibility and developed management skills, while for some the important factor was being part of a social group. Being on campus meant that the coach, a member of the University teaching staff, was able to give each player time in addition to the training sessions, take an interest in the players' development, to show respect for them as people. The coach acted as an educator who was aware of his influence and significance in the life of the player during that period. An 'open door' policy was developed and encouraged so that various forms of 'counselling' work took place.

Evaluation and goal setting

In order to achieve player development a purposeful evaluation of each player's performance in both practice and match situations was undertaken. This provided constructive feedback to the player as an individual and as part of a unit and a team. Aspects of physical conditioning, skill development and enhancement of tactical knowledge were included. The evaluation exercise was the basis for the goal setting programme. The system was devised to increase motivation and self-confidence whilst at the same time reducing anxiety and internal conflict. Open communication was encouraged and agreed realistic goals were set between the coach and the individual player. Short as well as long-term goals were set and an emphasis was placed on performance goals as opposed to outcome goals. The advantage of the latter approach in a game such as rugby football is that performance goals are within the player's control and some measure of success is possible, irrespective of the competitive outcome. Players respond best when they have goals to aim for and if these targets are realistic, they will show greater commitment in meeting them. At the same time the interaction between coach and player should be such that the latter is encouraged to use his own judgement in an intelligent way, thus adopting an approach where problem-solving by the player is the key. This should lead to the development of self-evaluation and subsequently self-coaching by the player with, of course, when necessary, supportive guidance from the coach.

Benefits of player development programme

As a result of this programme of individual development there was clear evidence of individual improvement - for example thirty eight players went on to become full internationals, seven of whom captained their country. Also commendable success as a club in university championships and other competitions resulted, as shown in Table 1. In the period 1969-1986, no less than 30 championships were won by 1st, 2nd and 3rd squads at national and international levels.

Table 1. Loughborough University Rugby Football Club achievements: 1969-1986

University Athletic Union 1st XV Championship:

Winners in 1971, 1973, 1974, 1975, 1977, 1978, 1979, 1984, 1985 and 1986.

2nd XV Championship:

Winners in 1969, 1972, 1973, 1974, 1975, 1977, 1978, 1979, 1980, 1982, 1983, 1985 and 1986.

3rd XV Championship:

Winners in 1984, 1985 and 1986.

Leicestershire Cup:

Winners in 1978, 1984 and 1985.

USA National Rugby Tournament:

Winners in 1979.

A further indication of the coach's change in function and sphere of influence from 1st team coach to club coach is shown by the winning of the Inter-University Championships by teams at all levels during the latter part of those years under discussion. The achievement of performance goals is related to the outcome of matches in rugby football where success is an expression of the effectiveness of the player, the unit and the team. This success led to an increase in enjoyment, self-confidence and motivation.

If winning the championship had been the sole criterion of success within the club, those teams who did not achieve that objective would have been judged as having failed. Therefore, by avoiding the equating of winning with success, and losing with failure, motivation was easier to maintain throughout the season, irrespective of competitive outcome.

Sensation

In order to meet a player's desire for sensation, in the form of sensory stimulation, and excitement, total rugby - 'a fifteen man approach' - was adopted. This produced rugby at its most exciting. Every player was encouraged to be involved by the overall style of play.

In tandem with this approach a physical fitness training programme was devised for each player according to his individual requirements, the demands of the game and positional needs. The training cycle covered the three or four years with appropriate schedules for out-of-season, pre-season, in-season and the recuperation phases (Fig.1).

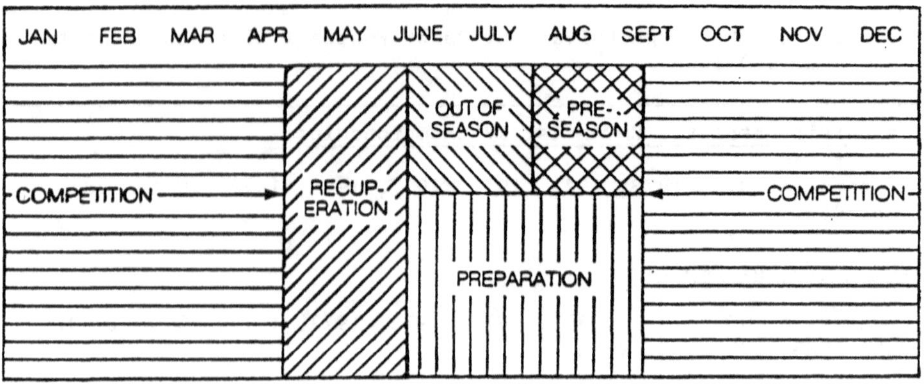

Figure 1. The all-year round training programme

The cycle allowed for 'peaking' at certain points during the playing season. It identified and worked on weaknesses as well as developing strengths during out of season and pre-season phases.

The situation was ideal for training and practice because of the available facilities and the keen positive attitude of the young players at this stage in their playing careers. Nevertheless a responsibility was recognised towards the players who devoted hours of their time to an activity they cherished, and resulted in carefully structured training sessions which provided coherence, variety and inclusiveness. The intrinsic enjoyment of these sessions was only too evident which was an encouraging reaction. The players appear to enjoy the sessions for their own sake in addition to their role of specific training for rugby football.

Conclusion

In conclusion practical coaching solutions were sought to develop those factors which are known to affect players' motivation for taking part in an activity like Rugby Union Football, namely affiliation, achievement and sensation. In seeking and implementing these solutions it became evident that there are very few players, who do not deeply appreciate help with their personal playing development. For the coach's own satisfaction and motivation - an important consideration - this is the most rewarding aspect of the work. Coaching is also concerned with quality control, the realisation of potential and the setting of appropriate standards of performance. However, to achieve these aims there is the need to create a happy environment where all members of the club are recognised for their own unique contribution.

INDEX

For Product Safety Concerns and Information please contact our EU representative GPSR@taylorandfrancis.com
Taylor & Francis Verlag GmbH, Kaufingerstraße 24, 80331 München, Germany

www.ingramcontent.com/pod-product-compliance
Lightning Source LLC
LaVergne TN
LVHW021002300926
849160LV00007B/219

9780415509275